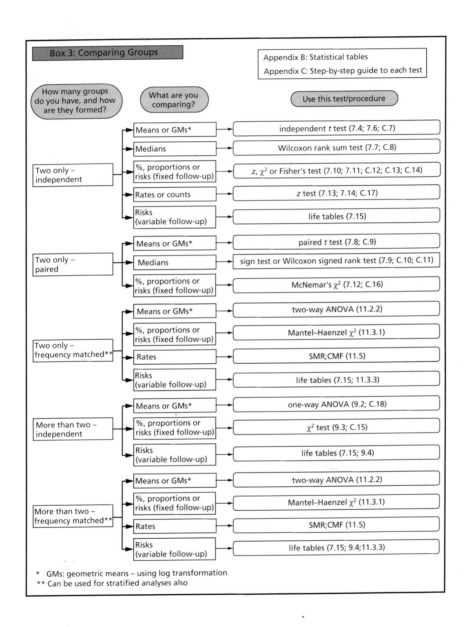

Box 3: Comparing Groups

Appendix B: Statistical tables
Appendix C: Step-by-step guide to each test

How many groups do you have, and how are they formed?	What are you comparing?	Use this test/procedure
Two only – independent	Means or GMs*	independent t test (7.4; 7.6; C.7)
	Medians	Wilcoxon rank sum test (7.7; C.8)
	%, proportions or risks (fixed follow-up)	z, χ^2 or Fisher's test (7.10; 7.11; C.12; C.13; C.14)
	Rates or counts	z test (7.13; 7.14; C.17)
	Risks (variable follow-up)	life tables (7.15)
Two only – paired	Means or GMs*	paired t test (7.8; C.9)
	Medians	sign test or Wilcoxon signed rank test (7.9; C.10; C.11)
	%, proportions or risks (fixed follow-up)	McNemar's χ^2 (7.12; C.16)
Two only – frequency matched**	Means or GMs*	two-way ANOVA (11.2.2)
	%, proportions or risks (fixed follow-up)	Mantel–Haenzel χ^2 (11.3.1)
	Rates	SMR;CMF (11.5)
	Risks (variable follow-up)	life tables (7.15; 11.3.3)
More than two – independent	Means or GMs*	one-way ANOVA (9.2; C.18)
	%, proportions or risks (fixed follow-up)	χ^2 test (9.3; C.15)
	Risks (variable follow-up)	life tables (7.15; 9.4)
More than two – frequency matched**	Means or GMs*	two-way ANOVA (11.2.2)
	%, proportions or risks (fixed follow-up)	Mantel–Haenzel χ^2 (11.3.1)
	Rates	SMR;CMF (11.5)
	Risks (variable follow-up)	life tables (7.15; 9.4;11.3.3)

* GMs: geometric means – using log transformation
** Can be used for stratified analyses also

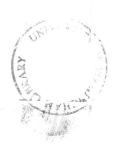
In memory of Professor James McGilvray (1938–1995)

Interpretation and Uses of Medical Statistics

LESLIE E. DALY

MSc, PhD, HonMFPHM
Associate Professor
Department of Public Health Medicine and Epidemiology
University College Dublin
National University of Ireland, Dublin

GEOFFREY J. BOURKE

MA, MD, FRCPI, FFPHM, FFPHMI
Emeritus Professor
Department of Public Health Medicine and Epidemiology
University College Dublin
National University of Ireland, Dublin
Formerly Consultant in Epidemiology and Preventive Medicine
St Vincent's University Hospital
Dublin

FIFTH EDITION

Blackwell
Science

© 2000 by
Blackwell Science Ltd
Editorial Offices:
Osney Mead, Oxford OX2 0EL
25 John Street, London WC1N 2BL
23 Ainslie Place, Edinburgh EH3 6AJ
350 Main Street, Malden
   MA 02148-5018, USA
54 University Street, Carlton
   Victoria 3053, Australia
10, rue Casimir Delavigne
   75006 Paris, France

Other Editorial Offices:
Blackwell Wissenschafts-Verlag GmbH
Kurfürstendamm 57
10707 Berlin, Germany

Blackwell Science KK
MG Kodenmacho Building
7–10 Kodenmacho Nihombashi
Chuo-ku, Tokyo 104, Japan

First published 2000

Set by Excel Typesetters Co., Hong Kong
Printed and bound in Great Britain by
MPG Books Ltd, Bodmin, Cornwall

The Blackwell Science logo is a
trade mark of Blackwell Science Ltd,
registered at the United Kingdom
Trade Marks Registry

DISTRIBUTORS

Marston Book Services Ltd
PO Box 269
Abingdon, Oxon OX14 4YN
(*Orders*: Tel: 01235 465500
         Fax: 01235 465555)

USA
Blackwell Science, Inc.
Commerce Place
350 Main Street
Malden, MA 02148-5018
(*Orders*: Tel: 800 759 6102
             781 388 8250
         Fax: 781 388 8255)

Canada
Login Brothers Book Company
324 Saulteaux Crescent
Winnipeg, Manitoba R3J 3T2
(*Orders*: Tel: 204 837 2987)

Australia
Blackwell Science Pty Ltd
54 University Street
Carlton, Victoria 3053
(*Orders*: Tel: 3 9347 0300
         Fax: 3 9347 5001)

A catalogue record for this title
is available from the British Library

ISBN 0-632-04763-1

22528725

Library of Congress
Cataloging-in-publication Data

Daly, Leslie E.
   Interpretation and uses of medical statistics /
Leslie E. Daly, Geoffrey J. Bourke. — 5th ed.
      p. cm.
   Previous editions entered under: Bourke,
Geoffrey J.
   Includes bibliographical references and index.
   ISBN 0-632-04763-1
   1. Medical statistics. 2. Medicine —
Research — Methodology. I. Bourke,
Geoffrey J. (Geoffrey Joseph) II. Bourke,
Geoffrey J. (Geoffrey Joseph). Interpretation and
uses of medical statistics. III. Title.

RA409 .B65 2000
519.5′02461 — dc21   99–045805

For further information on
Blackwell Science, visit our website:
www.blackwell-science.com

Contents

Note: An exclamation mark in square brackets after a chapter or section heading signifies material that is somewhat more difficult than that surrounding it.

Preface

For a difference to be a difference, it has to make a difference.

Gertrude Stein (1874–1946)

The first edition of this book appeared in 1969, and was designed to introduce the basic concepts of statistics and their medical application to readers who had no formal training in statistical theory or methods. The book emphasized interpretation rather than techniques of calculation, and sought to make readers familiar with the expressions and methods commonly employed in the analysis and presentation of data in medical research. Its success demonstrated the need for such a book, and a second edition, incorporating a number of revisions and extensions, was published in 1975. The third edition, published 10 years later, while retaining the basic aim of interpretation, entailed a comprehensive revision of the book's scope and content. Taking account of the developments in the range and sophistication of statistical techniques in medical research, and the need for a greater understanding of statistics by medical undergraduates and graduates, the book included details for calculation of the common statistical tests, and chapters on research design and methodology. The fourth edition (1991) greatly expanded on the material covered previously and more emphasis was placed on the use of confidence intervals.

In the past 9 years there has been further expansion in the use of statistical analyses in the medical literature, and a number of techniques and approaches rarely seen in the 1980s have come into common use. This fifth edition of our book takes account of some of these changes, though the new topics chosen for inclusion may of course not please everybody. The book has also undergone a major restructuring—with some sections totally rewritten – and it is now more logically organized and, we hope, substantially more user-friendly.

Included in the new material are descriptions of the box plot, the stem and leaf diagram and the dot plot, and we have provided a method for calculation of a confidence interval for a single median. The geometric mean is considered in some detail in the context of log-transformed data, with emphasis on the interpretation of significance tests and confidence intervals for the comparison of two geometric means. There is a new chapter, entitled 'Associations: Chance, Confounded or Causal?' which explains *without any formulae* the concepts underlying confounding, confidence intervals and p values, and the interpretation of associations observed in research investigations. We believe that understanding this descriptive chapter is central to the understanding of the place of statistics in medical research.

One change we have made, informed by our teaching, is in our explanation of sampling variation. Previously we illustrated this topic with the sampling distribution of the mean. This resulted in the usual confusion between the standard error of the mean and the standard deviation of the actual observations. In this edition, sampling variation is introduced in the context of the sampling distribution of a proportion or percentage, and we hope that this has made the explanations much more understandable.

Because of its paramount importance we have added an entirely new chapter on the calculation of sample size. This chapter considers sample size calculations in some detail and provides, in addition to the relevant formulae, useful tables that should give researchers an indication of the order of magnitude of the number of subjects they might require in different situations. A chapter on measurement in medicine includes some material from the previous edition, but much is new. In particular, we describe the quantification of agreement using the kappa statistic or the Bland and Altman techniques. Finally, for the benefit of the researcher, we have included a copy of the World Medical Association Declaration of Helsinki (1996) in an Appendix.

Given the increasing number of new statistical computer programs and the rate at which upgraded versions of existing software appear, we decided to dispense with the chapter on statistical computing altogether. Our experience is that discussion of computer software becomes out of date in a very short time. The reader would be best advised to consult with current users regarding suitable programs for biostatistical or epidemiological data analysis. Readers familiar with previous editions will note too the disappearance of the chapter on vital statistics. We felt that the techniques previously discussed in this chapter were better sited elsewhere throughout the book and that the topic did not warrant a chapter all to itself.

There are a number of features to this text book that make it unique, some of which are new to this edition. A major change is the addition of 'summary boxes' throughout the text. These boxes give the essence of the topic under consideration and should be a great aid in revision. All relevant formulae are summarized at the end of each chapter in such boxes also. Additionally, as a guide to first-time readers, some chapters or chapter headings have an asterisk in parentheses after them '[!]', signifying material that is generally a little more difficult than the material that surrounds it.

The reader should note too the new guide to the choice of a statistical test on the inside front and back covers. Appendix C, which was a feature of previous editions, also provides an overview of the statistical methods covered in the text together with a detailed step-by-step description of the computational approach for each test. This appendix should be useful to those who, having previously read the detailed description in the body of the book, just wish to select and carry out a particular procedure. Looking up statistical tables can also be confusing, and the tables in Appendix B were especially designed (for the third edition) with the end-user in mind. Each table is laid out in a standard format that greatly simplifies its use.

As in the previous editions, derivations of formulae are avoided and instead emphasis is placed on explaining their logic. Although alternative methods are available for some of the more advanced techniques discussed, we are of the view that confusion is avoided if one only is presented. In any event, with the wide availability of many excellent and easy-to-use statistical computing packages, the necessity for hand computation has decreased greatly over a number of years. Nevertheless many studies can still profit from a 'hand analysis', and computational details and formulae for tests or procedures are only given if they are feasible to undertake with a calculator. This allows researchers to perform some calculations without a computer and to gain a deeper understanding of what the computer is doing in particular situations. It also facilitates further calculation as an adjunct to computer output, where a software package might not perform all the requisite calculations (confidence intervals for some parameters of 2×2 tables for instance). On the other hand, for those using more advanced techniques, the book's concentration on the interpretation of results should help the readers understand the output from a computer package without burdening them with arcane formulae.

Despite the changes in the book over the past 30 years we hope that it will continue to appeal to those who, though less interested in the actual statistical calculations, seek a basic understanding of statistical concepts and their role in medicine. This book contains much more than a 'cookbook' of statistical techniques, and much less than the detailed and often difficult texts that cover advanced methods. We have tried to steer a middle course by introducing concepts slowly and carefully, by avoiding any proofs or unnecessary formulae, and yet going far enough to cover most of the important topics and techniques in what we hope is an understandable manner. Parts of the book may be skipped over by those who want only a basic introduction to statistics or who wish to understand what they read in the journals, while enough detail is given to enable it to be used as a practical guide to data analysis. It should be suitable as a textbook for a range of courses taken by medical and paramedical students at both undergraduate and postgraduate levels. To assist the reader, an overview of the structure of the book is included in the following pages.

Authors always appreciate feedback from their readers. While positive comments are of course always welcome, it is the suggestions for improvement, the identification of areas that are unclear, and the pointing out of mistakes, misprints and misspellings that can be most useful. We would therefore like to express our thanks to those readers who have written to us in the past, to our colleagues who made valuable suggestions, and particularly to those of our students who have made their views known. To help readers contact us about this edition of *Interpretation and Uses of Medical Statistics* we have set up a dedicated email address (**iums@ucd.ie**) and a web page (**http://www.ucd.ie/iums**). We will use the web site to post any corrections to the text and we will include links to other sites that may be of interest. Additionally we plan to include exercises based on material in the book – mainly from past examination papers that we have set.

Just as we were contemplating this new edition in late 1995, Professor James McGilvray, who had been a co-author, died suddenly. This book is dedicated to his memory.

L.D and G.J.B

Structure of the book

Chapter 1 introduces the reader to the different types of data, and to graphical methods used to present them. The mean, median and mode are described together with percentile indices and the standard deviation. Chapter 2 introduces the notion of probability and chance at a basic level and describes sampling techniques commonly employed.

Chapter 3 is a central chapter that, without any statistical formulae, introduces the notion of associations and their interpretation. The ideas underlying much of the remainder of the book—statistical significance and confidence intervals, confounding and its elimination and the meaning of causality—are considered. Chapter 4 introduces the reader more formally to estimation using confidence intervals. Methods for estimating a single proportion, mean, count and rate are described and the normal and Student's t distributions are introduced. Chapter 5 considers the general principles underlying hypothesis tests and statistical significance with an introduction to the concept of power. Applications in the one-sample case are described.

Chapter 6 of the book is concerned with research methodology and the design of studies in medicine and epidemiology. Cross-sectional, cohort and case–control studies are described, together with the measures commonly used in the analysis of such studies. The randomized controlled trial is discussed in detail.

Chapter 7 gives a detailed description of confidence interval estimation and hypothesis tests for the comparison of two groups. Paired and independent data are considered and the material covers all the procedures commonly encountered in the medical literature. Comparisons between arithmetic means, geometric means, medians, proportions (percentages, risks), counts and rates are discussed with consideration of the clinical life table also. Chapter 8 discusses in detail how sample sizes are chosen for research investigations and gives useful tables to allow indicative size to be determined. Concentration is on two-group studies.

Chapter 9 considers the comparison of more than two groups and introduces the reader to the analysis of variance. Computations for a one-way analysis of variance (ANOVA) and the test for a trend in proportions are detailed, while other methods are discussed more generally. Chapter 10 covers the topic of simple regression and correlation, with some computational details. Chapter 11 is perhaps the most difficult in the book. It considers the statistical control of confounding and multivariate analysis. Analysis of variance and covariance, multiple regression and logistic regression are discussed from the point of view of interpreting results but details of calculations are not given. Calculations are given however for the Mantel–Haenzel analysis of a series of 2×2 tables and for the standardization methods commonly used in vital statistics. The population life table is also considered. The concluding

Chapter 12 considers the whole question of bias and measurement error in medical investigations. Methods for quantifying measurement precision are described and the analysis of agreement is considered in detail. The concepts of sensitivity and specificity are introduced. The chapter concludes with some brief guidelines for critical reading of the medical literature and the setting up of a research project.

The book has four appendices. Appendix A details short-cut computational methods for some of the techniques discussed in the text. Appendix B contains a comprehensive set of statistical tables and Appendix C outlines, in step-by-step form, the computational procedures for each of the statistical tests described in the book. Appendix D reproduces the World Medical Association Declaration of Helsinki (1996).

1 Describing Data—A Single Variable

1.1 Introduction

In order to read a paper in a medical journal or to appreciate the results of a research project, it is necessary to understand how data are collected and how data are described and summarized. Though logically this book should start with the collection of data and the large question of study design, it is in fact easier to explain how to describe data first. This chapter introduces some of the basic methods used to achieve this end. Readers who understand the essentials of descriptive methods are well on their way to being able to interpret and use medical statistics.

1.2 Types of data

Usually medical research is performed on persons. Essentially a group of persons is studied and information about each individual is recorded. This information can arise from direct measurement (e.g. weight on a scales), from asking a question (e.g. 'where were you born?'), from observation (e.g. gender—usually obvious), from the results of a diagnostic test or tests (e.g. a diagnosis of coronary heart disease) or from a host of other data collection methods. Sometimes, however, the unit of observation is not an individual person. It may, of course, be an animal—which might give rise to a similar type of information as that available on people—but the unit of observation could also be a group of individuals. For instance, there may be interest in comparing a number of different hospitals in terms of efficiency or cost. The unit of observation would then be the hospital (including all its patients and staff) and the information would be obtained for each hospital in the study.

Suppose that one wanted to study certain characteristics in a group of medical students, such as age, sex, city of birth, socio-economic group and number of brothers/sisters. Each of these characteristics may vary from person to person and is referred to as a *variable*, while the values taken by these variables (e.g. 18 years of age; male; born in Dublin, etc.) are referred to as *data*. Data and the variables that give rise to them can be divided into two broad categories—qualitative and quantitative—based on the values the variable can take. Thus the description can apply either to the variable or to the data.

Qualitative data are not numerical and the values taken by a qualitative variable are usually names. For example, the variable 'sex' has the values male and female, and the variable 'city of birth' values such as London or Dublin. Some variables may seem to be numerical although in essence they are not. For instance, there are a number of systems for classification of people into socio-economic groups or social classes based on income, occupation, education, etc. In many of these, a numerical label is used to describe the different groups or categories. Thus social class 1 in Ireland corresponds to 'higher professional' occupations, while social class 6 corresponds to 'unskilled manual' work. The numerical unit is not a unit of measurement, however, but only a tag or label and socio-economic group cannot be considered to be a quantitative variable.

Some qualitative variables do have an intrinsic order in their categories. For instance, in some sense (income/social prestige) social class 1 is 'higher' than social class 6. Such variables are called *ordinal*. Be careful, however: the order intrinsic in the categories may not correspond to the order of a numerical label used to describe them. After all, six is higher in value than one!

Qualitative variables are also called *categorical* or *nominal* variables—the values they take are categories or names. When a qualitative variable has only two categories (alive/dead, male/female, hypertensive/normotensive), it is called a *binary*, a *dichotomous* or an *attribute* variable.

The variables 'age' and 'number of brothers/sisters' are examples of quantitative variables. They assume numerical values that have an intrinsic numerical meaning. Such variables are also called metric or just plain numerical variables. The values mostly arise from an actual measurement, as in the first variable above, or from a count, as in the second.

Sometimes a distinction is made between continuous and discrete quantitative variables. A *discrete* (quantitative) variable is one whose values vary by finite specific steps. The variable 'number of brothers/sisters' takes integral values only; numbers such as 2·6 or 4·5 cannot occur. A *continuous* variable, on the other hand, can take any value. Given any two values, however close together, an intermediate value can always be found. Examples of continuous variables are 'birth weight', 'age', 'time' and 'body temperature', while examples of discrete variables are 'number of children per family', 'number of hospital admissions' or 'number of tablets in bottles of different sizes'. In practice, variables that are continuous are measured in discrete units and data may be collected accurate to the nearest kilogram (for weight) or centimetre (for height), for example. The distinction between continuous and discrete variables is not that important, however. Though there are a number of different grouping systems that are used to categorize data and variables, the most important is that which distinguishes between qualitative and quantitative. In essence, qualitative data refer to qualities and quantitative data to quantities.

Variables and data come in two basic forms
- qualitative — also known as categorical or nominal
- quantitative — also known as metric, or numerical

A qualitative variable is called
- ordinal if there is an order in the categories
- binary, dichotomous or attribute if it has two categories

1.2.1 Scores, scales and binary data [!]

Interesting variables can arise in medicine from scoring systems or scales. Often the severity of a symptom or disease is classed as mild/moderate/severe, using perhaps subjective criteria, and there are many more formal systems, such as those used to categorize cancer into severity groups (stage I, stage II, etc.). Such variables with only a few categories are unambiguously qualitative and ordinal.

If a categorical variable is assigned categories described by numbers, it is important to realize that it cannot be dealt with as if it were a numerical variable. An important concept here is that of distance between categories. For a numerical variable, the distance between two values is obtained by subtracting one from the other. Thus, a 40-year-old person is 5 years older than a 35-year-old, and a 15-year-old is 5 years older than a 10-year-old. The distance between social class 1 and social class 2 (whatever that might mean) is not the same as the distance between class 5 and class 6, however.

Some clinical scoring systems can give a large number of numerical categories for a variable. A simple scoring system might be based on assigning a score of 1 for the presence of each of a number of symptoms and adding the scores up. More complex systems might assign different scores to different symptoms or base the assigned score on the severity of the symptom. The Apgar score, used to measure the degree of distress in a newborn infant, is an example of the latter. It assigns a score, depending on severity, of 0, 1 or 2 to five different signs, giving a total score that can range from 0 to 10 (Apgar, 1953).

Often *visual analogue scales* (VAS) are used to measure subjective responses. In part of the EuroQol questionnaire, for instance, respondents mark a position on a line to provide information on their subjective health status (Fig. 1.1). Similarly, assessment of pain is often by means of a VAS where the subject might be asked to mark a position on a line drawn between two extremes of 'pain as bad as it could be' to 'no pain at all'. The position of the mark would be used to assign a numerical score to the quantity being determined (health status or pain intensity in the above examples).

In situations like this, with a large number of possible numerical values based on a count (of symptoms) or a measurement (of a mark along a line), it

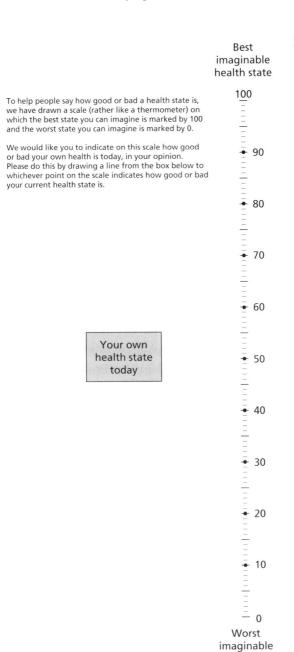

To help people say how good or bad a health state is, we have drawn a scale (rather like a thermometer) on which the best state you can imagine is marked by 100 and the worst state you can imagine is marked by 0.

We would like you to indicate on this scale how good or bad your own health is today, in your opinion. Please do this by drawing a line from the box below to whichever point on the scale indicates how good or bad your current health state is.

Best imaginable health state

Your own health state today

Worst imaginable health state

Fig. 1.1 The visual analogue scale in the EuroQol health questionnaire (copyright EuroQol© Group, with permission; for further information, email Frank de Charro: fdecharro@csi.com).

is not entirely clear whether the variable should be classed as a quantitative rather than a qualitative ordinal. Certainly some researchers treat such variables as numerical.

The position of a binary variable is interesting. In one sense, it is qualitative with just two categories, but it can always be considered ordinal also. It just requires that, on some level, it is decided that one category is 'higher' than the other. Thus, in the variable 'gender', for instance, one might consider that a female has a greater level of 'femaleness' than a male. It is a short step to then assigning a number to the categories of a binary variable (e.g. the value '1' assigned to female and '0' to male) and treating it as quantitative. Special techniques for the analysis of binary variables are considered later.

1.3 Qualitative data—simple tables and bar charts

Obviously, it is necessary to have some way of presenting data other than by means of a long list of the values for each variable looked at, in each individual studied. The basic rule for displaying qualitative data is to count the number of observations in each category of the variable and present the numbers and percentages in a table. The object of a table is to organize data in a compact and readily comprehensible form. A fault that is fairly common is to attempt to show too much in a table or diagram. In general, a table should be self-explanatory without the need for over-elaborate explanations, including 'keys' or notes. Examples have often been seen in which it is more difficult to interpret a table or diagram than to read the accompanying text, and this defeats the whole purpose of the presentation.

Table 1.1 presents the major indication for endoscopy in 193 patients who had undergone the procedure in a children's hospital. The variable ('major indication for endoscopy') has four categories—'Small-bowel biopsy', 'Abdominal pain', 'Vomiting' and 'Crohn's disease'. The number of persons falling into each category is counted. The figures, which appear in the body of the table, are referred to as the *frequencies* and record the total number of observations in each group or class; the sum of the frequencies in the column makes up the total frequency or the total number of observations. It is seen that percentage frequencies are also shown. Percentage or relative frequencies are usually given in tables and are particularly useful for comparative purposes.

Table 1.1 Major indication for endoscopy in 193 paediatric referrals (from Gormally et al., 1996).

Major indication	No. of patients	Percentage
Small-bowel biopsy	42	(21·8)
Abdominal pain	92	(47·7)
Vomiting	53	(27·5)
Crohn's disease	6	(3·1)
Total	193	(100·0)

1.3.1 Tables in practice

A problem that arises in practice when preparing tabular data is the number of decimal places to present in percentages. One decimal place is usually sufficient and the exact percentage should be rounded to one decimal place. In Table 1.1, for instance, there were 92/193 children with abdominal pain as the major indication for referral. This is 47·668%, which rounds up to 47·7%. The rules for rounding are fairly simple. If the second decimal place is 5 or greater, 1 is added to the first decimal place. If the second decimal place is 4 or less then the first decimal place remains the same.

Be careful, however, not to round twice—this rule must be applied to the original calculated percentage only. For instance, 3/87 = 0·03448 or 3·448%. Rounded to a single decimal place, this should be 3·4%. If the figure were to be rounded initially to two decimal places, giving 3·45%, and later rounded to a single decimal place, the incorrect result of 3·5% would be obtained.

The second problem that is commonly encountered is when the rounded percentages do not add exactly to 100%. In Table 1.1, for instance, the percentages add to 100·1%. There is no correct answer to this problem, but certainly one solution is to give the correct rounded values in the table with the total always showing 100·0% since that is what is expected. This is the solution adopted in this text. Some give the correct total (usually 100·1%, 100·0% or 99·9%) and others change one of the percentages in the table to force addition to 100.0%.

1.3.2 Bar charts and pie diagrams

Qualitative data can also be presented in a diagrammatic form, such as a *bar chart* (Fig. 1.2). The categories of the variable are shown on the horizontal axis and the frequency or, if required, the relative frequency is measured on the vertical axis. (Sometimes, the variable is shown on the vertical axis and the frequencies on the horizontal, with the bars going across the page.) Bars are constructed to show the frequency, or relative frequency, for each class of the attribute. Usually the bars are equal in width and there is a space between them. Figure 1.2 is a simple bar chart illustrating the data in Table 1.1. The height of the bar shows the frequency of each group and gives a useful 'picture' of the distribution. When bar charts are being constructed, it is important that the scale should start at zero; otherwise, the heights of the bars are not proportional to the frequencies, which is the essential thing. They could then be very misleading as a source of information.

Another method for displaying qualitative data is by means of a *pie chart* or *pie diagram*. Essentially, a circle is drawn whose total area represents the total frequency. The circle is then divided into segments (like the slices of a pie) with the area of each proportional to the observed frequency in each category of the variable under examination. Figure 1.3 shows a pie chart for the data in Table 1.1. While the pie diagram has its uses, in most cases the pictorial representation of a qualitative variable given by the bar chart is preferred. Moreover, the

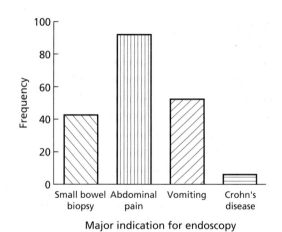

Fig. 1.2 Bar chart of data in Table
1.1.

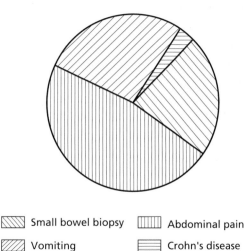

Fig. 1.3 Pie chart for data in Table
1.1.

bar chart is easier to construct and, with slight adaptations, extends to the
display of quantitative data, as discussed in the following section.

> Presenting qualitative data
> • count the number of persons in each category
> • use a table, bar chart or pie chart

1.4 Picturing quantitative data

1.4.1 Frequency distributions

It was explained in the previous section that the basic rule for displaying
qualitative data was to count the number of observations or units in each

category of the variable and to display these frequencies in a table or bar chart. The same rule can also be used for quantitative data, but categories may have to be created by grouping the values of the variable.

Table 1.2 and 1.3 show what are called the *frequency distributions* for two quantitative variables. Family size in Table 1.2 is a discrete variable and birth weight in Table 1.3 is a continuous variable. Since family size is a discrete variable and there are not too many different values, no grouping is required for the tabular presentation in Table 1.2, apart from the last category, which includes all families sized seven and over. Birth-weight data, however, being continuous, have to be grouped for tabular presentation. There are a few simple rules for grouping a continuous variable. First, the groups or classes should encompass the full extent of the data and should not be overlapping. In practice, somewhere between six and 20 groups is usually sufficient. In the birth-weight example, there are 14 classes: the first is from 1·76 to 2·00 kg, the second from 2·01 to 2·25 kg, and so on, as shown in Table 1.3. The limits for these classes (1·76, 2·00, 2·01, 2·25, etc.) are chosen so that each observation fits into one of the classes. There are some technical points relating to the choice of cut-off points for the tabular presentation of such continuous data, which are discussed in the next section, but the general approach should be

Family size	Frequency (numbers)
2	2
3	2
4	2
5	3
6	4
7 and over	7
Total	20

Table 1.2 Distribution of family size in 20 coronary heart disease patients who had at least one sibling.

Birth weight (kg)	No. of births
1·76–2·00	4
2·01–2·25	3
2·26–2·50	12
2·51–2·75	34
2·76–3·00	115
3·01–3·25	175
3·26–3·50	281
3·51–3·75	261
3·76–4·00	212
4·01–4·25	94
4·26–4·50	47
4·51–4·75	14
4·76–5·00	6
5·01–5·25	2
Total births	1260

Table 1.3 Birth-weight distribution of 1260 female infants at 40 weeks' gestation. Original data from Hayes *et al.* (1983), with permission.

clear. It is also advisable to have the width of each class (the *class interval*) identical. In the example, the class intervals each cover a quarter of a kilogram. Again, this is discussed in more detail later.

1.4.2 Class limits, class intervals and class mid-points [!]

The class limits presented in Table 1.3 are referred to as the tabulated class limits and actually take account of the accuracy to which the data were recorded. The birth-weight data were recorded to the nearest 0·01 kg. Thus, a value of 1·764 kg would have been recorded as 1·76 kg and a value of 2·008 kg would have been recorded as 2·01 kg. Values like 2·255 kg would have been recorded as 2·26 or 2·25 kg, according to the judgement of the person taking the measurements. (The sensitivity of the weighing scales would, in practice, probably not allow for a reading of exactly 2·255 anyway.) The upper tabulated limit of one class, 2·00 kg, say, is just 0·01 kg (the recorded accuracy of the data) below the lower tabulated limit, 2·01 kg, of the next class. All recorded values must fit into one of the tabulated classes.

The *true class limits*, on the other hand, are the limits that correspond to the actual birth weights included in each class. Thus, all weights from 1·755 to 2·005 kg (ignoring weights of exactly these values) are included in the class 1·76 to 2·00 kg; weights between 2·005 and 2·255 kg are included in the class 2·01 to 2·25 kg, etc. The tabulated limits depend on the accuracy to which the data are recorded, while the true limits are those that would have been employed if it were possible to measure with exact precision. The true class limits are the more important for later applications, although it must be remembered that these depend on the tabulated limits chosen, which in turn depend on the degree of accuracy in the recorded data (Table 1.4).

The *class interval* is the difference between the true upper class limit and the true lower class limit. Thus, the class 1·76 kg to 2·00 kg has true upper

Table 1.4 Tabulated limits, true class limits, class intervals and class mid-points for the birth-weight data (kg).

Tabulated limits	True class limits	Class interval	Class mid-point
1·76–2·00	1·755–2·005	0·25	1·88
2·01–2·25	2·005–2·255	0·25	2·13
2·26–2·50	2·255–2·505	0·25	2·38
2·51–2·75	2·505–2·755	0·25	2·63
2·76–3·00	2·755–3·005	0·25	2·88
3·01–3·25	3·005–3·255	0·25	3·13
3·26–3·50	3·255–3·505	0·25	3·38
3·51–3·75	3·505–3·755	0·25	3·63
3·76–4·00	3·755–4·005	0·25	3·88
4·01–4·25	4·005–4·255	0·25	4·13
4·26–4·50	4·255–4·505	0·25	4·38
4·51–4·75	4·505–4·755	0·25	4·63
4·76–5·00	4·755–5·005	0·25	4·88
5·01–5·25	5·005–5·255	0·25	5·13

and lower limits of 2·005 and 1·755 and a class interval of 2·005 − 1·755 = 0·25 kg. In the birth-weight example, all the class intervals are equal.

Another important concept is the *class mid-point*, the use of which will be referred to later. This is the value of the variable midway between the true lower class limit and the true upper class limit. It can be calculated by adding together these upper and lower limits and then dividing by 2. The mid-point for the first class in Table 1.3 is thus (1·755 + 2·005)/2 = 1·88 kg. The mid-point for the second class is 2·13, for the third 2·38, and so on (see Table 1.4).

Usually, measurements are rounded up or down, to give a particular degree of accuracy, and the true class limits are determined as described above, midway between the upper and lower tabulated limits of two adjacent classes. In medical applications however, age is often measured as 'age last birthday'. In this case, tabulated limits of 20–24 years, 25–29 years, etc. correspond to true limits of 20–25, 25–30, etc. and class mid-points of 22·5 and 27·5 years, respectively. The difference between the method for dealing with age compared with that used for most other variables often causes confusion, but it is still most important to understand how the accuracy to which data are recorded affects calculation of the true class limits and mid-points.

The notion of class intervals cannot be applied in quite the same way to discrete frequency distributions. Thus, in Table 1.2, the values 2, 3 and 4 cannot be interpreted as 1·5–2·5, 2·5–3·5 and 3·5–4·5. The variable takes only the integral values 2·0, 3·0 and 4·0, and there are no class intervals as such.

1.4.3 Histograms and frequency polygons

Quantitative data can be represented diagrammatically by means of a *histogram*. A histogram is a 'bar chart' for quantitative data. Figure 1.4 shows the histogram for the birth-weight data. For equal class intervals (0·25 kg in the example), the heights of the bars correspond to the frequency in each class but, in general (see below), it is the area of the bars that is more important. With equal class intervals, the area is, of course, proportional to the height. The total area of all the bars is proportional to the total frequency.

The main differences between a histogram and a bar chart are that in the latter there are usually spaces between the bars (see Fig. 1.2) and the order in which the bars are drawn is irrelevant, except for the case of an ordered qualitative variable.

The histogram gives a good picture of the shape of the distribution, showing it to rise to a peak between 3·25 and 3·50 kg and to decline thereafter. An alternative method of presenting a frequency distribution is by means of a *frequency polygon*, which in Fig. 1.5 has been superimposed on the histogram of Fig. 1.4. The frequency polygon is constructed by joining the mid-points of the top of each bar by straight lines and by joining the top of the first bar to the horizontal axis at the mid-point of the empty class before it, with a similar construction for the last bar. The area under the frequency polygon is then equal to the area of the bars in the histogram. Earlier it was mentioned that the

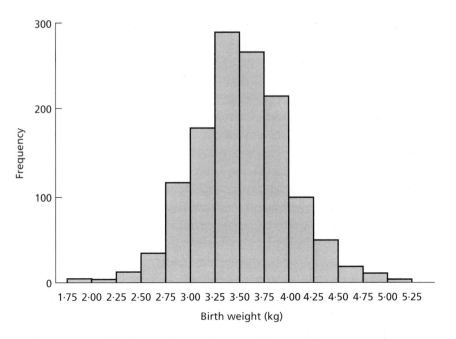

Fig. 1.4 Histogram of data in Table 1.3. Birth-weight distribution of 1260 female infants at 40 weeks' gestation.

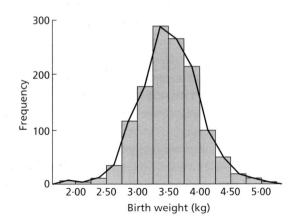

Fig. 1.5 Histogram and superimposed frequency polygon of data in Table 1.3. Birth-weight distribution of 1260 female infants at 40 weeks' gestation.

area of the bars of the histogram was proportional to the total frequency. It follows that the area enclosed by the frequency polygon is also proportional to the total frequency. Figure 1.6 shows the frequency polygon for the birth-weight data with the histogram removed.

1.4.4 Drawing histograms [!]

This section considers some of the points that must be observed when constructing frequency histograms in practice, and can be omitted at a first reading.

When preparing quantitative data for presentation, the chosen class

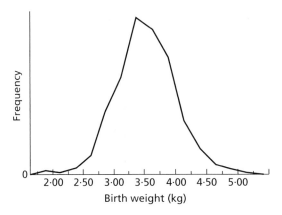

Fig. 1.6 Frequency polygon.
Birth-weight distribution of
1260 female infants at 40 weeks'
gestation.

intervals should not overlap each other and should cover the full range of the data. Depending on the total number of persons or units studied, the data should be divided into somewhere between five and 20 intervals. If too many intervals are employed, the resulting histogram may have too many peaks and valleys, instead of rising to a maximum and falling off, as in Fig. 1.4. This is most often due to small frequencies in each class and, when it occurs, a larger class interval should be employed. If too few intervals or classes are used, too much information may be lost. Creating appropriate classes is often a trial-and-error procedure. Sometimes the number of persons or units in a study may be too small for a histogram to be drawn.

The edges of the bars in the histogram should, ideally, be drawn on the true class limits, but for presentation purposes, to give 'nice' units on the horizontal axis, the bars are sometimes shifted over slightly. This should only be done, however, if the class intervals are much larger than the accuracy to which the data were recorded. In the birth-weight example, the accuracy, 0·01 kg, is 4·0% of the class interval of 0·25 kg and the bars are drawn at 1·75, 2·00 . . . instead of at the true class limits of 1·755, 2·005 . . . These differences could not be detected by the naked eye, but in other situations the true class limits may have to be employed.

In this example too, equal class intervals of 0·25 kg were used throughout and such a practice is to be strongly encouraged. If class intervals are unequal, problems can arise in drawing the histogram correctly. Note, too, that open-ended intervals, such as ⩾ (greater than or equal to) 4·76 kg, will also lead to problems and should be avoided if possible.

Suppose, for example, that the two classes 3·76–4·00 and 4·01–4·25 were combined. From Table 1.3, the frequencies in these classes were 212 and 94 persons, so there are 306 persons in the new combined class of 3·76–4·25. If the histogram were drawn with the height of the bar over this class as 306, Fig. 1.7 would be obtained. Something seems very wrong here and it is due to the fact, already noted, that the *area* of each bar should be proportional to the frequency, not its height. Since the class interval for this class at 0·5 kg is twice that for the other classes, the bar should only be drawn to a height of 306

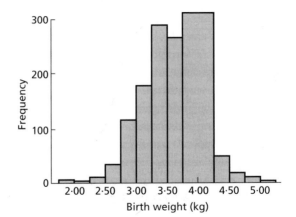

Fig. 1.7 Incorrectly drawn histogram due to non-allowance for unequal class intervals.

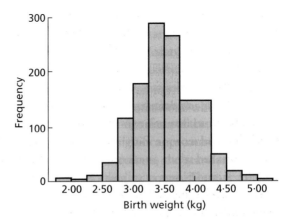

Fig. 1.8 Correctly drawn histogram allowing for unequal class intervals.

divided by 2, which equals 153. If this is done, the areas of each bar will be proportional to the frequencies in their corresponding classes and Fig. 1.8 is obtained. This is similarly shaped to the histogram obtained with equal class intervals, which shows that unequal class intervals do not distort the picture of the data. It is much easier, however, to draw histograms with equal class intervals.

If one has a histogram—or its corresponding polygon—created from data broken into many different-sized class intervals, it can be difficult to interpret the scale on the vertical axis. In fact, it is difficult to interpret the scale for any polygon without first knowing the class interval on which the original histogram was based. As has been said, it is area that is important and, for this reason, the frequency scale is often omitted from frequency polygons.

1.4.5 Frequency curves

As opposed to a frequency polygon (made up of segments of straight lines), reference is often made to a variable's *frequency curve*. This is the frequency polygon that would be obtained if a very large number of units were studied. Suppose that 20 000 female births had been studied, instead of the 1260 in the

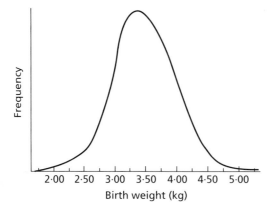

Fig. 1.9 Frequency curve for female birth weight at 40 weeks' gestation.

example, and that a histogram with class intervals of 0·05 kg instead of 0·25 kg were constructed. The histogram of this distribution would, in all likelihood be similar in shape to the earlier one and, although there would be many more bars, each bar would be much narrower in width—in fact, one-fifth as wide. In the same way as before, a frequency polygon could be drawn. However, because the mid-points of each class are much closer together, the frequency polygon would approximate much more closely to a smooth curve. In appearance, it might resemble Fig. 1.9.

By studying larger and larger groups and by continually reducing the class interval, the frequency polygon will approximate more and more closely to a smooth curve. Thus, when frequency curves are mentioned, it is usually the distribution of a variable based on a very large (infinite) number of observations which is being considered. In describing the shapes of distributions, frequency curves rather than polygons are often referred to.

1.4.6 Stem-and-leaf diagrams

Drawing a histogram can often be quite tedious and an alternative method can be employed when the raw (original non-grouped) data are available. Table 1.5 shows the ages at which 21 females were admitted to hospital with a hip fracture. A histogram could be drawn for these data, but the same end result can be achieved with the stem-and-leaf diagram. If the tens part of the age were taken as a 'stem' on which the units part of the age were to be attached like a leaf, Fig. 1.10 would be obtained.

The stem is written down in the first column and usually a vertical line is drawn to separate the stem from the leaves. Here the leaves are the units part of the age and the leaves belonging to each stem are put in the next columns. Thus, there is only one patient in her 50s at age 53 and the digit '3' goes in the first leaf column on to the stem '5'. There are two ages (62 and 67) that belong to the second stem of '6', and the units '2' and '7' go in the first and second leaf columns. In this way, the leaves are added to the stems to give the complete diagram.

Table 1.5 Ages of 21 females admitted to hospital with a hip fracture (years).			
53	76	84
62	78	85
67	78	86
71	82	87
73	84	87
73	84	94
73	84	98

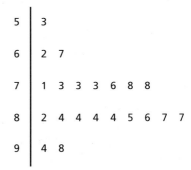

```
5 | 3

6 | 2 7

7 | 1 3 3 3 6 8 8

8 | 2 4 4 4 4 5 6 7 7

9 | 4 8
```

Fig. 1.10 Stem-and-leaf diagram of the ages (years) of 21 female patients with a hip fracture. See Table 1.5.

If the diagram is turned so that the stem is at the bottom it can be seen that a crude histogram of the data has been created. The classes correspond to the range of values implied by the stem—in this example, from 50 to 59 years, 60 to 69 years, etc. As long as the digits of the leaves are written in equal-width columns, the number of observations in each class is given by the length of the row, which corresponds to the height of the bar of the histogram.

The stem-and-leaf diagram is quite simple to draw and the digits for the leaves need not be put in ascending order. In Fig. 1.10, for instance, the '8' (for 98) could have been put in the first leaf column of the '9' stem and the '4' (for 94) could have been put in the second column. Thus, once the appropriate stem has been chosen, the leaves can be filled in easily by just going through the data without even having to order them.

For a given set of data, choosing an appropriate stem is sometimes a process of trial and error, but there are a few tricks that can ease the task. Usually the number of stems is between about five and 20 but this depends on having a sufficient number of values for each stem. Figures 1.11 and 1.12 display two further stem-and-leaf diagrams, which illustrate some of the possibilities. In Fig. 1.11, the diastolic blood pressures of 19 patients are shown. In this example, the stem consists of the tens digit, but each is duplicated; the first occurrence in the stem relates to units of 0, 1, 2, 3 and 4, while the second relates to units of 5, 6, 7, 8 and 9. The lowest diastolic blood pressures are then 70, 72 and 74 (first stem), followed by 75, 75, 77 and 78 mmHg in the second stem. This approach enabled the creation of six stems, while the use of the tens unit on its own would, for these data, have resulted in only three. Note that it is not possible to create three stems within a single tens digit, since the number of possible different leaves on each stem must be the same.

```
7 | 0  4  2

7 | 5  5  7  8

8 | 0  0  2  2  3  3

8 | 5  5  7

9 | 2  4

9 | 5
```

Fig. 1.11 Stem-and-leaf diagram for diastolic blood pressure (mmHg) in 19 patients.

```
24 | 2  3  5  8

25 | 0  1  2  7  9  9

26 | 2  4  8

27 |

28 | 4  6

29 | 0
```

Fig. 1.12 Stem-and-leaf diagram for serum cholesterol (mg/dL) in 16 patients.

In Fig. 1.12, which shows the serum cholesterol in mg/dL, two digits have been used for the stem. Note that there were no serum cholesterols in the 270s and therefore this stem appears without a leaf.

Without doubt, the stem-and-leaf diagram is a useful alternative to the histogram for determining what data look like. It is relatively easy to draw for small sample sizes and manages to display the values of the actual observations in a useful format. It cannot be used if the data have been collected in grouped form, however. The histogram, on the other hand, can display grouped data, but always hides the actual values. It is, however, the more usual approach for data presentation in the medical literature.

1.4.7 Dot plots

Figure 1.13 shows another diagram picturing the age data from Table 1.5. The *dot plot*, as it is called, is easy to draw with a relatively small sample size and does give a good picture of the data. Each dot on the diagram represents a single individual and the spread of the data is particularly easy to see.

1.4.8 Cumulated frequency polygons [!]

A further way of presenting quantitative data is by means of the *cumulated* (or *cumulative*) *frequency polygon* or *ogive*. In Table 1.6 the birth-weight data have been rearranged by a process of successive cumulation of the frequencies in Table 1.3. Thus, four infants weigh less than or equal to 2·0 kg, seven (4 + 3) weigh less than or equal to 2·25 kg, 19 (7 + 12) weigh less than or equal to 2·5 kg, 53 (19 + 34) weigh less than or equal to 2·75 kg, and so on. These are the

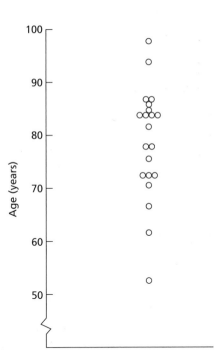

Fig. 1.13 Dot plot of the ages of 21 female patients with a hip fracture. See Table 1.5.

Table 1.6 Cumulated frequencies for the birth-weight data of Table 1.3. (The weights given should theoretically be increased by 0·005 kg—see text.)

Birth weight less than or equal to (kg)	Cumulated frequency
2·00	4
2·25	7
2·50	19
2·75	53
3·00	168
3·25	343
3·50	624
3·75	885
4·00	1097
4·25	1191
4·50	1238
4·75	1252
5·00	1258
5·25	1260

cumulated frequencies. The cumulated frequencies in Table 1.6 are given for values less than the upper tabulated limit for each class. This is done for convenience of presentation and the values in the first column should be more correctly given as the true upper class limits, which are 0·005 kg above the tabulated limits (see discussion in Section 1.4.2). In Fig. 1.14, the cumulated frequencies have been plotted in the form of a cumulated frequency polygon or ogive. When the points have been plotted, successive points are joined by straight lines. In principle, the ogive can be used to estimate the number of female babies weighing less than or equal to a certain number of kilograms, by

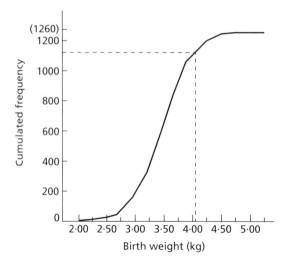

Fig. 1.14 Cumulated frequency polygon (ogive) for birth weight of 1260 female infants at 40 weeks' gestation.

interpolation. Suppose one wanted to estimate the number of babies weighing less than or equal to 4·1 kg. By drawing a vertical line from the relevant point on the horizontal scale, noting where it meets the polygon and moving horizontally across to the vertical scale, it can be estimated that about 1133 infants weigh less than or equal to 4·1 kg (see Fig. 1.14). Obviously, it would be possible to give a mathematical formula for estimating this number but the graphical method is sufficient for most practical applications. If the original (ungrouped) measurements were available, this calculation could, of course, be performed by direct counting.

1.4.9 Summarizing the picture

A major part of descriptive statistics is to summarize and describe the data that are available. The histogram, stem-and-leaf diagram, dot plot or frequency polygon gives a picture of a set of numerical data, but it is also possible to describe the picture in words and numbers. There are three major groupings into which a description of numerical data can fall. The first is the shape of the distribution, which is a verbal description of what the distribution looks like (numerical measures of shape are also available). The second grouping refers to the average value. Most readers are probably familiar with the idea of an 'average', which is used to describe the general level of magnitude of a particular variable. For example, it is common to refer to the average number of days spent in hospital by a given group of patients. There are a number of different ways in which the 'average' may be defined and measured and such measures are called *measures of central value* or *central location*. A measure of central value, as its name suggests, 'locates' the middle or centre of a collection of values; sometimes, however, as will be seen, extreme values may also be of interest. The third grouping for the description of a numerical variable relates to the dispersion or spread of the data. These three groupings are considered in turn.

A numerical distribution can be summarized by giving descriptions or measures of
- its shape (based on a histogram, a stem-and-leaf diagram or a dot plot)
- where its centre is
- how spread out it is

1.5 Shapes of distributions

There are three important concepts in describing the shape of a frequency distribution. The first question to ask is whether the distribution has one 'hump' or two 'humps'. Figure 1.15a shows a 'two-humped' frequency curve for a variable. The technical term for this is a *bimodal* distribution (see Section 1.6.4 below) and, although such distributions do occur, the *unimodal* ('one-humped') distribution is much more common. In a unimodal distribution, the frequency of observations rises to a maximum and then decreases again.

Unimodal distributions can be subdivided into *symmetrical* and *skewed* distributions. Symmetrical distributions can be divided into two halves by the perpendicular drawn from the peak of the distribution and each half is a mirror image of the other half (Fig. 1.15b).

Figures 1.15c and the 1.15d are skewed distributions. (This is a concept that really only applies to unimodal distributions.) Such asymmetrical distributions are said to be positively or negatively skewed depending upon the direction of the 'tail' of the curve. Figure 1.15c is a *positively skewed* distribution with a long tail at the upper end. Figure 1.15d is *negatively skewed*; there is a long tail at the lower end of the distribution. Since the curves shown are smooth continuous curves, the variable, which is plotted along the horizontal scale, must also be assumed to be continuous. Curves of frequency distributions may assume any particular shape, of which the four illustrated are common examples. When a distribution is positively skewed most of the observations are over to the left around the 'hump'. Some observations, however, are spread far out to the right (positive direction) with no corresponding values to the left (negative direction). Often one can anticipate

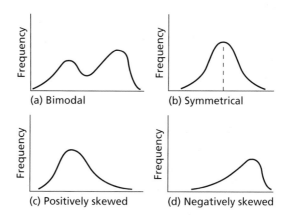

Fig. 1.15 Examples of frequency distributions: (a) bimodal; (b) symmetrical; (c) positively skewed; (d) negatively skewed.

whether skewness is likely to be present or not, even before examining the data. One such case is the variable 'length of in-patient hospital stay'. Most patients will have a stay of about 5 or 6 days; there will be some lower values than this (but none lower than 1 day!) and perhaps quite a few higher values for those in hospital for considerable lengths of time. This essentially means that, if the histogram of lengths of stay is drawn, it will have a definite positive skew.

Shapes of quantitative distributions
- symmetrical or skewed
- unimodal or bimodal (if symmetrical)

1.6 Measures of central value

1.6.1 The (arithmetic) mean

The most common measure of central value is the *arithmetic mean*; generally this is what is meant by the average of a series of numbers, though the word average is a general term that is applied to other measures also. Often the arithmetic mean is just called the mean. The arithmetic mean is calculated by adding up the values of each observation and dividing this total by the number of observations. The purpose of the arithmetic mean is to summarize a collection of data by means of a representative value.

Table 1.5 gives the ages of 21 females with a hip fracture. The sum of all the ages is $53 + 62 + 67 + \dots$, which equals 1659. Since there are 21 observations, the arithmetic mean is obtained by dividing 1659 by 21, obtaining exactly 79·0 years. (It is usual to present a mean to one more decimal place than the original measurements, rounding up if required.) If x represents the value of any variable measured on an individual, the mean is calculated by adding up all the x values and dividing by the number of persons studied, which is denoted n. A special symbol Σ (sigma — the capital Greek letter 's') is used as shorthand for 'add up all the', so that the arithmetic mean ($\bar{x}$, pronounced 'x-bar') of a variable is expressed as:

$$\bar{x} = \frac{\Sigma x}{n} \tag{1.1}$$

In the example above, $\Sigma x = 1659$, $n = 21$ and therefore $\bar{x} = 79\cdot0$ years. The symbol Σ is called the summation sign. When ambiguity can be avoided, the term 'mean' is often employed for the arithmetic mean.

The interpretation and use of the arithmetic mean require little comment, since the concept of the 'average' is widely used and understood. The mean provides a useful summary measure for a particular collection of data, as in the example above, and it is also useful for purposes of comparison. If, for instance, it is wished to compare the ages of two groups of patients, the most convenient form of comparison is in terms of the mean ages in the two groups. Comparisons of this kind are very important in statistical analysis, and they are discussed at greater length in subsequent chapters.

1.6.2 The grouped mean [!]

It is particularly easy to calculate the arithmetic mean from data such as those in Table 1.5. The actual age of each patient is known and it is a simple matter to add up all the individual ages and divide by 21. It has been pointed out, however, that quantitative data are often presented in a frequency distribution, and the exact value the variable takes for each person is not then known, but only the class into which each person falls. Table 1.7 repeats the frequency distribution of birth weight presented in Section 1.4.1. An estimate of the arithmetic mean birth weight can still be made by making a few assumptions.

Assume that the infants in each class all have a birth weight corresponding to the class mid-point. Thus, the four infants in the class 1·76–2·00 kg are assumed to have a birth weight of 1·88 kg, and the three infants in the next class are assumed to weigh 2·13 kg, and so on. Thus, the mid-point of each class is taken as being representative of all the values within that class. In doing this, it is not suggested that the four infants in the class 1·76–2·00 kg have an exact weight of 1·88 kg; it is suggested only that the *average* weight of these four infants will be about 1·88 kg and, since this is midway along the range of possible weights in this class, it seems to be a reasonable assumption to make.

Using this approach, the mean birth weight of the 1260 infants is estimated by adding up the four assumed weights of 1·88 kg, the three weights of 2·13 kg, the 12 weights of 2·38 kg, and so on, up to the final two weights of

Table 1.7 Birth-weight distribution of 1260 female infants at 40 weeks' gestation.

Birth weight (kg)	Class mid-point (kg)	No. of births
1·76–2·00	1·88	4
2·01–2·25	2·13	3
2·26–2·50	2·38	12
2·51–2·75	2·63	34
2·76–3·00	2·88	115
3·01–3·25	3·13	175
3·26–3·50	3·38	281
3·51–3·75	3·63	261
3·76–4·00	3·88	212
4·01–4·25	4·13	94
4·26–4·50	4·38	47
4·51–4·75	4·63	14
4·76–5·00	4·88	6
5·01–5·25	5·13	2
Total births		1260

5·13 kg. The sum of these weights is 4429·05 kg. Dividing by the total number studied, $n = 1260$, the mean birth weight of these infants is obtained as 3·52 kg. Of course, since the actual birth weight of each infant is not given, this is only an estimate, but, unless there is something peculiar about the distribution, this estimated mean should be very close to the true mean that would have been obtained if all the actual birth weights were known.

1.6.3 The median

Although the arithmetic mean is the most common measure of central value, there are several other measures that are widely used. One of these is the *median*. The median is the value of that observation which, when the observations are arranged in ascending (or descending) order of magnitude, divides them into two equal-sized groups. Consider the age data shown in Table 1.5. The 21 observations are already arranged in ascending order of magnitude (moving down the columns), so the middle observation or median is the eleventh one, which has the value of 82 years. This can be obtained either by counting up from the bottom until the eleventh highest observation is reached, or counting down from the top until the eleventh lowest observation is reached. Had the data not been in ascending order of magnitude, it would have been necessary to order them.

The median can also be calculated for data where there is an even number of observations, by taking the arithmetic mean of the two middle observations. In this case, the median is not one of the observations. Essentially, the median is the middle number.* Half the observations are less than the median and half the observations are greater than the median. This, of course, is not quite true when there is an odd number of observations, since one cannot talk about half the observations in this case. The basic idea, however, should be clear.

A more complex method must be employed to calculate the median if only a frequency distribution of the variable is available. Although a mathematical formula can be derived, the easiest approach is to construct the cumulated frequency polygon for the observations. Figure 1.16 gives this for the birth-weight data. (This was already presented in Fig. 1.14). The vertical scale can be given as a percentage of all the observations (i.e. 1260 corresponds to 100%) or, as previously, in terms of the number of observations. The median is the birth weight below which half or 50% of the values lie. Given the construction of the frequency polygon, this is obtained by drawing a horizontal line from the 50% point (or at $1260/2 = 630$ observations)† to the polygon. The value where the vertical line dropped from this point meets the bottom axis gives the median of the distribution. From Fig. 1.16, the median birth weight can be estimated as 3·51 kg. Thus, half the infants have birth weights

---

* If there are n observations, the median is the value of the $[(n + 1)/2]$th observation. If n is odd, $(n + 1)/2$ will be an integer. If n is even, $(n + 1)/2$ will involve the fraction 1/2.

† Note that, with this approach, the point on the axis corresponding to $n/2$ will define the median rather than $(n + 1)/2$ used with ungrouped data.

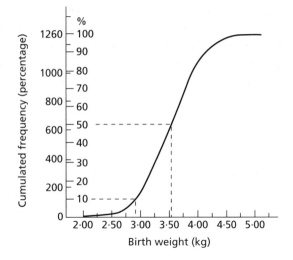

Fig. 1.16 Cumulated frequency polygon for birth-weight data.

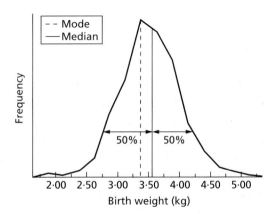

Fig. 1.17 Frequency polygon for birth-weight data showing the position of the median and mode.

below 3·51 kg and half have birth weights above this figure. The assumption underlying this approach for estimation of the median is that observations are distributed evenly within each class. In terms of a frequency curve or polygon, a vertical line from the median divides the area under the curve in half. Fifty per cent of the area lies below the median, representing 50% of the total frequency (Fig. 1.17).

To summarize, then, the median is calculated by arranging the observations in ascending (or descending) order of magnitude and the middle value of the series is selected as being a representative value for the variable. Thus, the median is an alternative to the arithmetic mean as a measure of the average for a given group of observations.

Although the median is quite simple to calculate and commonly used as a measure of central value, the arithmetic mean is generally preferred. The reasons for this are dealt with later, but at this stage it should be noted that, in general, the arithmetic mean and the median will be different in value. In the example of the ages of 21 patients with a hip fracture (Table 1.5), the arithmetic mean is 79·0 years and the median is 82·0 years. In the birth-weight

example, the mean is 3·52 kg, while the median is 3·51 kg. Whether the
median is less than, greater than or, in rare cases, equal to the mean depends
upon the general shape and characteristics of the particular distribution
concerned, a point which is discussed later in this chapter. However, for
fairly symmetrical distributions, the mean and the median will be close in
value.

1.6.4 The mode

A third measure of central value is the *mode*. The mode may be defined as the
most commonly occurring value, or as the value of the variable that occurs
with the greatest frequency. Among the 21 patients in Table 1.5, four were
aged 84 years. The next most frequent age was 73 with three occurrences.
Eighty-four years is the modal value for this distribution.

The mode can also be calculated for data arranged in a frequency distribution. Previously it was explained how a frequency distribution may be illustrated by means of a histogram or a frequency polygon. It was explained also
that, as the number of observations is increased and the class intervals are
reduced, the frequency polygon approximates more and more closely to a
smooth unbroken curve. The point at which this curve reaches a peak represents the maximum frequency, and the value that corresponds to this
maximum frequency is the mode.

In a histogram, the group into which most observations fall is the *modal
group* or, more generally, the *modal class*. In the birth-weight histogram, the
modal class is seen to be 3·26–3·50 kg, which has a total of 281 observations
(see Fig. 1.4). The value at which a frequency polygon reaches its maximum
gives a single estimate of the mode, though a more precise estimate of exactly
where the mode is within the modal class can be derived algebraically. In the
birth-weight data, the mode occurs at 3·38 kg—the mid-point of the modal
class (See Fig. 1.17). In the sense that the mode is the most frequently occurring value, it may be said to be a representative or average value, and may also
be used as a measure of central value, like the mean or the median. The mode
is usually different in value from both the mean and the median.

As a measure of central value, the mode is less commonly used than either
the arithmetic mean or the median. Moreover, some distributions do not have
a modal value, while other distributions may have more than one such value.
A 'one-humped' distribution with one mode is called unimodal, while a 'two-
humped' distribution is generally referred to as bimodal even if one of the
'humps' is higher than the other.

1.6.5 The weighted mean [!]

One should be careful in statistical calculations not to blindly employ techniques in situations where they may not be appropriate. One example of this is
the use of the ordinary arithmetic mean when a *weighted mean* should be
used. Table 1.8 shows the average length of stay observed in three wards of a

Ward	No. of patients	Average length of stay (days)
A	30	9·0
B	20	12·0
C	5	20·0

Table 1.8 Average length of stay of patients in different hospital wards.

hospital. It would be incorrect to calculate the overall average length of stay for all three wards by taking the mean of the three lengths of stay (9·0 + 12·0 + 20·0)/3 = 13·7 days.

The overall average length of stay should, in some manner, take account of the number of patients in each ward for which an individual length of stay was calculated. To calculate an overall representative value, each component length of stay in the average must be 'weighted' by the number of patients in the ward. The weighted average length of stay is then:

$$\frac{(30 \times 9\cdot0) + (20 \times 12\cdot0) + (5 \times 20\cdot0)}{30 + 20 + 5} = 11.1 \text{ days}$$

where one divides by the sum of the weights (patients). In notational form, a weighted mean can be expressed by:

$$\bar{x} = \frac{\sum wx}{\sum w} \tag{1.2}$$

where w represents the weights for each observation. In this example the weighted mean of 11.1 days is actually the mean length of stay that would have been calculated if the actual lengths of stay of all 55 patients had been available. Generally, it is incorrect to take an unweighted average of a series of means, and the approach outlined above should be used.

1.6.6 Comparison of mean, median and mode

Three different measures of central value have now been described—the arithmetic mean, the median and the mode. At this stage, it may occur to the reader that the concept of an 'average' or 'central value' is not at all precise, and this is in fact the case. Each of the measures described may be claimed to be an 'average' in some sense, and yet they will generally be different in value when used to describe the same data. Yet this is less confusing than it may seem, because the same ambiguities occur when the word 'average' is used in normal conversation, even though one may be quite clear what is meant when the term is used. If, for instance, it is said that the 'average' number of children per family is two, this does not mean that it is the precise arithmetic mean, which may be 1·8 or 2·3. What is probably meant is that two is the most commonly occurring family size—that more families have two children than have one, three or four, for example. In this case, the mode is being used as the 'average' value. In contrast, if it is said that the average age of a group is 32·4 years, probably the arithmetic mean age is being referred to. Or, again, if it was decided to say something about the average income of medical practitioners, the median might be preferred—this will indicate that half the doctors earn the median income or less and half earn the median income or more. In general, no hard and fast rules can be laid down about which measure to use—any one of the measures may be the most suitable in a particular instance. The mean, median and mode may be close together in value, or they may differ considerably in value; this depends upon the shape of the distribution.

In symmetrical distributions, the mean, median and mode all coincide; in asymmetrical or skewed distributions, the values of these measures will generally differ. The arithmetic mean is sensitive to extreme values, while the median and mode are not. For example, the mean of the following series of observations

$$4 \quad 5 \quad 5 \quad 5 \quad 5 \quad 5 \quad 75$$

is 14·9, which seems a poor representative value. The extreme value of 75 increases the mean, which uses all the observations in its calculation. The median, on the other hand, is not affected by the value of 75 and is seen to be 5. The median seems more appropriate as a central measure in this situation. In most practical situations, the mode is not a useful representative value. In the example above, the mode has the same value as the median (5), but many sets of data may have more than one mode (e.g. 1, 2, 2, 4, 4, 9 has modes of 2 and 4) or no mode (e.g. 1, 2, 4, 5, 9). Data with more than one mode are called *multimodal* or, as has been said, in the case of the two modes only, *bimodal*.

The example above with the extreme value of 75 is, in some sense, a very skewed distribution. If, now, the mean, median and mode are examined in terms of their positions in a skewed frequency curve, what is happening can be seen more clearly. Figure 1.18 shows a positively skewed frequency distribution, with some values far away from its 'centre' in the right-hand tail. The position of the mode at the peak of the distribution is easily found. Obviously, there is now a larger area to the right of the mode than to the left, so that the median, which divides the total area into halves, must be greater than the mode. Finally, the arithmetic mean is larger than either of the other measures because it is influenced by the extreme values in the upper tail of the distribution. (In a negatively skewed distribution the order of magnitude will, of course, be reversed to mean, median, mode—in alphabetical order!) Remember that the distribution of the ages of the hip-fracture patients was negatively

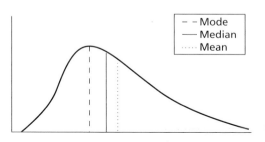

Fig. 1.18 A positively skewed
distribution.

skewed and that the mean, median and mode were, respectively, 79 years, 82 years and 84 years.

Looking at Fig. 1.18, it can be seen that, in highly skewed distributions, the median or mode may well be a more appropriate measure of central value than the arithmetic mean. (A further measure, especially suitable for positively skewed data, called the geometric mean, will be discussed below.) The arithmetic mean, however, remains the most commonly used measure of central value, partly because it is very amenable to further mathematical manipulations. Whatever measure is used however, its purpose is the same — to describe or summarize a collection of data by means of an average or representative value.

1.6.7 Data transformations [!]

It was pointed out in the previous section that, if data are skewed, the median may be a better representative value than the arithmetic mean. Though there are techniques suitable for the analysis of skewed data, there are advantages to working with data that are reasonably symmetrical in the first place. Data do not always behave as required, however, and sometimes the raw data are *transformed* prior to analysis to reduce the degree of skewness. Essentially, a transformation of the data is a change of scale. Thus, instead of working with a variable like length of stay in a hospital (which, as said above, usually has a markedly positive skew), one might instead take the square root of each observation and perform all analysis on the transformed variable. The square-root transformation will tend to reduce positive skewness and so the square root of hospital stay may be an easier scale to work with from the statistical point of view, even though logically it leaves a lot to be desired. Figure 1.19 shows diagrammatically how the square-root transformation tends to make the length of stay of seven patients more symmetrical than in the original scale. In the original data, it is the lengths of stay of 14 and 16 days that essentially skew this distribution, and the diagram shows how the square-root transformation brings these high values in the tail further back towards the left than lower-value observations. The transformation thus reduces a positive skew.

There are a number of different transformations that can be applied to data to reduce the degree of skewness, and Fig. 1.20 illustrates their use. In most

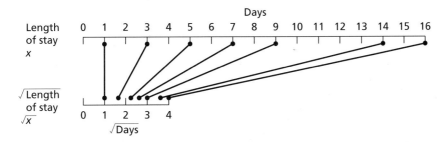

Fig. 1.19 The square-root transformation applied to seven lengths of stay.

Degree of skewness		Transformation	
Positive, low		Square root	$\sqrt{x}$
Positive, medium		Logarithmic	$\log x$
Positive, high		Reciprocal	$1/x$
Negative, low		Square	x^2
Negative, high		Cubic	x^3

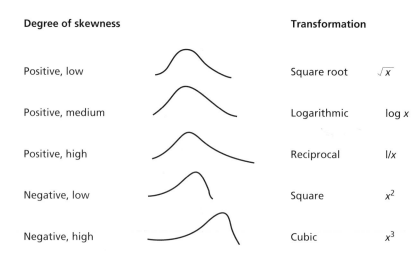

Fig. 1.20 Common transformations to reduce skewness (x is the original observation).

cases, it is a matter of trial and error by drawing the histograms of the transformed distributions to see which transformation works best. When a data transformation is employed, all analyses are performed on the transformed data. However, it can be quite difficult sometimes to understand what is happening and queries always arise on how to present any results.

The log transformation [!]

One of the commonest transformations of data in medicine is the log or logarithmic transformation. As can be seen in Fig. 1.20, it is used when the data have a medium level of positive skewness. In practice, the transformation is often used for any degree of positive skew, since it has some particularly nice properties. It is always wise, however, to check with a histogram (or stem-and-leaf diagram) of both the raw and transformed data to see if, visually at least, a degree of symmetry has been achieved with the transformation.

The log of any number is whatever power to which 10 must be raised to obtain it. For instance the log of 100 is 2 since 10^2 is equal to 100. Similarly the log of 1000 is 3. Though raising 10 to a fractional power might not seem to make much sense, mathematically it is a legitimate concept. For example, $10^{2.3}$ is in fact 199, and therefore the log of 199 is 2·3. Note that 199 (which has a log of 2·3) lies between 100 (which has a log of 2) and 1000 (which has a log of 3). The log of any positive number can be easily obtained by using a calculator.

The log transformation reduces the magnitude of large observations to a much greater degree than it reduces that of smaller observations, and thus, as pointed out, is suitable for making a positively skewed distribution more symmetrical. If any of the observations have a value of zero or less, the log is undefined and in this case the usual solution is to add a positive number to each of the original observations so that they are all above zero. The log of these values is then taken.

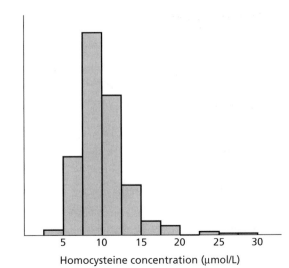

Fig. 1.21 Distribution of fasting plasma homocysteine in 797 normal subjects (μmol/L) (based on Graham *et al.*, 1997). See Table 1.9.

Homocysteine concentration (μmol/L)

Table 1.9 Fasting plasma homocysteine levels in normal subjects (based on Graham *et al.*, 1997). For original and transformed data, see Figs 1.21 and 1.22.

	Normal subjects
Number	797
Plasma homocysteine (μmol/L)	
Median	9·47
Mean	10·06
Geometric mean	9·67
Log plasma homocysteine	
Mean of logs	0·9855

As a simple illustrative example, suppose the original observations on a sample size of three were 2, 5 and 12. The positive skew in these data is fairly obvious. The logs of these three numbers are 0·301, 0·699 and 1·079, respectively, which are much more symmetrical.

Figure 1.21 shows a histogram of fasting plasma homocysteine levels in 797 normal subjects.* (The reader should not worry if he/she does not know what homocysteine is!) As can be seen, the distribution has a definite positive skew. Table 1.9, which gives some summary measures for these data, shows that the mean is greater than the median. In Fig. 1.22, the distribution of the log of each value in the distribution is shown. The distribution of the transformed variable is much more symmetrical and the log transformation has achieved its objective.

The geometric mean [!]

As was pointed out earlier, after a transformation one usually operates on the transformed data. Continuing with the simple example of the three observations 2, 5 and 12, the logs of these were 0·301, 0·699 and 1·079. Notationally,

* Based on data from Graham *et al.* (1997). A number of subjects in the original paper have been omitted from this illustrative example.

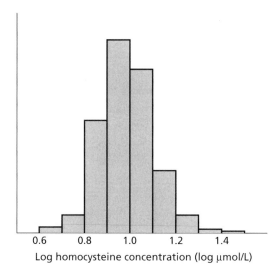

Fig. 1.22 Distribution of the log of fasting plasma homocysteine in 797 normal subjects (log μmol/L) (based on Graham *et al.*, 1997). See Table 1.9.

whereas x refers to one of the original observations, 'x prime' (x') is used to denote log (x). The arithmetic mean of these three logs is obtained by adding them up and dividing by 3, which gives 0·693. In general terms, the mean of the logs can be expressed as:

$$\bar{x}' = \frac{\sum x'}{n} \qquad (1.3)$$

This is the mean of the log-transformed data. To return to the original units of measurement, 10 should be raised to the power of this mean:

$$10^{0·693} = 4·93$$

In other words, the log of 4·93 is equal to 0·693 and 4·93 is just the mean of the logs transformed back to the original scale. This back-transformation is called the antilog. The value of 4·93, obtained by taking the antilog of the mean of the log-transformed data, is given a special name—the *geometric mean*. In general:

$$GM(x) = 10^{\bar{x}'} \qquad (1.4)$$

where $\bar{x}'$ is the mean of the log-transformed data given by Eqn. 1.3. The geometric mean is often used as a measure of central location in positively skewed distributions. In fact, for certain special distributions, the geometric mean is equal to the median, and considering it as an alternative to the median for positively skewed distributions should give a fair idea of its usefulness.*

As a further example the arithmetic mean of the 797 log-transformed

---

* If the distribution of the log-transformed data is perfectly symmetrical, then both the arithmetic mean and the median of the transformed data have the same value. Half of the transformed observations are above this value and half are below. But, by just back-transforming everything, half of the original observations are also above the back-transform of the value and half are below. Since the back-transform of this value is just the geometric mean, the geometric mean and median are identical in value as long as the log-transformed data are symmetrical.

Table 1.10 Calculation of the geometric mean of three observations.

Original observations		Log-transformed observations	
x	2, 5, 12	x'	0·301, 0·699, 1·079
Πx	$2 \times 5 \times 12 = 120$	$\Sigma x'$	$0·301 + 0·699 + 1·079 = 2·079$
GM(x)	$\sqrt[3]{120} = 4·93$	$\bar{x}'$	$2·079/3 = 0·693$
		GM(x)	$10^{0·693} = 4·93$

homocysteine values, whose histogram is shown in Fig. 1.22, is 0·9855 log μmol/L. The antilog of 0·9855 is $10^{0·9855} = 9·67$. Thus, the geometric mean homocysteine is 9·67 μmol/L (Table 1.9).

The reader may wonder why this measure is called the geometric mean. The reason is that an alternative explanation of its derivation exists. While the arithmetic mean is the sum of the observations divided by the total number of observations, the geometric mean is obtained by taking the product of the observations (i.e. multiplying them all together) and taking the nth root of the result, where n is the number of observations.[*]

$$GM(x) = \sqrt[n]{\Pi x} \qquad (1.5)$$

Here the symbol Π (pi—the capital Greek letter 'p') means 'multiply all the values', so that Πx means the product of all the x values.[†] For example, the product of the three observations discussed above is 120 ($2 \times 5 \times 12$). Taking the cube root of this gives 4·93 ($4·93 \times 4·93 \times 4·93 = 120$), which is the geometric mean obtained previously by back-transforming the mean of the logs (Table 1.10).

> Measures of the centre of a quantitative distribution
> • arithmetic mean (grouped and weighted mean)
> • median (used for skewed data)
> • mode
> • geometric mean (used for positively skewed data)

1.7 Other measures of location—quantiles

All the measures discussed so far are measures of central value; that is, they are designed to 'locate' the centre or middle of a distribution. However, it may also be of interest to locate other points in the distribution. Consider the polygon for the birth-weight data shown in Fig. 1.23. The vertical lines divide up its total area in certain proportions and the values (of birth weight) at which the lines are drawn are given special names—*percentiles*. Ten per cent

---

[*] The nth root of a number is that number which multiplied by itself n times gives the original number. For n equal to two and three, respectively, the terms 'square root' and 'cube root' are used.

[†] Like Σ meaning add up all the values.

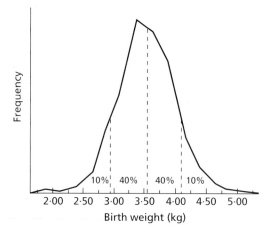

Fig. 1.23 The 10th, 50th and
90th percentiles of birth-weight
distribution.

of the area of the polygon lies below 2·91 kg and 2·91 kg is called the 10th percentile of the distribution. (It is seen later how to actually estimate these percentiles.) Since area is proportional to frequency, this can be interpreted to mean that, in the example, 10% of female infants at 40 weeks' gestation weigh less than (or equal to) 2·91 kg and 90% have birth weights above this figure.*

It has already been pointed out that the median divides a distribution in two halves so that 50% of infants weigh less than the median — 3·51 kg. For this reason, the median is also called the *50th percentile*. It is drawn in as the middle line in Fig. 1.23. Other percentiles are similarly interpreted. The 90th percentile of the birth-weight distribution, for instance, is 4·10 kg. Ninety per cent of infants w igh less than 4·10 kg and 10% weigh more. The 90th percentile is sometimes called the 'upper 10th percentile'. Like the 50th percentile (the median), the 25th and 75th percentiles are sometimes given special names — the *lower quartile* and *upper quartile*, respectively.

The percentiles divide the distribution into 100ths, but sometimes it is more convenient to refer to a different set of divisions. Thus, quartiles divide the distribution into quarters, quintiles divide the distribution into fifths and deciles divide it into 10ths. For example, the third quintile is the same as the 60th percentile and the ninth decile is the 90th percentile. Note that some people refer to percentiles as plain 'centiles' and that the general term for all such divisions is *quantiles*.

Quantiles can be used to create groups from a numerical distribution. Note, however, that the various quantiles define the cut-off points. Thus, for example, there are three quartiles (the 25th, 50th and 75th percentiles) which define group boundaries. The quartiles break the data into four groups, which are correctly called quarters. Similarly the (four) quintiles divide a distribution into fifths. It is incorrect to refer to the groups themselves as quartiles or quintiles, though it is often done.

* The question of whether an individual with the exact value given by a particular percentile should be included in the upper or lower group is, for all practical purposes, immaterial in continuous distributions.

The measures included in the example and their interpretation should illustrate, without requiring formal definitions, the meaning and purpose of percentiles. They are used to divide a distribution into convenient groups. The median or 50th percentile locates the middle of a distribution. The other percentiles similarly locate other points or values in the distribution. All these measures are called measures of location. The median, like the mean and the mode, is a special (i.e. particularly important) measure of location and is called a measure of central value or central location. Whilst measures of central location are the most important, other measures of location assist in describing a distribution more fully. In certain circumstances, measures like the fifth and 95th percentiles may be of greater interest than the median. By using the median in conjunction with these other measures, a compact description of a distribution can be made.

Quantiles divide a distribution so that a particular percentage or proportion of observations are below a given quantile
- percentiles (centiles) divide into 100ths
- deciles divide into 10ths
- quintiles divide into fifths
- quartiles divide into quarters
- tertiles divide into thirds
- the median divides into halves

1.7.1 Estimating percentiles in practice [!]

Percentiles can be difficult enough to calculate in practice, especially when dealing with small sample sizes. High and low percentiles (for example, the first or 99th) need a large number of observations and usually a computer is used to estimate them. A computer uses a mathematical method, similar to that described for the median, which is based on the ogive or cumulated frequency polygon. To estimate the 10th percentile of the birth-weight distribution, for instance, one would find the 10% point of Fig. 1.16, move horizontally across to the polygon, drop a vertical line from this intersection and read off the corresponding birth weight. It is, as already noted, approximately 2·91 kg.

There are special non-graphical methods for calculating the quartiles (25th, 50th and 75th percentiles). One such approach is described below, applied to the 21 ages of the fracture patients considered in Section 1.6 (Table 1.5).* The basic idea is simple. The quartiles break up a distribution into quarters, so the first thing is to break up the distribution into two halves and then break each of these halves into two also. The observations are divided into two halves based on the median, and the median of each of the two halves gives the other

---

* Other methods giving slightly different results are also used (see Frigge *et al.*, 1989).

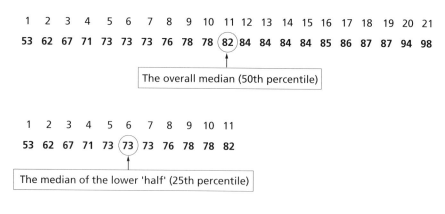

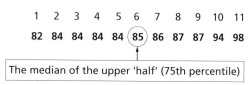

Fig. 1.24 Calculation of quartiles for the ages of 21 female patients with a hip fracture (years). The ranks of the observations are given in small numerals. See Table 5.1.

two quartiles. Though simple in concept, there is a slight ambiguity regarding how to split the observations based on the median.

For example, taking the 21 ages that are shown in Fig. 1.24, the median is the middle (11th) observation, which, because there is an odd number of observations, is actually one of the observed values. It is 82 years. What is required now is the middle observation of the half of the data below the median, and the middle observation of the half above the median. The question arises as to whether to include the original median (82 years) in either, both or neither of these halves. The solution suggested here is to include the median in each half of the data when moving to the next stage. Thus, the first quartile is the median of the 11 observations 53, 62 . . . right on up to and including 82. The first quartile is thus the sixth observation in this group: 73 (see Fig. 1.24). Similarly, the third quartile is obtained from the median of the observations starting with 82 and going on up to 98, which gives 85 years.

No ambiguity arises when there is an even number of observations, since the median is not one of the observations. Thus, with an even number of observations, exactly half the observations are below the median and half above it and it is clear which observations make up each half for the second median calculation.

1.7.2 The centile chart

The ability of percentile measures to summarize a frequency distribution is the basis of the *centile chart*. Figure 1.25 shows such a chart for the birth weight

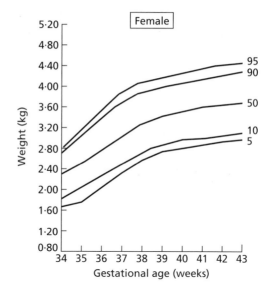

Fig. 1.25 Centile chart of birth weight for gestational age (from Hayes *et al.*, 1983, with permission).

of female infants by gestational age. The chart displays the fifth, 10th, 50th, 90th and 95th percentiles of birth weight at each gestational age from 34 to 43 weeks. The chart is used to make a judgement whether a newborn infant is heavier or lighter than would be expected. Suppose, for example, a female is born at 38 weeks weighing 2·9 kg. It can be seen from the chart that this weight is below the median (below 'average') but is well above the 10th percentile (about 2·68 kg) for this gestational age. Thus, the birth weight is not exceptionally unusual. On the other hand, a birth weight below the fifth percentile for a particular gestational age would suggest that an infant was much lighter than expected and would probably result in further investigation. Centile charts for height and weight by chronological age are also used to detect any growth retardation in children.

The centile chart in Fig. 1.25 was constructed by forming, for each gestational age (in completed weeks), the birth-weight distribution of a large number of female infants. The percentiles of each separate distribution were then calculated and plotted on the chart.*

1.7.3 The box plot

A number of pictorial representations of the distribution of a variable have already been described—the histogram, the frequency polygon, the stem-and-leaf diagram and the dot plot. Graphical methods can be very useful in explor-

---

* The birth-weight distribution at 40 weeks is based on the data discussed in this text (Table 1.3). The percentile values on the chart may, however, differ slightly from those obtained from these data; this is because a statistical 'smoothing' technique was employed to 'even out' the plotted percentile lines.

ing and examining data and in fact there is a whole area of statistics which is given the name exploratory data analysis (Tukey, 1977). One of the techniques used to describe data, which is being used more and more in medical applications, is the *box plot*.

Essentially, the box plot shows the distribution of a variable based on various percentile values. A rectangular box shows where most of the data lie, a line in the box marks the centre of the data (usually the median) and 'whiskers', which encompass all of or nearly all of the remaining data, extend from either end of the box.

Figure 1.26 shows the box plot for the 21 ages of the fracture patients. Each element is explained below. Note, however, that sometimes box plots are drawn vertically instead of horizontally. The quartiles on the diagram are denoted Q_1 (25th percentile—lower quartile), Q_2 (50th percentile—median) and Q_3 (75th percentile—upper quartile). The box is drawn with its boundaries at the lower and upper quartiles, with a line marking the median in the middle. Exactly half of the data is contained within the box and the median shows how spread out each half is. Look at Fig. 1.24, which shows the three quartiles for these data—73, 82 and 85 years.

Having drawn the box, the next step is to find where the 'fences' are. A fence is a boundary that in some sense defines limits within which most of the data should lie. It is not immediately clear what exactly 'most of the data' means and there are a number of different methods for constructing the fences (Frigge *et al.*, 1989). One in common use is described here. The difference between the upper and lower quartiles ($Q_3 - Q_1$) is called the *interquartile range* (IQR) (see Section 1.8.1). The fences are defined to be 1·5 times the IQR below the lower quartile and 1·5 times the IQR above the upper quartile. In

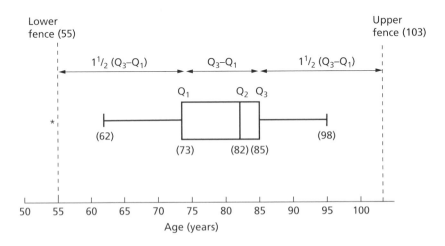

Fig. 1.26 Box plot of the ages of 21 female patients with a hip fracture. See Table 1.5. Note that only the box and whiskers (in thick lines) are actually drawn on a box plot and, in particular, the fences are not included. The arrows, lines, symbols and numbers in this figure are to show how the plot is created.

the example, the IQR is 12 years, 1·5 times the IQR is 18 years and the fences are at 55 (73 − 18) years and 103 (85 + 18) years.

Although the fences define a boundary within which most of the data should lie, the fences themselves are never actually drawn on a box plot. Instead, whiskers are drawn from the lower and upper quartiles, not to the boundary fences, but to the most distant data point *within or at the fences*. Thus, while the upper fence is at 103 years, the largest age observed was 98 years and the upper whisker extends only as far as this figure. The lower fence is at 55 years, but the smallest data point within the boundary defined by this is 62 years. The lower whisker then extends down to 62 years (see Fig. 1.26). Data points outside the fences (outliers) are marked in individually, as, for example, the age of 53 years in the figure just below the lower fence boundary. Outliers may be an indication of errors in the data and outlying values should probably be checked for accuracy.

Care should be taken when interpreting box plots in the literature (or on computer output), since the quartiles can be calculated in a number of different ways and different definitions can be used for the fences. (Multipliers of the IQR other than 1·5 are used and the fences are sometimes put at the 10th and 90th percentiles.) Overall, however, the box plot gives a succinct summary of a distribution. Skewness is immediately obvious from the position of the median in the box and the length of the whiskers, together with the position of outliers. The age data for hip fractures seems to have a negative skew — as was evidenced from Fig. 1.10 also.

Comparing stem-and-leaf diagrams with box plots

Stem-and-leaf diagrams and box plots are two relatively recently proposed graphical methods for exploratory data analysis and each has its strengths and limitations. The stem-and-leaf diagram is essentially a simplified histogram and gives a good picture of the overall shape of the distribution, particularly in the middle. Any problems with bimodality are easily seen.

The box plot hides any bimodality and concentrates more on observations at the extremes of the data. A box plot always identifies outliers, which may not be as obvious from a histogram or stem-and-leaf diagram. Box plots are particularly useful for the comparison of numerical data between groups, when a series of box plots can be drawn and direct contrasts of various percentile measures can be made. (See Chapter 7.)

1.8 Measures of dispersion

1.8.1 The range and interquartile range

When looking at a set of values or a frequency distribution, it can easily be seen if the observations are widely dispersed from the measure of central value or are scattered fairly closely around it, but it may often be desirable to describe the dispersion in a single summary figure. One method of doing this is to calculate the *range* of the values, which is the difference between the highest and lowest values in the set. For instance, the minimum age in the patients with a hip fracture was 53 and the maximum was 98 (see Table 1.5 or Fig. 1.24). The range for these data is therefore 45 years. It is also legitimate to say the range of these data is from 53 to 98 years, but statisticians usually prefer to use the term range for the single figure. Without doubt, the range is the most easily understood measure of variability or spread in data, but it suffers from the disadvantage that it is based only on the extreme values (i.e. highest and lowest) and ignores all the values in between.

Another measure of spread that has been met already (in Section 1.7.3) is the *interquartile range* (IQR). This is the difference between the upper (or third) quartile (75th percentile) and the lower (or first) quartile (25th percentile). The IQR for the age-at-hip-fracture data is 12 years, obtained from the upper and lower quartiles of 85 and 73 years, respectively. When the median is used as a measure of the centre of the data, the interquartile range is often used as the measure of spread.

1.8.2 The variance and standard deviation

The variance

The most commonly used, but perhaps least understood, measure of variability is the standard deviation. This measure takes account of all the observations in the data and has many uses in statistics. An intuitive justification of its derivation is now given.

Table 1.11 shows two sets of data, each with the same mean of $\bar{x} = 13.5$. The first set of data is far less spread out than the second, as can be seen by comparing the ranges. Concentrating on the second set of data, an initial approach to defining a measure of dispersion or spread might be to see how far each individual observation is away from the (arithmetic) mean. The deviations of the four observations from the mean are:

Table 1.11 The variance and standard deviation.

Observations	12 13 14 15	10 11 15 18
Mean ($\bar{x}$)	13.5	13.5
Range	$15 - 12 = 3$	$18 - 10 = 8$
Squared deviations from the mean $(x - \bar{x})^2$	$(12.0 - 13.5)^2(13.0 - 13.5)^2$ $(14.0 - 13.5)^2(15.0 - 13.5)^2$	$(10.0 - 13.5)^2(11.0 - 13.5)^2$ $(15.0 - 13.5)^2(18.0 - 13.5)^2$
Sum of squared deviations $\Sigma(x - \bar{x})^2$	5.0	41.0
Variance $S^2 = \dfrac{\Sigma(x - \bar{x})^2}{n-1}$	$5.0/3 = 1.66$	$41.0/3 = 13.66$
Standard deviation S	$\sqrt{1.66} = 1.29$	$\sqrt{13.66} = 3.69$

$$10\cdot0 - 13\cdot5, \quad 11\cdot0 - 13\cdot5, \quad 15\cdot0 - 13\cdot5, \quad 18\cdot0 - 13\cdot5$$

or

$$-3\cdot5, \qquad -2\cdot5, \qquad +1\cdot5, \qquad +4\cdot5$$

Now try taking an average of these deviations using the arithmetic mean. At this point, an important property of the arithmetic mean will be noted. This is that the sum of deviations from the arithmetic mean is always zero. The minus deviations cancel out the plus deviations; a measure of variation cannot be calculated algebraically as the average of the deviations, since their sum is always zero. In calculating the dispersion of values around the arithmetic mean, however, it is immaterial whether the deviations are plus or minus; only the numerical magnitude of the deviation is of interest. Hence, to avoid getting zero when the deviations are added together, try squaring these deviations.* The squared deviations are

$$(-3\cdot5)^2, \quad (-2\cdot5)^2, \quad (1\cdot5)^2, \quad (4\cdot5)^2$$

or

$$12\cdot25, \qquad 6\cdot25, \qquad 2\cdot25, \quad 20\cdot25$$

An average of these squared deviations would now appear to be a reasonable definition of variability. For reasons discussed in Section 4.6.3, the average value is determined by summing the squared deviations and dividing by one less than the total number of deviations. The resulting measure is called the *variance* and is given the symbol S^2. The sum of the squared deviations in the example is 41, so that the variance is $41/3 = 13\cdot66$. The variance can be expressed in terms of a formula:

$$S^2 = \frac{\sum (x - \bar{x})^2}{n - 1} \tag{1.6}$$

This formula is easy to understand: x is an individual observation, $\bar{x}$ is the arithmetic mean and n is the number of observations. The mean ($\bar{x}$) is subtracted from each observation or value (x), and the resulting deviation is squared. This is done for each of the values. Finally, the sum of the squares of the individual deviations from the mean is divided by the total number of observations less one ($n - 1$). Appendix A details an equivalent computational method to determine the variance.

Degrees of freedom [!]

The divisor, $n - 1$, for the variance is called the *degrees of freedom* for the statistic, which is a term that will be met with in a number of different contexts. The term essentially means the number of independent quantities making up

---

* Just ignoring the minus signs and averaging the absolute deviations also gives a measure of spread, but this is rarely used.

the statistic that are free to vary. The variance in the example considered is calculated from the four original observations and their mean, which, of course, is not independent of them. If, knowing nothing else, one were asked to guess at what the first observation might be, any value might be given. If one were asked to guess the second and third observations, again any values would suffice. However, given these three guessed values and the mean, the fourth value is predetermined. For instance, if one chose the values 11, 12 and 15, the fourth value would have to be 16 since the mean must be 13·5. Thus, there are three degrees of freedom for this variance, and in general the degrees of freedom for a variance are one less than the sample size. The degrees of freedom for any statistic can usually be determined as the number of independent quantities used in the calculation of the statistic (e.g. the n individual observation), less the number of parameters in the statistic estimated from them (e.g. the sample mean).

The standard deviation

To avoid working with 'squared' units, the square root of the variance can be taken and this is called the *standard deviation*. The square root of 13·66 is 3·69, which is the standard deviation of the four observations 10, 11, 15 and 18. The standard deviation can be defined in mathematical notation as

$$S = \sqrt{\frac{\sum (x - \bar{x})^2}{n - 1}} \tag{1.7}$$

(see Eqn. 1.6). The standard deviation is sometimes called the *root mean square deviation*.

Table 1.11 shows the standard deviations and variances for the example just considered and for the four observations 12, 13, 14 and 15, which have the same arithmetic mean but are less spread out. Their standard deviation is 1·29, compared with the value of 3·69 obtained for the observations 10, 11, 15 and 18.

The standard deviation has the expected properties of a measure of spread. If one distribution is more spread out than another, then it has a larger standard deviation. If a distribution has no variability or spread (i.e. all the observations have the same value), then the standard deviation is zero. (The reader should verify this from the formula for the standard deviation.) Unfortunately, at this stage, the reader can have no feel for the magnitude of the standard deviation and how to interpret the actual numerical value. This is discussed in Chapter 4, but misinterpretations abound in this area.

As might be expected, the standard deviation is the usual measure employed when the arithmetic mean is used as the measure of the centre, but the range is far easier to understand. None the less, because the standard deviation is used extensively in subsequent chapters of this book, the reader would be advised to make a special effort to grasp the meaning of the measure. The variance and standard deviation may also be calculated for a grouped frequency distribution. As for the mean, the calculation is somewhat longer and is presented in Appendix A.

1.8.3 The coefficient of variation

If one wants to compare the variability of some measurement in two groups, the standard deviation can be used. However, if the two groups have very different means, the direct comparison of their standard deviations could be misleading, particularly in cases when more variability in the group with the larger mean might inherently be expected. For instance, the standard deviation of the height of 17-year-old boys is around 5·9 cm and of 2-year-olds around 4·1 cm (*Geigy Scientific Tables*, 1984). The standard deviation is greater in the older group, suggesting more variability of height than in those aged 2 years. However, 17-year-olds are a lot taller than 2-year-olds (average heights of 174·3 cm, and 87·0 cm, respectively) and it might be useful to see what the variation in heights is *relative* to the mean. For this purpose the *coefficient of variation* can be employed. This is simply the standard deviation expressed as a percentage of the mean:

$$CV = \frac{s}{\bar{x}} \times 100 \qquad (1.8)$$

This is independent of the unit of measurement and is expressed as a percentage. The coefficients of variation of the heights of 2-year-olds and 17-year-olds are 3·4% and 4·7%, respectively, showing that the height of 2-year-olds is relatively more variable than that of 17-year-olds, though it is less variable in absolute terms.

Measures of the spread in variability of a distribution
- range
- interquartile range
- variance
- standard deviation
- coefficient of variation

1.9 Summary

In this chapter, the essence of descriptive statistics has been discussed. Distinctions have been made between qualitative and quantitative data, and diagrammatic presentations of quantitative data have been outlined. The histogram, frequency polygon, stem-and-leaf diagram, dot plot, cumulated frequency polygon and box plot have been described. Summary descriptions of a frequency distribution have been explained relating to shape, measures of location and measures of spread.

Statistic	Formula	Eqn. No.
Arithmetic mean:	$\bar{x} = \dfrac{\sum x}{n}$	(1.1)
Weighted mean	$\bar{x} = \dfrac{\sum wx}{\sum w}$	(1.2)
Median	middle number	
Mode	most frequent number	
Geometric mean	$GM(x) = 10^{\bar{x}'}$	(1.4)
	($\bar{x}'$ is the mean of the logs)	(1.3)
	$GM(x) = \sqrt[n]{\Pi x}$	(1.5)
Range	maximum − minimum	
Interquartile range	$IQR = Q_3 - Q_1$	
Variance	$S^2 = \dfrac{\sum(x - \bar{x})^2}{n-1}$	(1.6)
Standard deviation	$S = \sqrt{S^2}$	(1.7)
Coefficient of variation	$CV = \dfrac{S}{\bar{x}} \times 100$	(1.8)

2 Probability, Populations and Samples

2.1 Introduction

The first chapter of this book showed how data gathered in a study might be organized, summarized and presented. Such descriptive statistics form only a part of statistical analysis and the remainder of this book, for the most part, deals with what are called inferential statistics. In this chapter, some of the groundwork for the material to follow is presented and the reader is introduced to a number of ideas that underlie the research process.

Essentially, statistical inference embodies a methodology that enables something about a large population to be discovered on the basis of observing a subgroup or sample from that population. This chapter starts with a brief foray into the notion of probability and then the ideas underlying sampling are explored, with a discussion of sample survey techniques.

2.2 Probability

2.2.1 Definitions

Central to all statistical analysis is the mathematical theory of probability or chance. Interest in this area arose during the seventeenth century in the context of gambling, and since then the subject has been studied in depth and is a field of investigation in its own right. Although some purists might disagree, a fairly sound grasp of statistical concepts is possible without a deep understanding of probability theory. In line with the origins of the theory of probability, examples in this section tend to be from games of chance, such as cards or dice.

Intuitively, everyone has an idea of what probability is. The probability of a coin landing heads is 1/2; the probability of getting a 3 on the roll of a die is 1/6; the probability of drawing an ace from a pack of cards is 4/52. The truth of such probability statements will depend on whether the coin or die is un-biased (not a two-headed coin or a loaded die) or whether all the aces are actually in the pack and that it is well shuffled.

What can be deduced about probability from the above examples? Firstly, a probability is measured on a numerical scale ranging from 0 to 1. An event with the probability of 0, for all practical purposes, cannot occur; an event with a probability of 1 is a certainty (e.g. death). Between these two extremes, a probability can take any value from 0 to 1 and can be expressed as a fraction (1/6) or a decimal (0·1667). Probabilities can also be expressed in terms of percentages, e.g. a probability of 16·67%. The second point about the probability of an event is that it can be calculated if it is known how many times the event can occur out of all possible outcomes, *provided that each outcome is equally likely*. Thus, there are six equally likely outcomes to the throw of a die; one of these is the appearance of a 3 on the upper face, so that the probability of a 3 is 1/6. In a pack of cards, there are four aces in 52 cards. Of the 52 possible outcomes, all equally likely, four are favourable, so that the probability of an ace is 4/52. The caveat that each outcome must be equally likely is important. For instance, to determine the probability of obtaining two heads after tossing a €1 coin and a €2 coin, it would be incorrect to conclude that, because there are three possible outcomes (two heads, one head and zero heads) and only one is favourable, the answer is 1/3.* In fact, there are four *equally likely* outcomes for the €1 and €2 coin, respectively; these are H/T, T/H, H/H and T/T, where H/T means a head on the €1 coin and a tail on the €2 coin. Of these four equally likely outcomes, only one is favourable, so that the probability of two heads is 1/4.

The probabilities discussed above were all defined from outside the particular experiment (drawing of a card, tossing of a coin) and can, thus, be called *a priori* probabilities. Such probabilities have the property that, if the experiment were repeated a large number of times, the proportion of times the event would be observed would approach the *a priori* probability. If a coin is tossed three times, three heads might be obtained, but if it is tossed a million times or more the proportion of heads should be very close to 0·5 or 50%.

This gives rise to the frequency definition of probability, which is an event's relative frequency in a very large number of trials or experiments performed under similar conditions. This suggests that a probability could be estimated on the basis of a large number of experiments. For instance, to determine the probability of a live-born child being a male, one could examine a large series of births and count how many males resulted (ignoring the problem of hermaphrodites!). In Ireland in 1997, there were 52 311 live births, of which 26 855 were male. Thus, the best estimate of the probability of a male, on the assumption that the same underlying process in sex determination is appropriate, is 26 855/52 311 = 0·513 or 51·3%.

---

* The euro (€) is the single currency for eleven European Union member states. The old familiar terminology of 'heads' and 'tails' is retained here, though not all states have a head on one side of their coinage.

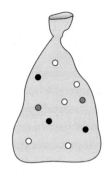

○ Red (5)
● Green (3)
◉ Blue (2)

Fig. 2.1 A bag of coloured marbles.

There is another type of probability, which does not fit into the framework discussed above. A person may say, for instance, that the probability of an outbreak of influenza this winter is 0·01 or 1% or that the probability of their passing the final medical examination is 0·9 or 90%. There is no way that such probabilities can be interpreted as an event's long-term relative frequency as described above, and such probabilities are referred to as subjective probabilities. In a loose sense, a subjective probability expresses one's degree of belief in a proposition. Such definitions are not considered in this book, although subjective probability can provide an alternative framework within which to view statistical inference.

2.2.2 Probability and frequency distributions

Having defined a probability in terms of an event's long-term relative frequency in repeated trials, it is now necessary to examine the relationship of probability to statistical calculations. A simple example will illustrate most of the concepts, and no mathematical rigour is attempted. Consider a bag of 10 coloured* marbles, five red, three green and two blue (Fig. 2.1), from which one marble is drawn. The *a priori* probability that this marble will be red is 5/10 = 0·5, that it will be green is 3/10 = 0·3 and that it will be blue is 2/10 = 0·2. If, now, it were not known either how many marbles were in the bag nor what colours they were, the proportions of each colour could be estimated by drawing one marble, noting its colour, replacing it and continuing in the same manner for a large number of trials. If a bar chart were drawn for the number of different times each colour was obtained, the results might be similar to those shown in Fig. 2.2, which is based on the results of 10 000 such draws: 4986 of the draws were of a red marble, 3016 were of a green marble and 1998 were of a blue marble. If each of these figures is divided by the total number of trials (10 000) relative frequencies for red, green and blue of 0·4986, 0·3016 and 0·1998, respectively, are obtained. These relative frequencies are almost identical to the actual *a priori* probabilities, as would be expected, given the original definition. When the number of observations on

---

* The illustration is in monochrome. The reader should have no difficulty in imagining the colours, however!

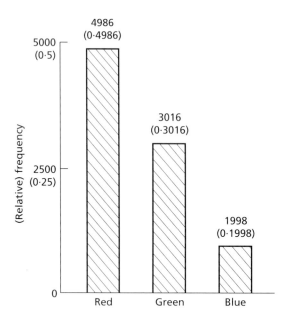

Fig. 2.2 A bar chart showing the colours obtained in 10 000 draws of a single marble (with replacement) from the bag in Fig. 2.1. Relative frequencies are given in parentheses.

the bar chart is replaced by the relative frequency, a relative frequency diagram is obtained, as also illustrated in Fig. 2.2. Note that the relative frequencies must sum to 1·0.

The experiment described, then, gives rise to a relative frequency diagram showing the distribution of colours in the bag of marbles. From the opposite point of view, however, given the relative frequency diagram in Fig. 2.2, the probability of obtaining a specific result in one draw of a marble from that particular bag could be known to a high degree of accuracy.

This example serves to illustrate the close connection between probability and frequency distributions. Instead of working with a bar chart, the frequency distribution of a quantitative variable, such as birth weight at gestational age 40 weeks, might be given, as in the last chapter. This may easily be transformed into a relative frequency distribution, when, instead of the total area under the curve being given the value of 1260, reflecting the total number of births studied, it is given a value of 1·0 or 100%. Whereas in the bar chart example the relative frequencies of a particular colour were represented by the height of the bar, in a relative frequency distribution of a numerical variable it is the area under the curve above a certain range of values that represents their relative frequency. (Remember—it was pointed out that it was the area of a bar that was important in a histogram, rather than its height.)

Figure 2.3 shows the relative frequency polygon for the birth-weight data. Note that the vertical axis is not given a scale, since it is relative areas under the curve that are of interest. As an illustration, the relative frequency of birth weights between 2·50 and 3·00 kg* is about 0·12 or 12%. Given this frequency distribution, it can be deduced that the probability of any one child in

---

* Actually 2·505 to 3·005 kg. See discussion in Section 4·2.

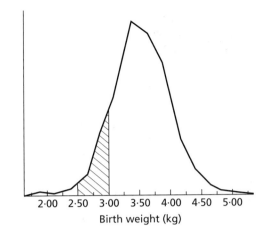

Fig. 2.3 A relative frequency
distribution of birth weight at
gestational age 40 weeks for
females. The shaded area is 12%
of the total area.

the study (female, 40 weeks' gestation) having a birth weight within these
limits is 0·12 or 12%.

Thus, the relative frequency distribution for a variable provides information on the probability of an individual being within any given range of values
for that variable. It should be noted that, with a continuous distribution, such
as weight, a probability cannot be ascribed to an exact weight of, say, 2·4 kg;
such an exact weight would really signify a value of exactly 2·40 kg — the zeros
continuing indefinitely — and the area over such a value is actually zero.
However, the probability of an individual having a value, for instance,
between 2·395 and 2·405 kg can be established, which is, in the example, as
accurate as the original measures were in the first place.

2.2.3 Combining probabilities [!]

Going back to the example of the bag of marbles, some simple rules of combining probabilities can be illustrated. Suppose that one wanted to determine
the probability of obtaining, in one draw from the bag, either a red marble *or*
a green marble. Of the 10 possible outcomes eight are favourable, therefore
the probability of a red *or* green marble is 8/10 or 0·8. This result, however,
could also have been obtained by adding together the separate probabilities of
a red marble (0·5) and a green marble (0·3). This gives rise to the general addition rule of probability; the probability of the occurrence of *two mutually
exclusive* events is obtained by adding together the probability of each event.
If A and B are two such events:

$$P(A \text{ or } B) = P(A) + P(B). \tag{2.1}$$

where P(event) means the probability of the event. Mutually exclusive means
that, if one event occurs, the other event cannot occur, and the additive rule
only holds under this condition. If a marble is red, it cannot be green at the
same time. On the other hand, to determine the probability of an ace or a
diamond in a pack of cards, the additive principle would not hold, since

the existence of the ace of diamonds makes the two events not mutually exclusive.

Suppose now that a marble is drawn and returned to the bag and then a second marble is drawn. What is the probability of obtaining a red marble first and then a green one? In this situation, the multiplicative rule of probability holds and the probability of the joint occurrence of two *independent events* is given by the multiplication of the separate probabilities:

$$P(A \text{ and } B) = P(A) \times P(B). \tag{2.2}$$

Thus, the probability of a red and a green marble is $0.5 \times 0.3 = 0.15$. The requirement of independence means that the occurrence of the first event does not affect the probability of the second event, and this is required for the multiplicative rule. Since in the example the marbles were replaced, the result of the first draw could have no influence on the result of the subsequent draw. If the events are not independent, a different rule must be used. This is:

$$P(A \text{ and } B) = P(A) \times P(B \text{ given } A). \tag{2.3}$$

where $P(B \text{ given } A)$ means the probability of the event B given that the event A has already occurred. An example of this more general rule follows. Suppose that the first marble was not replaced. What now is the probability of a red marble and a green marble? The probability of a red marble is 0.5, but if a red marble is drawn from the bag and not replaced, the probability of a green marble is not now 0.3. There are only nine marbles left after a red marble has been drawn: four red, three green, and two blue, and the probability of a green marble is, thus, 3/9 or 0.3333 if a red marble was drawn already. Thus, in this instance the probability of a red and a green marble in that order is $0.5 \times 0.333 = 0.1666$. Examples of the use of this rule in its application to the calculation of survival rates are seen in Section 7.15. $P(B \text{ given } A)$ is referred to as a *conditional probability* and the independence of two events A and B requires in probability terms that:

$$P(B \text{ given } A) = P(B). \tag{2.4}$$

2.3 Populations and samples

2.3.1 Statistical inference: from sample to population

When medical researchers collect a set of data, their interest usually goes beyond the actual persons or items studied. For instance, in the study of birth weights in the previous chapter, the purpose was to construct centile charts that would be applicable to future births. Because of this desire to generalize, describing the results of a particular study is only a first step in a statistical analysis. The second step involves what is known as statistical inference. In technical terms, a statistical inference is an attempt to reach a conclusion about a large number of items or events on the basis of observations made on only a portion of them. The opinion poll, which studies a small number of persons to estimate attitudes or opinions in a large population, is a good example of this. In the medical field, a doctor may prescribe a particular drug because prior experience leads him/her to believe that it may be of value to a particular patient. A surgeon too may use a particular operative technique because in previous operations it seemed to give good results. (As is seen in Chapter 6, however, such inferences may be erroneous, and the controlled clinical trial provides a sound scientific method to compare the efficacy of medical interventions.)

In statistical terminology, it is usual to speak of *populations* and *samples*. The term population is used to describe all the possible observations of a particular variable or all the units on which the observation could have been made. Reference may be made to a population of patients, a population of ages of patients at hospital admission or a population of readings on a thermometer. What is to be understood as the 'population' varies according to the context in which it is used. Thus, the population of patients in a particular hospital and the population of patients in the whole of Ireland are quite distinct populations. It is important to understand that the term 'population' has a precise meaning in any given context.

A population may be finite or infinite. The population of hospital patients in Ireland at or over any particular period of time is finite. On the other hand, the population of readings on a thermometer is infinite since, in principle, an infinite number of such readings can be taken. Many populations are so large that they may be regarded as infinite — for example, the number (population) of red blood cells in the human body.

In its broadest sense, a sample refers to any specific collection of observations drawn from a parent population. It is possible to have a sample of patients, a sample of temperature readings, and so on. The two properties required of any sample are that it be of reasonable size and that it be representative of the population from which it was taken. At one extreme, a sample may include all of the units in the parent population, in which case it is referred to as a *census*. In many countries, a census of the full population is taken at regular intervals. A census is, by definition, completely representative of the population. At the other extreme, a sample may consist of only one unit selected from the population. Although it is of theoretical interest, such a sample cannot in practice reveal very much about a parent population unless many assumptions are made. In this sense, a reasonably sized sample is somewhere between two units and all the population. Intuitively, however, it would be felt that sample sizes of two or three are also inadequate, and that the larger the sample, the more reliance can be placed on any inference made from it. Exactly what is an adequately sized sample depends on the precise nature of the study being carried out and on many other factors, which are considered at a later stage.

Why study samples at all? Why not always examine the full population, as in a census? There are two basic reasons that may be put forward. First, it is usually too expensive and time-consuming to study an entire population and in fact it may not even be possible to define the population precisely. What, for instance, is the population of patients with coronary heart disease? The second reason, just as important, is that a sufficiently sized representative sample can give information concerning a population to whatever degree of accuracy is required. Thus, a census is, in many instances, a waste of resources and effort although it is only with a census that the number of persons in a population can be determined precisely.

2.3.2 Non-representative samples

A large sample does not by itself, however, make for a representative sample. One of the best examples of this is taken from the early days of the opinion poll. In 1936, an American magazine, *The Literary Digest*, sampled telephone subscribers and its own readers to forecast the result of the forthcoming US presidential election. They received 2·4 million replies (out of 10 million selected for the sample) and predicted as a consequence that one of the candidates, Landon, would have a landslide victory over Roosevelt. Few people have ever heard of Landon, so what went wrong? A little thought might suggest that telephone subscribers and readers of a particular magazine could be of a different social class from the entire voting population, and that voting preferences might indeed depend on this factor. Such was the case, since few of the sampled groups were to have been found on the breadline or in the soup queues of those depression years. The voting preferences of the sample were not representative of the entire population and, in addition, the replies received (about 24%) were unlikely to have been representative of the sampled group. The survey drew an incorrect inference because of *bias*. A bias can be broadly defined as any factor that will lead to an erroneous conclusion, and the technical names for the two biases in this survey are selection bias and non-response bias.

The huge sample size made no difference to the validity of the study and in fact a smaller unbiased sample would have been greatly preferable. This was realized by an individual called George Gallup. He organized two properly conducted small surveys, one of only 3000 persons, from which he predicted that the *Digest* poll would show Landon as victor (before that magazine had time to even count the replies to their own poll), and a second of about 50000 persons, which predicted the correct result of the election. George Gallup was the eponymous founder of the famous polling company.

2.3.3 The simple random sample

How, then, is it possible to ensure that a representative sample is selected? An intuitive approach might be to uniquely identify all the units in a (finite) population and 'put all the names in a hat', mix well and draw out enough names to give a sample of whatever size is required. This is the principle used in the selection of winning tickets in a raffle or lottery, and it is the model underlying the *simple random sample*. This type of sample forms the theoretical basis for most statistical inference. A simple random sample is a sample chosen in such a way that, at each draw, every name in the hat has the same chance of being chosen. Everybody in the population has the same chance of getting into the sample.

Such samples are representative of the population in so far as no particular block of the population is more likely to be represented than any other. The general term 'random sample' refers to the situation when every member of the population has a known (non-zero, but not necessarily the same) probability of selection. Random is thus a term that describes how the sample is chosen, rather than the sample itself.

2.3.4 Sample statistics and population parameters

When any data are to be studied, it must always be remembered that they are (usually) a sample from a far larger population of observations and that the purpose of the study is to make inferences about the population on the basis of the sample. Any time a frequency polygon for a variable is constructed, it is being used to estimate the underlying population distribution of that variable. Although, in practice, it is never known precisely what this distribution looks like, one could imagine taking a measurement on everyone in the population and forming a population frequency curve. (With such a large number of observations and using very small class intervals, a curve rather than a polygon would be obtained.) For the population of all female births at 40 weeks' gestation, for example, a curve similar to that in Fig. 2.4 for birth weight might be obtained. This (population) curve would then have a mean and standard deviation. Similarly, when an association is examined, it is the underlying association in the population(s) from which the sample(s) came that is of concern.

Usually statistical inferences are made on quantifiable factors in a study. These include measures of position or spread for a single quantitative variable

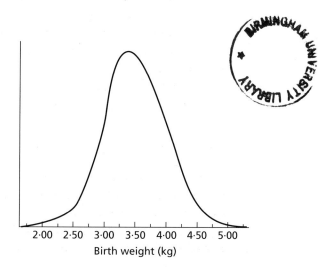

Fig. 2.4 The underlying frequency distribution of birth weight for the population of females at 40 weeks' gestation.

(means, medians, percentiles, standard deviations, etc.) and percentages in various categories for a single qualitative variable. In general, the underlying values of such measures, in the population(s), are symbolized by Greek letters, with the corresponding Roman letters denoting the factors in the sample. For example the mean and standard deviation of a sample were symbolized by $\bar{x}$ and S in the last chapter. The corresponding population measures are μ (mu — the lower-case Greek letter 'm') and σ (sigma — the lower-case Greek letter 's'). In a population such factors are technically referred to as parameters, while in a sample they are called statistics. (A good way of remembering this is that populations have parameters with a 'p' and samples have statistics with an 's'.) With this terminology, the purpose of statistical inference is to estimate or discover something about population parameters on the basis of sample statistics.

Population
- the large group that is of interest

Sample
- a sufficiently sized representative subgroup of the population

Simple random sample
- each member of the population has the same chance of being chosen in the sample

Statistical inference
- the process of drawing a conclusion about a population on the basis of a sample

---

2.4 Sample surveys

2.4.1 Simple random sampling

To draw a simple random sample from a given population, one needs to have some list of all the units in the population. Such lists are referred to as the sampling frame. Obviously, to put 'all the names in a hat' and draw a sample would, in practice, be a very tedious operation and fraught with potential biases, due to lack of mixing, for example. An alternative and equivalent method is, however, available. This requires the use of a table of random numbers. One page from such a table is given in Appendix B (Table B.1). Essentially, a table of random numbers can be thought of as being produced by someone sitting down in front of a hat containing the numbers 0 to 9 on 10 separate pieces of paper. He draws a number, notes it down, replaces it in the hat, mixes well and draws another number, repeating the process millions of times. Tables of random numbers are not, of course, produced by real humans but are generated by computers. They have the important property that every digit has a one in 10 chance of being present at any particular position in the table. Thus, such tables can be used to simulate the physical drawing of a sample from a hat. Suppose that a sample of size five is required from a population of 80 individuals. First, number the 80 units in the population from 01 to 80. Start at an arbitrary point (use a pin) in a table of random numbers and read down the nearest column. Since two digits are sufficient to identify any member of the population, read the first two digits of a column and continue reading down the column until five different two-digit numbers between 01 and 80 are obtained. Repeat numbers should be ignored, as should numbers outside this range. The numbers chosen in this way identify the particular members of the population who are in the sample. For example, start at the top of the sixth column in Table B.1. The first eight two-digit numbers are 72, 12, 90, 86, 15, 28, 28, 36; ignoring 90, 86 and the second 28 for the reasons stated, the remaining numbers identify the members of the sample.

2.4.2 Stratified random sampling and quota sampling

A refinement of the simple random sample is the *stratified random sample*. The population is divided into groups, or strata, on the basis of certain characteristics, for example age or sex. A simple random sample is then selected from each stratum and the results for each stratum are combined to give the results for the total sample. The object of this type of sample design is to ensure that each stratum in the population is represented in the sample in certain fixed proportions, which are determined in advance. For example, in determining the smoking habits of a national population, age and sex are obviously important factors, and it might be desirable to select a sample whose age and sex composition exactly reflects the age and sex composition of the whole population. With a simple random sample, it is unlikely that the age and sex composition of the sample would achieve this. However, by dividing the population into age/sex groups and selecting a random sample within each group whose size is proportional to the size of the group, it can be ensured that the age/sex distribution of the sample matches exactly that of the entire population. Although the sample proportions often reflect the proportions in the population, not all stratified random samples are selected in this way. Certain strata may be deliberately 'over-represented' in the sample, while others are 'under-represented'. The important point is that the sample proportions are predetermined. For this reason, stratified random samples are often preferred to simple random samples. If a stratified sample has been taken with some strata over- or under-represented, the sample as a whole will not reflect the population. If one wanted to estimate, for example, the population mean, a weighted mean of the within-strata means would be used with the weights equal to the size of the population in each of the strata (see Section 1.6.5).

Sometimes, a sampling survey is undertaken specifically to compare two or more groups. The most efficient comparison can be made when the same sample size is used for each group. If the groups in the population are not the same size, this requires a stratified sample, with equal sample sizes taken from each strata.

A sampling method similar to the stratified random sample, and commonly used in opinion polls and market research, is the *quota sample*. This, however, is not a random sample in the true sense of the word. In quota sampling, the main objective is to fill certain quotas of individuals in well-defined groups, such as males aged 25 to 34 years. The quotas are arranged so that the final sample mirrors the population exactly in relation to, say, age and sex groups, and to that extent a quota sample is similar to the stratified sample. However, one is free to choose anyone who will fit the requirements of the quotas, and obviously only cooperative individuals and easily contactable persons would be included. There is no guarantee that the persons chosen within a particular group are representative of the population in that group as regards the factors being studied, and large unquantifiable biases may occur. In a stratified random sample, however, every person in a particular stratum has the same probability of inclusion in the sample, and this ensures, in a probability sense, representativeness in terms of other variables.

2.4.3 Multistage and cluster random sampling

The *multistage random sample* is another sampling technique, which has the advantage that a full list of the population to be surveyed is not required. Suppose that schoolchildren in a certain area are to be sampled. Rather than obtaining (with great difficulty) a full list of all such children and taking a simple random sample of these, a list of the different schools in the area could be obtained, and a simple random sample taken of the schools. A simple random sample could then be taken from a list of the children in these schools only (much smaller than the full list of children in the population). The sampling would, thus, be accomplished in two stages, with a large reduction in the practical work involved. There are potential difficulties in multistage samples, however, and a statistician should be consulted before undertaking such a task. A variant on the multistage sample is the *cluster sample*, where a simple random sample of groups (e.g. schools) is taken, and everyone in the chosen group is studied. This method, too, should be used only with professional advice.

Different forms of sampling can be identified:
- the simple random sample
- the stratified random sample
- the quota sample (non-random)
- the multistage random sample
- the cluster random sample

2.4.4 Bias in sampling

Sample surveys of defined populations have an important part to play in medical research, and should be characterized by the care taken in choosing the sample correctly. Random samples refer to very specific techniques and should not be confused with haphazard sampling, when anyone and everyone can be included in the sample on the researcher's whim. The importance of a random sample is threefold: it avoids bias, most standard statistical inferential methods assume such sampling and, as is seen in the next chapter, precise statements concerning the likely degree of accuracy of a sample result can be made.

Apart from bad sampling, there are two main sources of bias in any sample survey. The *Literary Digest* poll discussed in Section 2.3.2 suffered from both. The first is that of non-response. To conduct any survey of people, one must eventually contact the individuals actually sampled. If some are uncooperative or impossible to trace, these exclusions from the sample may affect its representativeness. Non-response rates higher than 15–20% may cast doubt on any conclusion drawn from a particular study. The second source of the bias in a sample survey relates to the choice of the sampling frame (selection bias). It is very important not to draw conclusions about a different population from that actually sampled. It is always necessary to check the adequacy of the sampling frame (the population list) in terms of its coverage of the population, and care should be taken not to over-generalize the results. For instance, a medical researcher may sample rheumatoid arthritis patients who attended a particular teaching hospital, but would be in error to generalize any of the results to a target population of all rheumatoid arthritis patients. Rheumatoid arthritis does not necessarily lead to hospitalization and in a teaching hospital, in particular, a more severe type of arthritis may be seen. At best, the results of such a study should be generalized to rheumatoid arthritis patients in hospital.

Major sources of bias in sampling are:
- non-random sampling
- non-response bias
- selection bias

2.4.5 Non-random sampling

An approximation to the simple random sample, which, though requiring a list of the population, is much easier in practice, is the *systematic sample*. In such a sample, every nth person is chosen, where n depends on the required sample size and the size of the population. One starts at random in the list, somewhere among the first n members; thus, if every 10th member of a population is to be chosen, one would start by choosing a random number from 1 to 10—say 7—and include the 7th, 17th, 27th, etc. persons on the list. Such a method could be used advantageously for sampling hospital charts, for instance, when a simple random sample might prove very difficult indeed.

A major problem of medical research, however, is that, in many situations, random or systematic sampling is impossible, because the population of interest is not strictly definable. Many studies are performed on what are known as samples of convenience, or *presenting samples*. Typically, a doctor may decide to study 100 consecutive hospital admissions with a particular condition. There is no sense in which such individuals could be considered a random sample from a particular population, but it can be reasonably hoped that information on such patients might provide insight into other similar patients who may be diagnosed some time in the future. The best approach is to ask from what population the patients actually in the study could be considered a random sample, and to make a statistical inference about that hypothetical, and possibly non-existent, population. There are large departures from the theoretical assumptions underlying statistical analysis with this approach, but it still seems the only solution to the problem of definite non-random samples often met with in the medical situation.

Forms of non-random sampling include
- the systematic sample (which often approximates a random sample)
- the presenting sample (which does not)

2.5 Summary

In this chapter some background material, necessary for a complete grasp of the chapters to follow, has been introduced. A basic understanding of probability and its relationship to frequency distributions is central to most statistical inference. The distinction between populations and samples and the notion of making an inference about a population on the basis of a sample from that population is, of course, the core idea in statistical analysis, while, from the practical point of view, the different techniques that can be used in actually taking a random sample from a population are important.

The next chapter of the book examines in a non-technical way how the results from surveys are analysed and interpreted.

3 Associations: Chance, Confounded or Causal?

3.1 Introduction

The first chapter of this book showed how data gathered in a study might be organized, summarized and presented—one variable at a time. In the second chapter, the notion of sampling was introduced, together with the idea of making a statistical inference from a small subgroup to a larger population. This third chapter introduces the reader to many of the concepts central to the interpretation of scientific and medical research. The chapter is, as far as possible, non-mathematical and concentrates on the ideas involved. The more mathematical details will come later! This chapter suggests that the main thrust of research is determining the existence of associations between variables and then interpreting those associations. The ideas underlying formal statistical analyses (significance testing, confidence intervals), the problems of confounding variables and the notion of causality are considered. The chapter acts as a general introduction to the remainder of the book and as an overview of the scope and limitations of the research process.

3.2 Examining associations

In the first chapter, methods for describing and summarizing a single variable were considered in some detail and two main categories of variable were described—qualitative and quantitative. Though the distribution of a single variable may be of some interest, it is when two or more variables are considered together that some substantive conclusions can be drawn from a collection of data. With relatively few exceptions, most of the well-formulated research questions in medicine can be answered by determining if there is an association between two particular variables in a given study.

What is meant by an association? Essentially, it means that knowing the value of one variable in an individual gives some information about the likely value of the other. This can be expressed in many different ways: it can be said that the two variables are related, that the two variables are correlated, that they are not independent, that one variable is dependent on the other, that one variable influences the other, that one variable causes the other. The terms 'influence' and 'cause', however, suggest an interpretation of the association which may not be valid (see below), while the other terms are less prescriptive in their interpretation.

Readers should ask themselves what pairs of variables could be defined to help answer the following questions. Does consumption of folic acid prevent neural-tube defects? Does using a mobile phone cause brain cancers? Does blood pressure increase with age?

3.2.1 Means or medians in groups

The idea of an association between two variables is probably much clearer with a number of examples. For many questions of interest, one of the variables will be qualitative and the value of the variable will define membership of a particular group or, equivalently, possession of a particular attribute. The variables sex and smoking status are typical examples. In this context, a difference between groups regarding some factor corresponds to an association between the variable defining the groups and that factor. In simple terms, groups are being compared and, if there is no difference between the groups, there is no association.

If the variable being compared is quantitative, such as age or blood pressure, the presence of an association can be investigated by comparing the distribution of the variable between the groups. Such a comparison will often be summarized by presenting a measure of the centre, such as the median or mean, in each of the groups, while a more complete picture can be given by showing a box plot or a dot plot of the quantitative variable in each group.

Table 3.1 shows the mean, geometric mean, quartiles and interquartile range of plasma homocysteine levels in 746 patients with vascular disease and in the 797 normal subjects already presented in Table 1.9. Figure 3.1 shows

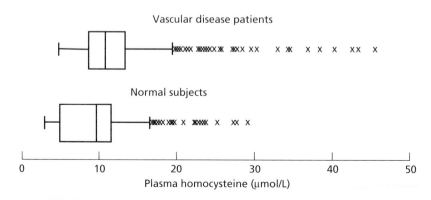

Fig. 3.1 Box plots of plasma homocysteine in 746 vascular disease patients and 797 normal subjects (based on Graham *et al.*, 1997).

Table 3.1 Plasma
homocysteine levels in
patients with vascular disease
and normal subjects (based
on Graham *et al.*, 1997).

	Vascular disease patients	Normal subjects
Number	746	797
Plasma homocysteine (μmol/L)		
Mean	11·93	10·06
Geometric mean	11·15	9·67
Median (Q_2)	10·79	9·47
Lower quartile (Q_1)	8·79	8·05
Upper quartile (Q_3)	13·22	11·44
Interquartile range	4·43	3·39

Summary measures of association*

Mean plasma homocysteine

Patients: 11·93 μmol/L

Normal subjects: 10·06 μmol/L

Difference

The mean homocysteine was 1·87 μmol/L (11·93 minus 10·06) higher in patients than in normal subjects

Ratio

The mean homocysteine in patients was 1·186 times (11·93/10·06) that in normal subjects

Percentage difference

The mean homocysteine was 18·6% (1·87/10·06) higher in patients than in normal subjects

* The mean is used for illustration even though the data are fairly skew

---

box plots of homocysteine in each group. A difference between the two groups in the distribution of homocysteine is apparent. Those with vascular disease have much higher homocysteine levels, and the whole distribution seems to have shifted upwards. Thus there is an association between homocysteine levels and the presence of vascular disease. Usually only one measure of the centre would be employed in group comparisons and in this situation, given the skewness in the data, either the median or the geometric mean would be appropriate.

If only two groups are being compared there are advantages to summarizing the comparison or association with a single figure, rather than presenting mean or median values in each group. When comparing a quantitative variable, the most commonly used measure is the difference between the means or medians. For simplicity, the arithmetic mean is used in the illustration, even though the skewness of the data might suggest use of the median or geometric mean as a summary measure. Thus, as shown in Table 3.1, vascular disease patients have a mean homocysteine that is 1·87 (11·93 − 10·06) μmol/L higher than that of normal subjects. Less usually, a ratio measure could be used and one could say that the mean homocysteine in patients was 1·186 times

Smoking status	Males		Females	
	n	(%)	n	(%)
Current smoker	669	(49·4)	499	(36·4)
Ex-smoker	328	(24·2)	215	(15·7)
Never smoker	356	(26·3)	657	(47·9)
Total	1353	(100·0)	1371	(100·0)

Table 3.2 Smoking status in males and females based on a study of 2724 persons (from O'Connor & Daly, 1983, with permission).

(11·93/10·06) that in normal subjects. Finally, the difference could be expressed as a percentage of one of the groups, so that one could say that the mean homocysteine was 18·6% (1·87/10·06 expressed as a percentage) higher in patients than in normals. Note that the 18·6% can also be derived from the decimal part of the ratio measure.

3.2.2 Percentages in groups

An association between two qualitative variables is examined by means of a *contingency table*, which is a table with the categories of the two variables making up the rows and columns of the table and the number of persons in each category combination given in each cell of the table. Table 3.2 shows the association between smoking status and gender in a population survey. Smoking has three categories—current, ex- and never—and gender has two— male and female. This table is called a 3 × 2 table, because it has three rows and two columns. An association between two qualitative variables can always be interpreted as a comparison of groups with regard to the qualitative variable whose percentage distribution is given in each of the groups.

Often it is not clear which way percentages in such a table should be presented. Taking the current example, should one give the percentages of males and females within each smoking group or give the percentages in each smoking group within males and females (as has been done here)? The answer will depend on the context of the study, how the data were collected and what the objective of the presentation is. Here it is legitimate to use either approach, since the study is cross-sectional, but, since the main interest is probably the difference in smoking habits between male and female, the table presented is more appropriate. See also Section 1.3.1, where the number of decimal places to present in tables is discussed.

Table 3.2 shows a difference in smoking status between males and females and thus the existence of an association between gender and smoking. Such data can be presented in a composite bar chart, as shown in Fig. 3.2. A composite bar chart will often, as here, be given with a percentage scale, rather than absolute numbers, to allow direct comparison of the groups.

The contingency table is one of the most important devices in statistics for examining associations. One of the reasons for the central place of the

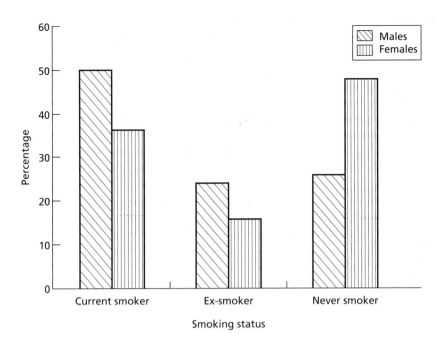

Fig. 3.2 Composite bar chart showing smoking status of males and females (based on O'Connor & Daly, 1983).

Table 3.3 Smoking status in males and females based on a study of 2724 persons (modification of Table 3.2).

Smoking status	Males		Females	
	n	(%)	*n*	(%)
Current/ex-smoker	997	(73·7)	714	(52·1)
Never smoker	356	(26·3)	657	(47·9)
Total	1353	(100·0)	1371	(100·0)

Summary measures of association
Smoking
    Males: 73·7%
    Females: 52·1%
Absolute difference
    21·6% = 73·7% − 52·1%
Relative difference
    Relative to females (41·5% more):
        41·5% = 21·6%/52·1% expressed as a percentage
    Relative to males (29·3% fewer):
        29·3% = 21·6%/73·7% expressed as a percentage
Ratio
    Relative to females:
        1·415 = 73·7%/52·1%
    Relative to males:
        0·707 = 52·1%/73·7%

contingency table is the fact that any quantitative variable can be grouped into a small number of categories and treated like a qualitative variable. Thus age is often analysed as a qualitative variable with a small number of (age) groups.

In general, there is no easy way to summarize an association between two qualitative variables in a single number. If, however, each variable has only two categories, there are a number of commonly used measures of the association in the resulting 2 × 2 table. In later chapters of this book, particular emphasis will be placed on the analysis of such tables, but mention will be made of the simpler measures here.

If no distinction were made between current and ex-smokers, Table 3.2 would become a 2 × 2 table comparing the percentage of (current or ex-) smokers between males and females (Table 3.3). The two figures to be compared are 73·7% and 52·1%. The association could be summarized in a single number by quoting the absolute difference in percentages—males have 21·6% more smokers than females (73·7% minus 52·1%)—or the ratio of the percentages—the percentage of smokers in males is 1·415 times that in females (73·7% divided by 52·1%).

Absolute and relative differences [!]

The reader should be careful, however, in interpreting percentage differences. Sometimes a relative percentage difference is presented instead of the absolute difference and it may not be clear which has been used. The relative percentage difference is the absolute difference in the percentages divided by the percentage in one of the groups. Thus the difference of 21·6% is 41·5% of the percentage smoking in females (21·6% divided by 52·1% and multiplied by 100).* This means that, relative to the percentage of smokers in females, male smoking is 41·5% higher. Unfortunately, this can be expressed in a statement such as, 'There are 41·5% more smokers among males than among females', and the percentage could be misinterpreted as an absolute difference. The use of an appropriate modifier such as 'relative' or 'absolute' can sometimes obviate this difficulty and the phrase 'a difference of 21·6 percentage points' can be used, which unambiguously refers to an absolute difference. In general, however, the oft-used term 'percentage difference' remains ambiguous when referring to a qualitative variable. No confusion arises for a quantitative variable, however.

When relative measures are presented, one should note which of the groups acted as the baseline or reference group. The female group was used in the discussion above. Had males been the reference group, one would have said that the percentage of smokers in females was 0·707 that in males (52·1% divided

---

* Note that, if unity is subtracted from the ratio of the percentages in the two groups, which was 1·415 in the above example, the figure of 415 is obtained. This is the relative difference expressed as a proportion rather than a percentage.

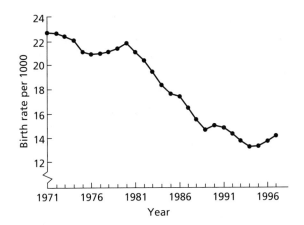

Fig. 3.3 Birth rates in Ireland, 1971–1997 (based on Department of Health, 1987, 1997).

by 73·7%). Similarly, compared with males, females had 29·3% relatively fewer smokers (21·6% divided by 73·7%). Note that $1·0 - 0·707 = 0·293$, showing the relationship between the relative percentage and the ratio measure when it is less than unity.

3.2.3 Graphs and scattergrams

Graphs and scattergrams essentially display the relationship or association between two quantitative variables. In fact, it is only by means of such diagrams that this type of association can really be examined and tabular presentations of such data do not help in seeing if an association is present. A fault that is fairly common is to attempt to show too much material in a graph. In general, it should avoid excessive information and detail and yet be self-contained, in the sense that it should present the essential points without the reader having to search the text for explanations. The lines of the graph should be capable of being easily followed to observe a change in the value of the vertical scale for a given change in the value of the horizontal scale. If the values of each variable tend to increase together, the association is called positive; if one variable increases while the other variable decreases, the association is called negative.

The choice of scale is important for interpreting what the graph is showing and one should be careful when a transformation of scale, such as the log transformation, has been used.

Figure 3.3 shows a graph of the birth rate (number of births per 1000 population) in Ireland from 1971 to 1997. This is an example where the unit of observation is a calendar year and the (quantitative) variable is a rate calculated for that year. It is easy to see from the graph the steady fall in the birth rate from the early 1980s and the small but definite rise that commenced in the mid-1990s. Note that, unlike the bar chart, it is not necessary to start either of the axes at the zero mark, and often the axis is shown with a break in this case.

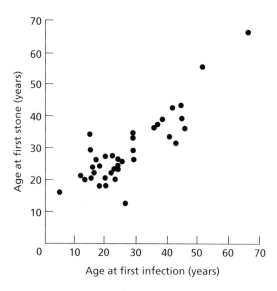

Fig. 3.4 Relationship between age at first stone and age at first infection in 38 women with two or more stone-associated urinary-tract infection (abbreviated from Parks *et al.*, 1982, with permission).

Figure 3.4 represents another important type of diagram, called a scatter-gram. Like the graph, it displays a relationship between two quantitative variables. Here the relationship is between 'age at first urinary-tract infection' and 'age at development of first renal stone' among a sample of women with two or more stone-associated urinary-tract infections. Typically, while graphs display how one variable may change over time with a line joining the corresponding points, a scattergram is designed more to show the association, or lack of association, between two general quantitative variables. For each subject, or whatever the unit of observation might be, the values for each variable are taken and a point is plotted in relation to the two values. For example, one extreme point can be seen in the upper right-hand corner of the diagram. This point corresponds to an age at first urinary-tract infection in a female of 68 years and an age at first renal stone, which is approximately the same. On the other hand, another isolated point will be seen corresponding to an age at first urinary-tract infection of about 25 years, in a female whose age at first renal stone was approximately 12 years. The spread of points on the scattergram shows an upward trend to the right. This indicates that there is a positive association or relationship between the two variables considered and that the older the women are at first infection, the higher the age at first kidney stone. In Chapter 10, various techniques for quantifying associations of this kind are explained.

The existence of an association between variables can be determined by examining
- means/medians in groups (a quantitative and a qualitative variable)
- percentages in groups (two qualitative variables)
- graphs or scattergrams (two quantitative variables)

3.3 Interpreting associations

As already pointed out, many, if not most, important questions in medical research can be answered by determining if an association exists between two variables. If an association is found in a particular study, then the important next step is to try and interpret what the association means. Before jumping to any conclusion that there is a causal effect, which is what one is presumably looking for, one must ask if there could be other explanations for the finding. There are two possibilities that must be considered. The finding may be due to chance or the finding may be due to bias or confounding. It is only when these two factors can be eliminated that the possibility of a causal effect should be contemplated. It could be said that the whole field of research design and statistical analysis relates to the determination of the roles of bias and chance as explanations for observed associations.

There are three possible explanations for an observed association between two variables
- chance
- bias or confounding
- a real (causal) effect

3.4 Associations due to chance

One explanation that must always be considered for an observed association is that it is due to chance alone. As has been pointed out, most studies are performed on samples of persons and problems can arise with small sample sizes. Results based on a small sample may not reflect the true situation in the population.

Much of the remainder of this book will be spent describing how to determine if chance alone could explain an observed finding, especially for the usual situations of sample sizes intermediate between a handful and a couple of million. This is the main purpose of a formal statistical analysis and will lead to consideration of the concepts of *statistical significance* and *confidence intervals*. The key question is whether a valid inference can be made from the sample result to the general population from which the sample was taken or whether the findings could represent a chance occurrence that does not reflect the true situation in that population. Some examples will be presented to illustrate the basic ideas.

3.4.1 Statistical significance or hypothesis testing

The example

A research group is interested in comparing the effects on 5-year survival in breast-cancer patients of two different drug preparations, drug B, which is the

Treatment	Alive	Dead	Total
Drug A	17 (68·0%)	8 (32·0%)	25 (100·0%)
Drug B	12 (48·0%)	13 (52·0%)	25 (100·0%)

Table 3.4 Five-year outcome in a trial comparing drugs A and B.

standard therapy, and drug A, which is potentially useful. They decide to put 25 patients on each of the two treatments and to follow the patients for 5 years to determine their mortality. Essentially, the study has been set up to determine if there is an association between the type of treatment and survival.

As described, this study would fit into the category of a clinical trial, but, as is seen in Chapter 6, the proper setting up of a clinical trial is more complex than outlined above. Postponing more detailed discussion to that chapter, however, assume for the moment that the two groups of patients (25 on drug A and 25 on drug B) are similar as regards all factors that might affect overall mortality, such as age or the severity of their disease. The only factor that differentiates the two groups is assumed to be the particular treatment that they have been given. On this basis, a comparison between the two groups should be valid in determining the drug effects.

Suppose, now, that at the end of the study the results shown in Table 3.4 are obtained. The 5-year survival rate with drug A is 68%, compared with only 48% with the standard therapy, drug B. What can be concluded about the effects of the two drugs?

Medical importance

The first step in a statistical analysis of a particular study is to examine the data to see if any association is evident. As already seen in the example, the absolute survival advantage of drug A-treated patients over drug B-treated patients was 20% (68% − 48%). Examining the results of any study requires, usually, only the application of the simple methods of descriptive statistics and is a task that may be carried out with an absolute minimum of specialist statistical knowledge. Amazing as it may seem, however, this task is sometimes overlooked by a researcher, who mistakenly thinks that a statistical analysis in the form of a hypothesis test (considered below) is all that is required. This point cannot be emphasized too strongly; examination of results, in terms of means, proportions, percentages or whatever, is a prerequisite for any formal statistical analysis.

In examining the results, the researcher must ask a question akin to 'Are my results medically important?' By this is meant 'Do the results as they stand suggest that an important new finding has emerged that will perhaps change medical practice, or alter one's view of a disease process, or have a major impact of some sort?' As discussed earlier, this can often be reduced to asking if an association is present in the data. Certainly, an absolute difference in mortality of 20%, as in the example above, would seem to be an important finding. On the other hand, if the two mortality rates had been 49% and 50%, respectively, the medical importance of the finding would be questionable, since the difference between the two treatments is so small. The question of what size of result can be considered important, however, is one for the clinician and practising doctor and not for the statistician to answer. If the results of a particular study are not deemed to be medically important, little more can be done. No amount of mathematical or statistical manipulation can make a silk purse out of a sow's ear. A study, for instance, that shows only a very small difference between two groups in the variable under examination (a small degree of association) is of little interest unless it is carried out to show the equivalence of the groups in the first place. Such is not usually the case.

If the results of a particular study do seem medically important, then further analysis, leading to a formal statistical hypothesis test, must be performed. The purpose of such a test is to enable a judgement to be made on whether or not reliance can be placed on the (important) result obtained. The precise form of this hypothesis test will depend on, among other things: the sample size in the study; the types of variables involved in the association; the number of groups being compared; how the groups were formed; the scale of measurement of the variable under analysis; and the precise hypothesis being tested. Rather than examining at this stage the particular hypothesis tests that might be appropriate for the data in the above example, a more conceptual approach to the problem is now considered. (These data are analysed in Section 7.10.1.)

The null hypothesis

The medical hypothesis the research group wish to test in the example is that, in terms of 5-year survival, drug A is better than drug B. There is no doubt, of course, that, in the patients studied, drug A is indeed better, but the basic question is whether or not it is legitimate to extrapolate from the particular situation of these 50 patients to the general situation of all patients. The problem is one of statistical inference and requires a decision to be made concerning drug effectiveness on the basis of a small group of patients. Certainly, if there had only been, say, 10 persons in this study, few would pay much attention to the results, since, even without any formal statistical analysis, extrapolation from a sample size of only 10 might seem a somewhat dubious procedure. On the other hand, if there had been 10 000 patients studied, few would doubt the reasonableness of accepting the result.

The notion of making a decision on the basis of a sample, and thus on incomplete evidence, is not unique to statistics. The holding of an examination to decide if an individual should obtain a degree is but one example. In essence, the individual student is 'sampled' on the day of the examination and performance in that particular examination will not necessarily reflect true ability; the student may have an off-day; the questions asked may be in his/her one weak area or, of course, the opposite could occur, with a bit of luck (chance). The decision, however, is made on the basis of the examination taken. The decision may be fair or it may not and an element of doubt always remains. This element of doubt is the price paid for incomplete information, and is the only reason that statisticians have a part to play in medical, or any other, research.

The first step in performing a statistical hypothesis test is to reformulate the medical hypothesis. In many situations, it is far easier to disprove a proposition than to prove it. For instance, to prove that (if it were true) all cows were black would require an examination of every cow in the world, while one brown cow disproves the statement immediately. Suppose, again, someone has found a landscape painting in an attic and wonders if it might be by, say, Constable.* They decide to send it to an art expert. The expert could never prove the painting was by this painter—the best she/he could do might be to determine that the frame and canvas were sufficiently old, that the style seemed to be like Constable's, that the signature looked like his and that other facts were not inconsistent with the supposition. On the other hand, a television satellite dish on the roof of a farmstead in the painting would disprove completely the hypothesis that Constable could have been the artist.

Similarly, taking another analogy: a wife could probably never prove her husband was totally faithful to her. Though she may never find any evidence, it would always be possible that he was being very careful. On the other hand, it would be easy to prove her husband was having an affair if he was careless and left enough incriminating evidence around. Faithfulness is easy to disprove but not easy to prove. In branches of mathematics too, such as geometry, many proofs commence with the supposition that the required result is not true. When a consequent absurdity occurs, the supposition is rejected and the result required is thus proved.

In statistical analysis, a very similar approach is used. Rather than trying to 'prove' the medical hypothesis (drug A is better than drug B), an attempt is made to 'disprove' the hypothesis that drug A is the same as drug B. This reformulation to what is essentially a negative hypothesis is central to an understanding of hypothesis tests. In fact, the reformulated hypothesis is generally referred to as a *null hypothesis* and in most cases the researcher wants to disprove or reject it. In general, such hypotheses refer to no association between the two relevant study variables in the population and in this example the null hypothesis states that there are no real differences in survival between the two treatment groups. Although in many situations the null hypothesis may not be explicitly stated, it is the cornerstone of every statistical test.

The (statistical) null hypothesis
- negates the existence of a true association between two variables
- states that the population groups are the same in a two-group comparison
- is the reverse of what the study is designed to show
- is such that the researcher usually wants to reject it

---

* John Constable (1776–1837) was a famous English landscape painter.

Having reformulated the original medical hypothesis in the form of a null hypothesis, the further premise that it can be 'proved' or 'disproved' in some way must be examined. Unfortunately, real life is not like geometry and, when dealing with biological variability and the uncertainty introduced by not being able to study everybody, proof or disproof of a proposition can never be absolute. This is why rejection or acceptance of a null hypothesis is referred to, rather than the proof or disproof of it. In fact, for reasons discussed later, it is preferable to refer to the non-rejection of a null hypothesis rather than to its acceptance. An interesting analogy may be drawn with the judicial process. An individual is assumed innocent until proved guilty. The assumption of innocence corresponds to the null hypothesis and 'proved guilty' (which corresponds to rejection of this hypothesis) does not refer to absolute truth but to the decision (possibly fallible) of a jury on the basis of the (possibly incomplete) evidence presented. Absolute truth is no more discernible in statistics than in a court of law.

The first step, then, in hypothesis testing requires that a hypothesis of medical interest must be reformulated into a null hypothesis, which, on the basis of the results of a particular study, will or will not be rejected, with a margin of error in whatever conclusion is reached.

A null hypothesis always makes a statement about reality or, in more technical terms, about a population or populations. The results of a study are based on a subset of (or sample from) the population(s) of interest. In medical situations, however, it is sometimes very difficult to identify the precise population(s) referred to in a null hypothesis, as in many situations the study groups are not random samples from fully specifiable populations. In the example, the null hypothesis that drug A has the same effect on 5-year survival as drug B refers, in a vague sense, to all patients similar to those included in the study. In some way, however, the results are important only in so far as they can be applied to patients in the future, while the study groups themselves are based on patients already diagnosed and treated in the past. As is discussed in Chapter 6, hypothesis testing in the context of a clinical trial such as this requires a slight alteration in the interpretation of the null hypothesis, but, for clarity, at this point it will be assumed that the two treated groups (drug A and drug B) are representative of two populations. The 25 persons on drug B are representative of the population of all patients with breast cancer if they had all been given the standard treatment, and the 25 persons on drug A are representative of the population of patients if they had all been treated with that particular drug. The fact that the populations do not exist in reality does not detract from the approach, and the conclusion of the study will relate to the question 'What would happen if all patients were treated with either one of the preparations?'

The above discussion may seem somewhat convoluted, but it is important to realize that the results of any study are useful only in so far as they can be generalized and that, for statistical analysis, the existence of certain populations may have to be postulated for valid application of the techniques.

Testing the hypothesis

Figure 3.5 illustrates the two states of reality implied by the null hypothesis. Reality, according to the null hypothesis, is that the two drugs are equivalent (in terms of 5-year survival). Corresponding to any null hypothesis there is always an alternative hypothesis, which includes all possible realities not included in the null hypothesis itself. In this example, reality according to the alternative hypothesis is that drugs A and B have different effects.

Of course, it can never be known what actually corresponds to reality, and the whole purpose of hypothesis testing is to enable a decision to be taken as to which of the two alternatives (a null hypothesis or the alternative hypothesis) should be decided upon. Important results, of course, immediately suggest that the alternative hypothesis is more tenable than the null hypothesis (which states there is no difference between the two groups). The main problem, however, is whether or not enough reliance can be placed on the results to actually reach such a conclusion. The question that should be asked is whether the results are spurious (due to chance) or whether they reflect a real difference between the effects of the two drugs. What is meant by spurious is best illustrated by examination of Table 3.5. This shows the number of heads and tails obtained by tossing a €1 coin and a €2 coin 25 times each. The figures are identical to those obtained in the clinical trial example (Table 3.4), with the coins replacing the two treatments and heads and tails replacing the outcomes of 'alive' and 'dead'.

Because the two coins were unbiased, a large number of tosses would in the long run have resulted in 50% tails for each coin (approximately). The results in Table 3.5 did, however, actually occur. Knowing how the results were obtained, it can be said with hindsight that the percentages of heads and tails do not indicate differences between the two coins and in that sense it may be

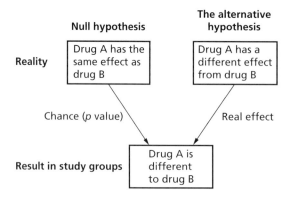

Fig. 3.5 Reality and results in hypothesis testing.

Table 3.5 Results of tossing two coins 25 times each.

Coins	Heads	Tails	Total
€1	17 (68·0%)	8 (32·0%)	25 (100·0%)
€2	12 (48·0%)	13 (52·0%)	25 (100·0%)

said that the observed result is spurious or due to chance. Since the figures obtained in the clinical trial, however, are identical to those of the coin-tossing experiment, it can only be concluded that they can throw no light on the efficacy of the drugs in question and that interpretation of the results is difficult. There is evidence that drug A could be better than drug B, but this observation could be due to chance and in reality the drugs may have identical effects. In statistical terms, there is no firm evidence to reject the (null) hypothesis that the two drugs are the same.

As well as illustrating the two possible states of reality, Fig. 3.5 also shows the sample results and how they might be achieved. If the null hypothesis were true, it would be expected that the results in the two groups would be fairly close and, if it were false, the observed results would be expected to reflect the true actions of the drugs.

Of course, the main problem is that the sample results obtained may not reflect reality precisely and it is, of course, necessary to work backwards from the results to reality. The reason that the observed results on a single sample may not reflect reality in the population is called *sampling variation*. Essentially, this means that the results obtained in any given sample would have been different if a different sample had been taken. Though the sample result should reflect the situation in the population, the sample result can vary depending on the sample actually chosen. This is why the backwards inference from the sample to the population is subject to chance variations.

If there is a large (important) difference between the groups, then one of two possibilities emerges. The null hypothesis could be false and there could be a true drug effect, which has manifested itself in the sample. Alternatively, the null hypothesis could be true and sampling variation would be the explanation for the observed spurious result. Hypothesis testing provides a method whereby it is possible to differentiate between these two alternatives.

The p *value and statistical significance*

The approach taken is to calculate (as described later in Chapter 5) the probability of obtaining the observed result or one even more at variance with the null hypothesis if, in fact, the null hypothesis were true. In the example, the probability of getting a survival difference between drugs A and B of 20% or greater, in a study of two groups of 25 patients on two similar drugs, would be calculated using a formula on the observed data. This calculated probability is called the *p* value.

The *p* value
- is a measure of the likelihood of the observed result, or one even more extreme, if in fact there is no association in the population
- is the probability of getting the observed result, or one even more discordant, if the null hypothesis were true
- is the chance of a spurious result being observed

If the size of this probability is large (usually arbitrarily set at 5% or greater), it is accepted that the result could be spurious and due to chance and that, therefore, the null hypothesis cannot be rejected. In the example, it was seen that the results of the trial could have been obtained in practice by tossing two coins, and it might therefore be predicted that there is a fairly large probability of this result being spurious. (The actual probability or p value for this example can be calculated as greater than 10%.)

If, on the other hand, the magnitude of this probability is small, it may be decided that, since the result is unusual, there is evidence to reject the null hypothesis and to accept the alternative hypothesis. Of course, to reject the null hypothesis could be wrong, but the smaller the calculated probability, the less the chance of making a wrong decision. Going back to the analogy with the judicial process, the jury must decide whether the evidence (corresponding to the observed result) is consistent with the accused being innocent (the null hypothesis). If the evidence is such that it is difficult to explain its existence if the person is innocent, then the jury will probably declare a verdict of guilty (rejecting the null hypothesis).

It has already been pointed out that, when the probability of a spurious result is large, it is not possible to distinguish between the realities postulated by the null and alternative hypotheses (between spurious and real results). Because of this ambiguity the statement 'do not reject the null hypothesis' is generally used, instead of the clearer but less accurate 'accept the null hypothesis'. This corresponds to the possible judicial verdict in Scottish law of 'not proven' rather than 'not guilty'.

The purpose of every statistical hypothesis test is to enable calculation of a p value under a specified null hypothesis

Rejection or non-rejection of the null hypothesis depends on the p value
    If the p value is small, the null hypothesis is rejected
        (meaning there is likely to be a real association)
    If the p value is large, the null hypothesis is not rejected
        (meaning that there might, or might not, be a real association)

The rule of thumb mentioned above, i.e. that a value of p less than 5% ($p < 0.05$) leads to a rejection of the null hypothesis, is fairly arbitrary but universally used. Cut-off points other than 5% can be taken and whichever is chosen is called the significance level of the test. Sometimes, a significance level of 1% is taken and the p value (chance of a spurious result) must be less than 1% before the null hypothesis can be rejected. The smaller the p value, the less likely that the sample results arose from the reality suggested by the null hypothesis, and the more likely that they reflect an underlying reality of the null hypothesis being false. However when a p value very close to 5% is calculated, it is obviously nonsense to reject the null hypothesis at, say, a p of 4·99% and to fail to reject it at a p value of 5·01%. The 5% level is purely a guideline.

In a statistical analysis, rejection of a null hypothesis is referred to as a *statistically significant result*. Thus, a statistically significant result is a result that is not likely to have occurred by chance.* The cut-off level used for the p value is called the significance level of the test. Although the significance level should be stated explicitly, usage often takes a 'significant result' to imply the rejection of a null hypothesis at a 5% level and a 'highly significant result' to imply a 1% level of significance.

A non-significant result means that the null hypothesis is not rejected (usually with $p > 5\%$). A non-significant result is always ambiguous and should not be taken to mean that there is no effect. A non-significant result means that the observation might be due to chance or it might be due to a real effect. There is no way of knowing. Just as it would be almost impossible to prove absolutely that a painting was by a particular painter or that a spouse was always faithful, the null hypothesis is never accepted; it is just 'not rejected'.

A statistically significant result means that:
- the observed result is unlikely to be due to chance
- the observed result is not compatible with the null hypothesis
- sampling variation is not sufficient to explain the observed result
- the null hypothesis can be rejected
- the alternative hypothesis can be accepted
- there is evidence to doubt the null hypothesis
- assuming the null hypothesis, the chance of the result being spurious is small: $p < 5\%$ or $p < 0.05$

For those persons unhappy about postulated populations to which the null hypothesis refers, an alternative interpretation of hypothesis tests can be suggested. As has been said, the reason for any statistical analysis in the first place is the problem of sampling variation or the uncertainty introduced into results due to the small number of subjects studied. If any given study were repeated on millions of subjects and showed the same results as obtained on the smaller, actual number studied, no statistical analysis would be necessary, since (apart from problems due to bias—see below) the results would speak for themselves. In this light, a significant result can be interpreted to mean that, if large numbers were, in fact, studied, similar results to those obtained in the smaller study actually carried out would be expected. A non-significant result, on the other hand, would mean that, if a study were to be performed on a very large

---

* Often the phrase 'significant result' is employed without the modifier 'statistically'. This is perfectly acceptable usage, and in fact the word significant should perhaps only be used with this meaning in any scientific or medical discourse. Also note that 'occurred by chance' should be taken to have the phrase 'if there were no association in the population' appended to it. The p value is calculated assuming that the null hypothesis is true.

number of subjects, there could be no certainty that the actual sample results would be observed in the larger study. For instance, if the two coins were tossed millions of times, the percentage of tails in each coin would be very close to 50%, unlike the percentages obtained in the small number of tosses in the example.

At this point, the difference between a statistically significant result and a medically important result must be reiterated. Medical importance relates to the magnitude of the observed effect, while significance refers to the statistical question of whether or not the result is spurious or likely to be due to chance. What is ideal in any situation is an important result that is also significant. An important result that is non-significant (as in the breast-cancer trial example discussed above) may provide some grounds for optimism but no reliance may be placed on the results. Non-important results, statistically significant (as they can be sometimes) or not, usually give very little information to the researcher.

Overview

The general form of a hypothesis or significance test thus runs as follows: a null hypothesis is postulated, and it is usually hoped to be able to reject it; the results of the particular study are examined; if medically important, they are subjected to further mathematical manipulation, which depends on the type of study, the measurements made and other relevant factors. This eventually leads to the calculation of a p value, which is the probability of the observed results (or results even more at variance with the null hypothesis) being spurious if the null hypothesis were true in the first place. If the p value is small (usually with $p < 5\%$), the null hypothesis is rejected and the result declared statistically significant. If the p value is large, it is concluded that the result is non-significant, and no decision can be made about whether or not there is a real effect. Therefore, the null hypothesis cannot be rejected.

3.4.2 Confidence intervals

As described above the purpose of hypothesis or significance testing is to determine if an observed association in data from a given study is likely to be real or to reflect a chance occurrence only. Hypothesis testing used to be the most common approach to statistical analyses, but in recent years an alternative, but complementary, approach has been widely adopted—that is, statistical analysis via confidence intervals.

Precision

Whenever one makes a measurement, there is a degree of error in the numerical value that is put on that measurement. If a person were said to have a height of 178 cm, few would assume that the person was exactly 178·0 cm tall.

In all probability the person's height would be somewhere between 177·5 and 178·5 cm, the quoted figure being obtained by rounding to the nearest centimetre. One might say 'plus or minus half a centimetre' explicitly to quantify the precision of the given figure.

The precision of a measurement is usually determined by the sophistication of the measuring instrument.* A simple instrument may not give a very precise result, whereas a more complex or expensive instrument might. If one were trying to measure the thickness of a hypodermic needle, the result given by a micrometer would be much more precise than that given by a ruler! Often the manufacturer of a particular measuring instrument will give details about the degree of precision that might be achieved with it—often by means of a '± error term'. This is usually interpreted to mean that the true answer is within the limits given by adding or subtracting the error term to the recorded measure.

It should be noted too that absolute precision is never required (and in fact is impossible to achieve) and the purpose of the measurement may dictate how precisely it should be made. For instance the distance between London and New York given as 5500 (±50) km is probably sufficient for the international traveller but may not be precise enough for an airline pilot.

Precision of a sample estimate

As discussed earlier, the purpose of a sample study is to make inferences about the larger population from which the sample was taken. When a study is performed, the sample taken can be seen as a measuring instrument used to measure something in the entire population. In this context, the term 'sample estimate' is used to refer to the measurement made by the sample. Thus, a sample mean is a measurement or estimate of the mean in the population from which the sample was taken; a percentage difference in a sample is an estimate of the percentage difference in the population. For example, the absolute difference in the percentage of smokers between males and females of 26·1% (see Table 3.3) is an estimate of the true percentage difference in the entire population from which the sample was taken. The absolute survival difference of 20·0% in favour of the drug A-treated group compared with the drug B group in Table 3.4 is an estimate of the true effect of treatment (in the population).

Just as any measurement has a certain degree of precision, so too a sample estimate has a certain degree of precision as a measurement of the corresponding population parameter. It would be surprising if the percentage difference in male–female smoking in the population were exactly 26·1%, but it is 'likely' to be 'somewhere around' that figure (assuming no bias in the study and that a proper random sample was taken). Similarly, in the population,

---

* Precision in this context essentially means how sharply defined the measurement is. See Chapter 12, where the concept of accuracy is considered and the whole topic of measurement error is discussed in detail.

drug A is likely to have a survival advantage of around 20·0%. A confidence interval for a sample result gives a direct measure of the precision of that result.

For instance, it is possible to perform a calculation on the smoking data discussed above to show that one could be 95% sure that the true difference in (current/ex combined) smoking percentages between males and females (in the population) was 21·6% ± 3·5% or somewhere between 18·1% and 25·1%.* The interval from 18·1% to 25·1% is the 95% confidence interval.

There are two central parts to the confidence interval. First, there is the level of sureness or confidence with which the statement can be made. This is usually set at 95%. Secondly, there is a range of possible values for the underlying situation in the population. Here, on the basis of this sample result, the percentage difference in the population could be as low as 18·1% or as high as 25·1%, and it is likely to be somewhere between these two figures. The sample cannot tell what the situation in the population is exactly, but it can give an estimate of it. The precision of that estimate is given by means of a confidence interval. Confidence intervals can be formed for any statistic that can be measured in a sample.

A confidence interval
- gives the precision of a sample estimate of a parameter
- is a range of values surrounding a sample estimate, within which, at a given level of confidence, the true value of the corresponding parameter in the population is likely to be found

---

In this example, there is an association between gender and smoking in the population. At a 95% level of sureness or confidence, smoking in males may be anything from 18·1% to 25·1% higher than in females and these figures can be interpreted as measures of the possible strength of the association in the population that is involved. Note that absolute certainty is impossible on the basis of a sample — the precision of a sample estimate depends on the level of confidence set. As has been said, this is commonly set at 95% and it is at that level of confidence that the existence of associations is usually determined.

Chance associations

What determines the precision of a sample estimate? What corresponds in sampling to using a micrometer rather than a ruler in measuring a thickness? The answer is intuitively obvious: the bigger the sample, the more precise the sample estimate is likely to be. Small samples may give quite imprecise results.

In the fictitious clinical trial comparing drug A and drug B, the observed survival advantage in favour of drug A was 20·0%. It has already been stated, on the basis of a hypothesis test, that this result could be due to chance or sam-

---

* Do not worry how this calculation was made; that will be considered in detail later in the book.

pling variation. What conclusion could be drawn from a confidence-interval approach to the same data? Again, without going into the formulae involved, it can be shown that the 95% confidence interval for the survival advantage is 20·0% ± 26·8%, or from −6·8% to 46·8%. The precision of the observed difference of 20·0% is low. At a 95% level of confidence, the survival advantage of drug A is likely to be between −6·8% (corresponding to survival being truly 6·8% *lower* under drug A) to 46·8% (corresponding to survival being truly 46·8% higher under drug A). Thus, a 0% difference (survival truly being the same in the two groups) is possible within the precision of the sample result and therefore the result allows for the possibility of there being no association between treatment and survival in the population of all patients. The confidence interval allows the conclusion that drugs A and B might have the same effects, with the sample results arising by chance.

Confidence intervals and hypothesis tests are two sides of the same coin and one can always infer the statistical significance of an association from a confidence interval on a measure of that association. If the confidence interval for the measure of the association includes the value corresponding to a lack of association (the null value), the observed association could be due to chance and is called non-significant. If the confidence interval excludes this particular value, the association is unlikely to be due to chance and can be declared statistically significant. Obviously, a 5% level of significance corresponds to a 95% confidence interval.

If a statistic is a measure of the degree of association between two variables
- its confidence interval can be used to determine whether the observed association could be due to chance
- a confidence interval that overlaps the null value (corresponding to no association) is equivalent to a non-significant result
- a confidence interval that excludes the null value is equivalent to a statistically significant result

---

3.5 Associations due to bias or confounding

A bias can be defined as any factor or process which leads to a conclusion that differs from the truth. Bias can occur at any stage of a study, from the initial study design and sampling, through the data collection and recording, to the inferences and conclusions that are drawn from those data, and finally to the publishing stage. Perhaps the most important bias that can arise is that due to confounding.

3.5.1 Confounding

Suppose that a study were done on consecutive male postoperative patients and that those with grey hair had a higher mortality than those without grey hair. Suppose too that a statistical analysis had shown that this observation was statistically significant and unlikely to be due to chance. Before jumping to any conclusion that grey hair causes a higher mortality, one must ask if there is another explanation for the finding.

In this example, the reader has no doubt concluded already that an association between having grey hair and operative mortality is not causal and could be explained by an age effect. It is fairly obvious that men with grey hair tend to be older than those without grey hair and that, since operative mortality increases with age, those with grey hair would in fact fare worse. A third variable, age, has acted as a *confounder* of the association between grey hair and operative mortality. In broad terms, a confounder is any extraneous factor that is related to both variables under study. A confounder can distort a true association or can (as in this case) create a spurious one. The possibility that any observed association between factors might be due to confounding is what makes the research process and the interpretation of research findings so fraught with difficulty. Typical confounders are age and sex.

There are two main strategies for controlling confounding in research. The first is to concentrate on study design and set up a study in such a way as to eliminate the effect of confounding variables from the beginning. This can be done by restriction, matching or randomization. The second method is to use analytic approaches to adjust, control or correct for confounders. Though both these topics will be considered in some detail later in the book, a brief outline of what is meant is given below.

A confounder
- is a third variable that distorts the association between two study variables
- is associated with each of the study variables
- can be controlled for by design or analysis

3.5.2 Matching and restriction

The problem with the operative mortality study, as described in the previous section, was that consecutive patients were taken and that therefore the grey-haired men were (naturally) older than the non-grey-haired subjects. If there were some way to compare grey-haired and non-grey-haired men *of the same age*, then age would not be an explanation of any association found. One way might be to confine the study to subjects in a single narrow age-group only and, in that age-group, compare mortality between those with and without grey hair. This process, called *restriction*, would allow examination of the effect of grey hair independent of age, though in the single age-group only.

The approach could be extended by including in the study all the grey-haired men undergoing an operation and for each taking a non-grey-haired man of the same age in the comparison group. This process of *matching* would ensure that the two groups had the same age and thus age could not explain mortality differences that might be found. (Different techniques for achieving matching of confounders will be considered in Section 6.7.2.) A factor can only be a confounder of a particular association if it is related to both factors under investigation and the association of the confounder with one of the factors can be removed through matching or restriction.

3.5.3 Randomization

A confounder arises in group comparisons when the confounding variable is related to both group membership and the outcome variable of interest. In the particular situation of evaluation of therapy, forming comparison groups in a certain way can essentially eliminate the action of confounders. Going back to the illustrative clinical trial example of 25 persons on drug A and 25 persons on drug B (see Section 3.4.1), the assumption was made that the two groups were similar except for the particular drug administered. In a clinical trial, the two groups are made similar by a process of randomization. Though the topic will be discussed in detail in Chapter 6, essentially this means that the two groups were formed by a process equivalent to the tossing of a coin ('heads' into one group, 'tails' into another), with nothing but chance dictating which patient went into which group. Thus there is no reason why any factor should appear more often in one group than in another, or why the distribution of any quantitative variable should differ between the groups. Thus, randomization ensures that there is no variable related to group membership. Randomization ensures that baseline differences between the two groups are only due to chance and that the only distinction between them is the administered treatment. Randomization is an extremely powerful method of eliminating confounders in the design of a study, but in reality it can only be used in the comparison of two treatments or interventions. In studies of harmful exposures—cigarette smoking, for example—it is impossible and unethical to randomize to smoking and non-smoking groups; so that the less efficient techniques of matching or restriction are required if design elements are to be employed to control for potential confounders. (See Section 3.6.2 and fuller discussion in Chapter 6.)

3.5.4 Stratified analyses

If confounders have not been controlled in the design of the study, it is still possible to adjust or correct for a confounding effect at the analysis stage. The most easily understood approach is a *stratified analysis*. (The more complex *regression* approaches are considered later in Chapter 11, where stratification is also considered in more detail.) Essentially, the data are broken up into categories defined by the confounder and comparisons are made within these categories. In the example of grey hair and operative mortality, one would create a number of age-groups or categories and compare grey-haired and non-grey-haired subjects within each age-group. If the age-groups are narrow enough and do not span many years, the effect of grey hair, independent of age, would be seen. Hopefully, in the example, within each age-group, the mortality would be the same in those with and without grey hair. Thus, the stratified analysis would show that, once age was allowed for, grey hair had no effect on mortality. A stratified analysis allows examination of the data as if it came from several studies, each performed on patients in a narrow age band (i.e. using restriction), with a final combination of the different studies to give an overall, age-adjusted, result.

Numerical example [!]

For readers who would prefer to see the mathematics of confounding and of a stratified analysis, Table 3.6 shows fictitious data relating to the association between operative mortality and grey hair.* To simplify the situation, only two age-groups are considered (less than 60 years and 60 years or older). A total of 1500 patients were studied and 50% had grey hair and 50% did not. Mortality in the grey-haired group was 4·8%, compared with 3·2% in the non-grey-haired. Over 90% of the grey-haired subjects were aged 60 years or older, compared with 40% in the other group. Thus the potential for confounding exists—grey hair and mortality are associated, but age is associated with grey hair and, as will be seen, is also associated with mortality.

The second part of the table shows the stratified analysis. The data are analysed separately in each of the (two) age-groups. In those aged under 60 years, mortality was the same, at 2%, irrespective of what colour hair

(a) Distribution of deaths and age in 750 grey-haired humans and in 750 non-grey-haired humans

Table 3.6 Fictitious example of age confounding an association between grey hair and operative mortality.

	Grey-haired persons	Non-grey-haired persons
Deaths *n* total	36/750	24/750
(%)	(4·8%)	(3·2%)
Age 60+ *n* total	700/750	300/750
(%)	(93·3%)	(40·0%)

(b) Mortality by age and grey hair (figures are 'number dead/total' with percentage mortality in parentheses).

Age (years)	Grey-haired persons	Non-grey-haired persons
<60	1/50 (2·0%)	9/450 (2·0%)
60+	35/700 (5·0%)	15/300 (5·0%)
Total	36/750 (4·8%)	24/750 (3·2%)

* In fact the association between grey hair and operative mortality shown here is statistically non-significant. This is irrelevant to the explanation of confounding illustrated by these data.

the subject had. Within the older group, mortality was again the same in those with and without grey hair, but was at the higher level of 5%. Thus, the stratified analysis shows that grey hair had, of itself, no effect on mortality and that the important factor was age. However, because those with grey hair were older, as a group they had a higher mortality. The reader should examine the table in some detail for a full appreciation of what has happened here.

In this example, the main finding was due totally to the confounding effect of age. In most real-life situations, only partial confounding may occur, where an association may be distorted and appear enhanced or diminished.

3.5.5 Other sources of bias

Though perhaps the most pervasive, confounding is not the only bias that can explain observed associations. Selection bias and non-response bias in sample surveys have been mentioned already and the reader will find many other biases mentioned in later parts of this book, particularly in the discussion of study design in Chapter 6 and in the discussion of measurement in Chapter 12. Many biases are in fact particular to specific study designs and it is not appropriate to delineate them here. Though it is possible to adjust or correct for (measured) confounders in a study, in general statistical analysis cannot correct for other forms of bias. Careful study design and data recording are what is required.

Control of confounding through design
- matching
- restriction
- randomization

Control of confounding through analysis
- stratification
- regression

3.6 Causal associations

When chance and bias have been ruled out (as far as possible) as explanations for a numerical association between two variables, the potential for a real cause-and-effect relationship must be examined. Considerations of causal explanations, however, require much more than numerical manipulations and good study design.

3.6.1 Risk

The concept of cause in medicine is not an easy one (see Rothman & Greenland, 1998), but at a simplistic level a causal factor can be thought of as a factor that increases the *risk* of disease, after allowance has been made for potential confounders. It is important to realize that, when considering causation of disease, there is no one-to-one correspondence in individuals between the cause and the effect and the elucidation of causation requires the examination of groups of people.

Risk is a concept that is applied to an individual but is determined from examination of a group of people. In essence, the risk of disease is similar to the probability of disease and it is determined by examining how many develop disease over a period of time in a defined group of persons. (See Section 6.5.1 for further discussion of the concept of risk.) Suppose a study were performed on 4000 smokers and that 80 developed lung cancer in a 15-year follow-up period. The 15-year risk of lung cancer in these smokers would be 80/4000 or 2%. It is on the basis of a study like this that one might say 'The risk of lung cancer for a smoker is 2% over 15 years.' The main assumption here is that the smoker whose risk is defined is similar to the smokers actually studied and that he or she will have a similar disease outcome. Obviously, it might be possible to refine such an estimate of risk by examining risk by exact age or even by amount smoked.

The risk of disease
- for a group is defined as the proportion of persons in that group who develop the disease over a time period
- for an individual is that individual's probability of developing disease over the period in question

---

3.6.2 Risk factors and risk markers

If a larger proportion of persons develop a disease among a group exposed to some factor than develop it in a group not exposed, then that factor is said to be a *risk factor* or *risk marker* for the disease. Thus, smoking is a risk factor for lung cancer because more lung cancer is seen among smokers than among non-smokers. The difficulty is in moving from determining that something is a risk factor for a disease to being able to declare it a cause of the disease. When a group exposed to a factor has a higher risk of disease than a non-exposed group, the difference may be due to confounding variables and thus the risk factor may only be identifying a group at higher risk and may not be a cause in itself. Grey hair is not a risk factor for operative mortality! For this reason many persons prefer the term 'risk marker' as an alternative to the more usual 'risk factor'. Thus 'carrying a box of matches or a cigarette lighter' is a risk marker for lung cancer, but certainly is not a causal factor.

Often two factors that are associated can cause the disease and disentangling the actual effects of either can be very difficult in such situations. (The reader will find further discussion of this point in Section 11.4.) One of the old arguments against cigarette smoking being causally related to lung cancer was that both were genetically determined. Those with the genetic trait were more likely to develop lung cancer and, at the same time, were constitutionally more likely to take up cigarette smoking. In this scenario, the genetic trait would be a confounder and there would be no causal effect of cigarette smoking *per se*. A risk factor or marker can only be declared causal if one is sure that confounding has not created the relationship.

The 'gold standard' investigation of causality would be by means of an experimental study randomizing individuals to an exposed group or a comparison non-exposed group (see Section 3.5.3). Though it is now universally accepted that cigarette smoking is a cause of lung cancer, the final unequivocal proof could be obtained by means of the following type of study. Suppose that the study population was to be all births in Ireland over the next year and that, at birth, a coin was tossed to determine if a baby should be placed into the 'smoking' or 'non-smoking' group. Babies in the smoking group would be exposed to cigarette smoke as soon as possible after birth, would be encouraged to smoke as soon as they could without burning themselves, would be smoking at least 10 cigarettes per day by the age of 5. Babies in the non-smoking group would never be allowed near a cigarette or any other source of tobacco. After a number of years, there would be more lung-cancer cases among those in the smoking group. The important point about this study is that exposure to smoking is determined by the researcher on the basis of chance alone—the toss of a coin or *randomization*. Because of this there should be no differences between the smoking groups, apart from cigarette smoking, regarding any potentially confounding factor, genetic or otherwise, that might be related to lung cancer. Thus, any difference in lung-cancer risk must be attributable to the experimentally manipulated exposure of cigarette smoking only.

Of course, ethically (and practically) such a study could never be done and, when examining causality, researchers can only observe what is happening and cannot experimentally manipulate it. Confounders are always a possibility in an observational study and much effort is put into designing studies in such a way that confounding effects are eliminated or into controlling for confounders at the analysis stage. Unfortunately, however, no observational study design or analytic method can absolutely guarantee that an effect is not confounded to some degree and proof of causality on the basis of observational research will always have its detractors.

3.6.3 Causal criteria

It was because of this that criteria were developed by which to judge if an observed effect could be considered causal (*Smoking and Health*, 1964; Hill, 1965). These are outlined below in the context of the causal link between cigarette smoking and lung cancer. These criteria include the *consistency, strength, specificity, temporality* and *coherence* of the association. An association between a risk factor and a disease that satisfies most of these criteria can be taken as a strong, if not absolute, indication of causality.

The consistency of an association requires that different methods of study design and studies in different populations all lead to similar conclusions. With few exceptions, all the studies of the association of cigarette smoking and lung cancer show a positive result. The strength of an association means that the effect of the risk factor is large. As discussed earlier this might be quantified by comparing the risk of disease between those exposed and not exposed to the risk factor using difference or ratio measures. (This is considered again in Section 6.5.2.) A dose–response effect is also related to the strength of an association and means that, in the example being considered, lung-cancer risk increases with the amount smoked.

In the original formulation, the specificity of the association between cigarette smoking and lung cancer demanded that most persons with lung cancer would be cigarette smokers and that most cigarette smokers would get lung cancer. Of course, most cigarette smokers will not get lung cancer—they may die of a lot of other (smoking-related) diseases also and the requirement of specificity for a causal relationship has been diminished greatly. Usually, specificity is now taken to refer to only one side of the relationship—that most people with lung cancer will have been smokers. Though lung cancer can arise in non-smokers, the specificity of the association with cigarette smoking is fairly clear. For a condition like coronary heart disease however, the specificity of the association with any single risk factor is not seen. Most patients with coronary heart disease will not have high blood pressure even though high blood pressure is accepted as a cause of heart disease. The problem is that coronary heart disease is multifactorial—has many causes—and most patients will not have a single particular risk factor. However, most patients with heart disease will have one, or more, of the major risk factors of high blood pressure, high cholesterol or cigarette smoking.

Before a risk factor for a particular disease can be judged causal, it must be certain that in fact the risk factor was present before the disease occurred. Although fairly easy to show for cigarette smoking and lung cancer, this temporality requirement can sometimes cause difficulties for some other observed associations. For an association to be coherent, it should not be at odds with known facts concerning the natural history and biology of a disease, and there should be a reasonable explanation for the association in this light. The known carcinogenic effects of tobacco smoke contribute to the coherence of the association between smoking and lung cancer. Coherence is also known as *biological plausibility*.

A further criterion sometimes applied to judge if an association is causal is that of *reversibility*. An association between an exposure and disease is reversible if the future risk of disease reduces when exposure is removed. Cigarette smokers who have ceased smoking for over 20 years have a lung-cancer risk indistinguishable from that of lifelong non-smokers (Wald & Watt, 1997).

These criteria are useful in coming to an informed decision regarding the interpretation of an association between an exposure and disease. Few associations will meet all the criteria, but they act as a reminder that a causal interpretation of an association goes far beyond statistics and study design.

> Criteria used for judging the causal significance of an association include
> - consistency
> - strength and dose–response
> - specificity
> - temporality
> - coherence (biological plausibility)
> - reversibility

3.7 Summary

In this chapter, some of the central concepts in medical research and statistics have been introduced without mathematical detail. It was shown that most research questions can be formulated in terms of an association between two variables, but the interpretation of such associations, particularly in observational studies, is hampered by the problems of chance and bias. The fact that spurious associations can arise due to sampling variation was discussed, as were the approaches to examining this, using hypothesis testing and confidence intervals. Eliminating or controlling for bias, especially that due to confounding, was considered and the criteria for determining if an association could be considered causal were described.

The next chapter of the book begins a more detailed examination of the role of chance and considers confidence intervals. This is followed by a chapter on hypothesis testing. Subsequent chapters expand on many of the other issues first touched on above.

4 Confidence Intervals: General Principles; Proportions, Means, Medians, Counts and Rates

4.1 Introduction

The first chapter of this book discussed various methods available for organizing, presenting and summarizing data obtained in a particular study and, as has been said, such descriptive statistics form the basis of any statistical analysis. The second chapter considered the notion of sampling from a population to draw an inference about that population on the basis of the sample results. Chapter 3 then, using a non-mathematical approach, considered the problems of interpreting observed associations as due to chance, confounding or a real effect. In particular, some of the ideas underlying confidence intervals and significance testing were introduced.

This chapter considers statistical estimation using confidence intervals in greater depth. First, the normal distribution, which is central to much statistical analysis, is introduced. The estimation of a single population proportion is then described in some detail, explaining the ideas underlying sampling distributions and confidence intervals. The extension of the approach to estimate means, geometric means, medians, counts and rates in single samples is described.

A prerequisite for this chapter is an understanding of frequency distributions.

4.2 The normal distribution

4.2.1 Properties of the normal distribution

In this section, one of the most important theoretical distributions in statistics—the *normal*, or as it is often called, the *Gaussian distribution*—is introduced. The term 'normal' applied to this particular distribution should not be taken to mean that the distribution is common or typical. In fact, most variables in medical research are non-normal (not abnormal!), but there is nothing wrong with them. It should also be mentioned that a normal distribution for a variable is not a prerequisite for many forms of statistical analysis, although approximate normality can be a great help.

The normality of a distribution always refers to the underlying distribution of a variable in a population, so that the mean and standard deviation of such distributions are denoted by μ and σ, respectively (see Section 2.3.4). The normal distribution has certain definite features: it is unimodal, symmetrical and bell-shaped, but this is not to say that all unimodal, symmetrical, bell-shaped distributions are normal. Since normal distributions are unimodal and symmetrical, the mean, median and mode are equal in value. A normal distribution is characterized completely by its mean and standard deviation; that is to say, two normal distributions with the same means and standard deviations are identical. Normal distributions can, of course, have different means and different standard deviations. Figure 4.1 illustrates (a) normal curves with the same standard deviations but different means and (b) normal curves with the same means but different standard deviations. What distinguishes normal distributions from other unimodal, symmetrical, bell-shaped distributions are their area properties, or, more precisely, specific relationships between their percentile values and their means and standard deviations.

(a)

(b)

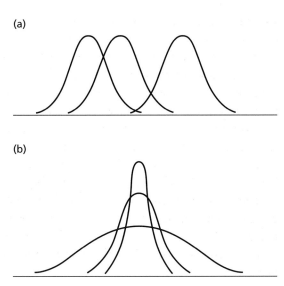

Fig. 4.1 Normal distributions: (a) same standard deviations, different means; (b) same means, different standard deviations.

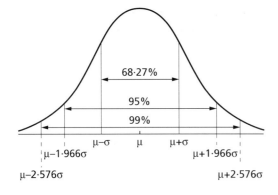

Fig. 4.2 Area properties of the normal distribution.

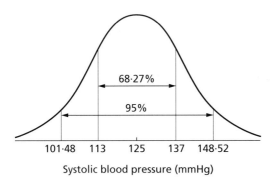

Systolic blood pressure (mmHg)

Fig. 4.3 Population distribution of systolic blood pressure in males aged 35–39: a normal distribution with mean 125 mmHg and standard deviation 12 mmHg (hypothetical example).

What are some of these properties? Figure 4.2 shows a typical normal distribution with a mean μ and standard deviation σ. Obviously, 50% of the area lies above the mean and 50% lies below the mean. Now, in a normal distribution it is also true that 68·27% (just over two-thirds) of the area lies between the values obtained by adding and subtracting the value of the standard deviation to and from the value of the mean, i.e. between $\mu - \sigma$ and $\mu + \sigma$ or within $\mu \pm \sigma$. Also, 95% of the area of a normal curve lies within $\mu \pm 1·96\sigma$. (The figures 68·27% and 1·96 in these relationships arise from the normality of the distribution and are specific to such distributions.) The area within which all (100%) of the area is contained cannot be stated since the two tails of the distribution continuously approach, but never reach, the horizontal axis.

Suppose, for example, systolic blood pressure is known to follow a normal distribution, with a mean of 125 mmHg and standard deviation of 12 mmHg, in males aged 35–39 years. Remembering that any area under a distribution curve can be interpreted as a proportion or percentage of the possible observations, it can be said that 68·27% of the blood pressures of the persons in this population will lie between 125 – 12 and 125 + 12 mmHg, that is to say, between 113 and 137 mmHg. Similarly, it could be said that 95% of the blood pressures will lie within 125 ± 1·96(12) or between 101·48 and 148·52 mmHg (Fig. 4.3). These results can, of course, be taken to mean that, if one person in this population is randomly chosen, there is a 68·27% chance that the blood pressure of this person will lie between 113 and 137 mmHg. These area properties are, of course, true for any normal distribution of a given mean and standard deviation and, essentially, are statements concerning percentiles of such distributions. For instance, $\mu + 1\cdot96\sigma$ gives the $97\frac{1}{2}$th percentile of a normal distribution, because 95% of the area is in $\mu \pm 1\cdot96\sigma$, leaving 2·5% in each of the two tails; $\mu - 1\cdot96\sigma$ gives the $2\frac{1}{2}$th percentile. In fact, any percentile of a normal distribution can be calculated by adding or subtracting a particular multiple of the standard deviation to or from the mean. These properties, of course, are valid only for normal distributions.

The log-normal distribution[!]

The log transformation was described in Section 1.6.7 as particularly suitable for making positively skewed data more symmetrical. If, in fact, the distribution of the log-transformed data is normal,* the original variable is said to have a *log-normal distribution*. Because of the essential symmetry of log-transformed data, the geometric mean of a log-normal distribution is equal to its median (see Section 1.6.7).

The normal distribution
- is a bell-shaped distribution
- has certain area properties
- in particular, 95% of observations in a normal distribution lie within mean $\pm 1\cdot96$ (standard deviations)

4.2.2 The standard normal distribution

Tables for the multiplying factors for the standard deviation that enable different percentiles to be calculated are widely available and a very abbreviated table is to be found in Appendix B (Table B.2).

Since these factors are independent of the mean and standard deviation of the distribution, the table conveniently gives the factors for a particular normal distribution of mean zero and standard deviation unity. This is called the *standard normal distribution*. For such a distribution, 68·27% of the observations lie between $\pm 1\cdot0$ and 95% are within $\pm 1\cdot96$ (e.g. with $\mu = 0$ and $\sigma = 1$, $\mu \pm 1\cdot96\sigma$ becomes $\pm 1\cdot96$). Table B.2 gives these factors (denoted z_c) for specified areas in both tails and also in the upper tail of the standard normal distribution. The table is given in terms of areas in the tails for later application, and much more extensive tables are to be found in some statistical textbooks. (It is worthwhile becoming familiar with one particular table of the normal distribution, since the layout and notation tend to change from book to book.)

To find the z_c value, which cuts off a particular area in both tails of a

---

* Of course the observed data would rarely conform to a normal distribution exactly.

standard normal distribution, look at the areas in the top row of the table. (Ignore for the moment the alternative description—two-sided significance level, etc.) The area is given as a proportion rather than as a percentage; thus 0·05 means 5%. The z_c value corresponding to each area is given in the last row. For example, in the standard normal curve, the values given by ± 2·326 cut off a total area of 2% in the two tails. For a normal distribution of mean μ and standard deviation σ, the figures that encompass 98% of the area are $\mu \pm$ 2·326σ. Note that, since the normal distribution is symmetrical, only the $+ z_c$ value is given in the table. The table also gives the z_c values that cut off particular areas in the upper tail of the normal distribution; thus, for example, 0·5% or 0·005 of the area is above 2·576 in the standard normal curve, or, in a normal distribution of mean μ and standard deviation σ, 0·5% of the values will lie above $\mu + 2 \cdot 576\sigma$.

The standard normal curve is obtained by a transformation of the observations in a general normal distribution. This is akin to changing the measurement unit, as, for example, from inches to centimetres in measuring height or from degrees Fahrenheit to degrees Centigrade in measuring temperature. If x has a normal distribution with mean μ and standard deviation σ, then $x - \mu$ has a normal distribution with mean zero and standard deviation σ, while $(x - \mu)/\sigma$ has the standard normal distribution of mean 0 and standard deviation 1. Often:

$$z = \frac{x - \mu}{\sigma} \tag{4.1}$$

is written as the equation for transforming a variable with a normal distribution to a variable with the standard normal distribution. The term $x - \mu$ measures how far the observation is from the mean and division by σ converts this to multiples of the standard deviation. Rather than being measured in the original units, each value is thus assigned a number that measures how many standard deviations it is away from the mean. The value z is often referred to as a *standard normal deviate*.

4.2.3 Normal ranges and the normal distribution

The statistical normal range

Though the terminology might suggest otherwise, extreme care should be taken in using the normal distribution to calculate normal ranges (reference ranges, reference intervals) for a biochemical or other test result. Often, it is not very clear what a normal range for a test means, but a common *statistical* definition might be: 'the limits within which 95% of the population have values'. The problem is how such a normal range should be calculated. It is very tempting to take a number of 'normal' individuals (whatever that might mean), perform the test and, using the sample mean and standard deviation, calculate 'normal' limits based on:

$$\text{mean} \pm 1.96 \text{ (standard deviations)} \qquad (4.2)$$

Unfortunately, this approach is only valid if the values of the test have a normal distribution and, as already pointed out, many variables in medicine have quite skew distributions and symmetrical distributions are not necessarily normal either. Unless one is sure that a variable has indeed got a normal distribution, the simplistic use of the above formula will fail to give the required normal range. More advanced texts give methods for determining if a variable has a near-normal distribution (see Altman, 1991), but, in general, it is safer never to make the assumption and to avoid using this approach altogether. How, then, should one calculate a statistical normal range? The answer is simple: estimate the appropriate percentiles of the distribution directly, using the ogive or an equivalent method (see Section 1.7.1). This was the principle behind the centile chart for birth weight in that section, which did not use the normal formula above.

Other normal ranges

By definition, the statistical normal range, as described above, forces a fixed 5% of the population to be abnormal. This, of course, is nonsensical. This normal range has nothing to do with disease status and, at best, can act, like the centile chart (see Section 1.7.2), as a warning bell for a perhaps unusually low or high value that might warrant further investigation.

Other definitions of a normal range are possible. Considering, for simplicity, an upper limit of normality only (i.e. no lower limit), a limit might be defined as the level above which some pathology may be present in an individual. Normal ranges based on this approach, which might be described as *clinical*, can be difficult to determine. A *prognostic* normal range, on the other hand, might define a test level above which an individual's prognosis is poor, while an *operational* or *therapeutic* normal range might define the point above which medical intervention might be of benefit. Special studies would be needed to determine such ranges. These four definitions of normal range (statistical, clinical, prognostic and therapeutic) are totally distinct and are likely to give very different values for any particular test. It should also be noted that, in practice, very little in life is black or white and for most tests there are grey areas that span the situation from health to disease. The topic of diagnostic tests is discussed further in Section 12.6.

4.3 Sampling variation — proportions

Some of the concepts are illustrated in this chapter, using a simple example. Suppose there were 130 smokers in a group of 200 male patients with peripheral vascular disease (PVD), representing a sample percentage of 65%. Assuming that it is meaningful to talk about the population of all such PVD patients from which this sample of 200 was drawn, the researcher wants to estimate the true (population) percentage of smokers in such patients.

Since the formulae cause less confusion if one works with proportions in a decimal representation instead of percentages (and is consistent in so doing), the problem is restated in those terms. Any final results that are in the form of a proportion can then be transformed back to percentages by multiplying by 100. The sample proportion of smokers, $p = 0.65$, could of course be used as an estimate of the population proportion, which shall be given the symbol π (pi—the lower-case Greek letter 'p'). This is called a *point estimate* and is the single best estimate available. It cannot be assumed, however, that the population proportion is exactly equal to this sample proportion. There is likely to be uncertainty or lack of precision in this measurement or estimate, since the whole population was not examined. Intuitively, however, it seems reasonable to make a statement such as:

'I am *fairly sure* that the true (underlying population) proportion π is *somewhere around* my sample result of $p = 0.65$.'

The theoretical considerations in the remainder of this chapter lead to a definition of a confidence interval by quantifying (putting figures on) the vague terms 'fairly sure' and 'somewhere around'.

4.3.1 The sampling distribution of a proportion

The difficulty with this, and any, sampling study is that the sample actually obtained is one of many (an infinite number of) possible samples that could have been taken, and a different sample would most probably have given a different proportion of smokers. Thus, the sample proportion on which the estimate of the population proportion is based is one of many possible sample proportions. *Sampling variation* refers to the fact that the sample proportion can vary with the particular sample chosen. The major question, then, is whether the single sample proportion actually obtained can reveal anything about the population proportion, since another different sample would have given a different result.

At this stage, it is necessary to do a 'thought experiment', which is basically the consideration of a 'what if' situation. It is important to realize that this experiment is never carried out in reality—only one sample is ever taken to estimate a population parameter. What would happen, though, if very many different samples, all the same size, were taken from the population? Many different sample proportions would be obtained. If these proportions were then considered as a collection of quantitative data, the distribution of these data could be examined using the methods described in Chapter 1. First, a frequency distribution of the proportions could be produced and a frequency polygon formed from the histogram, in the usual manner. If a large enough number of samples were taken (an infinite number—to be distinguished from the sample size, which is the number of persons in each sample), the frequency

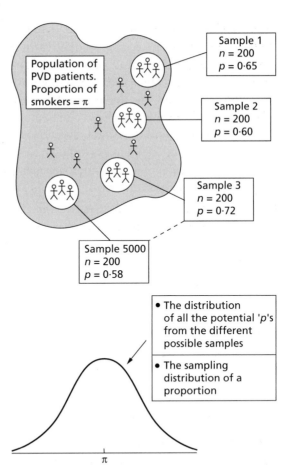

Fig. 4.4 The sampling distribution of a proportion.

polygon would become a smooth frequency curve and it would be possible to talk about the underlying distribution of these (potential) sample proportions. This underlying distribution is called the *sampling distribution of a proportion* (Fig. 4.4).

4.3.2 Properties of the sampling distribution of a proportion

The sampling distribution of a proportion has a number of important properties, which are discussed below. The descriptions in this section are not quite accurate but will give the essential idea of a sampling distribution. More precise considerations will come later.

Any distribution has a shape, a mean and a standard deviation, and obviously so does the special distribution here—the sampling distribution of a proportion. From studies in theoretical statistics, certain statements can be made about these factors, but no proofs are attempted in this book.

First, the sampling distribution of a proportion turns out to be a normal distribution. In other words, the possible sample proportions have a symmetrical, bell-shaped distribution, which has all the properties of the normal distribution described in Section 4.2. The second result is that the mean of the sampling distribution of a proportion turns out to be the unknown proportion in the population from which the samples were taken. Thus, as in fact might be expected, the different possible sample proportions are distributed symmetrically around the true population value, denoted π. A sample proportion is no more likely to be above than below this unknown population value. The third, and perhaps most important, question is 'how spread out is this particular normal distribution?'. It can be shown that the standard deviation of the sampling distribution of a proportion depends on π, the unknown population proportion, and n, the sample size (of each of the samples). The standard deviation of a sampling distribution is called a standard error and the standard error of a proportion is given by:

$$SE(p) = \sqrt{\frac{\pi(1-\pi)}{n}} \tag{4.3}$$

No attempt is made to justify this formula, except to note that the square root of the sample size is a divisor and that the larger the sample size, the smaller is the standard error of the proportion. In other words, the larger the sample size, the less spread out is the sampling distribution of the proportion. In more concrete terms, it means that for large sample sizes there is less variability in the possible sample proportions that could be obtained or that with large sample sizes an observed sample proportion is likely to be nearer the true population value than with small sample sizes. This is a general result pertaining to the standard error of any statistic or, in other words, to the spread of any sampling distribution.

The sampling distribution of a statistic
- is the distribution of potential values of that statistic that could be obtained in repeated samples of the same size from a population

The standard error of a statistic
- is the standard deviation of the sampling distribution of that statistic
- measures the precision of the sample value of that statistic as an estimator of the true population value; the smaller the standard error is, the more precise the estimate
- decreases with increasing sample size

4.4 Confidence intervals for a proportion

4.4.1 Confidence intervals using the normal distribution

Having looked at the theoretical properties of the sampling distribution of a proportion, it is now possible to return to the example of the 200 PVD patients. It can now be said that the sample proportion of smokers actually observed ($p = 0.65$) is one random observation from all the possible propor-

tions that could have been obtained with different samples sized 200 from the
population. These possible proportions have a normal distribution whose
mean is equal to the unknown population proportion, π, which is being estimated and whose standard deviation (the standard error of a proportion) is
equal to:

$$\sqrt{\frac{\pi(1-\pi)}{n}}$$

Since the actual value of π is not known, an estimate of this standard error can
be made by substitution of the sample value of the proportion, $p = 0.65$. Thus
the standard deviation of the sampling distribution of the proportion is
approximately equal to:

$$\text{SE}(p) \approx \sqrt{\frac{p(1-p)}{n}} \tag{4.4}$$

which is, in this case, $\sqrt{[0.65\,(1-0.65)/200]} = 0.034$. The 'wavy' equal sign in
the above expression means 'is approximately equal to' but, in general, the
quantity given by the expression is taken to be the same as the standard error
of a proportion, ignoring the fact that it is only an approximation.

From the properties of the normal distribution, it can be said that there is a
95% chance that the observed value of the proportion of smokers:

$$0.65 \quad \text{is within} \quad \pi \pm 1.96(0.034)$$

or:

$$0.65 \quad \text{is within} \quad \pi \pm 0.067$$

This statement can now be switched around to say that the following expression has a 95% chance of being correct:

$$\pi \quad \text{is within} \quad 0.65 \pm 0.067$$

or:

$$\pi \quad \text{is between} \quad 0.583 \quad \text{and} \quad 0.717$$

Instead of referring to this statement as having a 95% chance of being correct,
95% is taken as the degree of confidence that can be put in the statement. The
range 0.583 to 0.717 is called a 95% confidence interval for the unknown
population proportion π, and the figures of 0.583 and 0.717 are called the
95% confidence limits. The smaller figure is the lower confidence limit and the
larger figure is the upper confidence limit. The lower and upper confidence
limits for a parameter are denoted in this book by the subscripts l and u on the
symbol for the statistic. Thus, in the example:

$$p_l = 0.583 \quad \text{and} \quad p_u = 0.717$$

Earlier it was pointed out that the researcher might have intuitively stated, 'I am *fairly sure* that the unknown population proportion is *somewhere around* the sample value.' In this example, 'fairly sure' has now been quantified as '95% sure' and 'somewhere around' has been quantified as '±0·067' or as '±1·96 (standard errors)'. Translating back to percentages:

'I am 95% sure that the true percentage of smokers in PVD patients is 65·0% ± 6·7% or between 58·3% and 71·7%.'

In a scientific paper, the confidence interval is often written in parentheses after giving the point estimate: for example: 'The percentage of smokers in PVD patients is 65·0% (95% CI: 58·3% to 71·7%).' Note that it is preferable to use the word 'to' to reflect the interval rather than a dash '–', which can be confusing if a minus quantity is involved.

In terms of a formula, the 95% confidence interval for a proportion* can be estimated by:

$$p \pm 1{\cdot}96 \, SE(p)$$

or:

$$p \pm 1{\cdot}96\sqrt{\frac{p(1-p)}{n}} \qquad (4.5)$$

Note that, of necessity, the sample value is always inside the confidence interval. The confidence interval gives the precision of the sample estimate and thus the interval must surround the sample value of the statistic.

What if a higher level of confidence is desired—say 99%? What you gain on the roundabout, you lose on the swings: a 99% level of confidence would mean that the width of the confidence interval would be wider than that for 95% confidence. In Eqn. 4.5, the value 1·96 would be replaced by 2·576 (from Table B.2, 99% of observations in a normal distribution are within ±2·576 standard deviations of the mean), obtaining for a 99% confidence interval:

$$p \pm 2{\cdot}576\sqrt{\frac{p(1-p)}{n}} \qquad (4.6)$$

In the current example, the 99% confidence interval for the proportion of smokers is:

$$0{\cdot}65 \pm 2{\cdot}576(0{\cdot}034)$$

which gives 99% confidence limits of 0·562 and 0·738 or 56·2% and 73·8%.

Usually, only 95% or 99% confidence intervals are used, but with detailed tables of the normal distribution it is obviously possible to calculate confidence limits for any specified level of confidence.

---

* This formula should only be used for sample sizes above $n = 75$. See further discussion in Section 4.4.3.

A confidence interval (CI)
- gives the precision of a sample estimate
- puts a '±error' on a sample statistic*
- is a range of values surrounding a sample statistic within which, at a given level of confidence, the true value of the population parameter is likely to be found

* Sometimes the CI cannot be expressed simply as 'statistic ± error'

4.4.2 An exact approach using tables

The approach in the last section, using the normal distribution for estimating a confidence interval for a proportion, is only an approximation. It served, however, as an illustration of the central ideas of a sampling distribution for a statistic and the derivation of confidence limits based on the properties of that distribution.

In reality, the sampling distribution of a proportion is not normal; it follows a *binomial distribution* instead. This is, like the normal, a theoretical distribution and, based on it, it is possible to derive accurate formulae for the confidence limits for a proportion. Table B.11 in Appendix B gives the exact 95% and 99% confidence limits for all possible proportions in sample sizes ranging from $n = 2$ to $n = 75$. The table is straightforward to use. If the observed number of events or units with a particular characteristic in a sample size n is x, then the table is consulted for the sample size (n) at the top of the leftmost column and the observed number of events (x) in the next column. The third column gives the proportion of events ($p = x/n$) and the next two columns give the lower (p_l) and upper (p_u) 95% confidence limits for the population proportion. The final two columns give the 99% limits. Note that the exact confidence limits are not in general symmetrical around the sample proportion and cannot be put in the form of '$p \pm$ something'.

As a practical example, suppose that 23 histology slides from a sample of 40 were positive for a particular cancer. The sample proportion is $23/40 = 0.5750$ and a confidence interval for the population proportion of positive slides is required. To do this look up the table under $n = 40$. For $x = 23$, the proportion of positive slides is given as 0·5750, with a 95% confidence interval running from 0·4089 to 0·7296. On the basis of this sample of 40 slides, one can be 95% confident that the true percentage of positive slides in the population from which the sample was taken is between 40·89% and 72·96%. The 99% confidence interval is from 36·26% to 76·92%. (Usually the percentages would be quoted to one decimal place but the table gives the extra digit.)

Table B.11 gives exact confidence intervals for proportions based on the binomial distribution for sample sizes up to 75. For larger sample sizes, the formulae given in Section 4.4.1 are usually quite adequate.

4.4.3 Validity of the normal approximation [!]

Though the exact sampling distribution of a proportion is binomial, it so happens that as *n* (the sample size) increases, the binomial distribution becomes more like the normal distribution. This 'tendency towards normality' of the sampling distribution of a proportion is called the *central limit theorem*, and leads to what is called the normal approximation to the binomial. This approximation holds so long as $n(\pi)$ and $n(1 - \pi)$ are both greater than 5, where, as usual, *n* is the sample size and π is the proportion of units in the population with the required characteristic. Under these conditions, the sampling distribution of the proportion of individuals with the characteristic in repeated samples sized *n* is approximately normal, with the approximation improving with increasing sample size. The sampling distribution has a mean equal to the population parameter π and has a standard deviation (the standard error of the proportion) given by Eqn. 4.3.

The (95%) confidence interval formula:

$$p \pm 1\cdot96\sqrt{\frac{p(1-p)}{n}} \tag{4.5}$$

used in Section 4.4.1 is based on substitution of the sample proportion *p* for the population parameter π in this standard error. Equation 4.5 is the simplest expression for the confidence limits of a proportion, but a number of other methods are available that may be preferable with small sample sizes. These are reviewed by Newcombe (1998a). One, which is well-known, involves the use of a continuity correction. This is an extra term added to the standard error of Eqn. 4.5 to allow for the discrete nature of the binomial distribution. Many statistics related to the binomial distribution can have a continuity correction, but it is not recommended in this book. (See also discussion in Section 7.10.4 on mid-*p* confidence intervals.) The adequacy of the normal approximation depends on the magnitude of the population proportion π, which is unknown. However, the lower and upper confidence limits for π obtained from Eqn. 4.5 can be employed as a guide to the validity of the approximation instead. If these are denoted p_l and p_u, respectively, then the normal approximation to the binomial is quite acceptable as long as all the following quantities are greater than 5: np_l, $n(1 - p_l)$, np_u and $n(1 - p_u)$. In any case, even if the normal approximation is valid, it is more convenient and more accurate to use Table B.11 for samples sized 75 or less.

Taking the histology slide example, with 23/40 (0·5750) slides positive, the normal approximation for the 95% confidence interval is given by:

$$0\cdot5750 \pm 1\cdot96\sqrt{[(0\cdot575)(0\cdot425)/40]} = 0\cdot5750 \pm 0\cdot1532$$

which is from 0·4218 to 0·7282. These are quite close to the exact limits of 0·4089 and 0·7296 from Table B.11 (see Section 4.4.2), since the conditions for using the approximation hold.

Section C.2, Appendix C, summarizes the calculations of confidence intervals for proportions in the one-sample situation.

4.5 Sampling variation—means

Just as all the possible proportions from the different samples that could be taken from a population have a distribution, so too all the possible means have a sampling distribution. For what follows, think of the mean of a variable as a statistic measured on a sample, in the same way the proportion (of smokers) was a statistic.

Again, a simple example will be taken. The length of survival of 100 lung-cancer patients on a particular new therapy is determined. Overall, the patients—all followed to death—are observed to have a mean survival of 27·5 months, with a standard deviation of 25·0 months. The researcher is interested in estimating the true underlying (population) mean survival of these patients, denoted by μ. Assume for the moment that the standard deviation in the population, σ, is known to be exactly 25·0 months, even though, in reality, this is only the sample estimate.*

As in the case of the proportion, the distribution of all the possible sample means from samples of a given size (here $n = 100$) is examined. This is called the sampling distribution of the mean. Again, from theoretical considerations it can be determined that these possible sample means have a normal distribution, which has a mean actually equal to the unknown population mean, μ, and a standard deviation (called the standard error of the mean) equal to:

$$SE(\bar{x}) = \frac{\sigma}{\sqrt{n}} \tag{4.7}$$

where σ is the standard deviation of the variable in the population. In the survival example, then, the standard error of the mean is $25/\sqrt{100} = 2\cdot5$ years.

Two factors are noteworthy about the sampling distributions of the two statistics examined so far (the mean and a proportion). First, both sampling distributions are normal (or approximately so—see Section 4.5.1) and, secondly, the mean of each sampling distribution is the true value of the corresponding parameter in the population. As is seen below, these properties hold for the sampling distributions of a number of statistics and this explains the central role of the normal distribution in statistical analysis.

4.5.1 The sampling distribution of the mean [!]

The description above of the properties of the sampling distribution of the mean has simplified things somewhat, because the shape of the sampling

---

* The standard deviation here is much larger than the mean, but there is nothing unusual about this; survival times usually have quite a positively skewed distribution and one should not expect the properties of a normal distribution to hold.

distribution of the mean may not be quite normal in all situations. It is always so if the underlying distribution of the variable in the population (survival time in the example) is itself normal. However, variables with normal distributions are rare enough in medical applications and this situation rarely holds in practice. A normal distribution would be unusual for survival times, for instance. Non-normality of the variable, however, is not a major problem, due to an important theoretical result. As long as the distribution of the original variable is not very skewed, the sampling distribution of its mean is approximately normal and this approximation improves as the sample size increases. This is another example of the central-limit theorem, which, in fact, applies in a number of situations (see Section 4.4.3, where the theorem was introduced in the context of proportions).

The important point is that non-normality of the distribution of the variable under examination does not invalidate the use of the normal distribution for the sampling distribution of its mean. Unless the distribution of the variable is very skewed, sample sizes of over 30 are likely to be adequate for taking the sampling distribution to be normal. For very skewed distributions, confidence limits can be derived following a suitable transformation of the data (see Section 1.6.7 and Section 4.7 below).

The formula for the standard error of the mean

$$SE(\bar{x}) = \frac{\sigma}{\sqrt{n}} \tag{4.7}$$

involves both the sample size and the standard deviation of the population from which the samples are taken. As is the case for proportions, the standard error of the mean reduces with an increase in sample size and its magnitude varies inversely with the square root of this quantity. Often, when ambiguity can be avoided, the standard error of the mean is called just 'the standard error'.

It is possible to justify the formula for the standard error of the mean if one is willing not to question the explanation too much. If, for instance, samples sized one were taken from the population, the mean of each of these would be nothing more than the value of the observation on the individual unit chosen in the sample. The distribution of all possible means from different samples sized one would then be identical to the distribution of the variable in the original population. Thus, with a sample size of one, the standard deviation of the sampling distribution of the mean would be equal to the standard deviation in the population itself, σ. This agrees with Eqn. 4.7 when n is set equal to one. If now it is imagined that samples are taken whose size is the size of the original population, the mean of each of these samples (all identical) would be necessarily equal to the population mean, μ. In this case, there would be no spread of sample means around μ, and the standard deviation of the sampling distribution of the mean for sample sizes equal to the size of the population would be zero. For an infinite population, the sample size n would be infinite also and Eqn. 4.7 would give the standard error of the mean as zero also. This serves to explain the reasonableness of the equation. The standard error of the mean increases with increasing variability in the parent population and decreases with sample size.

4.6 Confidence intervals for a mean

4.6.1 Confidence intervals using the normal distribution

The same arguments employed for obtaining a confidence interval for a proportion can now be applied to the mean. In the lung-cancer survival example, the sample size is 100, so the skewed distribution of survival times should not invalidate the use of the normal distribution for the sampling distribution of the mean. The mean survival in the sample is $\bar{x} = 27\cdot5$ months and the population standard deviation, σ, is known to be $25\cdot0$ months.

The sampling distribution of the mean has a mean equal to the unknown population mean, μ, and a standard deviation (the standard error of the mean):

$$SE(\bar{x}) = \frac{\sigma}{\sqrt{n}} = \frac{25\cdot0}{\sqrt{100}} = 2\cdot5 \text{ years}$$

Since the sampling distribution of the mean has a normal distribution, 95% of possible sample means should lie within:

$$\mu \pm 1\cdot96(2\cdot5)$$

and there is therefore a 95% chance that the sample value actually observed ($\bar{x} = 27\cdot5$) is within these limits. This is then turned around to say that, with 95% confidence, μ is actually within:

$$27\cdot5 \pm 1\cdot96(2\cdot5)$$

or between $22\cdot6$ and $32\cdot4$ years. This is the 95% confidence interval for a mean based on the normal distribution. The mean survival is $27\cdot5$ months (95% CI: $22\cdot6$ to $32\cdot4$ years). In general terms, the 95% confidence interval is given by:

$$\bar{x} \pm 1\cdot96 SE(\bar{x}) \tag{4.8}$$

which is:

$$\bar{x} \pm 1\cdot96 \frac{\sigma}{\sqrt{n}} \tag{4.9}$$

The 99% confidence interval is given by:

$$\bar{x} \pm 2\cdot576 \frac{\sigma}{\sqrt{n}} \tag{4.10}$$

which, in the example, would give limits of $21\cdot06$ and $33\cdot94$ years. Appendix C (Section C.3) summarizes these calculations.

Equations 4.5 and 4.9 give 95% confidence interval formulae for sampling distributions of a proportion and the mean, respectively, under the assumption that both these sampling distributions are normal. It was also pointed out that the normal approximation is especially suitable for large sample sizes. In fact, the sampling distributions of many (but not all) statistics tend to normality with a large enough sample size, and a general formula for a 95% confidence interval is given by:

$$\text{statistic} \pm 1{\cdot}96 \text{ (standard error of the statistic)} \qquad (4.11)$$

This can be a useful formula in many situations.

> A general formula for a 95% confidence interval is often given by
> • statistic $\pm$ 1·96 (standard error of the statistic)

4.6.2 Standard deviations and standard errors of the mean [!]

There is always much confusion relating to the sampling distribution of the mean and the different 'standard deviations' that seem to be involved. There are three different distributions that become entangled together and the reader should try and distinguish between them. They are best described in the context of the example of survival times already discussed. The first distribution is the distribution of the variable in the sample. The particular sample of 100 lung-cancer patients has observed or measured survival times that can be formed into a frequency distribution whose (sample) mean, $\bar{x}$, is 27·5 months. The second distribution is the underlying distribution of survival times in the population of all such patients; it is not known what this distribution looks like and the purpose of taking a sample is to estimate its mean, μ. The third distribution of interest is a theoretical one. It is not a distribution of survival times; it is a distribution of mean survival times, each mean calculated from a different (potential) sample. Each potential sample has 100 persons in it and is one of the samples that could have been taken from the population of all lung-cancer patients. This third distribution is called the sampling distribution of the mean. Again, it must be emphasized that the only distribution which can actually be formed is the distribution of survival times in the sample actually chosen and that the sampling distribution of the mean, in particular, is a theoretical distribution, which exists only in the mind of the statistician, but exists none the less. Figure 4.5 summarizes the properties of these three distributions.

Now the standard deviations of these three distributions must be considered. The standard deviation is a measure of spread for any distribution. It is part of the description of the distribution. In the example, the spread of the sample was determined to be S = 25·0 months, and the assumption was made that the standard deviation of the population had the same value, σ = 25·0 months. On the other hand, the spread of the sampling distribution of the

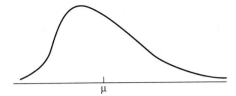

Original (underlying) distribution of a variable *x* in the population, with a mean μ and standard deviation σ (not necessarily normal).

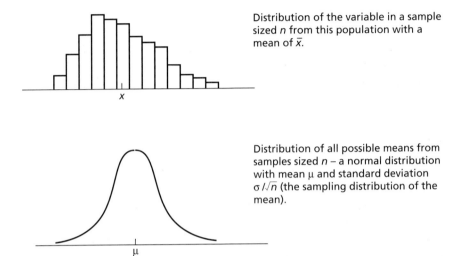

Distribution of the variable in a sample sized *n* from this population with a mean of $\bar{x}$.

Distribution of all possible means from samples sized *n* – a normal distribution with mean μ and standard deviation $\sigma/\sqrt{n}$ (the sampling distribution of the mean).

Fig. 4.5 The sampling distribution of the mean.

mean, which is called the standard error of the mean, is equal to $\sigma/\sqrt{n} = 2\cdot5$ months.

In describing a distribution, the mean and standard deviation are usually suitable measures of the centre and spread. Unfortunately, many persons tend to present the mean and standard deviation as, for example, $44\cdot3 \pm 17\cdot0$, with a note in the text that this signifies a mean plus or minus a standard deviation (or maybe $1\cdot96$ or two* standard deviations!) This should not be done. Such an expression can only be interpreted if the variable has a normal distribution. In this situation only (which is fairly rare):

mean ± standard deviation   contains about 68% of observations

mean ± 1·96 (standard deviations)   contains about 95% of observations

If the variable does not have a normal distribution, neither of these has any interpretation (see discussion of normal ranges in Section 4.2.3).

On the other hand, the mean plus or minus a multiple of the standard error (of the mean) has an interpretation (as long as the sample size is not too small), even if the variable does not have a normal distribution.

* Often 2 is used as an approximate multiplier instead of 1·96.

mean ± standard error	is a 68% confidence interval for the mean
mean ± 1·96 (standard errors)	is a 95% confidence interval for the mean

In other words, the (unknown) true, population mean is likely, at a 68% level of confidence, to lie within the limits given by the first expression and, at a 95% level of confidence, to lie within the limits given by the second expression.

Whether standard deviations or standard errors are presented depends on the purpose of the presentation. Just because they are smaller and therefore look better is not a sufficient reason to present standard errors!! It is also worthwhile noting, when reading the medical literature, how many times a mean ± something is presented with no statement as to what that something is. After all, it could be one standard deviation, two standard deviations, one standard error or two standard errors, and the interpretation of the expression is impossible without knowing which.

The standard error (of the mean)
- belongs to inferential statistics
- is the standard deviation of the sampling distribution of the mean
- measures the precision to which the sample mean reflects the population mean
- gives a 95% confidence interval for the mean:

$$\text{sample mean} \pm 1\cdot96 \text{ (standard errors of the mean)}$$

- does not describe the spread of a sample or population

The standard deviation
- belongs to descriptive statistics
- is a measure of spread (of a sample or a population)
- *in a normal distribution only* gives a range within which 95% of observations lie:

$$\text{mean} \pm 1\cdot96 \text{ (standard deviations)}$$

4.6.3 The Student's *t* distribution

So far, it has been assumed that the population standard deviation, σ, was known. This, of course, is an unrealistic assumption in most cases, and what happens when σ is replaced by the sample standard deviation, S, in the formula for the standard error is now examined. Remember that a 95% confidence interval for an unknown population mean was given by:

$$\bar{x} \pm 1\cdot96\,\sigma/\sqrt{n} \tag{4.9}$$

where $\bar{x}$ is the sample mean, σ is the population standard deviation, n is the sample size and $\pm 1\cdot96$ are the values that include 95% of the area under the standard normal curve.

It was realized that the above formulation, based on the normal distribution, would be inaccurate whenever S, the sample standard deviation, was substituted for σ, the population value, and especially so for small sample sizes. (As an aside, the population variance, σ^2, in a finite population of size N is correctly defined using a divisor of N rather than $N - 1$. The best estimate of this quantity from a sample sized n from an infinitely big population is given by S^2, however, with the $n - 1$ divisor. Hence this is the formulation used (see Eqn. 1.6).) It was not until 1908, however, that the solution to this problem was determined. In that year, a chemist-cum-mathematician, William Gosset, who was employed in the Guinness brewery in Dublin (Ireland), published a paper under the pseudonym 'Student', detailing the corrections which must be made in this situation. (Arthur Guinness Son & Co. did not allow Gosset to publish under his own name—possibly because they did not wish their competitors to realize just how useful statistics could be in sampling the quality of the brew!) Gosset's work was, essentially, to introduce what is now called the *Student's t* distribution, or the *t* distribution for short, for use in place of the normal distribution in the situation just described. The *t* distribution is, in fact, many different distributions, which are differentiated by their degrees of freedom (d.f.). Thus, there are *t* distributions with 1 d.f., 2 d.f., etc. Like the normal distribution, the *t* distribution is symmetrical, unimodal and bell-shaped, but it is more spread out and has different area properties. The fact that this distribution is more spread out allows for the increased variability introduced into the calculation of confidence intervals when only the sample value of the standard deviation is known. The degrees of freedom increase with sample size in the applications considered, and the Student's *t* distribution with a large number of degrees of freedom is pretty well identical to the standard normal distribution (see below).

The *t* distribution with any particular number of degrees of freedom is akin to the standard normal distribution, and Appendix B (Table B.3) gives a table of this distribution for degrees of freedom from 1 to 30 and some higher values. The table is laid out similarly to that for the normal distribution in Table B.2. Take, for example, the Student's *t* distribution with 8 d.f. The critical values of t, t_c, which cut off specified areas in the tail(s) of this distribution, are found on the row marked with d.f. = 8. It is seen, for instance, that 2·5% of the area is above $t = 2 \cdot 306$ while 1% of the area lies outside the limits defined by $t = \pm 3 \cdot 355$. Figure 4.6 illustrates these values for the *t* distribution with 8 degrees of freedom. In the normal distribution, the corresponding values would have been $\pm 1 \cdot 960$ and $\pm 2 \cdot 576$, respectively, thus illustrating the extra spread of the *t* distribution. Looking at Table B.3, it can also be seen that, as the degrees of freedom increase, the *t* distribution becomes closer to the normal distribution, and that at about 60 d.f., for instance, the values tabulated are indeed fairly close to those given for the normal distribution. (The entry for degrees of freedom equal to ∞ refers to an infinite number of degrees of freedom, when the *t* distribution and standard normal distribution coincide exactly.)

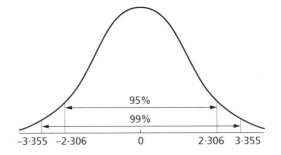

Fig. 4.6 The Student's *t*
distribution with 8 degrees of
freedom.

4.6.4 Confidence intervals using the *t* distribution

It was explained in the last section that, when the population standard deviation is not available, the sample standard deviation may be used in calculating confidence intervals, provided that the *t* distribution is employed instead of the normal distribution. An alternative derivation of the confidence interval formula (Eqn. 4.9) is to note that the standardized variable:

$$z = \frac{\bar{x} - \mu}{\sigma/\sqrt{n}} \tag{4.12}$$

with the usual notation, has a standard normal distribution. (See Eqn. 4.1, where the standard deviation of the sampling distribution of the mean is given by $\sigma/\sqrt{n}$.) Since 95% of the time z lies in ± 1.96, this can be reformulated to give the 95% confidence interval for μ as:

$$\bar{x} \pm 1.96\sigma/\sqrt{n} \tag{4.9}$$

which is the equation obtained before. Now, Student showed that:

$$t = \frac{\bar{x} - \mu}{S/\sqrt{n}} \tag{4.13}$$

had a *t* distribution with $n - 1$ d.f., where $\bar{x}$ is the sample mean, μ is the population mean, S is the sample standard deviation and n is the sample size. (The degrees of freedom for the *t* distribution relate to the degrees of freedom for the sample estimate of the standard error. Since this is based on the sample variance, $n - 1$ d.f. are used.) From this, a 95% confidence interval for the mean can be calculated as:

$$\bar{x} \pm t_c S/\sqrt{n} \tag{4.14}$$

where t_c is the *t* value on $n - 1$ d.f., which cuts off 5% of the area in the two tails of the distribution (e.g. for d.f. = 8, $t_c = 2.306$). It can be seen that, because the *t* distribution is more spread out, the confidence interval is wider than would be obtained with normal theory, when 1.96 would replace the 2.306 above. However, for large sample sizes ($n > 60$ is often suggested), the difference between the *t* value and that for the normal distribution is so small that the latter can be used with very little loss of accuracy.

Take a simple example. A research group studied the age at which nine children with a specific congenital heart disease began to walk. They obtained a mean figure of 12·8 months, with a (sample) standard deviation of 2·4 months. What are the 95% and 99% confidence intervals for the mean age of starting to walk in all children affected with this disease? There are 8 d.f. in this problem (one less than the sample size). The t value for a 95% confidence interval is, as noted above, 2·306. Thus, the researchers can be 95% sure that the mean age of walking for such children is:

$$12\cdot8 \pm 2\cdot306 \, (2\cdot4/\sqrt{9})$$

or:

$$12\cdot8 \pm 1\cdot84$$

that is to say, between 10·96 and 14·64 months. The 99% confidence interval is obtained by reading the t value corresponding to 1% of the area in both tails. For 8 d.f., the t value is 3·355, so that the 99% confidence interval is

$$12\cdot8 \pm 3\cdot355 \, (2\cdot4/\sqrt{9})$$

or:

$$12\cdot8 \pm 2\cdot68$$

This interval, of course, is wider than the 95% confidence interval. The quantity $S/\sqrt{n}$ is usually called the standard error (of the mean), even though it is only an estimate of this quantity, which is only known precisely when the population standard deviation, σ, is itself known. The formulae above (Eqns. 4.9 and 4.14) for the confidence interval for a mean both rely on the assumption that the population from which the sample was taken is not too skew, at least for small sample sizes. This must be checked on the sample data and, if necessary, a suitable transformation should be employed (see next section). Section C.3 in Appendix C summarizes the calculations of confidence intervals for means in the one-sample situation.

4.7 Confidence intervals for a geometric mean [!]

As explained in Section 1.6.7, the geometric mean for a distribution was obtained by taking the logarithms of each observation, getting the mean of these logs, and back-transforming to the original units of the observations:

$$GM(x) = 10^{\bar{x}'} \qquad (1.4)$$

where $\bar{x}'$ is the mean of the log-transformed data. In particular, for the homocysteine example, with a sample size of 797, the mean of the logs was 0·9855 and back-transforming this gave the geometric mean of 9·67 μmol/L.

How could a confidence interval be obtained for this? Essentially, one obtains confidence limits for the mean of the logs (i.e. for the mean of the transformed data) and then back-transforms these limits to get the confidence limits for the geometric mean. Remember that the major objective of any transformation in this context is to create a distribution that is more nearly symmetrical than the distribution of the original untransformed data. In this particular situation, the logs of the homocysteine measurements do have a fairly symmetrical distribution (see Figs 1.21 and 1.22). It is now quite reasonable to invoke the central-limit theorem and apply the standard methodology to the log-transformed data. On this basis, a confidence interval for the mean of the transformed variable is given by:

$$\bar{x}' \pm t_c \frac{S'}{\sqrt{n}} \tag{4.15}$$

where $\bar{x}'$ and S' are the sample mean and sample standard deviation of the log-transformed data.* This is particularly relevant for small sample sizes where the skewness of the original data would cause problems with a confidence interval for an untransformed mean. In any case, with fairly skewed distributions, the geometric mean is a more appropriate measure of the centre than the mean.

The 95% confidence interval for the mean of the transformed data is then (using 1·96 for the t distribution multiplier, since the sample size is so large):

$$0 \cdot 9855 \pm 1 \cdot 96(0 \cdot 1199/\sqrt{797})$$

or:

$$0 \cdot 9855 \pm 0 \cdot 0083$$

which is from 0·9772 to 0·9938. Thus, one can be 95% sure that the unknown population mean of the logs of homocysteine lies between 0·9772 and 0·9938. If the antilog of these limits is taken, the statement can now be made to read that one is 95% sure that the unknown population geometric mean lies between 9·49 and 9·86 μmol/L. This, of course, is the 95% confidence interval for the geometric mean (Table 4.1). In general terms, the confidence interval for a geometric mean is given by:

$$10^{\bar{x}' \pm t_c S'/\sqrt{n}} \tag{4.16}$$

Note that it is not correct to take the antilog of the 0·0083, adding and subtracting it from the geometric mean. One calculates the actual limits for the transformed data and back-transforms these limits. Note too that the confidence interval is not symmetrical about the geometric mean and therefore cannot be put in the form of 'geometric mean ± something'. In this particular example, to the degree of accuracy that the data are presented, the limits seem to be symmetrical, but this is not so in general. The point estimate of the geometric mean is 9·67 μmol/L (95% CI: 9·49 to 9·86 μmol/L).

---

* The antilog of S' is sometimes called the *geometric standard deviation*. It is difficult, however, to interpret what the geometric standard deviation is actually measuring and it is not correct to employ it directly to create a standard error for the geometric mean.

Table 4.1 95% Confidence limits for the geometric mean.

Sample mean of the logs 0·9855	I am 95% confident that	•	the population mean of the logs	•	lies between	0·9855 ± 0·0083 or 0·9772 and 0·9938
The antilog of the sample mean of the logs (geometric mean) 9·67	I am 95% confident that	•	the antilog of the population mean of the logs (population geometric mean)	•	lies between	$10^{0.9772}$ and $10^{0.9938}$ or 9·49 and 9·86

4.8 Confidence intervals for a median [!]

When the data are somewhat skewed, the arithmetic mean may not be the most appropriate measure of the centre of the distribution, and it is often preferable to employ either the median or the geometric mean—the latter for positively skewed data only. Calculation of confidence limits for the median requires a different approach from that used so far and is based on the ranks of the data. Essentially, the observations are ordered (ranked) from lowest to highest and numbered from 1 to n, where n is the sample size. If a number of observations are the same, for this application, they are still numbered with consecutive ranks.

The confidence limits are not based on a formula as such, but instead the ranks of the observations that correspond to the limits are determined. Table B.12 gives a table of the ranks determining 95% and 99% confidence limits for a median in sample sizes ranging from 5 to 100. Return to the hip-fracture data in Table 1.5. These data are shown in Table 4.2 with the ranks assigned to each observation.

The median is the middle or 11th observation, which is 82 years. Table B.12 shows that for a sample size of $n = 21$, the rank of the lower confidence limit, R_l, is 6. Thus the sixth lowest observation defines this limit, which is 73 years. The upper limit is given by the observation that is at rank:

$$R_u = n + 1 - R_l \qquad (4.17)$$

This upper limit can also be obtained by counting R_l observations backwards from the highest value. Thus the 95% upper limit is the 16th observation starting with the lowest or the sixth highest observation counting down from the top. This observation is 85 years. The median for these data is 82 years (95% CI: 73 to 85 years).*

For sample sizes above 100, an excellent approximation for the rank

---

* Because of the discrete nature of ranks, it is impossible to obtain a confidence interval in this manner with an exact confidence level of 95% or 99%. The approach here, following Conover (1998), gives the rank corresponding to the confidence level that is closest to the required nominal level. Different books may give different answers; in particular, some (e.g. Gardner and Altman, 2000) use a conservative approach, which gives the rank corresponding to the nearest probability equal to or above the nominal level.

Table 4.2 Ages at admission of 21 hip-fracture patients (see Table 1.5). From Table B.12, the ranks of the upper and lower confidence limits for the median are 6 and 16.

Rank	Age	
1	53	
2	62	
3	67	
4	71	
5	73	
6	73	← Lower 95% confidence limit
7	73	
8	76	
9	78	
10	78	
11	82	← Median
12	84	
13	84	
14	84	
15	84	
16	85	← Upper 95% confidence limit
17	86	
18	87	
19	87	
20	94	
21	98	

of the lowest 95% limit can be obtained from the following formula. First calculate:

$$R = \frac{n}{2} - 1{\cdot}96\frac{\sqrt{n}}{2} \tag{4.18}$$

where 1·96 is the appropriate multiplier from the normal distribution. R_l is then taken as R, if R is an integer, or otherwise by rounding up R to the next highest integer. As with Table B.12, the rank of the upper limit, R_u, is obtained from Eqn. 4.17, or by counting R_l observations backwards from the highest. In the homocysteine example (see Table 1.9), the median value in the 797 normal subjects was 9·47 µmol/L. Using Eqn. 4.15 for the 95% limit:

$$R = \frac{797}{2} - 1{\cdot}96\frac{\sqrt{797}}{2} = 370{\cdot}8$$

from which R_l is 371. Thus the lower limit is the 371st observation and the upper limit is the 427th observation or the 371st highest counting backwards from the highest value. From the raw data, these observations are 9·25 and 9·82 µmol/L, giving the required 95% confidence limits for the median homocysteine.

It is interesting to compare this answer for the median with that obtained for the geometric mean. With these skewed data, either measure of the centre could be considered suitable. The geometric mean for the same data in Section 4.7 was 9·67 µmol/L, with a 95% confidence interval from 9·49 to 9·86 µmol/L. The median and geometric means are similar in value and the confidence intervals could be compared by examining their widths. (The width is obtained by subtracting the lower limit from the upper limit.) The 95% interval for the geometric mean has a width of 0·37 μmol/L, while that for the median is somewhat wider at 0·57 μmol/L. The fewer assumptions underlying the median calculation explain why the precision of the median is lower.

These procedures for calculating the confidence limits for a single median are summarized in Section C.4 of Appendix C.

4.9 Confidence intervals for a count or rate [!]

4.9.1 Counts and the Poisson distribution

The sampling distributions of proportions, means and medians have been discussed in previous sections, and here the sampling distribution of counts is considered. This will allow confidence interval calculations for both counts and rates.

If one is counting the number of events over a period of time (number of attacks of angina in an individual over a 4-week period, for instance) or the number of items distributed in space (bacterial colonies on a Petri dish), the number of events or items will have a Poisson distribution (named after a French mathematician) under certain well-defined conditions, i.e. the sampling distribution of the count will be Poisson. This will happen only if the events or units have a random distribution and occur independently of each other.

Suppose that a patient is observed to have 18 attacks of angina over a 12-week period. This can be considered a sample in time of a 12-week period in the patient's history. Assuming that anginal attacks are random and independent (i.e. that one attack does not make the patient more liable to further attacks, or to the next attack being close in time to the initial one),* what is the underlying or true number of anginal attacks per 12 weeks for this patient? In other words, an estimate of the population number of anginal attacks per 12 weeks is required.

If the underlying number of anginal attacks in a 12-week period is μ (μ in this section denotes the number of attacks in a given period in the population and is not the population mean of a quantitative variable), then the number of attacks that would be observed in different periods of 12 weeks has a Poisson distribution, with a mean of μ and a standard deviation of $\sqrt{\mu}$. In other words, the sampling distribution of a count is Poisson, with a mean equal to the population value and a standard error equal to its square root. If a variable has a Poisson distribution, its variance is always equal to its mean, and this is one of the distinguishing features of the distribution.

Again, rather than detailing the somewhat complex calculations required

---

* Though this may not be fully true of angina, it is a reasonable assumption.

for confidence intervals based on the Poisson distribution, Table B.13 in Appendix B gives the exact 95% and 99% confidence intervals for a count based on such calculations. Note that the confidence interval is calculated for a count in an observed period, and the size of the period is irrelevant to the calculation. The count actually observed (not a figure converted to a count per week or whatever) must be used in the calculations. The table gives the observed count (denoted x) on the left-hand side, ranging from 0 to 100, and the 95% and 99% lower (x_1) and upper (x_u) confidence limits for that count. For the observed count of 18 anginal attacks in the example, the 95% confidence interval as given in the table is from 10·668 to 28·448. At a 95% level of confidence, the underlying number of anginal attacks (in a 12-week period) is between 10·7 and 28·4.

When the count is large, a normal approximation to the Poisson distribution is also available and the sampling distribution of the number of events or counts is normal, with mean μ and standard deviation (the standard error for a count) $\sqrt{\mu}$. On this basis, if x is an observed count, the 95% confidence interval for the number of counts is given by:

$$x \pm 1·96\sqrt{x} \qquad (4.19)$$

Applying this to the angina example, a 95% confidence interval of:

$$18 \pm 1·96\sqrt{18} \quad \text{or} \quad 18 \pm 8·316$$

which is from 9·684 to 26·316, is obtained. This is not a good approximation to the true interval of 10·668 to 28·448, because of the small count of 18. If the approximation is only used for counts above 100 (using Table B.13 for lower sample sizes), then the formula is reasonably accurate.

Although the discussion so far has been in terms of a count over a period of time, exactly the same principles hold if a count is made in a region of space. Suppose that a sample from a well-mixed suspension of live organisms were placed on a suitable nutrient in a Petri dish, and the resulting number of bacterial colonies were counted. The count could be expected to follow a Poisson distribution and a confidence interval could be calculated for the number of colonies.

4.9.2 Applications to rates

If one wished to express a count as a rate (e.g. the 18 anginal attacks in 12 weeks as a rate of 1·5 per week), the confidence limits for the observed count should be calculated and then converted to the rate. Using the exact limits, the 95% confidence interval for the weekly anginal rate is from 0·89 (10·688/12) to 2·37 (28·448/12) per week. Often, in a cohort study (see Chapter 6), an annual disease incidence rate is calculated by dividing the number of observed cases by the person-years of follow-up or person-years at risk. (A person-year of follow-up is one person followed for 1 year; 10 person-years of follow-up could be achieved by following 10 persons for 1 year each, five persons for 2 years each or one person for 10 years.) A confidence interval for such a rate is obtained by calculating the confidence limits for the number of cases and dividing these by the total person-years. This is also a useful approach for rates in vital statistics.

It is easy, using the normal approximation, to obtain a direct expression for the confidence interval for a rate. If the rate is denoted $r = x/PYRS$, where x is the number of observed cases and $PYRS$ is the person-years at risk or of follow-up, then substitution of the limits for the count (Eqn. 4.19) in the $PYRS$ definition of a rate gives a 95% confidence interval for a rate of:

$$\frac{x \pm 1{\cdot}96\sqrt{x}}{PYRS}$$

which is:

$$r \pm 1{\cdot}96\frac{\sqrt{x}}{PYRS} \qquad (4.20)$$

This can also be expressed as:

$$r \pm 1{\cdot}96\sqrt{\frac{r}{PYRS}} \qquad (4.21)$$

These two expressions are absolutely equivalent. Note, however, that the $PYRS$ figure must be expressed in the same units as the rate. In other words, if the rate is per 1000 person-years, then $PYRS$ should be given in thousands. With a little further substitution, however, the confidence interval can also be expressed without $PYRS$ appearing explicitly:

$$r \pm 1{\cdot}96\frac{r}{\sqrt{x}} \qquad (4.22)$$

The final formulation is useful in that the problems of the units in which $PYRS$ are expressed are avoided entirely. The rate r can be a rate per 1000, per 10000, per million or whatever, and the formula is still valid. Of course, the actual observed count of cases, x, which gave rise to the rate must be known.

As an example, suppose that 11 deaths from acute lymphatic leukaemia in children aged less than 15 years occurred in a small geographical area over a 12-year period. The average population aged 0–14 years over the period was 28560. From these data, the $PYRS$ would be $12 \times 28560 = 342720$. The average annual leukaemia rate in the region is then:

$$r = 11/342720 = 32{\cdot}10 \quad \text{per million}$$

Using Eqn. 4.20, the 95% confidence interval for this rate is:

$$32{\cdot}10 \pm 1{\cdot}96\frac{\sqrt{11}}{0{\cdot}34270} = 32{\cdot}10 \pm 18{\cdot}97$$

which is from 13·03 per million to 51·07 per million. The identical answer is, of course, obtained using Eqn. 4.21. Note that, since the rate 32·10 was expressed per million, the *PYRS* figure is given as 0·34270, which is in units of a million.

Using Eqn. 4.22 for the 95% confidence interval gives:

$$32.10 \pm 1.96 \frac{32.10}{\sqrt{11}} = 32.10 \pm 18.97$$

This, again, is the same answer, but the formula is considerably easier to use, since any possible confusion over the person-years value is avoided.

Rates or proportions? [!]

The astute reader will note that the concept of a proportion is very similar to that of a rate, and that in vital statistics one talks about, for example, an annual death rate calculated as the number of deaths in a year divided by the total population. The population here is essentially a person-year denominator. Without going into detail concerning the subtle distinctions between a rate and a proportion, it is easily shown that, for a very small proportion, the binomial distribution is approximated by the Poisson distribution. Equation 4.5 gave the 95% confidence interval for a proportion (using the normal approximation) as:

$$p \pm 1.96 \sqrt{\frac{p(1-p)}{n}} \qquad (4.5)$$

Now, if p is very small, $1 - p$ in the expression above will be near to unity and the formula above becomes:

$$p \pm 1.96 \sqrt{\frac{p}{n}}$$

If the proportion p is based on x events out of a sample size of *PYRS* ($p = x/PYRS$), this formulation for the confidence interval of a small proportion is seen to be identical to Eqn. 4.21 obtained for a rate, showing the equivalence of the binomial to the Poisson approach in this case. Section C.5 in Appendix C summarizes the calculation of confidence intervals for counts and rates.

4.10 Summary

This chapter concentrated on the estimation of population parameters, using statistics calculated on a single sample from the population. It was explained how theoretical considerations led to the concept of a sampling distribution of a statistic, which was the distribution of that statistic in repeated samples from a particular population. The important distinction between the standard error of the mean and the standard deviation was emphasized and the Student's *t* distribution was introduced. The estimation of confidence intervals was explained for proportions, means, medians, counts and rates. If a normal distribution approximates the sampling distribution of a statistic, a 95% confidence interval is given by:

$$\text{statistic} \pm 1.96 \text{ SE (statistic)}$$

The following chapter considers hypothesis testing as an alternative, but complementary, approach to statistical analysis.

Parameter	Confidence limits	(Eqn. no.)
Proportion	$p \pm z_c \sqrt{\dfrac{p(1-p)}{n}}$ (or use Table B.11)	(4.5)
Mean σ known σ unknown	 $\bar{x} \pm z_c \sigma / \sqrt{n}$ $\bar{x} \pm t_c S / \sqrt{n}$	 (4.9) (4.14)
Geometric mean	$10^{\bar{x}' \pm t_c S' / \sqrt{n}}$	(4.16)
Median	$R_l = smallest\ integer \geqslant \left(\dfrac{n}{2} - z_c \dfrac{\sqrt{n}}{2} \right)$	(4.18)
	$R_u = n + 1 - R_l$ (or use Table B.12)	(4.17)
Count	$x \pm z_c \sqrt{x}$ (or use Table B.13)	(4.19)
Rate	$r \pm z_c \dfrac{\sqrt{x}}{PYRS}$	(4.20)
	$r \pm z_c \sqrt{\dfrac{r}{PYRS}}$	(4.21)
	$r \pm z_c \dfrac{r}{\sqrt{x}}$	(4.22)

5 Hypothesis Testing: General Principles and One-sample Tests for Means, Proportions, Counts and Rates

5.1 Introduction

In Chapter 3, some of the concepts underlying *hypothesis testing* or, as it is often called, significance testing were considered. The null hypothesis was introduced in the context of a specific example and the important distinction between medical importance (based on the magnitude of an observed result) and statistical significance (based on a p value) was made. In this chapter, it is described how the p value is calculated in particular situations and some of the concepts underlying this approach to statistical analysis are considered in more detail. There is particular discussion of topics such as one- and two-sided tests, the relationship between confidence intervals and significance testing and the meaning of statistical power.

The examples considered are based on hypotheses concerning population parameters in studies consisting of one sample only, although most practical applications of hypothesis testing in medical statistics involve two samples. However, at this stage, the theory is best illustrated in the one-sample situation.

Prerequisites for this chapter include knowledge of the sampling distributions of means, proportions and counts.

5.2 The null and alternative hypotheses

The example which is taken has already been considered in Chapter 4 in the context of statistical estimation using confidence intervals. A sample of 100 lung-cancer patients on a new drug are observed to have a mean survival of 27·5 months, with a standard deviation of 25·0 months. Suppose, now, that from previous studies it is known that the mean survival of such patients (before the new drug was introduced) is 22·2 months. The investigators want to know if, on the basis of these data (the adequacy of which will be discussed in Chapter 6), they can conclude that the new drug prolongs survival.

The investigators' first step is to form a null hypothesis — in this case, stating that the new drug has no effect on survival. This is equivalent to saying that the population mean survival with the new drug is 22·2 months (the same as observed in a large series of patients who did not have this particular treatment) and that the sample value of 27·5 months arose purely due to chance. The population value for a parameter specified by the null hypothesis (here 22·2 months) is called the null value. Another way of looking at the null hypothesis is that it states that the 100 patients are a random sample from the population of all lung-cancer patients who, because the drug has no effect, have a mean survival of 22·2 months. Notationally, this may be written:

$$H_0 : \mu_D = 22 \cdot 2 \text{ months}$$

where H_0 means 'the null hypothesis is' and μ_D represents the mean survival in the population of patients treated with the new drug.

Having stated the null hypothesis, the investigators must then specify what the alternative hypothesis is. Without prior knowledge, they cannot be sure that the new drug does not actually reduce survival, so their alternative hypothesis is that the survival of patients with this drug is different from that of patients not so treated and:

$$H_A : \mu_D \neq 22 \cdot 2 \text{ months}$$

where H_A refers to the alternative hypothesis and $\neq$ means 'not equal to'. In most situations in medicine, the alternative hypothesis is stated in this simple way unless prior knowledge outside the study data suggests otherwise (see below). The alternative hypothesis is vague or diffuse, in that all survival times not equal to 22·2 months are included. As with the null hypothesis, the alternative hypothesis may be interpreted as implying that the 100 patients were a random sample from a population of treated lung-cancer patients whose mean survival was not 22·2 months. Since these 100 patients may have been the only group ever treated on the drug, a slight modification of the theory is required, in that they should be considered to be a sample from a hypothetical population of lung-cancer patients treated with this drug. The fact that the population only exists in the mind of the investigators does not matter, since the sample was treated and, of course, the inference is being made to a population of potentially treatable patients.

> The null hypothesis states
> - that there is no true effect in the population
> - that the observed sample result is due to chance alone
>
> The alternative hypothesis states
> - that some effect is present

5.3 The significance test

5.3.1 Calculating the p value

It was said in Chapter 3 that for a significance test one must calculate the probability (p) that a result such as the one obtained, or one even more unlikely, could have arisen if the null hypothesis were true. If this probability is less than the significance level, the hypothesis is rejected. This significance level should be stated before the test and it will be assumed here that it is set at the 5% level. The p value for this example can now be calculated.*

From the results of Chapter 4, it is known that 95% of all possible sample means, sized $n = 100$, from a population of mean $\mu_D = 22 \cdot 2$ (as specified by the null hypothesis) and standard deviation $\sigma = 25 \cdot 0$ will lie between:

$$\mu_D \pm 1 \cdot 96\sigma/\sqrt{n}$$

where $\sigma/\sqrt{n}$ is the standard error of the mean, and is equal to $25/\sqrt{100} = 2 \cdot 5$. (Note that it is assumed for the moment that σ is known exactly.) Thus, there is a 95% chance that a particular sample mean will lie between these limits, i.e.:

$$22 \cdot 2 \pm 1 \cdot 96 \, (2.5)$$

or:

$$22 \cdot 2 \pm 4.9$$

that is, between $17 \cdot 3$ and $27 \cdot 1$ (see Fig. 5.1). Alternatively, it could be said that there is only a 5% chance that the mean of such a sample is greater than $27 \cdot 1$ or less than $17 \cdot 3$, or, equivalently, more than $4 \cdot 9$ months away from the hypothesized mean. (Note that the addition law of probability (see Section 2.2.3) is used in making this statement.) It should be realized that $22 \cdot 2 \pm 4 \cdot 9$ is not a confidence interval. The value 22.2 is the (hypothesized) mean of the population and not the sample mean. In a significance test, a value for the population parameter is given (the null value) and this is used. The interval above, which does not have a particular name, surrounds the population mean, while the confidence interval always surrounds the sample mean.

---

* It is not correct to refer to a 95% significance level. The significance level—the chance of a spurious result—should be the small percentage (5%). The confidence level—the degree of sureness in the result—should be the large one (95%).

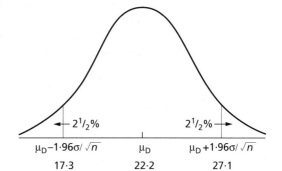

Fig. 5.1 Sampling distribution of the mean for samples sized $n = 100$ taken from a population of mean $\mu_D = 22\cdot2$ and standard deviation $\sigma = 25\cdot0$.

Now, in this case, the sample mean happens to be 27·5 (5.3 months above the hypothesized mean of 22·2) and thus it may be said that, if the null hypothesis were true, the chances of getting a sample result more than 5·3 months above or below 22·2 are less than 5%. But, by definition, this is the *p* value, so that, as a result of the calculation, it can now be stated, for this example, that *p* is less than 5% or $p < 0\cdot05$. Thus, statistical significance at a 5% level can be declared and the null hypothesis rejected, leading to the conclusion that sampling variation is an unlikely explanation of the observed sample result. In more medically meaningful terms, it might be said that the new drug gave a statistically significant increased survival in lung-cancer patients compared with that of previously available treatments.

The *p* value
- measures the chances of obtaining the observed result or one more extreme if in fact the null hypothesis were true
- measures the probability of the observed result or one more extreme being due to chance alone
- is based on how extreme a sample statistic is from the value specified by the null hypothesis

---

If, instead of a 5% level of significance, the researchers had decided to declare a significant result only if the *p* value was less than 1%, they could not have rejected the null hypothesis. Again, using the properties of the normal distribution, it is known that, if the null hypothesis were true, only 1% of possible sample means would lie outside:

$$\mu_D \pm 2\cdot576\sigma/\sqrt{n}$$

or:

$$22\cdot2 \pm 2\cdot576\,(2\cdot5)$$

and be less than 15·8 or greater than 28·6 months. The observed sample mean of 27·5 months does not lie outside these limits and therefore, by definition, *p* must be greater than 1%. Thus, the null hypothesis cannot be rejected at a 1% level of significance and a non-significant result must be declared at that level.

It can be seen from this that a result which is significant at one level may not be significant at a higher level. (A 1% significance level is usually referred to as a higher significance level than 5%.) To be more certain of the result, a more stringent criterion for rejecting the null hypothesis is necessary. On the other hand, a result that is significant at the 1% level is obviously also significant at the lower 5% level.

Values such as 17·3 and 27·1, as obtained in the example for the 5% significance level, are referred to as the *critical values* (lower and upper, respectively) for the test. Obviously, they depend on the actual study situation and the chosen significance level. If the test statistic, which for this formulation is the sample mean, falls between the two values, the null hypothesis is accepted at the defined significance level, and the interval from 17·3 to 27·1 is called the acceptance region for the test. The *critical region* for the test comprises all values below and including the lower critical value (17·3) and all values above and including the upper critical value (27·1). If the test statistic falls in the critical region, the null hypothesis can be rejected.

Significance level
- the cut-off value for p to declare a statistically significant result: $p < 0.05$ and $p < 0.01$ are often used

Test statistic
- the sample value of the quantity whose sampling distribution is known if the null hypothesis were true

Critical value(s)
- the minimum (or maximum) value the test statistic must achieve to declare a statistically significant result at a given level

Statistically significant
- unlikely to be due to chance
- a result with a sufficiently low p value
- null hypothesis can be rejected

5.3.2 What the p value is not [!]

The p value is essentially a measure of the unlikeliness of the observed result if in fact there is no real effect in the population—that is, on the assumption of the null hypothesis. If the observed result is unlikely to be due to chance—and 5% is typically taken as low enough to represent unlikely—then the null hypothesis is rejected. A significant result means that chance is an unlikely explanation of what was observed.

Many, however, misinterpret the magnitude of the p value. Rather than accepting it as a measure of the probability of the observed result *given the null hypothesis*, some (wrongly) take it as a measure of the probability of the null hypothesis itself *given the data*. It must be stressed that the p value does *not* measure the probability that the null hypothesis is true and in classical statistics this probability cannot be determined. The reader may have to give careful thought as to what the difference between these two probabilities is. Of course, the two probabilities are related and as one gets smaller so does the other; but they are different. At one level, it could be argued that this misinterpretation does not matter as long as the correct decision is made on the basis of the p value—rejection or non-rejection of the null hypothesis—and the correct interpretation is put on the decision—that chance is an unlikely explanation of the result or chance is a possible explanation.

An analogy may help. Suppose a woman has to drive home from work each evening and her husband always has the dinner ready waiting for her. She has been driving home on the same route for over 3 years and her husband knows to some degree of precision how long her journey takes. In fact, he has formed a frequency distribution of his wife's journey times and knows that, on average, she takes 45 minutes to get home. Not only that: he knows that 95% of the time she gets home within an hour, and in only 5% of her journeys over the past 3 years has she ever taken more than an hour. For 99% of the time, she has been home within an hour and a quarter. The variability in journey times has, of course, been due to normal traffic.

On this particular day, the husband is worried because his wife has not got home within the hour. Something unusual has happened, something that he knows, under normal conditions, happens less than 5% of the time. His mind immediately starts thinking about definite events that might have caused a delay, including things like car crashes. For argument's sake, assume that any delay not due to traffic is indeed due to an accident. In hypothesis-testing terms, the null hypothesis is that a crash has not happened and that the (observed) delay is due only to bad traffic (i.e. due to chance and not a real effect). The test statistic is the time taken to get home, and it has a known distribution under the null hypothesis. (If everything is normal, taking over an hour to get home happens less than 5% of the time.) Because of this unusual event, the husband rejects the null hypothesis at $p < 0.05$ and concludes that there has been a crash.

Now, the husband has no idea of what the probability is that his wife had an accident. The only way this could be worked out would be a detailed examination of accident statistics in the area related to time of day, length of journey, etc. He does know, however, that her late arrival is unusual under normal circumstances. Suppose she has not arrived within an hour and a quarter. This is most unusual if it is just a traffic delay ($p < 0.01$), and there is even more evidence to believe the worst. The probability of a crash, however, is still totally unknown. The decision is based on the probability of arriving so late if there had been no crash. In the same way, in a significance test, the probability of the null hypothesis remains unknown, and the p value measures the probability of the observed result if the null were true.*

---

* To set your mind at rest—the delayed wife arrived back 2 hours late. She had visited a friend in hospital! In study-design terms, rejection of the null hypothesis does not guarantee what the real 'cause' of the effect is. The fact that real causes of delay other than a crash were possible in the example corresponds to biases explaining an observed result, rather than the factor under study. See Chapter 3.

5.4 Relationship with confidence intervals

In the one-sample hypothesis test for a mean, it was stated that a result significant at the 5% level would be obtained if the sample mean ($\bar{x} = 27\cdot5$) lay outside the critical values given by:

$$\text{Hypothesized mean} \pm 1\cdot96 \text{ (standard errors)} \qquad (5.1)$$

which, in the example, were $17\cdot3$ and $27\cdot1$. When, in Chapter 4, the estimation of the population mean survival of all lung-cancer patients that could have been treated with the new drug was considered, a 95% confidence interval was calculated as (see Eqn. 4.11):

$$\text{Sample mean} \pm 1\cdot96 \text{ (standard errors)} \qquad (5.2)$$

which was from $22\cdot6$ to $32\cdot4$. This was interpreted to mean that it is 95% certain that the unknown mean survival lies between these values.

It is seen immediately that, if the population mean specified by the null hypothesis is outside the 95% confidence interval, the sample mean is outside the limits given by Eqn. 5.1. and, thus, an alternative approach to hypothesis testing is to declare a statistically significant result at the 5% level if the hypothesized mean (the null value) is outside the 95% confidence interval. This is quite logical and, in many cases, provides an acceptable alternative method of testing hypotheses. Note, however, that the confidence interval approach and the significance-test approach are not quite equivalent in all situations (comparing proportions, for instance) and the usual approach for significance testing is that outlined in Section 5.3. To reiterate the distinction, the hypothesis test is performed by seeing if the observed sample mean is further than $\pm1\cdot96$ SE away from the hypothesized mean (Eqn. 5.1). The confidence interval approach, on the other hand, is based on whether or not the hypothesized mean is more than $\pm1\cdot96$ SE away from the sample mean or is outside the 95% confidence interval.

Conversely, if the observed sample mean is within $\pm1\cdot96$ SE of the null value, the result is statistically non-significant, which is equivalent to the null value being inside the confidence interval. The two approaches happen to give identical results for the one-sample test described here, but in other situations there may be slight differences in conclusions if a confidence interval is employed instead of a formal significance test. This will only happen, however, in situations where the null value is close to the confidence limits and the p value (assuming 95% limits) is near to 5%. Thus, inferring statistical significance from a confidence interval is generally quite acceptable.

Statistically significant result at 5% level
- if the null value is outside the 95% confidence interval

Non-significant result at 5% level
- if the null value is included in the 95% confidence interval

---

5.5 One-sided and two-sided tests

The example which has been considered so far of a sample of 100 lung-cancer patients has been analysed with a null hypothesis of:

$$H_0 : \mu_D = 22 \cdot 2 \text{ months}$$

and an alternative hypothesis of:

$$H_A : \mu_D \neq 22 \cdot 2 \text{ months}$$

This alternative hypothesis does not distinguish between the situations where the new drug has a beneficial as opposed to a deleterious effect on survival. Consequently, the criterion for a significant result is whether or not the sample mean is further away from 22·2 months *in either direction* by 1·96 standard errors or 4·9 months. The ±1·96 SE is based on the areas in both tails of the normal distribution, adding up to the chosen significance level of 5% (see Fig. 5.1). For this reason, the test as described above is referred to as a *two-tailed* or *two-sided* significance test.

The two-sided significance test as outlined is appropriate to most medical applications when the direction of the anticipated results (i.e. greater or less than the value specified by the null hypothesis) cannot be determined beforehand. In the example, for instance, it would be dangerous if the researchers assumed, prior to the study, that the drug could only have a beneficial effect on survival. They were, therefore, correct in using a two-sided test, allowing for either increased or decreased survival compared with the hypothesized population value of 22·2 months.

In medical applications, it is rarely legitimate to employ a one-sided significance test (described below) and it is in fact difficult to find realistic examples where a one-sided test would be appropriate. In a one-sided test, it must be decided *before the data are even collected* that results in one particular direction could only have happened by chance and could never reflect a real underlying effect in the population. One possible very simplified example of such a situation is described below.

Suppose a study to examine the hereditary nature of cancer compared the maternal history of breast cancer between women who had a breast cancer themselves (cases) and a comparison or control group of similarly aged women who did not have breast cancer. (This is an example of a case–control study, to be discussed in Chapter 6.) A larger percentage with breast cancer among mothers of the cancer cases than among the mothers of the control women could be interpreted as evidence of some genetic effect. If would be very hard, however, to interpret a finding of fewer cancers in mothers of the cases. It is difficult to imagine any mechanism that would lead to less cancer in mothers of cancer patients than in mothers of non-cancer cases and therefore such an observation would have to be ascribed to chance. In this scenario, one might legitimately perform a one-sided significance test. For this example, a smaller percentage of maternal cancers in cases than in controls would always be interpreted as non-significant and due to chance (no matter how large the observed effect); evidence for a hereditary effect would be based on an *excess* of maternal cancers in cases only. In other words, interest would centre on an effect in one direction only. (The astute reader will spot that the illustration of the delayed wife and waiting house-husband in Section 5.3.2 related to a one-sided test!) A less realistic single-sample example is now given below to illustrate the calculations involved in one-sided tests in the one-sample situation.

Suppose that, in the general male population, the mean cholesterol level is known to be 6·5 mmol/L, with a standard deviation of 1·2 mmol/L. If researchers are interested in studying cholesterol levels in a group of 25 male volunteers on a prolonged high-fat, high-cholesterol diet, they might be justified in assuming that, whatever the mean cholesterol in this group may be, it cannot be below 6·5. They might thus decide on a one-sided significance test for the study. In such a case, the alternative hypothesis would be expressed as:

$$H_A : \mu_D > 6\cdot5 \text{ mmol/L}$$

where μ_D refers to the mean cholesterol level in the population of similar subjects on the same diet. The null hypothesis would be that the mean cholesterol is equal to 6·5 mmol/L. If the null hypothesis is rejected, only the alternative of mean cholesterol levels being greater than 6·5 mmol/L can be accepted. To continue with this example, suppose that the researchers discovered a mean cholesterol level of 6·9 mmol/L in their 25 volunteers: what can they conclude? In such a situation, it has been asserted beforehand that observed mean results less than 6·5 are due to chance and, therefore, spurious. It is only of interest to decide if mean values greater than 6·5 could be spurious or if they reflect a real difference in cholesterol levels of those on the diet. Again, using the properties of the sampling distribution of the mean, it can be asserted that, if the population mean cholesterol of those on the diet is 6·5 mmol/L, only 5% of possible sample means will lie above:

$$\mu_D + 1\cdot645\sigma/\sqrt{n}$$

or

$$6\cdot5 + 1\cdot645(1\cdot2/\sqrt{25}) = 6\cdot89$$

(see Fig. 5.2 and Table B.2 in Appendix B).

For a one-sided significance test, there is only one critical value. In this case, with the sample mean as the test statistic, it is the upper critical value of 6·89. The observed result obtained by the researchers was a sample mean of 6·9 mmol/L, which is just above the critical value, so that the null hypothesis may be rejected at a 5% one-sided level of significance. Subjects on this diet may be said to have statistically significant higher cholesterol levels than those observed in the general male population.

125

Section 5.6
One-sample z
test for mean

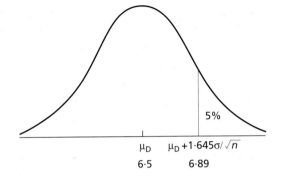

Fig. 5.2 Sampling distribution of
the mean for samples sized $n = 25$
taken from a population of mean
$\mu_D = 6 \cdot 5$ and standard deviation
$\sigma = 1 \cdot 2$.

Note that, if a two-sided test had been specified, the observed mean cholesterol level of those on the diet would have had to lie outside:

$$\mu_D \pm 1 \cdot 96 \sigma / \sqrt{n}$$

and be greater than or equal to $6 \cdot 97$ or less than or equal to $6 \cdot 03$. The observed sample value of $6 \cdot 9$ mmol/L is inside the acceptance region, so the result would be non-significant for a two-sided significance test.

In general, two-sided tests are more conservative than one-sided tests and make it harder to reject the null hypothesis. If in doubt, however, two-sided tests should always be employed, since definite prior information is required before the one-sided test is legitimate. The decision to perform a one-sided test must be made on *a priori* grounds before the data are examined. Note that, if the null hypothesis for the one-sided test had specified a difference in the opposite direction to that discussed above, the plus sign should be replaced by a minus sign and the critical region would be below the point defined by $\mu_D - 1 \cdot 645 \, \sigma / \sqrt{n}$.

5.6 General structure of a significance test: the one-sample *z* test for a mean

So far, two examples have been worked through in detail, showing how a particular null hypothesis could be accepted or rejected at a specified significance level. The examples taken dealt with the one-sample situation and hypotheses concerning means. As has already been stated, the particular hypothesis test used in a specific situation will depend on many factors, but the underlying approach is the same.

5.6.1 The test statistic

The one-sample test described in the previous sections will now be reformulated into a format that will be generally applicable in nearly all situations. This is achieved by changing the scale of measurement used in the example. It was seen in Section 4.2.2 that a normal variable with a given mean and standard deviation can be transformed so that the resulting variable has a mean of 0 and standard deviation of 1. This is achieved by using the equation:

$$z = \frac{\text{Value of variable} - \text{mean}}{\text{Standard deviation}}, \tag{5.3}$$

where z is the transformed or standardized variable (see Eqn. 4.1).

In the example of the lung-cancer patients (Section 5.2) the sampling distribution of the mean under the null hypothesis had a mean of $\mu_D = 22 \cdot 2$ and a standard deviation (called the standard error of the mean) of $2 \cdot 5$ calculated from $\sigma/\sqrt{n}$ with $\sigma = 25$ and $n = 100$. If, instead of looking at the distribution of possible sample means ($\bar{x}$), the distribution of

$$z = \frac{\bar{x} - \mu_D}{\sigma/\sqrt{n}} \tag{5.4}$$

is examined, it could be said that it follows a standard normal distribution of mean 0 and standard deviation 1. Thus, 95% of the time the value of z should lie between $-1 \cdot 96$ and $+1 \cdot 96$. In 5% of samples, z, calculated from Eqn. 5.4, would lie outside these limits. The z value corresponding to the sample mean of $27 \cdot 5$ is

$$z = \frac{27 \cdot 5 - 22 \cdot 2}{2 \cdot 5} = 2 \cdot 12$$

which is greater than $1 \cdot 96$. Thus, if the null hypothesis were true, a value of z as extreme as $2 \cdot 12$ would occur less than 5% of the time, so that the p value for the test is less than 5%. This is, therefore, a significant result and the null hypothesis that a population of patients treated with this new drug would have the same survival as all previous patients can be rejected. This, of course, is the conclusion that was reached before, using a slightly different but equivalent mathematical approach. In general, for a one-sample two-sided hypothesis test on a mean, the null hypothesis specifying the mean of a population to be μ_0 (a particular numerical value) may be rejected at a 5% level if:

$$z \geqslant 1 \cdot 96 \quad \text{or} \quad z \leqslant -1 \cdot 96$$

where:

$$z = \frac{\bar{x} - \mu_0}{\text{SE}(\bar{x})} \tag{5.4}$$

is the test statistic for this formulation of the test. Tests that employ the standard normal deviate (z) as a test statistic are generally called z tests. The critical and acceptance regions for this test are illustrated in Fig. 5.3. If $z \geqslant 1 \cdot 96$ it can be concluded that the true population mean is greater than that specified by the null hypothesis, while if $z \leqslant -1 \cdot 96$ it can be concluded that the population mean is, in fact, less than that specified by the null hypothesis.

127

*Section 5.6
One-sample z
test for mean*

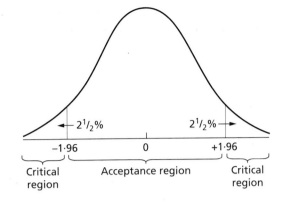

Fig. 5.3 The standard normal curve showing the critical region for rejection of H_0 and the acceptance region for non-rejection of H_0 for the z test at a two-sided significance level of 5%.

5.6.2 The z-test table

Going back to the properties of the standard normal distribution, it is known that ± 1.96 cuts off 5% of the area in the two tails. If a significance test at a 1% level is required, 1·96 would be replaced by 2·576, which corresponds to 1% of the area in both tails of a standard normal curve. Similarly, for a one-sided test, where the alternative hypothesis states that the population mean should be greater than that specified by the null hypothesis, a significant result at a 5% level would be obtained if $z \geq 1.645$, where 1·645 corresponds to a 5% area in the upper tail of the standard normal distribution. Table B.2 in Appendix B gives the critical values for various significance levels of one- and two-sided z tests. The table does not, however, allow for the calculation of an exact p value. In the example, for instance, with a z of 2·12 it was calculated that p was less than 5%. Obviously, if the area in the tails of the distribution outside ± 2.12 could be determined, the exact p value could be calculated. In fact, extensive tables of the standard normal distribution are available which would enable such an exact calculation, but the fact that p is less than 5% is sufficient for most practical purposes. Computer output usually gives the exact p value for a significance test and some journals insist on presenting exact values.

Note that the higher the absolute value of the test statistic, z, the smaller are the corresponding areas in the tails of the distribution and, thus, the greater the level of statistical significance achieved. Often, the results of a significance test may be expressed by giving a range within which the p value lies. Thus, using the table, if z were 1·72, the two-sided p value would be given as greater than 0·05 but less than 0·10. This could be written: $0.05 < p < 0.10$, which, of course, is not a significant result at the 5% level. The highest significance level achieved should be given if p happens to be less than 5%; thus 'p less than 1%' would be quoted rather than 'p less than 5%'. On the other hand, most researchers just write down NS (for non-significant) for all values of p above 5%, although it might perhaps be better if a more exact range were given. The results of a significance test are often written as $z = 2.12$; $p < 0.05$ or $z = 1.72$; NS. Use of the one-sample z-test is summarized in Section C.3 of Appendix C.

5.6.3 General structure of a significance test

As will be seen later, many test statistics are formulated in a similar manner to the one-sample z test as:

$$\frac{\text{Sample statistic} - \text{null value}}{\text{Standard error of statistic}} \tag{5.5}$$

and the format of the one-sample z test has general applicability to most statistical tests of significance. A null hypothesis is postulated, a significance level is set and a one- or two-sided test chosen. A test statistic is calculated on the basis of the sample data and null hypothesis. The particular statistic will, of course, depend on the data, the type of study and many other factors, but, whatever the statistic, it is known from theoretical considerations to have a specific distribution if the null hypothesis is true. Tables of this distribution are examined to see if the statistic lies in the acceptance region or inside the critical region for the particular test chosen. The critical region usually corresponds to areas in the tail or tails of the distribution in question. If the test statistic lies within the critical region, a significant result may be claimed. In practice, what is often done is to calculate the highest level of significance for the given statistic without prior setting of the level required. By convention, however, a significance level of 5% is usually assumed to be necessary for rejection of the null hypothesis.

General significance test	Example of one-sample z test
State the null hypothesis (H_0) ↓	$\mu_D = 22 \cdot 2$
Set the significance level ↓	5%
One- or two-sided test? ↓	Two-sided
Calculate the test statistic ↓	$z = \dfrac{\bar{x} - \mu_D}{\sigma/\sqrt{n}} = 2 \cdot 12$
Find the critical values of the distribution of the test statistic for the given (one- or two-sided) significance level ↓	Critical values are $-1 \cdot 96$ and $+1 \cdot 96$
If the test statistic lies within the acceptance region, do not reject H_0. If the statistic lies in the critical region, reject H_0 and claim a significant result	Acceptance region: $-1 \cdot 96 < z < 1 \cdot 96$ Critical region: $z \leqslant -1 \cdot 96$ or $z \geqslant 1 \cdot 96$ So H_0 rejected with $z = 2 \cdot 12$

5.7 Non-significant results and power: type I errors, type II errors and sample size

Having looked in detail at the calculation of significance levels and their interpretation in the context of the one-sample z test, the interpretation of non-significant results is now considered. This is sometimes referred to as 'the other side of significance testing' and leads eventually to the important question of determining adequate sample sizes for specific studies.

The example of the 100 lung-cancer patients and the one-sample z test will again be used to illustrate the ideas. As was seen, the level of statistical significance attained depends on the magnitude of the test statistic:

$$z = \frac{\bar{x} - \mu_0}{\sigma/\sqrt{n}} \qquad (5.4)$$

where $\bar{x}$ is the observed sample mean, μ_0 is the hypothesized mean, σ is the standard deviation in the population and n is the sample size. The larger the value of z, the greater the level of statistical significance achieved and the less likelihood that the observed result is spurious.

5.7.1 Factors affecting significance

What, then, are the factors that lead to statistically significant results? First, the magnitude of $\bar{x} - \mu_0$ is important; all else being equal, sample means far away from the hypothesized population value (the null value) will give significant results more readily than values close to it. This is an intuitively obvious result, in the sense that a sample with a mean very much larger (or smaller) than what was hypothesized tends to throw doubt on the hypothesis. So the degree of statistical significance depends, firstly, on the true (unknown) population value when the null hypothesis is false. The second factor that will affect the likelihood of a significant result is the population standard deviation, σ. Statistically significant results are more likely with small values of σ. Again, this is reasonable, since, if the spread or variation in the population is small, it should be easier to detect samples not originating from that population. The third and perhaps most important factor that will determine whether or not significance may be achieved is the sample size, n. For a given observed difference, $\bar{x} - \mu_0$, and given σ, larger sample sizes will more easily give significant results. In fact, it is easily seen from Eqn. 5.4 that any difference (no matter how small or unimportant) can be made statistically significant if the sample size is large enough. This highlights the distinction made in Chapter 3 between medically important and statistically significant results, and also justifies the claim that, with an important result based on large enough numbers, statistical analysis is almost entirely redundant.

From the opposite point of view, a non-significant result can be due to the true population mean lying very near the hypothesized value, too large a spread in the population, too small a sample size or any combination of these three factors. Although illustrated in the context of the one-sample z test, the above points may be taken as being generally applicable to most statistical tests of significance.

5.7.2 Type I and type II errors

Figure 5.4 illustrates the main elements of the decision process involved in hypothesis testing, using the one-sample drug trial as a practical example. At the top of the figure, two possible states of 'reality' are shown: either the null hypothesis is true and the (population) mean survival of patients treated with the drug is 22·2 months, or the null hypothesis is false. On the left side of the figure are noted the two possible decisions that can be made—rejection or acceptance of this null hypothesis. In the body of the figure are the implications of any particular decision for either of the two realities.

If the null hypothesis is true and a non-significant result is obtained, everything is fine and the correct decision has been made. If, however, the null hypothesis is true and a significant result is obtained, the decision to reject the hypothesis is incorrect and an error has been made. This form of error is called an alpha (α—the lower-case Greek letter 'a') error or type I error. The probability of making a type I error, denoted by α, is, by definition, the probability of rejecting the null hypothesis when it is in fact true. This, of course, is nothing more than the significance level of the test. (Remember, a significant result obtains if, traditionally, p is less than 0·05 and, by definition, p can be less than this value for 5% of the possible samples when the null hypothesis is true.) The p value for any result can be alternatively interpreted as the chance of making a type I or alpha error. Returning to Fig. 5.4: if the null hypothesis is false, a statistically significant result leads to a correct decision. If, however, in this situation a non-significant result is obtained, a decision error has again been made, and this is called the beta (β—the lower-case Greek letter 'b') or type II error. For non-significant results, it is, therefore, necessary to calculate the probability of making this error.

		REALITY	
		Null hypothesis true	Null hypothesis false (alternative hypothesis true)
		H_0: μ_D=22.2	$\mu_D \neq 22.2$
DECISION	Do not reject H_0 (non-significant result)	Correct decision	β or type II error
	Reject H_0 (significant result)	α or type I error	Correct decision

Fig. 5.4 Type I and type II errors in hypothesis testing.

Alpha (α)
- probability of making a type I (alpha) error
- probability of rejecting the null hypothesis when it is true
- significance level of the test

Beta (β)
- probability of making a type II (beta) error
- probability of not rejecting the null hypothesis when it is false

5.7.3 Factors affecting the type II error

The true value of the population mean

It has already been mentioned that a non-significant result should be expressed as a non-rejection of the null hypothesis rather than an acceptance of it, since, in this case, the two states of reality cannot be distinguished. The problem is, of course, that the alternative hypothesis (in the example, for instance) encompasses every possible mean survival not exactly equal to 22·2 months. If, in fact, the mean population survival of the drug-treated group was 22·3 months (3 days greater than in the group without the drug), it would be technically wrong to fail to reject the null hypothesis. Such an error, however, would not be very important, since an increase of mean survival of this magnitude would be irrelevant in cancer therapy. Obviously, if the true mean survival was as close to 22·2 months as above, it would be very difficult to obtain a significant result (the sample mean, $\bar{x}$, would most probably be very close to the hypothesized mean of 22·2) and there would be a high chance of a beta or type II error. On the other hand, if the true survival were much greater or less than 22·2, the chances of a type II error should decrease. This illustrates one of the important facts concerning type II errors: the chances of their occurrence depend on the true value of the population mean. The actual size of the β probability depends on the overlap between the sampling distributions of the mean under (a) the null hypothesis and (b) a specific alternative hypothesis for which the type II error is to be calculated. Figure 5.5 shows the sampling distribution of the mean for the reality specified by the null hypothesis, and a reality specified by one particular alternative hypothesis, suggesting a mean drug-group survival of 30 months. It has already been shown that the null hypothesis would not be rejected at the 5% level if the sample mean were less than 27·1 months, or did not lie in the lightly shaded area of the upper distribution.* If, however, the real population mean were 30·0 months (and thus the null hypothesis were false), a mean value of less than 27·1 could arise in a sample from this population. The probability (denoted β) that it would arise, with a consequent type II error, is given by the

---

* The critical region below 17.3 months (see Fig. 5.1) is not considered here since its overlag with the second distribution is negligible.

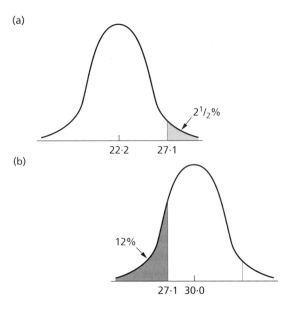

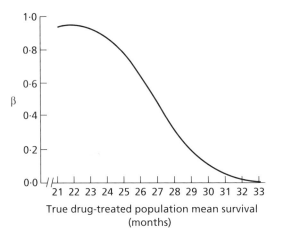

Fig. 5.5 Sampling distributions of the mean for (a) the null hypothesis, $\mu_D = 22.2$, and (b) a specific alternative hypothesis, $\mu_D = 30.0$.

Fig. 5.6 Operating characteristic curve for a two-sided 5% test of significance of the null hypothesis that the mean survival in the treated group is 22.2 months for samples sized 100 and population standard deviation of 25.0 months.

dark shaded area in the second curve. This can be calculated to be about 0.12 or 12%. The calculations are not detailed in this text.

Imagine now sliding the bottom half of Fig. 5.5 to the right or left, corresponding to different values for the alternative hypothesis. The area of the curve lying below the critical value of 27.1 (which corresponds to the magnitude of the β error) changes. Figure 5.6 shows a graph of calculated β values for various alternative survival times in the drug-treated population, with a sample size of 100 and a two-sided significance level of 5%. Such a graph is called the *operating characteristic curve* for a test. From this, it can be seen that if, for example, the true mean survival is 24 months, then β equals 0.9 and thus there is a 90% chance of making a type II error. For a mean survival of 30 months, however, the probability of a type II error reduces, as was said above, to about 12%. Sometimes, the value of $1 - \beta$ is quoted, rather than the value of β itself; $1 - \beta$ is called the *power* of the test. For a true mean survival of 30 months, the power of the test is $1 - 0.12 = 0.88$ or 88%. The power of a test increases as the difference between the hypothesized null value of the mean and the real value increases, and a high power means a low chance of a type II error or, alternatively, a large chance of detecting (significantly) a particular result. In general terms, the more discrepant reality is from the null hypothesis (i.e. the greater the 'effect' is in the population), the greater is the power of the significance test.

- The power of a significance test increases as the true size of the effect increases
- Large departures from the null hypothesis are easier to detect

---

The significance level of the test

How, then, can the probability of a type II error be reduced? Looking at Fig. 5.5, it can be seen that there are two main possibilities. First, the significance level could be reduced to greater than 5%, thus increasing the light shaded area in the upper curve. This, in turn, will decrease the dark shaded area in the lower curve, corresponding to the β probability. This is a fairly general result: for a given sample size and a specified difference between the true population mean and the hypothesized mean, increases in α will decrease β and vice versa. What you lose on the roundabout, you gain on the swings. However, since the α value or p value of the test is usually specified beforehand, decreasing the type II error in this manner is not to be encouraged.

The sample size

The other way of reducing β is by reducing the spread of the sampling distribution of the mean, thus reducing the overlap of the two curves. Now, remember that the spread of the sampling distribution of the mean is determined by the standard error of the mean or $\sigma/\sqrt{n}$. The population standard deviation, σ, cannot be controlled, but the sample size can be increased, thus reducing the standard error. This is another important result: for a given significance level and specified difference between the hypothesized population mean and the true population value, the β error may be reduced by increasing the sample size.

5.7.4 Presenting non-significant results

The further analysis required for negative or non-significant results can now be explained. So far, the interdependence of four quantities has been seen: the significance level (α); the probability of a type II error (β); the sample size (n); and the difference between the hypothesized mean μ_0 and that actually obtaining in the population sampled. Given three of these factors, the fourth may be calculated, assuming that the population standard deviation is known.

If the study gives a significant result, then quoting the significance level is sufficient, since it gives the probability of the only error that could have been made—the type I error (see Fig. 5.4). If, however, the study gives a non-significant result at a specified level (usually 5%), the reader should be told what the chances of missing a real result were, i.e. the β probabilities should be presented for a range of possible values for the mean of the population from which the sample was taken. This may show that, in fact, the chances of missing a result where the true mean lay a fair distance from that given by the null hypothesis were quite high and that, from the beginning, the study could have been judged inadequate to detect important medical findings. This is often expressed by saying that the power $(1 - \beta)$ of the study was too small. With non-significant results, the presentation of a confidence interval indicates clearly the precision achieved by a study and whether the sample size was adequate as determined by the range of possible true values included in the interval.

5.7.5 Sample sizes

The usual reason for missing important results is that the sample size is too small, and investigations have shown that many medical studies with non-significant results were too small to detect anything but the most marked departures from the null hypothesis. When the sample size is too small, it is impossible to distinguish between real and spurious results. The solution, of course, is to estimate the required sample at the beginning of a study, in the planning stages. This topic is considered in detail in Chapter 8.

Usually, the requirements needed to calculate a sample size are a specification of the significance level, the chance one is willing to take in making a type II error (β), the size of the effect one does not want to miss (i.e. the magnitude of what would be considered an important result in terms of departure from the null hypothesis) and an estimate of the population variability, σ. (This last requirement is not necessary when estimating sample sizes for comparing proportions.) From these factors, a required sample size can usually be calculated. Unfortunately, sample sizes often turn out to be much larger than expected by the investigator, and the final size of the study is often a compromise between the numbers required from the statistical point of view and the practical situation relating to the resources available. In this situation at least, whatever sample size is chosen, the investigator can know what the chances are of detecting an important result, and if these prove to be too low the study should probably not be undertaken in the first place.

Sample size calculations are based on the interdependence of
- the sample size
- the degree of departure from the null hypothesis
- the power of the study
- the significance level

5.8 The one-sample *t* test for a mean

So far in this chapter, it has been assumed that the population standard deviation, σ, is known, and this led to the derivation of the one-sample z test. The other assumptions underlying this test were that a random sample in the population of interest had been taken and that this parent population was not very skewed (see also Section 4.5.1). As discussed in Section 4.6.4 in the context of confidence intervals, the Student's t distribution should be used in place of the normal distribution (z) when the sample standard deviation, S, is used instead of the population standard deviation, σ, for sample sizes of less than 60 or so. In this more realistic situation, the appropriate one-sample test statistic is, instead of Eqn. 5.4:

$$t_{n-1} = \frac{\bar{x} - \mu_0}{S/\sqrt{n}} \tag{5.6}$$

where $\bar{x}$ is the sample mean, μ_0 is the hypothesized population mean, n is the sample size and S is the sample standard deviation. The t_{n-1} indicates that it is necessary to look up a table of the t distribution on $n - 1$ degrees of freedom, rather than the table of the normal distribution, for obtaining the critical values. The resulting significance test is called the t test.

The one-sample t test will be illustrated using the example already discussed in Section 4.6.4. In that example, a researcher studied nine children with a specific congenital heart disease and found that they started to walk at a mean age of 12·8 months, with a standard deviation of 2·4 months. Assume now that normal children are known to start walking at a mean age of 11·4 months. Can the researcher conclude that congenital heart disease influences the age at which children begin to walk? Since the sample size is much less than 60 and only a sample estimate of the standard deviation is available, a t test must be employed. The null hypothesis is that children with congenital heart disease start to walk at a mean age of $\mu_W = 11\cdot4$ months, and a two-sided significance level of 5% is chosen. The test statistic is from Eqn. 5.6:

$$t = \frac{12\cdot8 - 11\cdot4}{2\cdot4/\sqrt{9}} = 1\cdot75$$

on 8 degrees of freedom (d.f.). Looking up Table B.3 for the Student's t distribution, it is seen that the critical values for a two-sided 5% level of significance are $\pm2\cdot306$. The calculated t of 1·75 falls within the acceptance region for the test and thus the null hypothesis cannot be rejected. The effect of the congenital heart disease on mean age at starting to walk is non-significant ($t = 1\cdot75$; d.f. = 8; NS). The one-sample t test is summarized in Section C.3 of Appendix C.

5.9 The one-sample *z* test for a proportion

The significance test for comparing an observed sample proportion with some hypothesized value is similar in form to the one-sample *z* test for means. If the population proportion specified by the null hypothesis is called π_0 and the proportion observed in the sample is denoted by p, then an appropriate test statistic that has the standard normal distribution is:

$$z = \frac{p - \pi_0}{\text{SE}(p)} \tag{5.7}$$

where $\text{SE}(p)$, the standard error of the sample proportion, is given by Eqn. 4.3. Thus:

$$z = \frac{p - \pi_0}{\sqrt{\dfrac{\pi_0(1 - \pi_0)}{n}}} \tag{5.8}$$

where n is the sample size. Note that, assuming the null hypothesis is true, an exact expression for the standard error of the sample proportion can be given, rather than the approximation with the confidence interval approach, where Eqn. 4.4 was used instead and p was substituted for π. Note that the restriction mentioned in Section 4.4.3 on the adequacy of the normal approximation to the binomial distribution applies here as well. Both $n\pi_0$ and $n(1 - \pi_0)$ must be greater than 5 for the valid use of the *z* test on proportions.

As an illustration of this approach, the study of smoking in the 200 peripheral vascular disease (PVD) patients will be considered again (see Section 4.4.1). Based on the 130 smokers, the observed proportion of smokers was 0·65. Suppose now that the researcher wants to perform a test to see if the proportion of smokers is significantly different from the known proportion in a general population of the same age-group, which is 0·38 or 38%. From Eqn. 5.8, the test statistic is

$$z = \frac{0.65 - 0.38}{\sqrt{\dfrac{0.38(1 - 0.38)}{200}}} = 7.87$$

The null hypothesis states that the proportion of smokers in PVD patients is 0·38. Since the two-sided 5% critical values for the *z* test are ±1·96 and the 1% critical values are ±2·576, the hypothesis may be rejected at a 1% level ($p < 0.01$). Smoking among PVD patients is significantly different from that in the general population. The one-sample *z* test for a single proportion is summarized in Section C.2 of Appendix C.

5.10 The one-sample χ^2 test for many proportions [!]

Sometimes researchers may have sample values of a qualitative variable taking on more than two values, which they wish to compare with a known population distribution. For instance, a survey of the smoking habits of 250 female nurses gave 108 (43·2%) current smokers, 24 (9·6%) ex-smokers and 118 (47·2%) never smokers. Are these percentages significantly different from those obtained in females in the general population—36·4, 15·7 and 47·9%, respectively? (Assume that these define the population distribution exactly. See Table 3.2.) Since this smoking variable has more than two categories, the test described in the last section for single proportions cannot be applied. A special test is available for this situation, however. It is called the chi-square test and is denoted χ^2 (χ, chi—the Greek letter corresponding to 'ch'). The formulation of this test is quite different from anything encountered so far. The test is based on calculating expected numbers in the different categories of the variable if the null hypothesis were true, and comparing these with the numbers actually obtained (the observed frequencies).

5.10.1 The test statistic

In the example, the null hypothesis would specify that the percentages in the nursing population of current, ex- and never smokers were 36·4, 15·7 and 47·9%, respectively. Of the 250 nurses sampled, it would therefore be expected that 36·4% or 91·0 (250 × 0·364) would be current smokers, 15·7% or 39·25 (250 × 0·157) would be ex-smokers and 47·9% or 119·75 (250 × 0·479) would be never smokers. These are called the expected numbers. (In statistics, fractions of people are often allowed to end up in different categories, and this should not worry you!) Table 5.1 shows these expected numbers (E) and the numbers actually observed in the sample (O). The expected numbers will add up to the total sample size. The hypothesis test is now based on the discrepancy between the observed and expected values. If the observed and expected values are close, it would be reasonable to think that there would be little evidence to reject the null hypothesis. On the other hand, large discrepancies may make it possible to reject it. In fact, it is the relative differences that are perhaps more important, and the test statistic that compares these quantities and has a known theoretical distribution is χ^2. χ^2 is obtained by subtracting each expected quantity from each observed quantity,

Table 5.1 Calculations for the one-sample χ^2 test.

Smoking category	Observed numbers (O)	Hypothesized proportions	Expected numbers (E)	$(O-E)$	$(O-E)^2/E$
Current smokers	108	0·364	91·00	17·00	3·176
Ex-smokers	24	0·157	39·25	−15·25	5·925
Never smokers	118	0·479	119·75	−1·75	0·026
Total	250	1·0	250·00	0·00	9·127

$\chi^2 = 9·127$; d.f. = 2; $p < 0·05$.

squaring the answer, dividing by the expected number and adding the result over the categories of the variable:

$$\chi^2 = \sum \frac{(O - E)^2}{E} \tag{5.9}$$

This calculation is illustrated in Table 5.1, where a χ^2 value of 9·127 is obtained. Note that the $O - E$ quantities themselves always sum to zero.

5.10.2 The χ^2 table

The critical values of the chi-square distribution must now be looked up in tables, just as for the z and t tests in previous sections. Table B.4 in Appendix B gives such a table of critical values for χ^2 and the actual properties of this distribution are not of concern here. Note from the table that, like the t distribution, the chi-square distribution also has many different degrees of freedom. How are these degrees of freedom to be determined in the example? In the t test, the degrees of freedom depended on the sample size; in the one-sample χ^2 test, however, the degrees of freedom depend on the number of categories in the variable being examined, and the appropriate degrees of freedom are given by one less than the number of categories. For the χ^2 test on tabular data (see Section 7.10.3), the degrees of freedom relate to the number of cells in the observed table that are free to vary, given the total sample size. The degrees of freedom thus increase with the number of $(O - E)$ quantities in the expression for χ^2 and the greater the number of these, the higher the value of chi-square. A chi-square distribution with high degrees of freedom has higher critical values than a chi-square with lower degrees of freedom. Here, since smoking had three categories, the χ^2 test with 2 d.f. is appropriate for the example.

A further point to note about the chi-square distribution is that the critical values are all positive; this is because χ^2 must itself be positive, due to the squared term in Eqn. 5.9. The critical values given must then be exceeded for a significant result. For this one-sample test, only two-sided significance levels are appropriate, as the specification of differences in one particular direction has no real meaning. For a 5% two-sided test on 2 d.f., the critical χ^2 value is 5·991 from the table. The calculated χ^2 value of 9·127 is greater than this, so it can be concluded that there is a significant difference between the smoking habits of nurses and those of the general female population ($\chi^2 = 9·127$; d.f. $= 2$; p < 0·05).

The one-sample χ^2 test as described above requires that theoretical population proportions are hypothesized without reference to the sample values. Such situations will often arise in genetic calculations, for example. The one-sample χ^2 test can also be used in slightly different situations to test the goodness of fit of (grouped) data to a theoretical distribution, such as the normal. In these situations, the degrees of freedom are calculated differently, however, and a more advanced text should be consulted.

The χ^2 test requires that the actual sample frequencies observed in the different categories of the variable be known; it is not sufficient to know only the percentages or proportions occurring in the sample. The test is limited in that it does not easily lead to confidence interval estimation, but, with only two categories of a qualitative variable, it is mathematically equivalent to the one-sample test for proportions discussed in the last section. (The chi-square distribution with 1 d.f. is the square of the standard normal distribution.) This test should only be used if not more than 20% of the expected frequencies are less than 5 and no single expected frequency is less than 1. If these assumptions are not met, combination of adjacent categories may increase the expected frequencies to the required levels. The one-sample χ^2 test is summarized in Section C.6 of Appendix C.

5.11 The one-sample *z* test for counts or rates

If the normal approximation to the Poisson distribution is valid, then a significance test to check whether or not an observed count x (in a particular time period or spatial area) could have come from an underlying (population) with a true count of μ_0 is given by:

$$z = \frac{x - \mu_0}{\sqrt{\mu_0}} \tag{5.10}$$

where $\sqrt{\mu_0}$ is the standard error of the count and can be specified exactly under the null hypothesis. Note that, like the situation for a proportion, the standard error used for the confidence interval is based on the observed data (i.e. $\sqrt{x}$ — see Eqn. 4.19).

Suppose that 11 deaths from acute lymphatic leukaemia in children aged under 15 years occurred in a small geographical area over a 12-year period and also that, based on the population size and national figures, 5.45 cases would have been expected. Could the observed figure have been due to chance? Using Eqn. 5.10, the significance test is:

$$z = (11 - 5 \cdot 45)/\sqrt{5 \cdot 45} = 2 \cdot 38$$

The critical 5% two-sided z value is 1·96 and the result can be declared significant at $p < 0·05$:

The one-sample significance test for a rate will be illustrated on the same data as above, which were also used in Section 4.9.2. If the average population age 0–14 years in the geographical region were 28 560, the person-years at risk (*PYRS*) would be 12 times that figure, or 342 720 (remember the observation period was 12 years). The average annual leukaemia rate in the region is then 11/342 720 or 32·10 per million. Suppose also that the average annual rate nationally were 15·90 per million. The null hypothesis states that the true population rate (θ) in the region is $\theta_0 = 15·90$, while the observed rate is 32·10. The form of the significance test for a rate is:

$$z = \frac{r - \theta_0}{\sqrt{(\theta_0 / PYRS)}} \qquad (5.11)$$

where θ_0 is the hypothesized rate, r is the observed rate and $PYRS$ is the person-years at risk, expressed in the same units as the rate. The expression $\sqrt{(\theta_0/PYRS)}$ is for the standard error of the rate under the null hypothesis. Note that with this notation $\mu_0 = \theta_0 (PYRS)$ or $5{\cdot}45 = 15{\cdot}90 \times 0{\cdot}3427$ (i.e. the null-hypothesis count is obtained by multiplying the person-years at risk by the hypothesized rate).

In this example, $PYRS$ must be expressed in millions, since the rate is expressed per million. Thus:

$$z = \frac{32{\cdot}10 - 15{\cdot}90}{\sqrt{(15{\cdot}90/0{\cdot}3427)}} = 2{\cdot}38$$

which, of course, is identical to the value obtained when the same problem was analysed using counts. There is a significant difference between the rate of $32{\cdot}10$ per million found in the study region and the national rate of $15{\cdot}90$, based on a two-sided 5% significance level. The methods of this section are summarized in Section C.5 of Appendix C.

5.12 Small sample sizes and the validity of assumptions [!]

5.12.1 Form of the sampling distribution

A fundamental requirement for valid application of tests of significance is that the sampling distribution of the statistic of interest (sample mean, proportion or count, for example) has a theoretical distribution whose properties are known.

Theoretically, the sampling distribution of the mean is normal only when the distribution of the variable in the population is itself normal. However, if the distribution of the variable in the population is not too skewed and the sample size is large enough, the central-limit theorem assures us that the sampling distribution of the mean will closely approximate a normal distribution. For moderately skewed data, sample sizes above 30 or so are sufficient. The same points apply for the t distribution, which is used instead of the normal when the population standard deviation is not known. (The use of the t distribution instead of the normal has nothing to do with whether or not the parent population is normal or not; the choice depends totally on whether an exact or estimated standard error is used. With sample sizes above 60 or thereabouts, the t distribution is closely approximated by the normal on the basis of examining the critical values, but this is a separate question from that of dealing with skewed data.)

The distribution of the sample is the only guide to the population distribution and, if it is very skewed, a transformation of the data (see Section 1.6.7) may be advisable prior to performing the z or t test for a mean. The test is then performed on the transformed data. *Non-parametric tests*, which make no assumptions about the distribution of the data, are also available, and such tests for the two-sample situation will be discussed in Chapter 7.

When the sampling distribution of proportions or counts is in question, slightly different problems arise. The sampling distributions of proportions and counts are binomial and Poisson, respectively. The tests discussed in Sections 5.9 and 5.11, however, made use of the normal approximation to these distributions. For small proportions or low counts, the approximations given in this text may not be accurate enough. An acceptable alternative, however, is to perform the significance test using the confidence interval approach.

5.12.2 *p* values using confidence intervals

As discussed in Section 5.4, a two-sided 5% significance can be inferred if the null-hypothesis value for the mean lies outside the 95% confidence interval for the mean (see also Section 7.5.1). If the null-hypothesis value is included in the confidence interval, the result is equivalent to non-significance. Much the same result holds when dealing with tests for proportions or counts. If the normal approximation is being used for both the significance test and the confidence interval, slight differences between the two approaches can arise, however. This is because, for proportions and counts, the standard error is actually a function of the population proportion or count. Thus, if the null hypothesis is true, the exact standard error is known. There is no pre-specified population value for a confidence interval, however, and the standard error must be approximated by the sample value. (Other more complex confidence interval estimates are available when this approximation is not made, but are not considered in this text.) The fact that different expressions for the standard error are employed for hypothesis tests from those for confidence intervals explains why the two procedures are not exactly equivalent. The discrepancies are small, however, and differences in interpretation will only arise when a result just achieves or fails to achieve significance at whatever level is being considered, and the corresponding confidence interval just fails to include or just includes the null value.

In any case, for small sample sizes, the normal approximation to the binomial or Poisson distribution as given in this text may not hold and, unless the result of the z test for a proportion or count (or rate) is very definitely significant or non-significant, an alternative approach is suggested. This is to use the tables for the exact binomial or Poisson confidence intervals, as described in Sections 4.4.2 and 4.9.1 and to infer significance at the appropriate level if the (exact) confidence intervals exclude the null value of the hypothesis test. This is a perfectly acceptable procedure and is recommended for small sample sizes. Note, however, that one-sided tests cannot be performed with this method, since the equivalence of the usual confidence interval is with a two-sided significance test.

5.13 Summary

In this chapter, the development of the one-sample normal (z) test was described in detail to illustrate the underlying structure of hypothesis tests. The relationship of confidence intervals to hypothesis tests was discussed, as were the concepts of one- and two-sided tests and the principles underlying power and sample size calculations. Later sections in the chapter detailed calculations for the more widely applicable one-sample t test. The z test for a single proportion, count or rate and the χ^2 test for many proportions were also described. The computational steps are summarized in Appendix C.

The next chapter of the book moves away from formal statistical analysis and examines common study designs in medical research. This puts the material of Chapter 7 in context, and that chapter details tests and confidence intervals for the comparison of two samples, which is the most common application area. The general principles discussed above, however, in the context of the one-sample test are applicable to all tests of hypotheses and are necessary for a full grasp of that and succeeding chapters.

Hypothesis test on	Test statistic	(Equation no.)
One mean:		
σ known	$z = \dfrac{\bar{x} - \mu_0}{\sigma/\sqrt{n}}$	(5.4)
σ unknown	$t_{n-1} = \dfrac{\bar{x} - \mu_0}{S/\sqrt{n}}$	(5.6)
One proportion	$z = \dfrac{p - \pi_0}{\sqrt{\dfrac{\pi_0(1-\pi_0)}{n}}}$	(5.8)
Many proportions	$\chi^2 = \sum \dfrac{(O-E)^2}{E}$	(5.9)
One count	$z = \dfrac{x - \mu_0}{\sqrt{\mu_0}}$	(5.10)
One rate	$z = \dfrac{r - \theta_0}{\sqrt{\theta_0/PYRS}}$	(5.11)

6 Epidemiological and Clinical Research Methods

6.1 Introduction

Medical research covers a wide field and it is often divided into three components: basic, epidemiological and clinical. Basic research is usually carried out in a laboratory and can involve biochemical, immunological, genetic and other types of investigation. Such research is often carried out on samples from patients but also includes animal experimentation. Epidemiological and clinical research tend to be more patient- and subject-centred. Epidemiology can be broadly defined as the science concerned with the distribution and determinants of disease in populations and, of course, clinical research deals directly with patients who have a disease or condition.

As discussed in Chapter 3, most questions in medical research can be answered by examining whether an association exists between two variables.

An association can arise purely due to chance, because of confounding or bias or because of a real, perhaps causal, effect. Statistical analysis, by means of hypothesis testing or confidence intervals, tackles the question of chance associations, and the analysis of single-sample studies was considered in detail in Chapters 4 and 5. The problem of confounding can be solved to a certain extent through stratified analyses and more complex analytic approaches, which are considered later in this book. However, as discussed in Section 3.5, avoidance of bias and confounding is best achieved through careful and appropriate study design. This chapter considers the standard designs employed in clinical and epidemiological research, describing the common measures of effect employed and emphasizing approaches to bias and confounding. Subsequent chapters deal in greater detail with the formal analyses of data arising from the designs considered. The material introduced in Chapter 3 is a prerequisite for the full understanding of the present chapter.

6.2 Observational and experimental studies

Most epidemiological or clinical studies involve the comparison of groups and can be broken up into two broad categories, distinguished by the design approaches taken to control for possible confounders of the comparison (see Section 3.5). *Experimental* studies are based on a process of randomization, whereby subjects are assigned by the investigator to the comparison groups (see Section 3.5.3. Control of confounding through randomization is perhaps the 'gold standard' of research designs, but for ethical reasons such studies are usually confined to the analysis of the effects of treatment or intervention. Experimental studies of treatment are variously called *clinical trials* or *randomized controlled trials*.

When comparison groups are not formed by a process of randomization, the resulting study is classed as *observational*. The researcher has no control over what subjects are in what groups and just observes and analyses the existing situation. Comparisons in observational studies are therefore fraught with the problem of confounded effects, which must be dealt with through appropriate analysis, restriction or matching. Observational studies can be further subclassified into three basic groupings—the *cross-sectional* study, which takes a snapshot in time, the *cohort* study, which follows subjects forward in time from cause to effect, and the *case–control* study, which proceeds backwards in time from effect to cause. These descriptors for different study designs are commonly used, but there can be confusion in terminology, which is discussed later, in Section 6.10.2.

Although case reports and clinical observations do not fall into the framework of designed studies, they form the basis and foundation-stone for most medical research. Clinical observations and 'hunches' often provide the initial ideas which may eventually lead to a formal study and to new knowledge being scientifically tested. Perhaps one of the best-known examples of this process started with the observation of Gregg (1941), an ophthalmologist, who noted an unusual number of congenital cataracts appearing in Australia. He suggested that this might be related to the exposure of the pregnant mother to German measles, of which there had been a severe epidemic in the previous year. This clinical observation eventually led to the implication of rubella virus in congenital malformations. A more recent example involves the discovery of acquired immune deficiency syndrome (AIDS) on the basis of an initial report of a few young men in Los Angeles with a rare and serious form of pneumonia (Gottlieb *et al.*, 1981).

> Experimental studies
> * randomized controlled trials
>
> Observational studies
> * cross-sectional studies
> * cohort studies
> * case–control studies

6.3 The cross-sectional study or survey

Essentially, a cross-sectional study is a snapshot in time and takes no account of the temporal relationship between any of the factors studied. Usually, it involves the examination of a cross-section of a particular population at one point in time. Cross-sectional studies may be based on a random sample from a defined population, or on a presenting sample of patients with a particular condition. The entire discussion of sampling techniques in Section 2.4 and the biases that can arise in sampling are particularly relevant to the cross-sectional study. If a study is hospital-based, one must be careful not to overgeneralize results and be wary of the selection biases that lead to hospital admission (see also discussion in Chapter 12).

Cross-sectional studies may be employed to study associations between different diseases or factors, but they cannot determine which might have occurred first. In terms of explaining disease aetiology (cause of disease), they provide only limited information. The *prevalence rate* of a disease can be defined as the proportion of persons in a population who have the disease in question at a particular point in time (point prevalence) or over a short time period (period prevalence).

$$\text{Prevalence rate} = \frac{\text{Number of existing cases of disease}}{\text{Population size}} \qquad (6.1)$$

Cross-sectional studies are ideally suited for studying prevalence. Such studies also have a use in estimating health needs or health attitudes and behaviour in a community, and the results of cross-sectional surveys may be a help in planning services or appropriate health education programmes. Screening programmes also fit into this category. (These programmes, however, are not designed for research purposes, but are set up to identify persons in the community who may have early evidence of a particular disease. The object of these studies is to commence early treatment of such persons and all persons at risk should be investigated. Sampling is not an appropriate approach.)

Although cross-sectional surveys are not as common in medical research as cohort or case–control studies, they are widely used in public health and many areas of social research, including, for example, government surveys of household budgets and unemployment. The opinion poll itself is also, of course, a cross-sectional survey.

Cross-sectional studies
- single examination of a cross-section (often a random sample) of a population at a single point in time

Used for
- studying prevalence
- estimating community needs, attitudes and behaviour
- limited examination of associations between factors and diseases

---

6.4 The cohort study

The essence of the cohort study* is that a group of subjects are examined and then followed over a period of time, looking at the development of some disease or end-point. In its simplest form, subjects are classified, at the initial examination, into (typically) two groups, one exposed and the other not exposed to some factor, and the objective of the study is to see if there is an association between this exposure and the end-point (Fig. 6.1). In rare situations, the exposure groups can be identified before study commencement and samples are taken from exposed and non-exposed groups separately.

The word exposure is to be taken here in its most general sense and can include personal characteristics (e.g. sex), behaviour (e.g. smoking) and exposures in the proper sense of the word (e.g. radiation). The follow-up period may be as short as 24 h, as for example in a study of operative mortality, or as long as 50 years or more. Follow-up can be *active*, where each subject is examined periodically, with the presence or absence of the end-point determined at each follow-up. If the end-point is mortality, follow-up can, in some countries, be *passive*, where the occurrence of the end-point is based on a notification of death to the investigators by the national authorities. At the end of the study, the occurrence or non-occurrence of the end-point should be known for all subjects.

Often the end-point of a cohort study is binary and signifies the occurrence

---

* The term cohort, which originally described a division of Roman soldiers (600 of them), now generally means a defined group followed over a period of time.

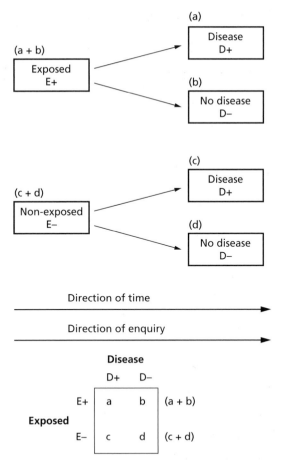

Direction of time

Direction of enquiry

Fig. 6.1 Schematic structure of a cohort study with component 2 × 2 table.

or non-occurrence of the event of interest. If it is possible for the end-point to recur, as, for example, a second heart attack or a further cancer, then the end-point is usually defined as the *first occurrence of the event*. Analysis of recurrent events and non-binary end-points (such as different causes of death) can be difficult and is not considered in this book.

There are two main types of cohort study, depending on their follow-up structure. The more straightforward is when all subjects are followed for the same length of time (fixed-time follow-up). Essentially, this means that the cohort study starts with a cross-sectional survey at a particular point in calendar time, with subsequent follow-up for a defined period. Variable-time follow-up will be considered in Section 6.6. In the fixed-time follow-up cohort study, the simplest presentation of the data is by means of a 2 × 2 table, which compares the percentages who develop disease between the exposed and non-exposed groups (see Fig. 6.1).

Cohort studies have two main areas of application. The first is in the study of *disease aetiology*. In this type of study, subjects without disease are followed forward in time and the risk of developing the disease of interest (or death) is compared between the exposed and non-exposed groups (see Section 3.6.2). The term *incidence* can also be used instead of risk to describe the onset of disease in a cohort study. Incidence (as opposed to prevalence, which refers to existing cases) is loosely defined as:

$$\text{Incidence rate} = \frac{\text{No. of new cases of disease (in a time period)}}{\text{Population size}} \quad (6.2)$$

The precise definition of population size in this context will be considered in Section 6.5.1, but for the moment incidence and risk can be considered synonymous—that is, the proportion of subjects who develop a disease in a given time period.

The second application area of the cohort study is in the study of *prognosis*, or, as it is sometimes called, the natural history of disease. In a prognosis study, patients with a specific disease are followed to see what factors are related to further morbidity (illness) and/or mortality. Prognosis studies should ideally start at a definite time in the natural history of the disease and usually commence at the diagnosis of a particular condition.

Cohort studies
- follow-up over time of a group of individuals to relate initial factors to the development of a specific disease or end-point
- future risk of disease is compared between exposed and non-exposed groups
- usually the exposed and non-exposed groups are identified only after the start of the study and are not an explicit part of the design

Used for studying
- incidence
- aetiology
- prognosis

6.4.1 The Doll and Hill and Framingham studies

Two famous and long-running studies to determine risk factors for specific diseases deserve mention. They were the first major cohort studies to be carried out and, apart from their contribution to knowledge of disease causation, deserve a place in history in their own right. The Doll and Hill smoking study, as it is generally called, surveyed in 1951 all the 59 600 doctors on the medical register who were resident in the UK. Postal questionnaires were used, and nearly 41 000 usable replies were received. The questionnaire elicited very simple information regarding the respondents' cigarette-smoking habits; each person was asked to classify himself/herself as a current smoker, a person who had smoked but had given up or a person who had never smoked at all. Current and ex-smokers were asked the age at which they started to smoke and how much they smoked. Ex-smokers were asked the age at which they ceased, and all respondents were requested to give their age at the time of the survey. Subsequent to the receipt of these questionnaires, all deaths among the

doctors were notified to the study team through medical associations and the
Registrar-General (who is in charge of death certification in the UK).

The study still continues, and a 40-year report was published in 1994
(Doll *et al.*, 1994). This study has shown, very conclusively, that the smokers
were at much higher risk of death from lung cancer and, indeed, all causes
than non-smokers, with the ex-smokers in an intermediate position. Risk
also increased with increasing use of tobacco. A large sample size was required for this study, since the death rate from lung cancer was relatively
low, and a sufficient number of deaths had to be obtained. Note that the
study was not based on a random population sample and the generalization
of the results requires that the *relationship* between lung cancer and smoking
be judged the same in the general population as in doctors. The very long
duration of this study is also noteworthy, although initial results were
available a few years after the study commenced. As has been said, the important point about any cohort study is that the presence or absence of the
end-point (death or development of disease) be determined in all subjects. The
Doll and Hill study employed routinely available records, in that the basic
source of information was the death certificate. Stringent confirmation of
cause of death was sought, however, and error checks on the time of death
were also made.

The second famous cohort study is the Framingham Heart Study (Dawber,
1980). This study commenced in 1948/1949, with a random sample of nearly
5000 male and female residents, aged 30–59 years, in the town of Framingham, Massachusetts (USA). The purpose of this study was to determine the
risk factors for coronary heart disease (CHD). Subjects underwent an initial
comprehensive medical examination, which concentrated on the suspected
risk factors for CHD. Subjects were examined every 2 years to determine the
change of risk factors with time and also the occurrence of the many manifestations of CHD. This study, which is also still ongoing, has provided much of
what is now known about the aetiology of this condition.

6.5 Measures of association in cohort studies

6.5.1 Risk, rates and ratios [!]

There are some terms in epidemiology and medical statistics that are often
used interchangeably and there is often some confusion about their use.
It is not possible to clear up all this confusion and only a brief mention of
the problem is given here. At various times, the reader will have met the
terms probability, percentage, proportion, risk, rate and ratio. First, the
term ratio is the most general of the terms and just means one number divided
by another. All the other terms are, or are expressed in terms of, ratios. Thus,
the proportion of males in a group (say 20 out of a total of 50, which equals
0·4) is a ratio under this definition, and so is the male:female ratio (20 to
30 = 0·66).

The terms 'percentage' and 'proportion' have the same interpretation and are essentially interchangeable. The baseline, however, is different. Each is made up from the number of persons with a characteristic divided by the total number of persons. Thus a proportion of 0·4 is the same as a percentage of 40% — 40 out of 100. A probability is the chance of something happening and is usually expressed as a proportion or as a percentage (see Section 2.2.1).

The difficulty really comes with the notion of risk and rate. Depending on context, the word rate has a number of meanings. A risk, however, is always the same as a probability and the risk of an event is the same as the probability of that event over a time period (Section 3.6.1). Risks can sometimes be expressed without reference to time and, based on a cross-sectional study, finding two persons with angina out of 1000 smokers, one could say that the risk of a smoker having angina is 0·2%. Risks can, of course, be expressed with any baseline and usually the base is chosen to eliminate (too many) figures after the decimal point. The risk here might be best expressed as 2·0 per 1000. Many, however, would refer to this as the prevalence (rate) of angina in smokers (see Eqn. 6.1). Technically this is not a rate, however.

In its purest meaning, the word rate refers to the amount of change per unit time (for example, the rate of acceleration of a car or the rate at which one's debts seem to increase), but everyday usage has, to all intents and purposes, expanded the use of the word beyond these confines.

In a cohort study with a fixed-time follow-up, the risk of the end-point or disease is:

$$\text{Risk} = \frac{\text{No. of persons who develop disease during follow-up}}{\text{No. of persons disease-free at start}} \quad (6.3)$$

which is defined over a particular time period. This is the usual meaning of risk: it is the probability of an event occurring over a defined period of time. It is often called the *absolute risk*, to distinguish it from other risk measures, to be discussed below. Most epidemiologists would define an incidence rate for the above study as:

$$\text{Rate} = \frac{\text{No. of persons who develop disease during follow-up}}{\text{Average population during the period}} \quad (6.4)$$

so that the difference between the rate and the risk is the denominator of the expression. For a mortality rate, the average population would be essentially the average of the number alive at the start of the study and the number alive at the end. In vital statistics, annual rates are usually calculated by counting the number of deaths in a year and dividing by the average population, obtained from census data (see Section 11.5.1). Though a risk must always lie between zero and one (or whatever baseline is used), a rate can have a value above one. For instance if 350 died in a 3-year follow-up study of 500 persons, the average population would be half of 500 (population at the start) and 150 (population at the end) which is 325, giving a rate of 350/325 = 1·08 deaths per person over 3 years. This can never happen with a risk, which, in this case, is $350/500 = 0.7$. If the rate is expressed as an annual rate, it becomes, of course, $1.08/3 = 0.36$ deaths per person per year.

The concept of rate, however, is perhaps best explained in the context of a rate 'per person-year of follow-up' (*PYRS*).* One person-year is one person followed for 1 year; 10 person-years is 10 people followed for 1 year each, or five persons followed for 2 years each or even one person followed for 10 years. In fact, the rate defined by Eqn. 6.4 is essentially a rate per person-year. On the assumption that the mean time to death is halfway through the follow-up period, the average population multiplied by the length of follow-up is in fact the total *PYRS* for the study. Thus the rate of 0.36 calculated in the last paragraph is a rate per person-year. It would often be expressed as a rate of 360 per 1000 person-years.

Though this would seem to be the essential difference between a rate and a risk in epidemiology, even in the case of cohort studies, the definitions do not necessarily hold well. For instance, the risk, as defined by Eqn. 6.3, is also called the cumulative incidence *rate*. However, unless otherwise stated, it is probably safe to assume that in epidemiology risks are defined per persons alive at the start of the study and rates are defined per person-year of follow-up.

At the end of the day, however, the reader should not get worried by all of this. In a low-mortality/incidence situation, the numerical difference between the rate and the risk is not important and in that situation the interpretation of any result is not affected by whether the actual calculation was of a rate or a risk. It is only in the high-incidence/mortality situation that there will be any numerical difference and in such a situation risk is probably a more understandable concept.

6.5.2 Comparative measures of risk

A number of different comparative measures of risk are available for the cohort study and they will be illustrated on data from a study of prognosis after a heart attack (Daly *et al.*, 1983). A total of 368 male patients who had suffered a heart attack and who had been cigarette smokers at that time were categorized into two groups: those who continued to smoke after their heart attack and those who had stopped smoking. These patients were then followed up for 2 years to examine the relationship between smoking cessation and mortality.[†] Note that this analysis excludes patients who did not smoke cigarettes at the time of their heart attack and that, in the terminology

---

* The concept applies equally to 'person-months', etc.

† Six patients who were not followed for this 2-year period are excluded from this illustrative analysis. See Section 6.6.4, where the complete results on 374 patients are presented. Note that the starting-point for this study is the time of categorization into continued or stopped smokers. This, in fact, took place 2 years after the initial heart attack. Thus the patients included in this analysis had already survived 2 years and the results relate to *subsequent* 2-year mortality.

Table 6.1 Risk comparisons in a cohort study. Subsequent 2-year mortality related to cessation of cigarette smoking in 368 survivors of a first heart attack.

	Survival at 2 years		
	Dead	Alive	Total
Continued smokers (E+)	19 (a)	135 (b)	154 (a + b)
Stopped smokers (E−)	15 (c)	199 (d)	214 (c + d)

Absolute risks of death (over 2 years)

    Continued smokers $\quad\quad R_{E+} = 19/154 = 12{\cdot}3\%$

    Stopped smokers $\quad\quad R_{E-} = 15/214 = 7{\cdot}0\%$

Odds of death (over 2 years)

    Continued smokers $\quad\quad \text{Odds}_{E+} = 19/135 = 0{\cdot}1407$

    Stopped smokers $\quad\quad \text{Odds}_{E-} = 15/199 = 0{\cdot}0754$

Comparative measures

    Relative risk $\quad\quad \text{RR} = \dfrac{12{\cdot}3\%}{7{\cdot}0\%} = 1{\cdot}76$

    Risk difference
    (attributable or excess risk) $\quad\quad \text{RD} = 12{\cdot}3\% - 7{\cdot}0\% = 5{\cdot}3\%$

    Attributable risk per cent $\quad\quad \text{AR}\% = \dfrac{5{\cdot}3\%}{12{\cdot}3\%} = 43{\cdot}1\%$

    Odds ratio $\quad\quad \text{OR} = \dfrac{0{\cdot}1407}{0{\cdot}0754} = 1{\cdot}87$

---

previously introduced, continuing to smoke cigarettes corresponds to 'exposed' (E+) and ceasing to smoke corresponds to 'not exposed' (E−). The outcome or end-point of the study is 2-year mortality. Table 6.1 presents the data in a 2 × 2 table, which is typical for the analysis of a cohort study (see Fig. 6.1).

The absolute risk of a continued smoker dying within the 2 years of the study period is given by the number of deaths in this group, divided by the total number in the group:

$$R_{E+} = a/(a+b) = 19/154 = 12{\cdot}3\% \tag{6.5}$$

The absolute risk for a stopped smoker is, similarly:

$$R_{E-} = c/(c+d) = 15/214 = 7{\cdot}0\% \tag{6.6}$$

Relative risk

These risks of 12·3% and 7·0% in continued and stopped smokers may be compared in a number of different ways. The measures of association in a general contingency table were discussed in Section 3.2.2, but the specific application to the cohort study is described here. Their ratio can be taken and the *relative risk* (also called the *risk ratio*) of death for continued smokers relative to stopped smokers over 2 years can be derived as:

$$RR = \frac{R_{E+}}{R_{E-}} = \frac{a/(a+b)}{c/(c+d)} = \frac{12\cdot3\%}{7\cdot0\%} = 1\cdot76 \qquad (6.7)$$

This means that a continued smoker has 1·76 times the risk of death of a stopped smoker. A relative risk of greater than unity means the risk is greater in exposed than in non-exposed; a relative risk of less than unity means that exposure is protective. A relative risk of unity means that the risks are the same in the two comparative groups. This relative risk measure is the most commonly employed comparative measure of risk.

Risk difference (attributable or excess risk)

The relative risk, however, does not take account of the magnitude of its two component risks. For instance, a relative risk of 2·0 could be obtained from the two absolute risks of 90% and 45% or from the two absolute risks of 2% and 1%. For this reason, an alternative comparative measure between two risks is also used. This is simply the subtraction of the two risks and is called the *risk difference*, the *attributable risk* or the *excess risk*:

$$RD = R_{E+} - R_{E-} = 12\cdot3\% - 7\cdot0\% = 5\cdot3\% \qquad (6.8)$$

Thus, continued smokers have an excess risk of death of 5·3% relative to stopped smokers. The term attributable risk is used because, all else being equal (i.e. assuming no confounders or other biases), continued smokers, had they not continued, would have experienced a risk of 7·0% so that the 5·3% excess can be attributed to their smoking. Obviously, if there is no difference in risk the excess risk is 0%.

Attributable risk per cent

Another comparative measure that is sometimes used is the attributable risk per cent. This is the attributable risk (defined above) as a percentage of the absolute risk in the group exposed to the risk factor (in this case, exposed to continued smoking). In this case:

$$AR\% = \frac{RD}{R_{E+}} = \frac{5\cdot3\%}{12\cdot3\%} = 0\cdot431 = 43\cdot1\% \qquad (6.9)$$

This can be interpreted to mean that, again all else being equal, 43·1% of the total risk of death in a continued smoker is attributable to smoking.

Which of these or any of the many other comparative risk measures (not discussed here) to employ depends on the purpose of a particular analysis. The relative risk is generally accepted as the best measure of the strength of an association between a risk factor and disease in the context of causation. It is less likely than the attributable risk to be influenced by unmeasured confounding or nuisance variables. A relative risk above about 2·0 is generally accepted as a strong risk factor (see Section 3.6.3). The attributable risk, on the other hand, is a more useful and direct indicator of the impact of prevention. For instance, on the basis of the above study continued smokers would have reduced their 2-year risk by 5·3% if they had given up the habit. Just over 40% of their risk of death could be eradicated if they had been persuaded to stop smoking; or, in other words, 40% of the deaths among continued smokers were, in theory, preventable.

> In a cohort study the absolute risks in exposed (R_{E+}) and unexposed (R_{E-}) can be compared using
> - the relative risk ($RR = R_{E+}/R_{E-}$)
> - the risk difference (attributable or excess risk) ($RD = R_{E+} - R_{E-}$)
> - the attributable risk per cent ($AR\% = RD/R_{E+}$)

6.5.3 Odds and odds ratios

Though absolute risk is usually the preferred measure in a cohort study with fixed-time follow-up, there is another measure, which will be introduced here. The odds of an event are defined by the number of occurrences divided by the number of non-occurrences, rather than divided by the total, as is done for the risk (compare Eqn. 6.3):

$$\text{Odds of disease} = \frac{\text{Number of persons who develop disease during follow-up}}{\text{Number of persons who do not develop disease}} \qquad (6.10)$$

The odds of disease and the risk of disease are two different measures of the same underlying process. If the risk of disease is low (less than a few per cent), then the odds and risk tend to be very similar numerically. For instance, if there are three cases in 150 persons, the risk is $3/150 = 0·02$, while the odds of disease are $3/147 = 0·0204$. The two measures are similar because, in the low-risk case, the denominators of the expressions for risk and odds are themselves quite close. When risk is high, however, the odds will have a quite different numerical value from the risk. Odds tend to be expressed as proportions, rather than percentages. The following expression shows the relationship between the odds of an event and the risk (expressed as a proportion):

$$\text{Odds} = \text{Risk}/(1 - \text{Risk}) \qquad (6.11)$$

Now, just as two absolute risks can be compared using their ratio (giving the relative risk or risk ratio), two odds can be compared with the *odds ratio*. Again, comparing an exposed and non-exposed group:

$$OR = \frac{\text{Odds of disease in exposed}}{\text{Odds of disease in non-exposed}}$$

$$= \frac{\text{Odds}_{E+}}{\text{Odds}_{E-}} = \frac{a/b}{c/d} = \frac{a \times d}{b \times c} \qquad (6.12)$$

Again, in a low-risk situation the odds ratio is numerically quite close to the relative risk, and with low enough risk is indistinguishable from it. In the example from the last section, with continued smokers taken as exposed and stopped as non-exposed and disease corresponding to death (Table 6.1):

$$\text{Odds}_{E+} = a/b = 19/135 = 0{\cdot}1407$$

$$\text{Odds}_{E-} = c/d = 15/199 = 0{\cdot}0754$$

These odds are not far off the values of the absolute risks in the two groups of $0{\cdot}1234$ and $0{\cdot}0701$, even though the risk is considerably more than a few per cent. The odds ratio:

$$\text{OR} = 0{\cdot}1407/0{\cdot}0754 = 1{\cdot}87$$

is also not too different from the relative risk of $1{\cdot}76$. If the risks were low, the values of relative risk and odds-ratio measures would be, to all intents and purposes, identical. Thus, in the low-risk situation, the odds ratio is an excellent approximation to the relative risk. Of course, in the cohort study there is no reason to use the odds ratio instead of the relative risk, but the fact that one can approximate the other will be seen below to have extreme importance.*

Equation 6.12 also shows that the odds ratio can be formulated in terms of ratio of the cross-products on the diagonal of the component 2×2 table, and the *cross-product ratio* is another term used for this measure:[†]

$$\text{OR} = \frac{a \times d}{c \times b} = \frac{19 \times 199}{15 \times 135}$$

It is unwise, however, to calculate the odds ratio using this expression, since it is easy to make a mistake about which cross-product goes over which. It depends on the orientation of the table and the order in which the categories are presented. It is safest always to use the direct ratio of the relevant odds in performing a calculation.

Further rearrangement of the cross-product ratio gives the important result that the odds ratio can also be expressed as:

$$\text{OR} = \frac{a/c}{b/d} = \frac{19/15}{135/199} = \frac{\text{Odds of exposure in those with disease}}{\text{Odds of exposure in those without disease}} \tag{6.13}$$

See Table 6.1 for where these odds come from, remembering that disease corresponds in the example to death. Thus, the odds ratio (which is interpreted as the ratio of the odds of disease in exposed to that in non-exposed) can be calculated on the basis of the odds of exposure in those with and without the disease or end-point. This, though only of mild interest in a cohort study, has

---

* Odds and odds ratios are sometimes used in cohort studies instead of risks and relative risks, because some analytic techniques (see Section 11.3.2) work best with these measures.
† The two sets of diagonal numbers in the 2×2 table are 19 and 199, and 15 and 135. The cross-products are then defined as 19×199 and 15×135.

major implications in the analysis of case–control studies, discussed in the next section.

> The odds ratio in a cohort study
> - is a good approximation to the relative risk in a low-risk situation
> - $OR = \dfrac{\text{Odds of disease in exposed}}{\text{Odds of disease in non-exposed}}$
> - $OR = \dfrac{\text{Odds of exposure in those who have disease}}{\text{Odds of exposure in those who do not have disease}}$

6.5.4 Independent risk factors — synergy, antagonism and effect modification [!]

In a cohort study, one might often be interested in the joint effect of two or more risk factors on the end-point being considered. Table 6.2 shows the (hypothetical) risk of developing a disease X in groups defined by drinking and smoking habits. An important question in relation to such data is whether or not the combined effect of both factors is greater than that expected on the basis of their individual effects in isolation. A *synergistic* effect is said to be present if the observed effect is greater than expected, and an *antagonistic* effect obtains if the effect is less than expected. Variables that interact in this way can also be called *effect modifiers* and are discussed further in Section 11.4. In the example, the observed effect of drinking and smoking is given by an absolute risk per 100 000 of 250, and the main question is how to calculate the expected effect. There are at least two methods of doing this, and they are best illustrated on a more concrete example.

Table 6.3 shows the same numerical data, but this time relating the price of a cup of tea or coffee to whether it is drunk on the premises or bought to take away. The price of a cup of coffee to drink at a table is not given, however. What would it be expected to be, on the basis of the prices displayed? It could be argued that, since it costs 40c extra (160c − 120c) to drink tea at a table, it should also cost 40c extra to drink coffee at a table.* Thus, the cost of coffee at a table should be the cost of coffee to take away plus this 40c or 180 c + 40c = 220c. The same result could be obtained by noting that coffee (to take away) costs 60c more than tea (to take away), so that coffee at a table should be 60c dearer than tea at a table, i.e. 160c + 60c = 220c. For obvious reasons, this is considered an *additive* model for the expected price of coffee at a table.

	Non-drinkers	Drinkers
Non-smokers	120	180
Smokers	160	250

Table 6.2 Risks (per 100 000) of developing a disease X in groups defined by drinking and smoking status.

* The euro (€) is divided into 100 cents (c).

	Tea	Coffee
To take away	120	180
To drink at a table	160	–

Table 6.3 Costs in cents of buying tea and coffee either to take away or to drink at a table on the premises.

An alternative method of calculating the expected price of drinking coffee at a table is to note that drinking tea at a table costs 1·333 times as much as taking it away (160c/120c = 1·333), so that the expected price of drinking coffee at a table would also be one-third greater or 180c × 1·333 = 240c. Again, the same result can be obtained by noting that (take-away prices) coffee is 1·5 times as dear as tea, so that the same should hold for prices on the premises. This gives coffee at a table as 160c × 1.5 = 240c. This is the expected price under a *multiplicative* model. The expected effect depends on whether one uses an additive or multiplicative model and which to use, even in the restaurant example, is not clear.

Going back to the same data as representing risks, the expected risk of disease X in smoking drinkers can be calculated at 220 per 100000 on an additive model, or 240 per 10000 on a multiplicative model. Looking at the data, it can be seen that the expected risk in the additive model is based on equality of attributable or excess risks for one variable at each level of the other. The excess risk due to smoking is 160 − 120 = 40 per 100000 in the non-drinkers and is 220 − 180 = 40 in the drinkers (using the additive expected risk of 220). In the multiplicative model, the expected risk is based on equality of relative risks. Thus the question of antagonism or synergy depends on what measure (relative or excess risk) is employed to quantify the effect of a risk factor. It is in this context that the idea of effect modifiers is relevant and, rather than asking about synergy or antagonism, one asks if the presence of a second risk factor modifies the effect of the first—remembering that the answer is dependent on what measure of effect is used.

There is no definite answer as to which of the two models should be used for calculating the expected effect or, equivalently, which measure (relative or excess risk) is more appropriate. In line with the fact that the excess risk measures the public-health importance of a factor or the effect of intervention, the additive model is perhaps the best in terms of assessing the impact of joint exposures. Up to recently, however, most epidemiological analyses worked with relative-risk type measures and risk factors were considered independent if there was no synergy (or antagonism), on a multiplicative scale.* In the

* There is much looseness in talk about independent risk factors for disease, and the terminology leaves much to be desired. Two risk factors can be considered independent under any of the following scenarios: (i) the factors are not associated with each other; if a person has one risk factor, he/she is neither more nor less likely to have the other; (ii) one factor works irrespective of the presence or absence of the other; or (iii) the presence of one factor does not modify the effect of another factor. This last is the sense used above and means that the factors do not act synergistically or antagonistically. This criterion depends on the effect measure employed.

example, the observed risk of 250 per 100 000 is greater than that expected on either model, so that a synergistic effect of tobacco and alcohol consumption can be claimed unambiguously. In other situations, model choice may affect the interpretation of results on the combined effect of two risk factors and with one choice risk factors could be synergistic, while with another they could be antagonistic.

6.6 Risk with variable-time follow-up [!]

6.6.1 Variable-time follow-up

The cohort study of prognosis in the last section was analysed in terms of a fixed follow-up for all patients. Each individual was known to be either alive or dead at 2 years from study commencement, and the 2×2 table (Alive/Dead by Continued/Stopped) formed the appropriate basis for analysis. Risks were calculated directly as the proportion who died over the period of follow-up. With many cohort studies, however, a fixed period of follow-up is not available for each individual and special methods must be employed to estimate and compare risks. Use of the methods described in the last section are not valid. Two common situations where variable-time or variable follow-up arises are described below.

In a study of occupational mortality, for instance, employees of a particular firm may enter observation at the time of their first employment and be followed up until death or a particular point in calendar time. Of interest is mortality in relation to the type of work or exposure of the employees. Unfortunately, each individual will be followed up for different periods from the time of his/her first employment to the date the study has to be analysed (this is typical for an *occupational cohort* study). Thus, for an analysis undertaken now, an employee who started work 5 years ago would have only 5 years of follow-up, compared with a much longer period for an individual who commenced, say, 12 years ago.

The second common situation where variable follow-up arises is in the context of a clinical trial or a cohort study of prognosis. Suppose a cohort study of mortality commenced in 1990. (The end-point of interest can, of course, be an event other than death, but for simplicity mortality, or equivalently survival, will be discussed here.) Patients enter into the study at diagnosis, but, in calendar time, this occurs over a 10-year period. As in the occupational cohort study, however, the analysis must take place at a fixed point in calendar time. If analysis is performed at the start of the year 2000, patients will have experienced various lengths of follow-up. The end-point for many patients will be known, because they have died, but an individual alive in January 2000 will die subsequently at an unknown date in the future. A follow-up terminated in this way due to the practical requirements of data analysis is referred to as a censored follow-up, and data from such a study are called *censored data*. Patients alive at the analysis stage of a study before experiencing the end-point of interest are called *withdrawals*. (Withdrawals should be distinguished from losses to follow-up—patients whose follow-up was terminated *before* the analysis date, due to loss of contact, missed visit or whatever.)

6.6.2 Erroneous approaches

Many erroneous approaches have been used to analyse data arising from variable follow-up. The approach described earlier of calculating mortality at a fixed time from study entry (e.g. 5 years) is only valid when each subject is known to be actually alive or dead at this time point. To use this fixed follow-up approach in a variable follow-up study requires that data collected on many patients be discarded. (This is further discussed in Section 7.15.) The calculation of a 'total study mortality', by dividing all the observed deaths by the total number studied, is not a mortality rate in any sense of the word, since it takes no account of the time over which the events occurred. With a follow-up of everyone to death, this figure would eventually reach 100%! Sometimes, a mean 'length of survival' is calculated by averaging the time of death of the decedents and the time to last follow-up of withdrawals. The resulting figure, however, measures the average length of follow-up rather than anything else and is totally dependent on the study duration. It is not a suitable summary measure of survival or mortality either.

Apart from discarding many of the data and using the fixed follow-up approach, two techniques are available for the analysis of variable follow-up data. The first is used mainly for an occupational cohort study.

6.6.3 Person-years of follow-up

For such data, a mortality rate per person-year of follow-up can be calculated (see Section 6.5.1.) For example, 20 deaths might be observed among 600 employees. The person-years of follow-up of these 600 are obtained by determining the length of follow-up of each employee and adding them up. If the total person-years of follow-up were calculated at 5400 years, the mortality rate would be expressed as 20/5400 or 3·7 deaths per thousand person-years, without explicit note of the number of individuals involved. A basic assumption of this method is that the mortality rate is not related to length of follow-up and so remains constant over time.

6.6.4 The clinical life table

For the analysis of variable follow-up data in a cohort study or clinical trial, the person-years of follow-up method can be employed, but in this situation what is called the *clinical life table method* is preferred. Many variants of this are available and a brief description follows. The method is described in detail in Section 7.15.

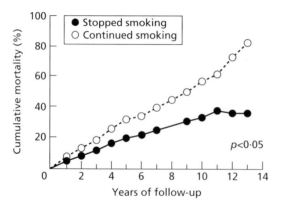

Fig. 6.2 Cumulative mortality in 157 continued smokers who survived a first heart attack by at least 2 years (from Daly *et al.*, 1983, with permission).

Essentially, the entire study period is subdivided into small intervals of time. In each interval, the number of patients alive at the start, the number of deaths and the number withdrawn alive or lost to follow-up are used to estimate a 'within-interval' mortality. These interval mortalities can then be combined to give a mortality risk (rate) for any time since study commencement. The clinical life table approach gives an unbiased estimate of mortality at yearly intervals (or whatever size intervals are chosen) from study commencement, and thus gives a far more complete picture of what is happening than the usual 2×2 table, which compares mortality at a single fixed time point only. The clinical life table is either a table or a graph showing the percentage mortality (or survival) at each time point from study commencement. These are sometimes called cumulative mortality or survival rates. Figure 6.2 shows the cumulative mortality over a 13-year follow-up of the continued and stopped smokers in the study of heart-attack survivors, discussed in Section 6.5. Although most of the patients were not followed for the full 13 years, the clinical life table method allowed calculation of the 13-year mortality, which was around 82% in the continued smokers and 37% in those who ceased. Mortality at all times from the start of the study can easily be read off the graph, and the visual presentation shows clearly how the two mortality curves diverge over time.

In addition to presenting a clear and unbiased picture of mortality over time, the clinical life table utilizes all the available data without discarding any of them. Losses to follow-up, as long as there are not too many, can also be accounted for by the method, given certain fairly reasonable assumptions. Though somewhat complex, life table techniques are central to the analysis of many cohort studies.

> Cohort studies with variable-time follow-up can be analysed using
> * person-years of follow-up
> * clinical life tables

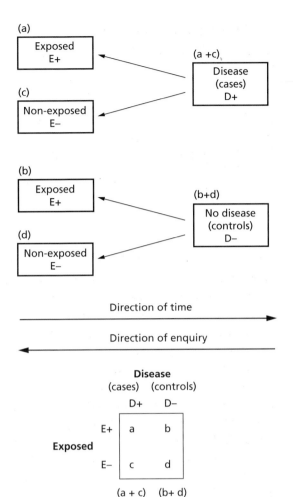

Fig. 6.3 Schematic structure of a case–control study with component 2 × 2 table.

6.7 The case–control study

One of the purposes of the cohort study is to determine associations between risk factors measured at the start of the study and subsequent morbidity or mortality. In essence, a cohort study goes forward from a risk factor to the development of the end-point of interest. An alternative to the cohort study for the elucidation of associations between risk factors and disease is a *case–control* study. The case–control study starts with the end-point and moves backwards in time to the identification of risk factors.

A group of persons with a particular disease (the cases) is studied as regards factors to which it was exposed in the past, and the results are compared with those obtained in a comparison group (the controls) without the disease. If the factor is associated with the disease, then it should appear more commonly in the cases than in the controls (Fig. 6.3). The investigation of Herity *et al.* (1981) into the association between smoking and drinking and the development of cancer of the head and neck will be taken as an example of this

		Cases	Controls
Ever smoked?	yes	175 (*a*)	152 (*b*)
	no	25 (*c*)	48 (*d*)
		200 (*a* + *c*)	200 (*b* + *d*)

Table 6.4 Relationship between smoking and head and neck cancer in a case–control study (abbreviated from Herity *et al.*, 1981, with permission).

type of study. Table 6.4 shows the basic results for this study, where it can be seen that there were more smokers among the cases than among the controls. A case–control study divides into four stages: the selection of cases, the selection of controls, the measurement of the risk factor and the analysis of the association.

> **Odds ratio**
>
> $$OR = \frac{a \times d}{b \times c} = \frac{175 \times 48}{25 \times 152} = 2{\cdot}21$$

> Case–control studies
> - cases (with the disease) and controls (without the disease) are examined for their prior history of exposure
> - the control group is an explicit part of the design
> - past exposure is compared between those who now have the disease and those who do not
>
> Used for
> - studying aetiology

6.7.1 Selection of cases

To avoid bias, cases in a case–control study should be newly diagnosed. Although this reduces the numbers available for a study, a group containing a mixture of newly diagnosed cases and long-standing chronic cases can cause great difficulty in interpreting the results. The main problem is that inclusion of late cases means that subjects who die soon after diagnosis may be under-represented. If the risk factors for occurrence of disease in the first place are also related to early mortality, the apparent effect of the risk factor may then be diluted. This is a particular problem in using a case–control study for heart disease, when early deaths in the community can usually not be included. The diagnostic criteria for defining a case must be explicit and clear. This enables the study to be replicated elsewhere and avoids ambiguities of interpretation. Often persons with other concurrent disease are excluded from the cases. Usually, in a case–control study, a presenting sample, to a particular hospital or unit, of newly diagnosed cases is taken. It must be remembered, however, that cases admitted to a hospital are not necessarily representative of all cases in the community at large. In the study of head and neck cancer, a presenting sample of 200 new patients attending a particular hospital over a 2-year period for treatment of cancer of the head and neck formed the case group. The definition of head and neck cancer is given in the original report.

6.7.2 Selection of controls

The selection of controls is, without any doubt, the most difficult part of a case–control study. Usually, the same number of controls as cases is taken and this is the most efficiently designed study. However, if the number of cases is limited or it is very expensive to identify cases, two or more controls can be taken for each case. This requires a larger total sample size than the equivalent equal-sized study and more than four controls per case is not worthwhile. (See Section 8.6.4, where this topic is considered in detail.)

Source of controls

The controls are usually said to represent the general population without the disease. However, this criterion needs slight adjustment and the requirement is that the controls should be taken from, and ideally be a random sample from, the *same population that gave rise to the cases*. This is important, particularly when the risk factor or exposure under investigation may be localized geographically.

If exposure to a certain chemical were being investigated and the case–control study was being carried out in a hospital close to the only factory that used that chemical, controls taken from the national population would be unsuitable. With such controls, the factory could be erroneously implicated in the disease. Cases from the area would be likely to include workers in the factory (even if exposure were not related to disease), while the controls, representative of the national rather than the local population, would be unlikely to include such workers. Controls are therefore usually sourced from the catchment area of the hospital in which the cases were diagnosed. Controls should not have the disease under investigation. Perhaps the best criterion for the choice of a control is that someone is eligible to be a control if that person would have been included in the study as a case, had he/she got the disease. Practical considerations usually dictate that controls are taken from patients in the same hospital as the cases. Such controls should not have the disease under investigation or a disease related to the risk factor being studied. One further advantage of this approach is that the same factors that determined hospitalization of the cases in a particular hospital may also have been likely to determine the hospitalization of the controls.

There are two difficulties with hospital controls, however. First, there is a possible bias related to the probability of an individual being admitted to hospital depending on both his/her disease and risk-factor status. The mechanism of this, which is called Berkson's bias, is complex and the reader is referred to Sackett (1979) for an explanation. The second problem, of course, is to what extent hospital controls may be judged representative of the general population that gave rise to the cases. Sometimes, case–control studies use community controls from family-doctor lists, population screening programmes or other sources.

Care must also be taken in the actual choosing of each individual control. Ideally, the person selecting the control should not know the nature of the risk factor being studied or subtle selection biases might occur. For instance, if cigarette smoking was one of the risk factors being studied, a potential control with a packet of cigarettes on his/her bedside locker might be deliberately avoided! As in any study, careful training of interviewers is necessary.

Matching

Apart from the source of the controls, the next problem arises in their selection. A random sample from the hospital patients not affected by the disease in question could be taken, but it is then possible that cases and controls would differ as regards confounders of the association between the putative risk factor and disease, such as age and sex. These variables could be controlled for in the analysis stage but are better adjusted for in the design of the study. (See discussion in Section 3.5.) A confounding effect is avoided if the controls are chosen to have the same distribution as the cases in terms of the confounders. This procedure, as discussed in Section 3.5, is called *matching* and is usually done for at least age and sex. Two different methods are available to achieve this. The first approach is called *paired matching*. Typically, a control of the same sex and age (to within a specified number of years) is individually matched to each case. Each case in the study has his or her own control without the disease. An alternative to pairing is *frequency matching*, whereby the distribution of, say, age and sex in the controls is forced to be identical to that in the cases, but not by individual matching. Usually, this is achieved by determining the age/sex distribution of the cases in, say, 10-year age-groups. If there were then 15 males aged 45–54 years in the cases, 15 males in the same age-group would be chosen for the controls. With frequency matching, there is not a one-to-one link between an individual case and a corresponding control, although the confounder distributions are forced to be equal.

What factors to match for in case–control studies often causes problems. Variables that are known to be associated with both the development of the disease and exposure to the risk factor are the prime candidates. As has been said, age and sex are two such factors. It should be noted, however, that matching for too many factors can lead to serious difficulties. Matching must not take place on variables related to the risk factor only, since this will tend to ensure equal distribution of the risk factor in cases and controls, and hence no result. Factors intermediate in the causal pathway between the risk factor and disease should not be matched for either, as again this will tend to reduce differences between the cases and controls. One can, however, match on variables related to the disease but not to the risk factor of interest, if the influence of such variables is not to be analysed and a small effect of a different variable is being investigated. Since over-matching cannot be adjusted for at the analysis stage, it is perhaps safest to match on age and sex only and adjust for other confounders through analytic strategies. In practice, also, it can be very tedious to match for a number of factors and, of course, any variables matched for cannot be analysed for a relationship with the disease.

In the study of head and neck cancer, the controls, frequency-matched to the cases for age (in 10-year age-groups) and sex, were chosen from patients attending the same hospital 'for the treatment of non-smoking-related cancers and benign conditions' during the same period in which the cases were hospitalized.

6.7.3 Measurement of exposure

Once cases and controls have been chosen, exposure to the risk factors must be determined. Unfortunately, this depends either on the patient's memory or on available records. *Recall bias* is due to cases recalling exposures to risk factors more accurately than controls. This is often because newly diagnosed patients often ask 'why me?' and think about possible exposures more than do controls. It is important that cases and controls are interviewed in the same manner and by the same person. Ideally, the interviewer should not know if the individual is a case or control, in order to avoid a biased response as a result of leading questions or a more careful interviewing of cases. In practice, this is nearly impossible to achieve. Also, if the case knows the purpose of the study, he or she might overemphasize or minimize exposure to the risk factors, thus biasing the results in this way. Some case–control studies are based on hospital charts and records only, and exposure information based on these may be quite dubious. Often such records are incomplete, and no mention of a particular factor either means that the factor was not present or that exposure was never ascertained or recorded.

In the head- and neck-cancer study, a predesigned questionnaire was administered by one of the investigators, and details of sex, age, occupation, education, tobacco and alcohol consumption and dental care were recorded.

Cases in a case–control study
- should be newly diagnosed

Controls in a case–control study
- should be matched to cases for at least age and sex
- should be taken from the same population that gave rise to the cases

---

6.8 Measures of association in case–control studies — the odds ratio

After collection of the data, the association between the risk factor and the disease must be examined. In the cohort study, the risk of disease is compared between the exposed and non-exposed groups using a relative risk or excess (attributable) risk measure. In the case–control study, however, no measure of absolute risk is possible, since patients are not followed forward in time. Though Table 6.4 has a similar layout to that for a cohort study, it is not legitimate to suggest that, since there are $175 + 152 = 327$ smokers, the risk of a smoker getting head and neck cancer is $175/327$. Three hundred and twenty-seven patients were not followed up and therefore they cannot form the denominator for a risk. If, in fact, two controls per case had been taken, the corresponding figure would be totally different. It is only possible to calculate risk in a study where subjects have been followed forward in time.

6.8.1 Non-matched case–control data

Since the absolute risk of disease is not calculable from a case–control study, neither are the odds. It would therefore seem than none of the comparative measures of risk are calculable either. However, a method is available to calculate the odds ratio from a case–control study and two different justifications can be used. The first is somewhat intuitive, and the second is more formal.

If the data from Table 6.4 had been from a cohort study with smokers and non-smokers followed up, the odds ratio for disease would be calculated from Eqn. 6.11 as:

$$\text{`OR'} = \frac{a/b}{c/d} = \frac{175/152}{25/48} = 2{\cdot}21$$

where the quotation marks signify that this is not really the required odds ratio. Now, suppose the study had been performed with two controls per case and that the proportion of smokers remained the same. The number of smoking and non-smoking controls would just double and the 'odds ratio' would then be:

$$\text{`OR'} = \frac{175/(2 \times 152)}{25/(2 \times 48)} = 2{\cdot}21$$

It is immediately obvious that the 'odds ratio' calculated in this way is the same, no matter what the ratio of controls to cases is. Now, suppose a cohort study had been performed in the population that gave rise to the cases. Those who developed the cancer would be the cases actually observed in the case–control study. Those who did not develop disease would be the group the controls were taken from. In this hypothetical cohort study, the ratio of 'controls' to cases would be very large, but the odds ratio calculated from the 2×2 table would be exactly the same as that calculated above (ignoring sampling variation). Thus, the odds ratio calculated from Eqn. 6.11 in a case–control study is the same as that which would have been obtained if a cohort study had been performed in this community.

The second argument for the estimability of the odds ratio from case–control data, which is more rigorous, relies on the fact, noted in the context of a cohort study in Section 6.5.3, that the cross-product ratio (Eqn. 6.12):

$$\frac{a \times d}{b \times c}$$

(where a, b, c and d are defined as in Fig. 6.1 or Table 6.1) estimates two different quantities. In a cohort study, it estimates the ratio of the odds of disease in those exposed to the odds to those non-exposed (Eqn. 6.11). However the cross-product ratio also estimates the ratio of the odds of exposure in those with disease to the odds in those without disease (Eqn. 6.13). Now, the odds of exposure in those with disease and in those without disease are each directly obtainable from a case–control study (because it samples each group—the cases and the controls—separately). Therefore, the cross-product ratio in a case–control study, which legitimately estimates the ratio of the odds of exposure, must also be a valid estimate of the ratio of the odds of disease—which is, of course, the quantity being looked for.

The importance of this result cannot be overemphasized. In a case–control study, even though measures of absolute risk are not available, the odds ratio is estimable. Additionally, since most case–control studies deal with rare diseases, the odds ratio is an excellent approximation to the relative risk. This is why it is often said that the relative risk is obtainable from a case–control study and many papers refer to the relative risk in such studies. This is perfectly legitimate and useful (since it is easier to think in terms of relative risks), as long as it is remembered that the estimation is based on the calculation of the odds ratio. Thus, in the current example, the risk of developing head and neck cancer is 2·21 times greater in those who smoke than in those who do not.

6.8.2 Pair-matched case–control data [!]

The calculation of the odds ratio as described above is not applicable to a pair-matched case–control study. In such a study, the data layout must take account of the pair matching, and Table 6.5 shows the unusual structure required. With paired data, the table must display the distribution of the matched pairs. There are four possibilities for each pair. The case and its (paired) control could both be exposed, they could both be non-exposed, the case could be exposed and its paired control not exposed, or finally the case could be non-exposed and the control exposed. These four categories are labelled a, d, c and b in Table 6.5. The best estimate of the odds ratio from such paired data turns out to be:

$$OR = \frac{c}{b} \tag{6.14}$$

which only involves the pairs in which there was a discrepancy between the case and control regarding exposure. Pairs in which the case *and* the control were both exposed or both non-exposed do not contribute to the estimate of the odds ratio. This is not an intuitive result and the justification for this estimate is too complex for this text. As for the unmatched situation, however,

	Cases	
	Exposed	Non-exposed
Controls		
Exposed	a	b
Non-exposed	c	d

Table 6.5 Data layout for
pair-matched case–control
data. Entries in the table are
the number of pairs.

> **Odds ratio**
>
> $$OR = \frac{c}{b}$$

this odds ratio is a valid estimate of the relative risk between exposed and non-exposed if the disease is rare.

> In a case–control study
> - absolute risk cannot be estimated
> - the odds ratio can be estimated and is the usual measure of association
> - if the disease is rare, the odds ratio is an excellent approximation to the relative risk

6.9 The analysis of cohort and case–control studies [!]

This section gives a very brief overview of the statistical analysis of the cohort and case–control study. The techniques are detailed in subsequent chapters, which should be consulted for a more complete discussion.

6.9.1 The cohort study

Usually, in a cohort study, the main analysis is a comparison of two groups—the exposed and the non-exposed. In the majority of cohort studies, the exposure groups are defined by measurements taken at the initial cross-sectional study and the two groups are not matched. The techniques for the comparison of two independent groups, discussed at length in Chapter 7, are appropriate for this type of data. If a variable-time follow-up is involved, life table techniques should be used (see Sections 6.6.4 and 7.15).

If the analysis has to take account of potential confounders of the association between exposure and the end-point, then a stratified analysis or *logistic regression* can be employed. In a stratified analysis, the measure of association (relative risk or excess risk, for example) is examined at different levels of the confounding variable (within different age-groups, for example) and a summary average measure (an adjusted measure) is calculated. Statistical significance tests are available to account for the stratification. Logistic regression offers an alternative but more complex methodology, and both these approaches are discussed in Chapter 11.

If, unusually, some form of matching has been used in the formation of exposed and non-exposed groups, the analysis should ideally account for this. Essentially, with frequency matching, a stratified analysis should be performed, with strata defined by the matching variable. This will give a statistically more efficient analysis than would be obtained by ignoring the matching and performing a simple two-group comparison. However, the overall estimate of effect should be similar, whether or not a stratified analysis has been used, since the influence of the confounder is removed by the matching process. Pair matching is extremely rare in a cohort study.

6.9.2 The case–control study

Analysis of the case–control study is based on a similar philosophy to that of the cohort study, remembering that the usual measure of association is the odds ratio. With frequency matching, a stratified analysis should be employed to give the most efficient approach (see Chapter 11). Using methods for the comparison of independent groups leads to a loss of power in the analysis, but the overall odds ratio should not be biased by the matching variable. If a pair-matched case–control study is being analysed, the analysis must take account of the pairing and the methods for the comparison of paired data should be employed, as described in Chapter 7. As already pointed out (Section 6.8.2), the calculation of the odds ratio must also take account of the pairing.

For general control of confounding, as in the cohort study, either a stratified analysis or logistic regression can be employed.

6.10 Comparisons of cohort and case–control studies

6.10.1 Strengths and weaknesses

It is worth comparing the cohort and case–control studies as methodologies for examining the causation of disease. Without doubt, all else being equal, cohort studies have major advantages over case–control studies. First, the time relationship of the exposure or the risk factor with disease is more clear-cut, since exposure is ascertained prior to disease development. Sometimes, a risk factor is determined from a blood test and a major difficulty of the case–control study is that usually the blood can only be taken after the disease has arisen and therefore blood levels are perhaps influenced by the disease onset itself. This is certainly true of heart disease, where an actual heart attack can change the levels of serum cholesterol, for example. Another major advantage of the cohort study is its ability to make standardized and uniform measurements of exposure before disease develops. This avoids some of the biases of exposure determination in the case–control study, including recall bias and biases due to measurement variation (including interviewer bias) and the availability of the data in the first place. In the cohort study, too, the comparison groups are based on exposure and are not biased by knowledge of future disease status. Mention has already been made of biases involved in control selection and matching in the formation of the comparison groups in the case–control study. Generally, in terms of bias, the cohort study is vastly superior to the case–control study. Sackett (1979) discusses this in detail. Sections 12.2 and 12.3 further discuss the biases that can arise in these studies

In terms of end-points also, the case–control study has limitations. In essence, it is confined to a single end-point (that which defines the cases), while the cohort study can examine a huge range of end-points with no difficulty. Of course, the biggest problem is that the case–control study cannot measure absolute risk of the end-point and analysis is confined to determining an approximate measure of relative risk (the odds ratio).

None the less, the case–control study does have some major strengths. One is the time frame in which the study can be completed and some answers obtained. A cohort study may take many years or decades of follow-up, while the case–control study deals with existing cases and looks back in time, and the only delay is that due to recruiting cases and controls. In addition, losses to follow-up create a difficulty with the cohort study that does not affect the case–control design. The sample sizes required for a cohort study are typically orders of magnitude higher than for a case–control investigation. The cohort study must be large enough for a sufficient number of end-points to develop in the exposed and non-exposed groups. Cohort studies with sample sizes of many thousands are not at all uncommon and the rarer the disease or end-point, the larger the sample needed. The case–control study, on the other hand, identifies cases who have the disease and compares them (most efficiently) with a similar-sized control group. Sample sizes in the hundreds are more usual and for a very rare disease the case–control study is probably the only type practicable. At the end of the day, what all of this means is that the case–control study is cheaper and easier to do, but that it has many disadvantages, particularly regarding possible biases.

Cohort studies for aetiology

Strengths
- exposure is measured before disease occurs
- control and standardization of exposure measure are possible
- multiple end-points can be studied
- absolute risks are estimable
- few biases

Weaknesses
- difficult for rare diseases
- slow to complete
- large sample size
- high cost
- losses to follow-up

Case–control studies
Strengths
- quick to complete
- small sample size
- low cost
- ideal for rare diseases

Weaknesses
- bias in determining exposure
    recall bias
    interviewer bias
    missing data
    lack of standardization of prerecorded data
    measures affected by disease onset
    use of non-newly diagnosed cases
- bias in choosing controls
    inappropriate source
    Berkson's bias
    over-matching
- no estimate of absolute risk
- only one end-point (disease)

6.10.2 Terminology

Unfortunately, though the essential concepts are relatively clear, there is much confusion in the literature relating to the nomenclature of observational study design in medicine. The comments here are an attempt to shed some light on the situation, but are not exhaustive and do not consider all the possible descriptive terms. What is meant by a cross-sectional study is usually clear enough, but it is the description of the investigations that have been called here 'cohort' and 'case–control' that gives rise to difficulty. Though adaptations and modifications to these two basic designs are possible (some of which have been given special names), most non-cross-sectional studies can be classed into one or other grouping.

What distinguishes the cohort and case–control designs is the *direction of enquiry*. The cohort study starts with exposure and the *subsequent* development of disease is determined in the exposed and non-exposed groups. The case–control study starts with the disease and *prior* exposure is determined in cases and controls. Generally, there is broad agreement on these definitions of cohort and case–control as descriptions of study designs.

The main confusion arises with the use of the terms *retrospective* and *prospective*, the former term related to looking backwards in time and the latter term related to the future. Some authors therefore refer to the cohort study as a prospective study and the case–control study as a retrospective study, where the terms relate to the direction of enquiry. However, others like to use the descriptors to describe, not the direction of enquiry, but the timing of the data collection or subject identification with respect to the commence-ment of the investigation.

Thus, a case–control study could be performed prospectively by identifying cases as they are diagnosed—subsequent to the calendar date the study com-menced—choosing controls and (because it is a case–control study) looking for exposure in the past history of the subjects. A case–control study can also be performed retrospectively by identifying cases who were diagnosed in the past (prior to study commencement) and using perhaps recorded data to determine the prior exposure of the subjects.

A cohort study is usually performed prospectively, in that the cohort is chosen (alive and disease-free) at the start of the study and follow-up takes place subsequent to study commencement over the next number of years. However, in certain situations, a cohort study can be performed retrospec-tively. This often happens in an occupational setting when good records have been kept of a group of employees. The cohort is defined as those, for example, working in a particular industry 50 years ago. These can all be iden-tified from employment records, and the cohort is followed up to the present, using employment and pension data to monitor exposure (often type of work) and the end-point (usually mortality). The direction of enquiry is forward, making it a cohort study, though all the data are collected retrospectively. One can therefore have retrospective prospective studies and prospective retro-spective studies and total confusion reigns. Part of the difficulty is exacerbated by the undoubted advantage of the cohort study design (also called prospec-tive), so that, if possible, the word prospective is attached to a study descrip-tion to enhance its standing! The bottom line is that the terms retrospective and prospective can be used in different ways and there is no sure method of knowing what is being referred to. A detailed description of a study design is usually needed to see what type of study is in question. At least the terms cohort and case–control unambiguously define the essential type of study and they are the preferred terms in this text.

As mentioned, there are a number of other terms used to describe a study design. Cohort studies can also be called *follow-up studies, incidence studies* or *longitudinal studies*. This final term, however, is sometimes taken to mean non-cross-sectional studies and therefore includes the case–control design also. The *historical cohort study* is a cohort study performed retrospectively and the case–control study can also be referred to as a *case–referent study*. One particular type of case–control study is called a *nested case–control study*. This is essentially a case–control study done within a cohort study. A typical situation for such a design arises when a new risk marker for disease, based on a measurement in blood or serum, is proposed. In many cohort studies, blood samples are taken at initial examination and stored for this very eventuality in freezers. The end-point of interest may be known from the cohort study and the risk marker measured on the stored blood can give a measure of prior exposure. A nested case–control design means that those who developed the condition of interest in the study are compared with a control sample (often the same size as the case group) of those who did not develop the end-point. This is much more efficient than finding the level of the new risk marker on everyone and means a huge saving in blood-assay costs, since not all bloods must be analysed. The substudy, however, is now essentially a case–control study (performed retrospectively on a cohort study). The design relies on the existence of stored samples but overcomes the usual case–control problems with the time sequence of exposure determination based on blood levels. Also, the overall absolute risk of the end-point is known from the cohort data.

6.11 The randomized controlled trial

This section considers the design of the experimental trial in medical research. The purpose of the experimental trial is to evaluate the effectiveness of some intervention or therapy. What distinguishes the experimental trial from the observational studies discussed so far in this chapter is that the researcher has direct control over many aspects of the investigation and, in particular, over the allocation of individuals to different treatment groups. This section is not intended to be a handbook for the clinician wishing to undertake a trial, but merely a guideline to the principles and practices of such trials.

6.11.1 Treatment and control groups

One of the most important questions facing any practising physician or surgeon is 'What treatment shall I use?' It is vital that the doctor (and patient) knows the effectiveness of the different treatments available, and thus what may be best in a particular situation. Advances in medicine require a detailed knowledge of treatment efficacy, and the experimental trial provides the only valid procedure for achieving this. Many therapeutic regimes commonly used in the past were seen to be worthless or even dangerous when evaluated in such a proper and scientific manner. Any proposed new therapy, be it medical or surgical, should be tested by means of a trial unless the results are so startlingly obvious that a formal evaluation is not necessary, such as a successful treatment for a condition that was 100% fatal.

'I have a wonder cure for the common cold. If you take this preparation for one day only, your symptoms will be cleared within a week.' Faced with a claim such as this, the most important question is 'What would happen to my cold symptoms if I did not take this preparation?' The claim of effectiveness only stands up when a comparison can be made with the situation pertaining without the treatment. This is the foundation-stone for the evaluation of any therapy. Its effectiveness must be compared with the results of either no treatment or the best treatment available before its introduction.

To evaluate a new therapy, then, requires comparing results on a group of treated patients with the results on a group with the same disease not so treated. These two groups are usually called the treatment and control groups, respectively. The control groups can receive either no treatment or an established treatment that has been shown to be effective. Many early evaluations of therapy used what are called *historical controls*. The results on a series of patients on the new treatment were compared with the results obtained on 'similar' patients in the past who did not have the 'benefits' of the newer approach. The word 'similar' is in quotations because the main problem with historical controls is that they are likely to be quite different from patients treated in the present. Historical controls may, in the first place, have had a better (or worse) outlook than the treatment group. Between the time when the historical controls were seen and treated and the present, there may have been changes in the natural history of the disease, general management may have improved, diagnostic criteria may have changed, and the historical controls may not have had as much attention and care as the treated group (who may be getting special attention because they are receiving the new therapy). For these and other reasons, a comparison between the results obtained on a treated group and a historical control group could be seriously biased, and any differences in outcome noted may not reflect a true treatment effect. A further problem with historical controls is that reliance is placed on past records to evaluate their prognosis, and missing or unrecorded information on some patients may further bias the results. In short, for a valid evaluation of therapy, a concurrent control group must be used. Note that, by its very nature, an experimental trial is a cohort investigation in that individuals must be followed forward in time to determine the effect of a therapy, and usually individuals are entered into a trial over what is sometimes an extended period of time.

Experimental (clinical) trials
- patients who have been allocated a treatment are followed up and compared with patients who have not been allocated the treatment
- the future risk of the end-point is compared between the treatment and control groups

Used for
- evaluating the effect of any treatment or intervention

6.11.2 Types of trial

The experimental trial in medicine may be employed in three main situations, distinguished by the type of individual studied and the effect of the treatment or intervention involved. In the *clinical* or *therapeutic* trial, the study groups consist of persons with a particular disease or condition and the treatment is therapeutic. The purpose of such trials is to determine if treatment can effect a 'cure' or remove manifestations of a disease already present in the patients. The total sample size for such trials is often in the region of 20 to 100 patients if the treatment is even moderately effective. Examples of such trials abound in the medical literature. Trials, for instance, of antihypertensive agents to reduce blood pressure and analgesics to alleviate pain fit into this category. The term 'clinical trial' is often applied loosely to the two categories below also.

In *secondary* and *primary prevention trials*, the treatment or intervention under investigation is prophylactic, in that its purpose is the prevention of a particular manifestation of disease which is not present at the start of the trial. In secondary prevention trials, the subjects already have the disease in question or have suffered one event, and it is hoped to prevent or delay a further event. Examples are trials of chemotherapy regimes in patients with cancer, where the end-point is often cancer recurrence or death. Drug treatment of patients who have had a heart attack and coronary bypass surgery in patients with angina can also fit into this category.

The primary prevention trial, on the other hand, is performed on subjects free of disease, with a view to preventing the first occurrence of an event. Cholesterol-reducing drugs have been tested in this manner to evaluate their effectiveness in preventing coronary heart attacks, and trials evaluating the usefulness of risk-factor modifications, such as the cessation of cigarette smoking, have also been carried out in this area (see Section 6.13.4, which discusses community intervention trials).

Since both primary and secondary prevention trials are concerned with the prevention or delay of a particular event, rather than the elimination of a condition which is present, very large sample sizes and an extensive period of follow-up may often be required. This is because a reasonable number of events must occur in the study population before an evaluation of the intervention can be made, and often the rate of events that can be expected in the study group is so small that large numbers are needed for this. Secondary prevention trials can require up to and over 1000 subjects, while primary prevention trials may require 10 000 or more subjects in order to have any chance of detecting an important result. (Chapter 8 discusses the calculation of sample sizes for clinical trials and other studies.)

6.11.3 Avoiding bias and confounding in trials

The salient features of the experimental study remain the same, no matter whether it is a therapeutic, secondary prevention or primary prevention trial. Without loss of generality, an illustrative example of a well-run and well-designed trial will be used to illustrate these features. This trial was one of the early secondary prevention trials evaluating a particular drug therapy (timolol—a beta-blocker) in reducing mortality among patients who had had a heart attack (myocardial infarction) (Norwegian Multicentre Study Group, 1981). Beta blockade remains one of the important secondary prevention interventions in such patients.

The essence of this and any experimental trial is the comparison of two groups—a group which has received the new therapy and a group which has received a different or no treatment. As has been discussed in Section 3.3, an observed difference between the two groups could be ascribed to chance, bias/confounding or a real treatment effect. Formal statistical analyses take care of the problem of chance but, as for any comparison, the effects of bias and/or confounding have to be accounted for. The question is whether there are differences between the groups, other than the intervention, that might explain the results. In the experimental trial, such differences could arise due to intrinsic differences between the groups regarding some factors related to outcome or through differences in the way the groups were managed (other than the treatment under consideration). Other differences between the groups could be spurious and due to measurement or observer variation. (This topic is considered in some detail in Chapter 12.)

In the observational study confounding can be controlled for by either design (typically through some form of matching) or analysis (stratified or regression approaches—to be discussed in detail later in this book). Though preference was expressed for a design approach to eliminate confounders, the problems of over-matching and practicality often dictate that only age and sex are accounted for in the design of observational studies—particularly in the case–control study. Analytic approaches require a belief in mathematical manipulation and prior measurement (and therefore knowledge) of potential confounders. The problem of the unmeasured confounder always remains in observational research.

In the experimental trial, however, the problem of confounders (known and unknown, measured and unmeasured) essentially disappears. A properly run trial is designed in such a way that confounding effects due to group differences of any sort (apart from the intervention under investigation) can be excluded as an explanation of any differences in outcome that might be found. Note that it is the design of the trial and the implementation of that design that eliminate confounding and bias. The following sections consider the three central design elements to achieve this in the experimental trial in medicine—randomization, single-blinding and double-blinding.

A difference in outcome between a treatment and a control group can be due to
- chance
- confounding or bias due to
    differences between the groups
    differences in handling the groups
- the true effect of intervention

Confounding and bias are avoided in the design of a trial by
- randomization
- single-blinding
- double-blinding

6.11.4 Randomization

How, then, can it be ensured that the treatment and control groups are as similar as possible regarding factors that may influence their eventual outcome? (Assume that only one treatment is being tested, although trials with more than two groups are possible.) The best method is by a process of *randomization (random allocation)*, which was introduced in Section 3.5.3. After a patient is deemed to be eligible for entry into the trial (see below), a coin is tossed. If it lands heads, the patient is allocated to the treatment group, if it lands tails, to the control group. This process is the essence of randomization, although admittedly, if used in practice, it would probably irrevocably damage any confidence the patient might have had in his physician (but see the discussion of informed consent in Section 6.14.3).

Allocation bias

Randomization by the tossing of a coin (or any equivalent method) ensures that the physician running the trial is not consciously or unconsciously allocating certain patients to a particular group. Thus, randomization can eliminate group differences due to selection or allocation bias. Without randomization, for instance, trials of a surgical versus medical technique are wide open to this problem. Low-risk cases are much more likely to be assigned to the operative group, leaving high-risk patients to be managed by the physicians. Assigning volunteers to the treatment group and those who do not volunteer to the control group is also likely to result in a biased comparison — volunteers will be quite different, in many respects, from patients who do not volunteer.

Often, it is suggested that patients be allocated to treatment or control groups alternately or on alternate days. The problem with such methods is that referring doctors may know which day corresponds to which group allocation and refer accordingly, or that the doctors running the trial may exclude certain patients if they know beforehand which group they are being assigned to. This latter problem can also arise if randomization according to birth date is employed (e.g. patients with an even birth year are assigned to one of the groups and the remainder to the other). The process of randomization, embodied in the idea of tossing a coin (after patient eligibility has been determined), is the only way to ensure that there has been no bias in treatment allocation. Note that a bias may not necessarily be present with any of the other methods, but the problem is that it might be. The results of a controlled trial based on a possibly biased method of group allocation are always open to doubt.

Long-run balance between the groups

The second important reason for randomization is that it ensures, in the long run, balance between the two groups as regards all factors, measured and unmeasured, that might confound the results. Note that it is not claimed that in practice balance will be actually achieved through randomization, but randomization does ensure that the two groups will differ only by chance. Significance testing, by its very nature, will allow for *chance* differences between the groups, and the *p* value allows for such differences when a significance level is assigned to a particular comparison. In a *randomized controlled trial* (to use perhaps the best descriptor for this type of study), it is wise, however, to check whether the measured confounders have similar distributions in the treatment and control groups, and a more powerful comparison (more likely to detect differences between the effects of treatments if they exist) is obtained if statistical adjustment is made for any observed differences. However, if a treatment effect is only apparent after such statistical adjustment, the results of the trial may not be widely accepted. As long as subjects are randomly allocated to the two groups, possible differences in unmeasured confounders are still allowed for, even without statistical adjustment.

In the trial of timolol, which is being used as an example, randomization was employed to allocate the post-myocardial-infarction patients to the timolol treatment or control group. Several hundred comparisons were made between the two groups, and the researchers concluded that the differences in these measured factors tended to be small. The final analysis, however, did include adjustments for the largest differences and other factors considered prognostically important, and it was noted that these adjustments did not materially affect the conclusions based on the unadjusted analysis.

Statistical assumptions [!]

The third and perhaps more subtle reason for requiring randomization in a controlled trial pertains to the assumptions underlying significance testing. Most trials are based on a presenting, non-random sample, and the difficulties regarding the assumption that the treated and control groups are random samples from specified (hypothetical) populations have already been mentioned in Section 3.4.1. Suppose, for example, that a randomized controlled trial resulted in 12 persons being allocated into one group and 13 into the other and that the difference in mean blood pressures was being analysed. Though this is a two-group study, the traditional analytic approach is similar to that used in the one-sample case discussed in Section 5.3. Assuming random sampling from two populations and assuming equality of means under the null hypothesis (which states that there is no group difference), the theoretical sampling distribution of the difference in the mean blood pressures is determined. The chance of the observed difference or larger can then be estimated from appropriate tables of this distribution, giving a *p* value for the comparison. If the *p* value is sufficiently small, the null hypothesis is rejected and a group difference more than that expected due to chance is accepted. (The details for this two-group analysis are considered in detail in the next chapter.)

With randomization or random allocation, however, the assumption of random sampling from populations is no longer required. Assuming that treatment did not have an effect in the trial above (the null hypothesis), the two groups should—apart from chance—have similar distributions of blood pressure. The observed blood pressures can then be taken to be just observations made on a particular set of 25 indistinguishable patients. The actual grouping observed, with 12 particular patients in one group and the remaining 13 in the other, gave the mean blood pressure difference actually observed in the trial. If a different allocation had been made (with a different 12 patients in one group and the remaining 13 in the other), then the mean blood pressure difference corresponding to this allocation (assuming patients had kept the same value for their blood pressures) could be found. Each possible allocation of the 25 patients into two groups of 12 and 13 corresponds to a particular mean blood pressure difference. The blood pressure difference observed is one of many possible differences that could have been obtained from the random allocation of the 25 patients into two groups of 12 and 13. There is a total of 5 200 300 possible different outcomes from such a randomization, and it is possible to determine, with the aid of a computer, the distribution of all the possible mean differences. It is then simple to determine directly how unusual the actual blood pressure difference obtained really is—simply on the basis of random allocation of these 25 patients. This is the *p* value for the comparison—the chances that the observed difference, or one larger, arose from chance alone. If the difference is far enough out in the tails of the distribution, then random allocation or chance is an unlikely explanation of the observed difference and the assumption of no treatment effect can be rejected. This, of course, means a statistically significant result. With this approach, the rejection of the null hypothesis means that, *for these 25 patients*, chance allocation is an unlikely explanation of the observed blood pressure difference and that the treatment effect is likely to be real.

Such *randomization tests* can be performed on a computer (albeit with some difficulty) and are an alternative to the statistical significance tests to be discussed in the next chapter. It so happens, however, that, in most cases, the *p* value from a randomization test will be the same as that given by the more traditional significance test (using a known theoretical distribution). This means that, in essence, random allocation obviates the need for convoluted arguments concerning random sampling from larger populations. The statistical inference, however, relates only to the individuals entered into the study, and generalizing results to a larger population involves issues relating to the representativeness of the trial group to the general body of patients affected with the particular disease being studied. The generalizing of trial results is discussed in Section 6.12.

Importance of random allocation (randomization)
• avoidance of allocation bias
• ensures long-run balance between the groups
• statistical theory assumes it

6.11.5 Randomization methods

Unrestricted randomization

Having cited the reasons for randomization—avoidance of bias in allocation, ensuring balance in the long run between the groups and compliance with statistical assumptions—the practice of randomization must be examined. Obviously, randomization by means of a coin is impractical and, as any conjurer will know, bias is even possible here! What is done is to make use of a table of random numbers to simulate the tossing of a coin. The use of such tables to take a random sample from a defined population has already been discussed (Chapter 2) and the tables are used in a different context here. Usually, the total sample size of a trial is fixed beforehand and a randomization schedule is made out before the trial commences. In practice, a table of random numbers is entered at a random point. Start at the top of column 2 in Table B.1, for instance. Go down the column in order, assigning each consecutive patient to the treatment or control group according to whether the digit in the table is odd or even. Assigning even numbers to the treatment group, the first 10 patients would be assigned as follows (in order, where T = treatment, C = control): T, T, T, C, C, T, C, T, C, T, since the first 10 numbers in the column are 4, 4, 8, 3, 9, 6, 5, 4, 3, 6. Continue in this way until a schedule is made out for all the patients to be entered into the trial. Since even and odd numbers appear at random in the table and since, on average, 50% of the digits are even, this satisfactorily simulates the tossing of a coin. (If there are more than two groups in the trial or if it is required, unusually, to allocate in a different ratio from 1 to 1, modifications of this procedure will have to be adopted.)

One problem immediately manifests itself: in randomizing the 10 patients, there are six in the treatment group and four in the control group. This type of result is to be expected with *unrestricted randomization* as described, and using this method it is not possible to ensure equal numbers in the two groups. This is not a major worry with large trials, but with a small total number of patients in a typical therapeutic trial such an imbalance of numbers is not desirable.

Restricted randomization

A solution to this problem is to use a *restricted randomization* procedure. It is decided, beforehand that, of every *n* individuals randomized, half will be in one group and half in the other. Suppose that, of every 10 consecutive patients, five are to be randomized to the treatment group and five to the control group. The tables of random numbers would be used as before, but after five persons are allocated to one group or the other the remaining patients in a block of 10 are assigned in such a way as to ensure that there are five in each group. Starting, for instance, at the top of column 5, the sequence C, T, T, C, C, C, C is obtained from the numbers 7, 4, 8, 5, 9, 9, 3. Stop at this point, because five out of the seven patients have been allocated to the control group, and allocate the remaining three patients out of this block of 10 to the treatment group, irrespective of the next numbers in the random-number tables obtaining finally C, T, T, C, C, C, C, T, T, T. This procedure, if continued, ensures balance of patients in multiples of 10 and is advisable even for large sample sizes. The timolol study used restricted randomization in blocks of 10. As well as ensuring balance of numbers in the trial as a whole, restricted randomiza-tion ensures, when interim analyses are being performed before the end of the trial proper, that, if only a portion of patients has been entered, the balance is still achieved. Restricted randomization also guards against imbalances due to a time trend in the type of cases admitted to a trial.

Stratified randomization

It has already been mentioned that randomization, in the long run, ensures valid comparability of groups and that any imbalance of confounding vari-ables can be adjusted for at the end of the trial. However, it is preferable to employ a design that aids comparability on known confounders than to adjust for these at the analysis stage. *Stratified randomization* achieves this purpose. If a few variables are known to be related to prognosis, then prior to randomization patients can be stratified into groups according to the values of these variables. Randomization then takes place separately within each group. This ensures balance with regard to these factors. In many trials too, the required sample size is so large that many different centres may have to participate. Such *multicentre trials* randomize separately within each centre to avoid imbalance of patients allocated from different centres, who may differ in various respects. Too many strata should not be used in stratified random-ization, however, because the trial may become administratively difficult to run and, paradoxically, with too many strata balance may be difficult to achieve. Restricted randomization must always be employed in each stratum to ensure that the numbers are balanced; otherwise the objective of the stratified randomization would not be achieved. In practice, stratified ran-domization is performed by forming a separate randomization schedule for each stratum in the trial. If a stratified randomization has been used, then the statistical methods employed in analysis should take this into account (see Chapter 11).

In the timolol trial, eligible patients were first assigned to one of three risk groups, and randomized separately within each group. In risk group I, 178 patients were allocated to timolol and 174 to the controls. In risk groups II and III, the numbers in the treated and control groups were 547 and 543, and 220 and 222, respectively, giving 945 patients on timolol and 939 in the control group. Thus, the treatment and control groups were well balanced as regards numbers and the distribution of the three risk groups. The timolol trial was also multicentre, with 20 centres participating, and the above procedure was carried out separately in each centre.

Randomization methods
• unrestricted
• restricted
• stratified (and restricted)

Randomization in practice

As has been stressed, the randomizing doctor must not know to which group the patient is to be allocated until after he/she has been judged eligible for entry into the trial. To avoid this allocation bias the schedule of randomization should not be known beforehand. This is often achieved by a sealed envelope technique, where a separate set of sealed opaque envelopes is prepared for each stratum within which randomization is to take place. The envelopes are numbered consecutively, and inside each is a card detailing the group to which each particular patient is to be allocated. Thus, in each centre of the timolol trial, there were (presumably) three sets of envelopes for each of the three risk groups. If an eligible patient was in risk category I, the next envelope in the appropriate set was opened and the patient's randomization group determined. As long as the size of the randomization block (for restricted randomization) is not known to the doctor, there is almost no way for the allocation group of any patient to be determined prior to the actual randomization. This implies, of course, that the randomization schedule is made out by an individual (usually the statistician or a member of the trial organizing committee) who is not directly involved in the actual process of the randomization. An alternative method of randomization, often employed in multicentre trials, is to telephone a central office once a patient is deemed eligible and to let them assign the patient from a prepared schedule. This has the advantage that, at any time, the actual number of patients entered into a trial is known by the central organizing committee.

The distinction between random sampling and randomization (random allocation) must be stressed. The purpose of the former is to choose a group that is representative of a larger population, and random sampling is not usually employed in controlled trials. The purpose of randomization, on the other hand, is to divide a single group into groups that differ only by chance. Randomization is the only way to ensure that individuals entered into a trial are not allocated to the treatment or control groups in a biased manner. (Although the above discussion has been in the context of randomizing individuals, it should be noted that some primary prevention trials have been based on the randomization of individual communities or factories into an intervention or control group. See Section 6.13.4.)

> Randomization (random allocation)
> - to create two groups as alike as possible that differ only due to chance
>
> Random sampling
> - to obtain a group representative of a larger population

6.11.6 Single- and double-blind trials

Single blinding and placebos

Once an individual has been entered into a trial, biases can still occur subsequent to randomization. If a patient knows to which of the two groups he/she has been assigned, this, in itself, may introduce subtle biases in evaluating the eventual outcome. For instance, patients who know that they are on a 'new wonder drug' may, for that reason alone, apart from any real effect of the treatment, experience a good prognosis. This is known as the *placebo effect*—in essence, this is the effect that an intervention may have on an individual totally independently of the true pharmacological or surgical effect of the particular intervention. In the last world war, injured soldiers injected with saline only (because of lack of availability of morphine), who thought they were being given morphine, experienced considerable relief of pain. Also, if a patient knows which group he/she is in, the stated response to the treatment may be biased one way or the other, due perhaps to the desire to 'please the nice doctor'! A *single-blind* trial is one in which the patient does not know to which of the two groups he/she has been allocated.

In a trial of a drug, for instance, single-blindness can be achieved by giving persons in the control group tablets of a similar size, colour, taste and smell as the active treatment but which contain an innocuous or inactive substance, such as starch or flour. Such a preparation is called a *placebo*. It should have no pharmacologically active ingredient related to the drug being studied, and its only purpose is to 'blind' the patients as to their allocated group.* A placebo treatment is easiest in a trial comparing a new treatment with no treatment at all, and there have been trials carried out using placebo surgical procedures by making a small skin incision but not performing the operation. Needless to say, there would be many ethical problems using such an approach (see Section 6.14.2). If, as is often the case, a drug trial is designed to test a new treatment against the usual standard treatment, then, if the trial is to be single-blind, either the two drugs must be presented as similarly as possible or a 'double-placebo' procedure must be used, where each group receives one of the active drugs and a 'look-alike' placebo of the other. Single-blindness, of

---

* In a placebo–drug trial, randomization can be carried out, not through a sealed envelope method, but by preparing bottles of tablets to be given to consecutive patients. The bottles would contain either the placebo or the active treatment, as the randomization schedule required.

course, should also mean that all the patients in a trial are managed similarly, with the same number of check-ups, out-patient visits and diagnostic procedures. In some situations, of course, a single-blind trial is not possible, as for instance in comparing a surgical and medical intervention. If a trial is not single-blind, however, biases may result.

Double-blinding

In addition to the patient being blinded as to treatment allocation, it is also desirable that the doctor be blinded. In a *double-blind* trial, neither the patient nor the doctor managing the patient or evaluating any response to treatment is aware of which group the patient has been randomized into. The purpose of the double-blind trial is to eliminate the possible biases caused by one group receiving better overall care (because they are known to be in the treatment group) or by the doctor unconsciously evaluating the patients in one group more stringently than in the other. In trying to be 'fair', for instance, a doctor may overcompensate, and thus judge individuals in the treatment group more harshly than if they were in the control group. For end-points that are subjective, in that they require a judgement in their interpretation, a double-blind trial is definitely required. Thus, a trial of antidepressants, with an end-point evaluated by means of an interview concerning depressive symptoms, would need to be double-blind to avoid possible biases in patient response and doctors' evaluation of that response. It could be argued that, if a trial had mortality as an end-point, double-blindness is not required. True, there is no room for bias in determining if an individual is dead or alive, but, if a specific cause of death is the end-point, there could be biases in assigning that cause to a decedent.

One obvious problem with a double-blind trial arises if the doctor is worried about whether or not a particular symptom exhibited by the patient is a side-effect of the active treatment, and whether the treatment should be stopped and the patient withdrawn from the trial. In such cases, the doctor may have to break the blindness of the study for the individual patient's welfare, and a record of the randomization schedule should be available. The term 'breaking the code' is sometimes used when a patient's group is determined in this manner, and should always be allowed for in the planning stages of the trial. In fact, a full list of the criteria for withdrawing a patient should be made out beforehand, and once a patient meets any of these criteria he/she should be withdrawn from the trial before the code is broken, even if it transpires that the patient was in the placebo group. Often, a safety monitoring committee is set up to review general safety aspects of a trial.

In the timolol trial, the controls received a placebo tablet similar in shape, size and colour to timolol, but differing slightly in taste. Although the end-point being evaluated was death, this trial was also double-blind and the cause of death was classified by a steering committee who were unaware of the randomization group of any individual. Very definite criteria for withdrawing a patient from the trial were laid down beforehand.

> Single-blind trials
> - the patient does not know which group he/she has been allocated to
>
> Double-blind trials
> - neither does the investigator

6.11.7 Measures of effect in trials

The results of a randomized trial usually consist of the event rates or risks in the treatment and control groups. Table 6.6 shows the simplified results of the timolol trial. The main analysis presented included end-points occurring when the patients were actually on treatment or within 28 days of withdrawal from treatment (see discussion in Section 6.12.1). Table 6.6 shows a summary of the mortality results at 33 months.* Mortality in the control group was 17·5% and in the timolol group 10·6%.

Relative risk and risk reduction

The usual measures of association for a cohort study can be employed to quantify the effects of treatment (Section 6.5.2). However, it is usual to give the result in the treatment group relative to that in the controls. Since the control group usually has the higher risk of the particular end-point, the relative risk is usually less than unity. From the table, the relative risk of death in those on timolol compared with placebo is (compare Eqn. 6.7):

$$\mathrm{RR} = \frac{R_T}{R_C} = \frac{10\cdot6\%}{17\cdot5\%} = 0\cdot61 \tag{6.15}$$

where the subscripts T and C refer to the treatment and control groups, respectively. The risk difference, which in this case is a reduction (and sometimes called the *absolute risk reduction*), is calculated as (compare Eqn. 6.8):

$$\mathrm{RD} = R_C - R_T = 17\cdot5\% - 10\cdot6\% = 6\cdot9\% \tag{6.16}$$

This, of course, is the excess risk in *the control group*. Treatment reduces mortality by 6·9%. As a percentage of the control mortality, this can be given as a relative reduction of (see Section 3.2.2):

$$\frac{6\cdot9\%}{17\cdot5\%} = 39\cdot4\%$$

This is often called the *relative risk reduction*, which means the risk reduction relative to the control value, not the reduction in relative risk. Note however that the measure is 1–RR, expressed as a percentage.

---

* The mortality given in this table is based on a life table analysis with variable follow-up, rather than on a fixed-time follow-up. The interpretation of the figures, however, is unchanged. (See Sections 6.5 and 6.6.)

Group	Number	Per cent mortality
Timolol	945	10·6
Control	939	17·5

Table 6.6 Mortality at 33 months in the randomized trial of timolol.

Relative risk	$RR = \dfrac{10\cdot6\%}{17\cdot5\%} = 0\cdot61$
Risk difference	$RD = 17\cdot5\% - 10\cdot6\% = 6\cdot9\%$
Number needed to be treated	$NNT = \dfrac{100}{6\cdot9} = 14\cdot5$

Number needed to be treated (NNT)

A useful measure, not suitable for observational studies of exposure, has been proposed to quantify a treatment benefit. Though only interpretable in the context of evaluating an intervention, it allows comparisons between different studies in a meaningful way and translates the results of a trial directly into clinical practice. It is based on the absolute risk reduction.

In the timolol trial, the background mortality is 17·5% (over 33 months) without treatment. Thus, if there were 100 patients, 17·5 deaths would be expected without treatment. If these 100 patients were treated, then 10·6 deaths would be expected. Thus, treatment of 100 patients prevents 17·5 – 10·6 = 6·9 deaths. How many should be treated to prevent one death? Divide both sides of this by 6·9 to find that it requires treatment of:

$$\frac{100}{6\cdot9} = 14\cdot5$$

patients to prevent one death. This is the definition of the *number needed to be treated*—the number of patients that one requires to treat in order to prevent a single death (or whatever the end-point might be). As is easily seen, it is calculated simply as the reciprocal of the absolute risk reduction (expressed as a proportion):

$$NNT = \frac{1}{R_C - R_T} \tag{6.17}$$

This has now become a standard measure to present the results of an interventional trial.

6.12 Applicability versus validity of trial results

6.12.1 Validity

The *validity* of trial results relates to whether or not the observed results of the trial are true or whether bias of one form or another affected these results.

Double-blindness with randomization is vital to achieving this end, but other factors are also relevant.

Sample size

The sample size of the trial should be adequate to detect an important treatment effect at a given significance level. This question was discussed in Section 5.7, but its importance cannot be overstressed. The sample size required for a trial must be estimated beforehand. Chapter 8 gives some sample size formulae that will suffice in many situations, but a statistician should be consulted concerning this and other aspects of a trial at its planning stages. A note of warning to those planning a trial: the version of Murphy's law for the controlled trial states 'if bias can occur, it will', but another law also holds; 'if the annual supply of suitable patients when the trial is being designed is n, when the trial commences it will reduce to $n/10$' (Lasagna's law)! The trial organizers are invariably over-optimistic about how many patients will be available for a study.

Many trials are undertaken with sample sizes that are too small to detect even an enormous treatment effect, and such trials result in non-significant differences between the comparison groups. Again, it must be stressed that statistical non-significance does not imply a lack of medical importance, it just means that chance is a possible explanation for the effect. Often, sample sizes required for trials may seem excessive and in many cases will require many centres to enter patients. As already mentioned, the timolol trial entered a total of 1884 patients (945 on timolol and 939 on placebo), but the original report does not give details of how this figure was arrived at. However, the fact that the trial did produce significant results suggests that care had gone into prior sample size calculations.

End-points and follow-up

In any trial, the end-points on which the effect of treatment is to be judged must be stated clearly, or the trial's validity may be suspect. These end-points, and there may be more than one, should be specified at the start of the trial; a particular end-point not considered at the start of the trial but which subsequently turns out to be greatly affected by treatment could relate to a chance occurrence, and positive results for such sought-for end-points are always a little suspect. The more objective an end-point is, the better, but, when necessary, subjective end-points have few disadvantages provided that the study is double-blind. (See also discussion of measurement accuracy and validity in Chapter 12.). As mentioned above, the major end-points for the timolol trial were mortality, both cause-specific and total, and non-fatal reinfarction. Events occurring when the patient was on therapy (active or placebo) or within 28 days of withdrawal from the study formed the basic end-points, although events in withdrawals were recorded up to the end of the study.

The validity of any trial is seriously compromised by inadequate follow-up of any of the patients entered. Many trials may run into years of patient entry and subsequent follow-up, and losses to follow-up can seriously bias the results. The follow-up of patients, however, is not an easy task, and its difficulty should not be underestimated. What happens to patients during follow-up is also very important. Withdrawals from the study due to adverse effects of treatment must be followed up as stringently as those who remain in the trial (see below). Treatments and interventions during follow-up, other than that being evaluated, should also be recorded. Some measure of patient compliance with the treatment (and placebo) regime is also required if treatment is long-term. Definite decisions as to what information is required at each follow-up must be made at the planning stage of the trial and, if a mortality end-point is included, cause and date of death must be ascertained from the appropriate sources. In the timolol trial, patients were seen at 1, 3 and 6 months following discharge from hospital, and thereafter every 6 months until the trial completion date. Patients were entered between January 1978 and October 1979, and analysis was based on a variable follow-up of all patients until October 1980. Thus, all participants had at least 1 year of follow-up, with early entrants having just under 3 years. The withdrawal criteria were carefully determined beforehand and reasons for individual withdrawals completely documented. Compliance with the treatment regime was based on a count of remaining tablets in the supply given regularly to each patient.

Statistical analysis

Appropriate statistical analysis of trial data is a *sine qua non* for the validity of results. Many trials will necessarily involve a variable length of follow-up of trial participants, and thus life table methods will be appropriate for an end-point such as death or other definite event (see Sections 6.6 and 7.15). In trials where the end-point may occur within a short period of time, each participant can be followed up for the same period and more standard analytic techniques applied. Great care must be taken, however, in the analysis of data based on variable follow-up.

Even though the trial may have included stratified randomization, the two groups should be assessed in terms of comparability with regard to prognostic factors and, if necessary, statistical adjustment techniques used in the analysis (see Chapter 11). One must be wary, however, of over-analysing a clinical trial. By searching hard enough, subgroups of patients in whom the treatment appears to work well will always be found. Unless these subgroups are defined beforehand and a stratified randomization is made within each subgroup, such treatment differences could easily be chance occurrences or due to imbalances of other prognostic factors. Little credence can be placed on results in subsets of patients when the groups are retrospectively determined, even if such results are statistically significant. The timolol trial employed Cox's regression model (Section 11.3.3) to correct for possible confounding variables, but presented the final results in terms of unadjusted clinical life tables, since the adjustment did not materially affect the results.

In nearly all trials, there will be individuals who, for one reason or another, did not receive any or all of the treatment required in the group to which they were randomized. Patient withdrawals due to side-effects, poor compliance and losses to follow-up all fit into this category. Should such persons, for analysis purposes, be included or excluded, or even changed from the treatment to the control group? The answer to this question depends on the purpose of the trial. If the purpose of the trial is to determine if the treatment can work or has an effect (an 'explanatory' trial), then non-compliers and withdrawals can be excluded from the analysis and end-points counted only in the patients on active therapy or placebo. Although answering the specific question as to whether or not the treatment can work, the explanatory trial will not answer the perhaps more important question: 'Will this treatment work if employed in practice on a group of patients?' The analysis of such a 'management' trial requires that the groups be analysed as randomized (i.e. according to the intention to treat, rather than what actually happened), with all events in each group counted. This is the more true-to-life situation, where in any group of patients there will be drop-outs and withdrawals from treatment. What is being evaluated in a management trial is a policy of using a particular treatment. The management trial is thus far more relevant to clinical practice. In the timolol trial, both methods of analysis were employed. As discussed in Section 6.11.7, the main analysis presented in the report only included end-points occurring when the patients were actually on treatment or within 28 days of withdrawal from treatment; an analysis including all end-points, however, was also performed on the intention-to-treat basis, showing only a slightly smaller effect of timolol on survival. Thus, there seemed to be no bias in the results due to selective withdrawals from treatment.

The most important of the factors that determine the validity of a controlled trial ('are the results true?') have now been covered. These factors include double-blindness, randomization, adequate sample size and clearly defined end-points. Completeness of follow-up is essential in terms of the end-points being analysed and other factors which may relate to them. Finally, an appropriate statistical analysis must be performed. In all of this, only the suspicion of bias is enough to put a question mark on the results. The onus is on the investigator to show that bias was as far as possible avoided, not on the reader of the trial report to show that it actually existed.

6.12.2 Applicability

Patient selection

The question now arises of the applicability of trial results, which relates to whether or not the results of the trial can be judged useful in clinical practice. This is determined almost totally by the type of patients selected for inclusion in the trial and the type of treatment tested, although obviously it also relates to which end-points were studied. Many explanatory trials restrict patients studied to those at high risk of experiencing the end-points. This has obvious advantages in reducing the required sample size (end-points would be more numerous), but the generalization of results to subjects who are not high-risk is questionable. Explanatory trials can show that the treatment works for some, but will not show that adopting this policy of treatment will have any real effect on the patient population at large. A management trial, on the other hand, is, as has been said, designed to see how the treatment works in practice, and thus low-risk cases should not generally be excluded.

In a trial, the patients entered are not a random sample of all patients. They are usually a presenting sample of such patients. The generalization of results to the patient population at large requires knowledge of how the patients were actually chosen for trial participation. Many trials will exclude patients with serious diseases other than that being studied, thus reducing the applicability of the end results, while ensuring, on the other hand, that imbalance of groups with 'awkward' cases is avoided. Diagnostic inclusion and exclusion criteria should, however, be clearly defined for any trial. The careful reading of a trial report may be a guide as to what kind of patient the trial may be generalized to. Trials based on volunteers are always suspect, because volunteers with a particular condition are likely to be quite unrepresentative of the full patient population.

Ideally, a trial should carefully present the sources of the patients studied; if they are hospital cases or cases in a specialized centre, results may be hard to generalize. The presentation of the timolol trial is exemplary as regards this point. Male and female patients aged between 20 and 75 years who were admitted to one of the participating centres with a suspected myocardial infarct were registered as potential trial entrants. Altogether, 11 125 patients were registered, of whom 4155 (37·3%) were diagnosed as having a definite myocardial infarction according to the defined criteria. Of these, 1884 (45·3% or 16·9% of the total registered) were eventually entered into the trial. Exclusions were due to early deaths, contraindications to timolol treatment, requirements for concomitant treatment or other factors that could have caused problems in randomizing to a placebo group, together with likely difficulties with successful follow-up. It should be noted again that the entry criteria should be satisfied prior to randomization and exclusions made before this takes place. If this is not done, serious imbalance of the groups may result. In the timolol trial, even ignoring selection biases causing admission to the particular centres, only 17 patients out of every 100 with a suspected myocardial infarction could be judged suitable for timolol and likely to survive long enough to take it. The results must be interpreted in this light. Mitchell (1981) discusses this aspect of the timolol trial in great detail.

Treatment regime

Another feature of trials relating to their applicability is the question of the actual treatment regime studied. Most trials use a fixed treatment dosage when drug therapy is in question, but to what extent this mirrors real clinical practice is a moot point. Often, in real life, the dose of a drug is adjusted to meet the individual patient's requirements or condition. Thus, a trial of a fixed dose of an antihypertensive drug may not prove instantly applicable to clinical practice. On the other hand, it must be said that trials allowing variable dosage are administratively difficult and cause problems in determining the validity of the results. It is impossible, for instance, to adjust the dose of a placebo, so blindness is lost to a large extent. The timolol trial employed a fixed dosage of timolol and placebo, with treatment started immediately after randomization (5 mg, twice daily for 2 days, and then 10 mg twice daily until trial completion).

The timolol trial was, without any doubt, well designed, well executed and well presented. Many trials do not fit into this category or are so poorly presented when published that it is impossible to judge their validity or applicability. A clear and concise presentation of all the factors discussed so far in this section is required if the results of clinical trials are to be correctly interpreted and, needless to say, all the factors need to be considered when a trial is being designed in the first place. Standardized reporting methods for clinical trials have been proposed (Begg *et al.*, 1996).

6.12.3 Meta-analysis

Directly related to the entire question of the applicability of trial results is the topic of *meta-analysis*. In recent years a large number of research groups have published articles that have been variously referred to as 'overviews', 'pooling', 'syntheses' or 'systematic reviews' of clinical trial results. These meta-analyses—which is now the preferred term—attempt to draw together results from *all* of the research into a particular therapy and to summarize the findings, usually by giving an overall measure of effect. This measure is often a summary relative risk or odds ratio based on a type of averaging of the results of the individual studies examined. Central to a good meta-analysis is that all the relevant studies (published and unpublished, positive and negative) are included. The objective is to obtain an unbiased view of how the particular therapy has worked in different situations, populations, etc. Marked differences in the effect of therapy between different studies may say something about the applicability or generalizability of trial results. The overall summary measure of effect takes account of all the investigations in the area and, of course, is based on a very large sample size—in essence, that of all the studies combined.

Meta-analyses are not easy to undertake and require careful attention to detail. Essentially, a meta-analysis is a study in itself, with the units of observation being other studies rather than patients. Inclusion and exclusion criteria are important to ensure that the trials examined give a true representation of what is known about a therapy, and an exhaustive search is needed to avoid biases resulting from missed studies. Though the idea of such formal summaries is attractive and forms the cornerstone of *evidence-based medicine*, the approach has its detractors, whose main argument is that meta-analyses do nothing more than average 'apples and oranges', giving uninterpretable results. The reader who is interested in further discussion of this should refer to Chalmers and Altman (1995).

Validity ('truth') of trial results depends on
- randomization, blindness
- adequate sample size
- appropriate end-points and complete follow-up
- appropriate statistical analysis

Applicability ('usefulness') of trial results depends on
- source of patients
- treatment regimes studied
- clinically relevant end-points

6.13 Alternative trial designs

The secondary prevention trial of timolol described and discussed in the previous sections was based on a fixed-sample size design, to compare a single treatment and placebo in two separate groups of patients. Other designs for randomized controlled trials can be used, and three of the most common are described below. The community intervention trial is also discussed.

6.13.1 The sequential trial

The *sequential trial* design avoids the sample size being fixed beforehand in the comparison of two groups, and in general enables the trial to be completed with a minimum of patients consistent with a statistically significant result. The fixed-sample size trial, on the other hand, cannot be evaluated until all patients have been entered, unless allowances have been made in the sample size calculation for interim analyses (see Section 8.2.1). Keeping the sample size in a medical trial at a minimum may be desirable on ethical grounds, but unfortunately a sequential trial can only be employed in certain situations. The more commonly used sequential trial design is described below. The basic idea behind the sequential trial is that patients enter in matched pairs, one member in each pair receiving (at random) the treatment to be tested and the other a placebo (or comparative treatment). Success or failure of the treatment is determined on each pair of patients sequentially as soon as the results become available and eventually, when a sufficient number of pairs have been entered into the study and evaluated, a statistically significant or non-significant result is obtained. At this stage, the patient entry is terminated, with no greater number entering the trial than is required to achieve a definite result. Analysis of the data takes place continually throughout the period of the trial, instead of being contingent upon the entry and completed follow-up of a fixed number of patients.

The usual sequential trial, however, can only be used to compare two groups, and one end-point only can be evaluated. This end-point is usually defined in terms of treatment success or failure, or in such a way that one of the treatments can be judged superior to the other in each patient pair. The sequential trial also will only achieve its aim of reducing the number of patients required if patient response to treatment can be determined fairly quickly after the commencement of therapy. If there is a long delay, many pairs of patients may already have been entered into the study unnecessarily when the trial is stopped. The statistical techniques involved in sequential trial (sequential analysis) are somewhat complex, but a brief outline of the method is given in Section 7.12.5.

6.13.2 The crossover trial

A second alternative to the standard two-group randomized controlled trial is the *crossover trial*, which uses a matched design with each patient as his/her own control. Treatments are compared on the same patients in different time periods. Self-paired experiments such as this ensure that the treatment or control groups are identical as regards patient characteristics and thus require a smaller total sample size than an independent two-group comparison. In a comparison of two treatments (A and B), the patient is first randomly assigned to, say, treatment A for a specified period. The effect of treatment is evaluated and the patient is withdrawn from the treatment for a time until any residual effect disappears. After this wash-out period, the patient is 'crossed over' to receive treatment B, and again the treatment effect is evaluated after a second period. Patients entering the trial are thus randomized to A and then B or to B and then A.

Unfortunately, the crossover trial can only be used in situations where the treatment effect is fairly immediate and also disappears after the withdrawal of treatment. The crossover trial can be used, for example, in testing antihypertensive therapy or anti-inflammatory drugs for arthritis. In both these examples, the 'symptom' returns after treatment withdrawal, so that a second treatment can be applied after the first. It is sometimes difficult, however, in the crossover trial to disentangle real treatment effects from a possible carryover effect from the last treatment, even with a long wash-out period, or from changes in response with the passage of time. To distinguish it from the crossover trial, the standard two-group trial is sometimes called a *parallel* trial.

6.13.3 The factorial trial

The third randomized trial design which is considered in a sense answers two questions for the price of one. If one wished to compare the separate effects of two different treatments (A and B) against a placebo, a *factorial trial* should be considered. It might be tempting to design a three-group trial with perhaps,

	Urokinase	No urokinase	Total
Warfarin	100	100	200
No warfarin	100	100	200
Total	200	200	400

Table 6.7 A factorial design for evaluating the effects of urokinase and warfarin in colorectal cancer.

randomization to A, B or the placebo, but it can be far more efficient to have four groups in such a comparison. Patients would first be randomized to receive either treatment A or the placebo. Within each of these groups, a second randomization would be made to either treatment B or placebo. Four groups would result: A and B; A only; B only; and neither A nor B. In the first International Urokinase/Warfarin Trial in Colorectal Cancer (Daly, 1991a), patients with operable colorectal cancer were randomized into receiving post-operatively either an intravenous drip containing urokinase or a saline drip (the placebo). Within each of these groups, patients were again randomized to receive either long-term warfarin therapy or no such treatment. The trial design required 100 patients in each of the four groups, and the end-points were survival and recurrence-free survival. Table 6.7 shows the required number of patients in their randomized groups. A factorial design, such as this, is analysed for the effects of the two treatments separately. The effect of urokinase, for example, is determined by comparing the 200 persons on urokinase with the 200 persons not on this treatment, irrespective of their warfarin therapy. The comparison is not biased by the warfarin therapy, because half of each group is on this drug, so that it cannot act as a confounder. Similarly, the effect of warfarin is analysed without reference to the allocation to urokinase. The sample size requirements for a factorial design like this are the same as for a normal two-group comparison, so, in essence, the extra result is free. The only problem arises if there is a synergistic effect (see Section 6.5.4) between the two treatments, and the group randomized to receive both has a better result than that expected on the basis of either therapy in isolation. Apart from this, the factorial design provides a useful adjunct to the usual two-group trial.

6.13.4 Community intervention trials

It was mentioned in Section 6.11.2 that the randomized trial could be used for the evaluation of a primary prevention intervention, such as the reduction of risk factors for Coronary heart disease (CHD). An alternative to this approach is also used. The problem with primary prevention is that it generally requires individuals to change their behaviour or lifestyle. In practice, this can best be achieved by, in addition to individual counselling, a community approach through a process of health education and promotion, whereby the community adopts healthier behaviour patterns. For example, cessation of smoking can be aided greatly by general publicity and the creation of 'smoke-free' zones. This type of intervention cannot be evaluated by the randomization of individuals, because the intervention is in the population at large. Community intervention trials are an attempt to tackle this problem. Typically, one community receives a health promotion programme, supplemented by individual interventions. A control or comparison community does not receive such an intervention. The success of the intervention is judged by comparing random samples of each community to assess changes in risk factors and behaviour and by the careful monitoring of end-points (such as heart attacks) in the entire populations.

The difficulty with such evaluations is that there may be differences between the communities, other than the intervention, that give rise to variation in the end-points. The lack of randomization introduces the major problem of confounded effects. Some trials have randomized a number of communities to intervention and non-intervention groups, but this does not overcome the difficulties.* The community intervention trial, however, seems the only way to examine the effect of health promotion in primary prevention. The earliest community intervention trial in CHD was in North Karelia in Finland (Puska *et al.*, 1981).

Alternative trial designs
- sequential
- crossover
- factorial
- community intervention

6.14 Ethical considerations for trials

Many ethical problems are raised in the context of the randomized controlled trial in medicine, and in this section some of the issues involved are indicated. Such ethical issues are still hotly debated in the medical literature and there are no hard and fast answers to many of the problems raised. However, ethical questions are distinct from medico-legal ones, and no attempt to consider the latter is made. The Declaration of Helsinki, adopted by the World Medical Assembly in 1964 and amended in various years up to 1996, provides general guidelines on biomedical research involving human subjects and is a cornerstone for the ethics of the randomized trial. The main points of the declaration (which is given in full in Appendix D) are included in the discussion below.

---

* Any form of randomization that randomizes groups rather than individuals is called *cluster randomization*. Cluster randomization must be used for any interventions that take place in a group setting and the analysis of such studies requires special techniques.

6.14.1 The nature of evidence

To turn the basic question on its head, it might be asked whether it is ethical not to perform randomized controlled trials on proposed new therapies. In the history of medicine, many therapies commonly employed simply did not work or resulted in more harm than good. Most of these therapies could have been determined as useless far sooner if subjected to a formal trial, and indeed many such therapies were abandoned as a result of their being tested scientifically. It is essential to know if a particular treatment is beneficial and the randomized controlled trial is, in essence, the only way by which this knowledge can be obtained. Clinical judgement on a haphazardly selected group with partial follow-up is not a firm basis for the evaluation of treatment. If the randomized controlled trial were to be considered unethical in all cases, then many patients would be condemned to unproved and worthless interventions and the advance of medical science would be halted almost completely.

Although one hopefully agrees with the above point, dilemmas still remain in accepting the existence of experimental trials in medicine. There are conflicts between an individual patient's welfare in the trial itself and the welfare of all patients with the particular condition in the future. There are conflicts between the doctor as healer and the doctor as investigator. In a trial, patients are allocated into two groups, one of which will receive the new treatment under investigation, while the other will receive the best treatment available or, in certain instances, no treatment at all. The first question that is asked is whether it is ethical to withhold a potentially good treatment from some individual patients for the eventual good of a larger group. Herein lies the crux of the controlled trial; if the treatment is *known* to be good, a trial cannot ethically take place, but, on the other hand, a trial cannot take place either without there being some suspicion that the treatment may be good. This leads to the conflict between knowledge and possibilities, and what may be firm 'knowledge' in one doctor's mind may be just a vague hope in another's. From the doctor's point of view, the individual patient's welfare must be of paramount importance and, if doctors have evidence that a new therapy is beneficial, they are not justified ethically in involving themselves in a trial of that treatment. Other doctors, however, may view the same evidence differently.

It would seem to be impossible to define universal criteria for what could be considered as evidence in favour of employing a particular therapy, apart from a well-designed and well-executed randomized controlled trial. On the other hand, there is no real argument against the doctor who says, 'I tried it out on 10 of my patients, and it really worked. I won't allow any of my patients to be entered into a trial.' It is interesting, however, that some doctors may feel far less uneasy using a possibly inferior therapy through ignorance than they do in submitting a possibly beneficial treatment to the rigours of a controlled trial.

The subjective nature of what evidence is required to form knowledge is thus a major problem in determining whether or not a particular trial is ethical. As healers, doctors must do what they think best for the individual patient; as investigators, they also have a responsibility to that individual patient to determine what indeed is the best therapy. It would seem, then, that, from the point of view of participating doctors, a trial is only ethical is so far as those doctors accept that they do not know which of the two treatments is better and have no preference for either.*

The question of exactly when a trial should be undertaken is relevant to this whole question. It is ethically easier to commence a trial at the introductory stages of a new therapy, since there would be little or no knowledge about its effects. However, a trial at the early stages of a new intervention is more likely to miss its full usefulness if it takes time (as with a new surgical procedure, say) to get the treatment 'just right'. If, on the other hand, one waits too long, the procedure may become generally accepted as worthwhile (without formal evaluation), making a trial ethically difficult to perform.

A similar problem arises once a trial is under way. If particular doctors see the results as they accrue and a trend in favour of one of the treatments becomes apparent, some may wish to change all their patients to that treatment because of their 'knowledge' of its better effect. Early trends in a trial, which will generally be statistically non-significant, may be very misleading; often, an early trend will settle itself out after a time to give an entirely different result at the end of the trial, when the validity and statistical significance of the results can be determined. It may, in fact, be unethical to stop a trial on the basis of early positive results that do not achieve significance, since the trial would not then have achieved its purpose. It must be stressed, however, that the patient's welfare comes first and that, if a doctor, for any reason, feels it better to withdraw a patient or change treatment, ethical considerations demand that this be done, irrespective of trial requirements.

In multicentre trials, this dilemma of early trends is often overcome by letting a steering committee, only, examine results as they come in. Trial participants will not be informed of results until the study has been completed, unless very definite trends are apparent. The ethical problem is thus switched from the participating doctors to a steering committee.

Patients have the right to expect individual and personal treatment from their doctors and it must be asked if this individual right can be sacrificed for the benefit of humanity and the progress of knowledge. This right of the individual patient seems to be sacrificed if the doctor has no choice over which therapy is to be given, which, of course, would be determined by the 'toss of a coin'. However, when there is an honest lack of knowledge about which is the better treatment, the patients do not lose out. Outside the trial, the chosen therapy would be, necessarily, at the whim of the doctor, and the fact that

---

* One criterion for making this judgement has been suggested and that is the answer to the question 'Would I allow a member of my family to enter the trial and be randomized to one or other of the treatments?'

the treatment is chosen by the 'toss of a coin' instead surely does not make a difference.

The question, then, of whether a randomized controlled trial is in itself ethical relates to the nature of evidence required to form knowledge. In most cases, a large body of doctors will agree on the necessity for a trial, although there will always be dissidents. As long as particular doctors are sure of their 'ignorance', the trial is, for them, ethically justified and patient's rights would not seem to be abrogated if they enter a trial. Indeed, rather than querying whether it is ethical to withhold a potentially good treatment from patients in the control group, it should perhaps be asked whether it is ethical to withhold the standard treatment from patients in the treatment group.

6.14.2 Trial design

Once the hurdle of determining whether it is ethical to undertake a particular controlled trial in the first place is overcome, ethical problems still remain, relating to the design and conduct of the trial itself. Firstly, the treatment to be investigated must be safe. Safe, however, is a relative term, since no therapy is without risk. The right balance must be struck between potential benefit and possible harm. Nor can the design and analysis of the trial be divorced from ethical questions. It is not ethical to enter patients into a trial whose eventual results may never be accepted because of failure to avoid bias in the setting up and execution of the trial. Also, if the sample size of a trial is too small to detect important results, it should probably not have been started in the first place. Nor, of course, should more patients than necessary be entered into a trial. The sequential trial is designed to avoid some of these problems, but, as already noted, its applicability is limited. Other little-used designs have also been proposed to reduce the number of patients on an inferior treatment. These *adaptive designs* require that a greater proportion of patients be randomized into the group showing the more favourable result at any time. Such trials, however, are limited in their scope and are in fact less appealing than they appear to be at first sight.

From the point of view of patient selection, ethical considerations will often demand certain exclusion criteria. The exclusion of pregnant women from most drug trials is universal, and ethical considerations must take precedence over the requirement of applicability of trial results.

The use of placebos and double-blind procedures in a trial also raises ethical problems. Unless the condition being studied is fairly innocuous, like the common cold, for instance, or no proved therapy is available, the control group should receive a standard therapy. Single-blindness can still be achieved by using the double-placebo procedure, and no control with a serious condition for which, treatment is available should be given a placebo only. How far one should go with placebos is a moot question. There are some examples in the early literature of placebo surgery. Ligation of the internal mammary arteries, for instance, used to be a common procedure for the relief of angina, but a clinical trial showed this treatment to be useless. Those in the control group had a placebo surgical skin incision made, but without further operative intervention. Would the results of this trial have been accepted without the placebo procedure?

In general, blinding of patients to their particular treatment does not seem to raise serious ethical problems, so long as informed consent has been obtained. As discussed previously, the double-blind trial refers to the blindness of the patient and of the doctor managing the patient and evaluating any responses to treatment. There is no problem, however, in allowing the doctor who is managing the patients to know to which treatment they have been allocated, so long as patients in the treatment and control groups are looked after similarly. In any case, if the patients' doctor is 'blind', the treatment code should always be easily available. The doctor evaluating the patients' response should, however, be 'blind'. Again, it must be stressed that doctors have the right and duty to withdraw a patient from a trial if they see fit.

6.14.3 Informed consent

The largest ethical problem with the randomized controlled trial today, however, is that of informed consent. This topic is discussed well in a report of the Cancer Research Campaign Working Party on Breast Conservation (1983). It can be a particular problem in the case of minors. In most countries, informed consent is a legal requirement of any trial in medicine. As with all ethical questions, that of informed consent does not have a simple 'yes' or 'no' answer. There is no doubt that patients have a right to know that they are participating in an experimental trial and that the therapy being tested is unproved. The problem is, however, that many patients may not wish to exercise this right. Informed consent may demand that some patients know more about their illness and their prognosis than they wish to; many prefer to put trust in their doctor that the best possible care will be given them. Is it ethical to burden such patients with the knowledge that in fact it is not known what is the best treatment, and with all the ancillary information that would be required for them to give an informed consent? (There may be an argument in certain situations that a person should not be asked to participate in a trial because of this.) The extent of information to be given is a major question that must be decided by trial organizers in the context of the particular situation.

If informed consent is to be obtained, what should it include?* This, again, is a debatable issue. Patients cannot be expected to understand everything about their disease and, in fact, one of the reasons for the trial in the

---

* It would seem that, from the ethical point of view, verbal informed consent is just as good as a written and signed statement. Written informed consent is often obtained for legal purposes only, though it does help to ensure that all points have been explained to the individual patient.

first place is that doctors do not know the best therapy themselves. Informed consent, however, does demand that the relevant facts concerning the trial and its purpose be explained as fully and clearly as possible. The two treatments should be described, as should also their possible benefits and side-effects. If the study is blind, this should be explained also. Some doctors, however, baulk at explaining that they will not be choosing the treatment but that the patient will be randomized. This, of course, is central to the trial itself, but it may result in destroying the doctor–patient relationship. Whether randomization is to be included in the description of a trial, for the purposes of informed consent, must also be left to the individual trial organizers to decide.

An important element in the process of seeking informed consent is the pressure that the doctor may, unconsciously, place on the patient to participate. Patients must fully realize that they are under no obligation to do so and that failure to become involved in the trial will not compromise their position with the doctor in any way whatsoever.

A trial design has been proposed by Zelen (1979) which neatly avoids the problem of obtaining informed consent to randomization and the consequent reduction of patient participation due to refusals. The resulting trial is controlled and (partially) randomized, but the design is not commonly used.

As has been seen, the randomized controlled trial poses many ethical questions, all of which are related to holding sacrosanct the welfare of individual patients and recognition of their rights. A very general principle could be proposed—that no patients in a trial be worse off than if they were not in the trial in the first place. The interesting fact is, however, that patients in a clinical trial often get better overall care and much more careful assessment and follow-up than the ordinary patient on standard therapy.

6.15 Summary

In this chapter, the scope and applications of the various research designs in medicine have been outlined. The basic design elements of cross-sectional, cohort and case–control studies were considered, and the important concepts of risk and comparative risk measures were introduced. The importance of randomization in the evaluation of therapy was considered in detail and the avoidance of bias in standard randomized controlled trials was described. Different trial designs were briefly introduced, with a concluding section on the ethics of medical experimentation.

The remaining chapters in the book consider in detail the statistical analyses of data arising from the research designs discussed. Chapter 7 considers the analysis of two-group comparative studies and this is followed by a chapter on the estimation of appropriate sample sizes. Chapter 9 extends the discussion to the comparison of more than two groups and Chapter 10 examines the analysis of relationships between two quantitative (numerical) variables. Chapter 11 describes the statistical techniques used to adjust for confounding effects and, finally, Chapter 12 considers various biases in medical research, particularly those related to the problems of measurement and diagnosis.

7 Confidence Intervals and Hypothesis Tests: Two-group Comparisons

7.1 Introduction

In one sense, medical research is all about examining associations between variables. When group membership is considered a qualitative variable, then comparing means in groups is the examination of an association between a quantitative and a qualitative variable, and comparing proportions in groups is the examination of the association between two qualitative variables. When the qualitative variable has only two categories, the situation reduces to the comparison of two groups or samples. Two-group situations are exceptionally common in medical research—for example, comparing cases and controls in a case–control study or a treatment and a control group in a clinical trial—and it is often more convenient to reduce an analysis to a two-group comparison by combining categories of a variable.

This chapter describes hypothesis tests and confidence intervals for the comparison of means, medians, proportions (risks), counts and rates in the two-group situation. The construction and comparison of life tables are also considered. It should be noted that, in the comparison of two groups, confidence intervals are preferably calculated for a single summary measure of the comparison or association (e.g. the difference between two means or a relative risk), rather than for each of the component statistics (e.g. the two separate means or risks). The techniques considered here are among the most common in the medical literature and it is hoped that this 'cookbook' chapter will be of practical use to researchers who wish to analyse their own data.

Since all the methods described are based on the same underlying philosophy, detailed discussion is avoided and the formulae are not derived formally. Therefore, a good grasp of the concepts of the confidence interval and significance test, as described in the earlier chapters, is necessary for the material that follows. Some understanding of the comparative risk measures (e.g. odds ratio, relative risks) is also needed for appreciation of the application areas of some of the techniques.

7.2 Independent and paired comparisons

One of the most common errors in statistical hypothesis testing is a failure to take cognizance of how the data were collected in the first place. Statistical analysis is not simply a tool applied to numbers; it is a methodology for examining real data, which a researcher may have spent many months or years gathering together.

This chapter considers the comparison of two groups and is, therefore, in essence, concerned with the analysis of two samples taken from corresponding populations. Apart from issues relating to the accuracy of data collection and whether or not the resulting numbers are truly a measure of what is being studied (see Chapter 12), the way in which samples are chosen from the populations is of vital importance.

7.2.1 Independent groups

Suppose that a sample has been taken from a population and it is of interest to compare blood pressures in alcohol drinkers and abstainers. Each of these groups can be considered to be a sample from one of the two populations defined by drinking and non-drinking. This is a common situation in medical research, where the comparison groups are defined by the value of some qualitative variable (such as drinking) in a single study group. Sometimes, however, the sampling from population groups is more explicit. Separate samples may, for instance, be taken of schoolchildren from rural and urban areas to compare IQs. The samples may be of equal size or may reflect the distribution of urban and rural children in the country as a whole (stratified samples).

Both of these examples have one important factor in common: the samples are *independent samples* from the populations being studied. By independent it is meant, in simple terms, that the actual selection of individuals for one sample group is not affected by the individuals already selected for the other group. It is vital to understand this notion of independence if the correct statistical test is to be chosen, and, before undertaking any statistical analysis, a researcher must be sure whether or not the comparison groups are independent.

7.2.2 Paired groups

At the other extreme from the comparison of independent samples is the comparison of *paired samples* or *individually matched* samples. A paired sample arises in two-group comparisons when every individual in one of the groups has a unique match or pair in the other group. This commonly arises in the case–control study, where controls can be chosen individually matched to cases for potential confounding variables, such as age or sex (see Section 6.7.2). This technique is sometimes called *artificial pairing*.

In animal experimentation, littermates often provide the experimental material. Two treatments may be compared in a group of rats by assigning one animal to one treatment and one of its littermates to the other treatment. Thus, every animal in one group would have a littermate in the other group. Such situations result in what is called *natural pairing*.

A third form of pairing is *self-pairing*, when the same individuals belong to both comparison groups. This can arise when, say, a new chemical is being tested for allergic reactions and compared with a non-allergic preparation. The chemical might be applied to a person's right arm and the other preparation to the left arm. The arms of the people under study would be compared and, for every right arm, there is a left arm. A further example of a self-paired situation is when some variable is measured before and after a particular therapy. The measurements made before the therapy are matched with the measurements on the same individual after the therapy. The same situation

205

*Section 7.3
Parametric/
non-
parametric
tests*

arises when two different treatments are tested on the same individuals on two different occasions, as in the crossover trial (see Section 6.13.2).

Although the examples of paired data above were for two-group comparisons, similar data may arise with more than two groups, although this is relatively uncommon in the medical literature. A point to note also is that, in a paired situation, the sample size in each of the groups must necessarily be the same, while this need not be so for independent comparisons.

7.2.3 Frequency matched groups

Between the extremes of independent data and paired data lie what are called *frequency matched* data. These arise when the distribution of a variable, or variables, is forced to be the same in the two groups. For example, each group might end up with the same proportions of individuals in a number of age categories, without any matching of individuals. This can typically arise in a case–control study or a clinical trial with stratified randomization. The analysis of frequency matched data is akin to a stratified analysis (see Section 3.5.4 also) and will be considered in Chapter 11. The techniques of this present chapter are only applicable to independent or paired data.

If one fails to account for pairing or matching in an analysis, the statistical test loses power and is more likely to miss a real difference if it exists. Thus, a test for independent data should not be used on paired groups. Occasionally, however, when suitable statistical methods are not available, matching or pairing can be ignored, with a consequent loss of power.

In two-group comparisons the groups can be
- independent
- paired
- frequency matched

This should be accounted for in the analysis

7.3 Parametric and non-parametric significance tests

Apart from how the data were collected, the measurement scale of the variable being studied can also determine the statistical hypothesis test to be used. In the discussion so far, it was sufficient to distinguish between quantitative and qualitative variables. In the medical literature, the vast majority of significance tests compare either proportions or means, operating on qualitative or quantitative data, respectively.

7.3.1 Scales of measurement

It was noted in Section 1.2 that a qualitative variable can have categories without an intrinsic order (e.g. diagnosis) or have ordered categories, which will often take a numerical label or tag although the concept of distance between these categories does not arise. On this basis, a hierarchy of variables can be created: qualitative variables with no intrinsic order; qualitative variables with order; and quantitative variables based on measurement. For convenience, these three types of variables will from here on be referred to as nominal, ordinal and quantitative variables, respectively. It is important to note that a quantitative variable, such as age, can be expressed in ordinal form (e.g. by ranking from youngest to oldest) or in nominal form (e.g. by categorizing into young, middle-aged or old and ignoring order). This means, essentially, that a significance test suitable for a low level of measurement can be applied to any higher level, if the scale of measurement is adjusted appropriately. Thus, tests suitable for nominal data can be applied to ordinal or quantitative data, and tests for ordinal data can also be applied to quantitative data.

7.3.2 Test assumptions

One of the rules of good statistical analysis, all else being equal, is to use the highest level of test available for the data; but usually all is not equal and, in particular, many tests suitable for quantitative data make large assumptions about the distribution of variables in the populations being compared. It was seen in Chapter 5, for instance, that an underlying assumption of data that were not too skew was required for a valid application of the one-sample t test, but that with a large sample size violations of this assumption could be tolerated. Significance tests that make assumptions about population parameters (and skewness can be considered a parameter!) of the variable being analysed are called *parametric tests*. Sometimes, assumptions can be made valid with a suitable transformation of the data (see Section 7.4.4).

In some situations, it is not possible to check whether such assumptions are true, particularly when the sample size tends to be small, and there is often doubt about whether or not a particular test is valid for a set of quantitative data. As has been said, however, quantitative data can be analysed as ordinal data, and most of the statistical tests of ordinal data are assumption-free. Such tests are called *non-parametric, distribution-free* or *rank tests* and provide a useful fall-back in many situations.

A further point about many of the rank tests is that they test a null hypothesis relating to median values, rather than mean values. The median, however, is much more appropriate for skewed data (see Section 1.6.6) and is close to the mean if the data have a nearly symmetrical distribution in the first place.*

---

* Though this book considers the non-parametric tests as essentially tests of differences in medians, an important underlying assumption about most of these tests must be mentioned. The tests assume that any group difference has arisen through a shift of the entire distribution of the variable upwards or downwards. In real data, statistically significant results can sometimes arise due to other differences between the groups.

It must be pointed out, however, that, in general, parametric tests are somewhat more powerful (in the sense of Section 5.7) in detecting differences between populations when the underlying assumptions hold, and many of the more complex parametric tests do not have a non-parametric equivalent. In general, too, the non-parametric tests are not useful for estimation purposes, and confidence intervals for estimates are usually difficult to calculate. Confidence intervals related to the non-parametric tests are not considered in this book.

In the two-sample situation, however, non-parametric tests can be exceptionally useful in the analysis of quantitative data. With small sample sizes, many of the underlying assumptions of parametric tests may be invalid, and the non-parametric tests are probably the only valid ones to use. For this reason, such tests are sometimes called *small sample tests*, and, in fact, tables for the non-parametric tests in this text are only given for studies of up to moderate size. With fairly large sample sizes, on the other hand, many of the assumptions for the parametric tests may hold approximately, and they can be employed with a large degree of confidence. For large sample sizes too, the non-parametric tests are computationally more tedious.

The remainder of this chapter outlines the application of the more common parametric and non-parametric significance tests for two-group comparisons. Confidence interval estimators are described for commonly used measures of association. Statistical tables are given in Appendix B, and Appendix C summarizes the application of each test for easy reference.

Parametric tests
- used for quantitative data
- test hypotheses about means
- make assumptions about parameters in the population

Non-parametric tests
- called also rank, distribution-free, small sample tests
- used for quantitative or ordinal data
- test hypotheses about medians
- make few assumptions
- useful and easy for small sample sizes
- confidence intervals difficult

7.4 Comparison of two independent means

7.4.1 The independent *t* test for two means

The parametric *t* test used for the comparison of means in two samples is one of the most commonly used tests in medical statistics. The test to be described in this section is for independent samples only and should not be used when the data are paired or frequency matched (see Section 7.2). Failure to take note

	Contraceptive-users	Controls
Sample size	20	20
Sample means	5·20	4·81
Sample standard deviations	0·53	0·48
Difference between means	0·39 mmol/L	
95% CI for difference	0·07 to 0·71 mmol/L	

Table 7.1 The independent *t* test comparing cholesterol levels in users and non-users of oral contraceptives.

$t = 2·439$; degrees of freedom (d.f.) = 38; $p < 0·05$.
CI, confidence interval.

of this is an oft-repeated error and results in a loss of power in the comparison. In other words, an independent *t* test performed (incorrectly) on paired data will increase the chances of declaring a non-significant result when, in fact, the null hypothesis is false.

Suppose 20 regular users of oral contraceptives were studied to determine if cholesterol levels in such women are significantly different from those of women who do not use oral contraceptives. Because the cholesterol levels in the population were not known, a comparison or control group of 20 similarly aged women who were not on the 'pill' was also taken, without pairing or matching. The results of the study are shown in Table 7.1. The mean cholesterol levels in the contraceptive-users and controls were 5·20 and 4·81 mmol/L, respectively, with corresponding standard deviations of 0·53 and 0·48 mmol/L. It is assumed that, on examination of the sample, there is no evidence of a major degree of skewness in the population.

The test statistic

The null hypothesis is that the mean cholesterol levels in the populations of oral contraceptive-users and non-users are the same. The results of the samples suggest a difference of 0·39 mmol/L between the two groups. Could this be due to chance or does it reflect a real difference?

The statistical approach is similar to the situation with one sample only. If there really was no difference between the two groups, it would be expected that repeat samples, sized 20, from each group would generate a series of mean differences distributed around the value of 0 (the null value). As in the one-sample case, a test statistic is calculated based on the difference — the degree of departure from the null value — obtained (0·39 mmol/L), divided by a factor that is the standard error (SE) of this difference (see Eqn. 5.5). This test statistic has a known distribution from theoretical considerations, and tables can be used to see if the calculated value lies in the tails of the distribution. Moreover, since no prior knowledge is available concerning the direction of the difference in cholesterol levels, a two-sided test must be employed.

The actual test statistic to employ is defined:

$$z = \frac{\bar{x}_1 - \bar{x}_2}{\mathrm{SE}(\bar{x}_1 - \bar{x}_2)} \tag{7.1}$$

where $\bar{x}_1$ and $\bar{x}_2$ are the means in the groups being compared and $\mathrm{SE}\,(\bar{x}_1 - \bar{x}_2)$ is the exact standard error of the difference between the means.

The standard error of a difference

In general, the standard error of a difference between two statistics (if they are independent) is calculated as the square root of the sum of the squares of the individual standard errors:*

$$\mathrm{SE}(y_1 - y_2) = \sqrt{\mathrm{SE}(y_1)^2 + \mathrm{SE}(y_2)^2} \tag{7.2}$$

where y_1 and y_2 are any statistics. This result will be used throughout the chapter, and here:

$$\mathrm{SE}(\bar{x}_1 - \bar{x}_2) = \sqrt{\frac{\sigma_1^2}{n_1} + \frac{\sigma_2^2}{n_2}} \tag{7.3}$$

where σ_1 and σ_2 are the population standard deviations and n_1 and n_2 are the two sample sizes.

When, as is usual, the population standard deviations are not known, the sample values S_1 and S_2 must be used instead. These are not substituted into Eqn. 7.3 directly, however. If it can be assumed that the two population standard deviations are equal, then what is called a *pooled variance* is calculated as the weighted average of the two sample variances:†

$$S_p^2 = \frac{(n_1 - 1)S_1^2 + (n_2 - 1)S_2^2}{n_1 + n_2 - 2}. \tag{7.4}$$

The t test

An appropriate test statistic for the comparison of two means is then obtained by substituting S_p^2 for each of the two population values in Eqn. 7.3

---

* This is based on the fact that the variance of a difference between two quantities is the sum of their individual variances. The square of a standard error is the variance of the sampling distribution of the mean, so that the standard errors for each of the two means must first be squared, giving the variances of the two different sampling distributions; these are then added together, giving the variance of the sampling distribution of the difference between the means, and the square root of this quantity gives the standard error. Note that, even though the difference between the means is being examined, the variance is given by a sum. The variability actually increases when two quantities are subtracted. The variance of a sum is also the sum of the variances.

† For technical reasons, a weighted average of the variances, rather than the standard deviations, is calculated and the assumption is usually stated in terms of equality of the variances. The statistical term for this is homoscedasticity!

$$t = \frac{\bar{x}_1 - \bar{x}_2}{\sqrt{\dfrac{S_p^2}{n_1} + \dfrac{S_p^2}{n_2}}} \qquad (7.5)$$

This has a t distribution on $n_1 + n_2 - 2$ degrees of freedom. The denominator of this expression is generally referred to as the standard error of the difference between means, even though it is only a sample estimate of that quantity. When the sample sizes are equal ($n_1 = n_2 = n$), this reduces to the simpler expression:

$$t = \frac{\bar{x}_1 - \bar{x}_2}{\sqrt{\dfrac{S_1^2 + S_2^2}{n}}} \qquad (7.6)$$

on $2n - 2$ degrees of freedom. Note that this equation is not to be used with unequal sample sizes.

In the example, the two sample standard deviations are fairly close in value and, since the sample sizes are equal, Eqn. 7.6 is an appropriate test statistic. (An example with unequal sample sizes can be found in Section 7.6.1). Substituting in the sample values:

$$t = \frac{5 \cdot 20 - 4 \cdot 81}{\sqrt{\dfrac{(0 \cdot 53)^2 + (0 \cdot 48)^2}{20}}} = 2 \cdot 439$$

This value must now be looked up in the tables of the t distribution for 38 degrees of freedom. Table B.3 does not give values for 38 degrees of freedom, but 40 is near enough for a valid approximation.* The critical 5% (two-sided) level for t is $2 \cdot 021$ and the statistic exceeds this, so $p < 0 \cdot 05$. Note, too, that the critical 1% value is $2 \cdot 704$ and that the result, although achieving a 5% level of significance, does not reach the 1% level. It can therefore be concluded that chance is not a likely explanation of the observed differences between the cholesterol levels of users and non-users of oral contraceptives at a 5% significance level.

7.4.2 Confidence intervals for a difference in independent means

The most common measure employed in the comparison of means is, in fact, the difference between the means. The confidence interval for the difference between two population means is given by:

$$(\bar{x}_1 - \bar{x}_2) \pm t_c \mathrm{SE}(\bar{x}_1 - \bar{x}_2) \qquad (7.7)$$

---

* If the critical t value for particular degrees of freedom is not available in the table, the entry for the degrees of freedom next above the required number should be used. This will be perfectly acceptable as long as the calculated t statistic is not just below this critical value. If this case arises, a more complete t table will have to be obtained.

In the most general unequal sample size situation, this is:

$$(\bar{x}_1 - \bar{x}_2) \pm t_c \sqrt{\frac{S_p^2}{n_1} + \frac{S_p^2}{n_2}} \qquad (7.8)$$

where $\bar{x}_1$ and $\bar{x}_2$ are the means in the two groups, n_1 and n_2 are the sample sizes, S_p^2 is the pooled variance given by Eqn. 7.4 and t_c is the appropriate critical value of the t distribution with $n_1 + n_2 - 2$ degrees of freedom. In the equal sample size situation, the standard error term can be simplified, with the denominator of Eqn. 7.6 used instead. In the cholesterol example, the standard error is 0·160. The degrees of freedom for the test are 38, but, since Table B.3 does not include an entry for this, the critical t_c value for 40 degrees of freedom must be chosen. This will give a slightly wider interval than with the correct t_c value, but this is an acceptable approximation. The critical t_c value for 40 degrees of freedom and a 95% confidence interval is 2·021, so that the confidence interval for the difference in mean cholesterols between the contraceptive users and non-users is:

$$0·39 \pm 2·021 \, (0·160)$$

$$0·39 \pm 0·32$$

$$0·07 \text{ to } 0·71$$

Thus, it is 95% certain that the mean cholesterol level in contraceptive users is at least 0·07 mmol/L higher than in controls and could be as much as 0·71 mmol/L higher.

The independent t test and confidence intervals for differences between means are summarized in Section C.7 of Appendix C.

7.4.3 Assumptions for the independent t test

A few words need to be said concerning the assumptions underlying this particular application of the t test. The first assumption, of course, is that the two samples are random and independent. The two-sample t test, like the one-sample test, also assumes that the populations from which the samples were taken are not too markedly skewed. The final assumption is that the standard deviations in the two populations are the same. If there is reason to doubt this assumption, it is not valid to pool the two sample variances into a single estimate; instead, it is necessary to calculate:

$$t' = \frac{\bar{x}_1 - \bar{x}_2}{\sqrt{\frac{S_1^2}{n_1} + \frac{S_2^2}{n_2}}} \qquad (7.9)$$

using the separate sample values for the variances. This statistic does not have a Student's t distribution and, although some approximate solutions involving the t distribution, with a complex formula for the appropriate degrees of freedom, are available, they are not given here. If the sample sizes are large enough (over 50 in each group), it is suggested that a normal approximation setting $t' = z$ be used. If the assumptions for the t test are not satisfied, a transformation of the data might provide a solution.

7.4.4 Data transformations

Skewness can be reduced, using the suggestions of Section 1.6.7, and sometimes these transformations can also achieve equality of variances in the two groups. In particular, the transformations for positively skewed distributions can be useful. Usually, with unequal variances, the standard deviation tends to increase with the size of the mean. The easiest way to determine which transformation may be most appropriate is to examine the ratios of the standard deviation (S) to the square root of the mean ($\sqrt{\bar{x}}$), to the mean itself ($\bar{x}$) and to the square of the mean ($\bar{x}^2$) in the two groups. Whichever set of ratios is closest in value in the two groups indicates whether the standard deviation is increasing in proportion to $\sqrt{\bar{x}}$, $\bar{x}$ or $\bar{x}^2$. The best transformation to use on each data observation (x) is then:

$$S \propto \sqrt{\bar{x}}: \text{use } \sqrt{x} \text{ (square root)}$$
$$S \propto \bar{x}: \quad \text{use } \log x \text{ (logarithmic)}$$
$$S \propto \bar{x}^2: \text{use } 1/x \text{ (reciprocal)}$$

where $\propto$ means 'is proportional to'.

The large advantage of using data transformations is that the independent t test can then be employed for what might have been originally quite skewed data. The test is just applied to the transformed data and the significance level obtained in the usual manner. The null hypothesis is that the two groups are the same, and rejection of the null hypothesis on the transformed data is equivalent to rejection on the original data. Thus, a significant effect on a transformed scale means that the groups differ by more than chance. Unfortunately, however, complexities arise if a confidence interval approach to data analysis is used. In general, confidence intervals for a difference on a transformed scale do not translate back to the original scale easily, and it is usually only in that scale that the results have any meaning. The major exception to this is the logarithmic transformation, where confidence intervals do have a useful and valid interpretation. This is why it is the most commonly used transformation for positively skewed data in medical contexts. Section 7.6 will consider this topic in detail.

7.5 Inferring significance from confidence intervals

7.5.1 Significance from a single confidence interval

There are a number of general points that can be made based on the particular comparison of means in the previous section. In two-group significance testing, the objective is to reject or not reject the null hypothesis of group equality with regard to the distribution of some variable. When that variable is quantitative, the significance test is usually based on the sampling distribution of the difference in means (see previous section). In theory, the sampling distribution of any comparative measure could form the basis of the hypothesis test, but usually the most convenient one is taken which satisfies the tenable assumptions.

When it comes to confidence intervals, however, a number of issues arise. The first is that the appropriate confidence interval in the context of a two-group comparison should be for some single measure of association between the variable and group membership. In general, it is not useful to estimate confidence intervals for the means (or other measure of the centre) in each group separately. Secondly, there are always a number of different contenders for this measure of association. In comparing means, for instance, there are at least two possibilities—the difference between the means or their ratio. The choice is usually determined with reference to the utility of the measure in the context of the study design, to the variable itself and/or to the assumptions needed to estimate the confidence interval in the first place. (Confidence intervals for a mean difference are considered in Section 7.4.2 above and the intervals for the ratio of two (geometric) means are discussed in Section 7.6.2 below.)

Similar to the one-sample situation (see Section 5.4), significance testing of the null hypothesis that two groups are equal can be inferred by examination of the confidence interval for a measure of association between the groups. In the example of the last section on cholesterol levels, the 95% confidence interval for the difference between the means is:

$$0{\cdot}07 \text{ to } 0{\cdot}71 \text{ mmol/L}$$

The null value (corresponding to no difference between the groups, or no association of oral contraceptive use and cholesterol) is that of a zero difference between the mean cholesterols. Thus, significance at the 5% level can be inferred from the fact that the interval does not include this null value. This is the main reason why it is more appropriate to calculate a confidence interval for a measure of association than for, in this case, the means in the two groups separately.

7.5.2 Significance from confidence intervals in each group [!]

It is, in fact, possible to be misled when confidence intervals are presented for each of the two means, rather than for the difference between the means. With separate intervals, it is very tempting to try and infer significance by seeing if they overlap—if the intervals do not overlap, it seems reasonable to conclude that the means differ more than you would expect by chance. This is a legitimate argument: statistical significance can be claimed if confidence intervals for a parameter in each group being compared do not overlap. Unfortunately, the converse is not the case. A difference may be statistically significant even if the confidence intervals for the component parameters do overlap.

Taking the cholesterol example, the mean cholesterols with their 95% confidence intervals, were, respectively, in contraceptive users and controls (using Eqn. 4.14 with 19 degrees of freedom for each expression):

$$5{\cdot}20 \pm 0{\cdot}248\,mmol\,/\,L\ (4{\cdot}95\ to\ 5{\cdot}45)$$
$$4{\cdot}81 \pm 0{\cdot}225\,mmol\,/\,L\ (4{\cdot}59\ to\ 5{\cdot}04)$$

Thus the 95% intervals overlap, while the difference is actually statistically significant and the 95% interval for the difference between the means excludes the null value of zero difference. This illustrates the problem. A judgement can be made if intervals fail to overlap, but overlapping intervals cannot easily be interpreted.

It is possible, however, with a bit of calculation, to determine approximate significance from confidence intervals calculated for some parameter in each group separately. Essentially, the confidence interval for the difference can be formed from the two confidence intervals for the parameters themselves.

The confidence intervals in groups 1 and 2 are each given by:

$$\bar{x} \pm t_c \frac{S}{\sqrt{n}} \qquad (4.14)$$

with different values for $\bar{x}$, S, n and t_c in each group. Given only the confidence limits and the relevant sample sizes, the values of S, the standard deviation in each group, can be determined. These estimates can then be used in Eqns. 7.4 and 7.8 to obtain the confidence interval for the difference in means. This, however, is rather tedious and a simple approximation, which holds in many situations, is given below, with a crude derivation.

Suppose the 95% confidence intervals for groups 1 and 2 are given by:

$$\bar{x}_1 \pm U_1 \qquad (7.10)$$

$$\bar{x}_2 \pm U_2 \qquad (7.11)$$

where U_1 and U_2 are the relevant standard errors multiplied by the appropriate t-distribution critical value. U_1 and U_2 are each half the total confidence interval width or half the difference between the upper and lower confidence limits. Using similar arguments to those used in deriving Eqn. 7.2, the 95% confidence interval for the difference between the means can be shown to be approximately:

$$(\bar{x}_1 - \bar{x}_2) \pm \sqrt{U_1^2 + U_2^2} \qquad (7.12)$$

Significance can then be inferred by noting whether or not the interval overlaps the null value of zero.* Use of this interval-width method is, in

---

* Using this approach, the reader should be able to derive the confidence interval for a difference between means, assuming the population standard deviations are known. The formula will be given by Eqn. 7.7, where z replaces t_c, and the standard error is based on Eqn. 7.3.

general, somewhat approximate, but it does make for an easy calculation. As an illustration, the confidence interval for the difference in mean cholesterols between contraceptive-users and non-users will be derived from the confidence intervals on the individual means. From the 95% confidence intervals for the means, U_1 and U_2 were 0·248 and 0·225, respectively. Thus, the 95% confidence interval for the difference between the means should be:

$$0·39 \pm \sqrt{(0·248)^2 + (0·255)^2}$$

$$0·39 \pm 0·33$$

The more accurate solution, using Eqn. 7.8 directly, gave ±0·32. It must be stressed that this approach is approximate. It works best for large and fairly equal sample sizes, when the variances can be assumed equal. The method could also be used for parameters other than the mean, but only if the confidence intervals are symmetrical.

7.6 Comparison of two independent geometric means [!]

7.6.1 The independent *t* test for log-transformed data

Section 1.6.7 illustrated the derivation of the geometric mean through a log transformation of the positively skewed plasma homocysteine data in 797 normal subjects and a confidence interval was given in Section 4.7. In Section 3.2.1, the comparison of this result with that for 746 vascular-disease patients was discussed. Table 7.2 repeats the basic results. In the original scale of μmol/L, the mean homocysteine level in patients is higher but, not only are the data positively skewed, the standard deviation is also considerably higher in patients than in normal subjects. Both the skewness of the data and the lack of equality of the measure of spread between the two groups suggest that a

Table 7.2 Plasma homocysteine levels in patients with vascular disease and normal subjects (based on Graham *et al.*, 1997). Original and transformed data.

	Vascular disease patients	Normal subjects
Number	746	797
Plasma homocysteine (μmol/L)		
Mean	11·93	10·06
Geometric mean	11·15	9·67
Standard deviation	5·17	3·06
Log plasma homocysteine		
Mean of logs	1·0471	0·9855
Standard deviation of logs	0·1524	0·1199

Ratio of geometric means: 1·15.
95% confidence interval: 1·12 to 1·19.

standard *t* test comparing the arithmetic means might not be appropriate for significance testing.* Remember that the assumptions underlying the *t* test are equality of variances and near-symmetrical populations.

Since a log transformation can reduce positive skewness and make standard deviations more similar, it is used on these data to accord with these assumptions.[†] The results of the transformation are also shown in Table 7.2. The log of each data value was taken and the means and standard deviations of the transformed data are given. As can be seen, the standard deviations of the transformed data are more nearly equal and, as was seen in Section 1.6.7, the transformed data are much more symmetrical.

The *t* test is applied to the transformed data simply by applying Eqn. 7.5 to the logs of the observations. Since the sample sizes are unequal, the pooled variance must be calculated first. Equation 7.4 gives an expression for the pooled variance of the log-transformed data, $S_p'^2$, with the 'prime' notation signifying the statistics estimated on the transformed data:

$$S_p'^2 = \frac{(n_1 - 1)S_1'^2 + (n_2 - 1)S_2'^2}{n_1 + n_2 - 2} \tag{7.4}$$

$$S_p'^2 = \frac{745(0.1524)^2 + 796(0.1199)^2}{1541} = 0.01865$$

The *t* statistic is then derived from:

$$t = \frac{\bar{x}_1' - \bar{x}_2'}{\sqrt{\dfrac{S_p'^2}{n_1} + \dfrac{S_p'^2}{n_2}}} \tag{7.5}$$

which becomes:

$$t = \frac{0.0616}{0.0070} = 8.80$$

Now, the degrees of freedom are 746 + 797 − 2, which is 1541. This is very large and the critical value for infinite degrees of freedom can be taken. This, of course, is 1·96 for a two-sided 5% test and 2·576 for a two-sided 1% test. The difference between patients and normal subjects in plasma homocysteine is (highly) statistically significant ($p < 0.01$). The null hypothesis — that the populations from which the groups had been taken had the same homocysteines — is rejected.

There are no particular difficulties, then, in performing a *t* test on transformed data and the calculations proceed as in the untransformed case, no

---

* Because of the large sample size here, the skewness of the data is less acute a problem than the non-equality of the variances or standard deviations. In any case, as already mentioned, both problems often go hand in hand and the solution to one may also be the solution to the other.
† Using the rule of thumb on transformations in Section 7.4.4, a reciprocal transformation might also be suitable. However, because of its ease of interpretability, and for didactic reasons, a log transformation is employed here.

matter what transformation was used. The data transformation is simply to ensure that the assumptions underlying the test are valid. Note that the significance test ignores any interpretational issues relating to the transformation used. The procedure here is summarized in Section C.7 of Appendix C, which deals with the independent *t* test in general.

7.6.2 Confidence intervals for a ratio of geometric means [!]

Things become a little more complicated when confidence intervals are used for transformed data. In the single-sample case, a confidence interval was obtained for the transformed quantity and the back-transformation of the confidence limits gave confidence limits for the back-transformed point estimate (see Section 4.7). A similar approach is used in the two-sample situation. Starting with a confidence interval for the difference between the means of the log-transformed data, Eqn. 7.8 gives the limits as:

$$(1.0471 - 0.9855) \pm 1.96 \ (0.0070)$$

where 1·96 is taken as the critical *t* value, given the large numbers of degrees of freedom, and the standard error term is from the denominator of the expression for the *t* test given above. The confidence limits for the difference in the means of the logs are then:

$$0.0616 \pm 0.0137$$

or 0·0479 and 0·0753. The obvious next step is to back-transform the point estimate of the difference between the mean logs and these confidence limits by calculating their antilogs.*

In the single-sample case, the antilog of the mean of log-transformed data is defined as the geometric mean:

$$GM(x) = 10^{\bar{x}'} \tag{1.4}$$

where $\bar{x}'$ denotes the mean of the logs of the original data. In the two-group case, the transformation of the difference in the means of the logs is:

$$10^{\bar{x}'_1 - \bar{x}'_2} = \frac{10^{\bar{x}'_1}}{10^{\bar{x}'_2}} = \frac{GM(x_1)}{GM(x_2)} \tag{7.13}$$

Thus, the back-transformation of the difference in the means of the logs is the ratio of the geometric means in the two groups. The log is the only transformation for which the back-transformation of a difference is an interpretable measure. In the present example:

$$10^{1.0471-0.9855} = 10^{0.0616} = 1.15$$

which, of course, is the ratio of the two geometric means of 11·15 and 9·67 μmol/L in Table 7.2. The back-transforms or antilogs of the confidence

* Taking 10 to the power of each quantity.

limits for the difference in the mean of the logs give the confidence limits for the ratio of the geometric means:

$$10^{(\bar{x}'_1 - \bar{x}'_2) \pm t_c \text{SE}(\bar{x}'_1 - \bar{x}'_2)} \tag{7.14}$$

where the standard-error term is given by the denominator of Eqn. 7.5 above—using Eqn. 7.4 calculated on the transformed values. In the example, the 95% confidence limits for the ratio of the geometric means are:

$$10^{0 \cdot 0479} = 1 \cdot 12$$

$$10^{0 \cdot 0753} = 1 \cdot 19$$

In other words, the ratio of the geometric means in vascular disease patients compared with normals is 1·15 (95% CI: 1·12 to 1·19). Since the confidence interval does not overlap the null value for the ratio of unity, statistical significance at the 5% level can be inferred. This procedure is summarized in Section C.7 of Appendix C.

7.7 Comparison of two independent medians

In many situations, especially with small sample sizes, the assumptions underlying the parametric independent *t* test described in the last section may not hold. Instead of using a transformation of the data, a non-parametric alternative is available. Also, if the measurement scale of the data is ordinal and not quantitative, the mean values are uninterpretable and the *t* tests cannot be used.

7.7.1 The Wilcoxon rank sum test for independent medians

Suppose that systolic blood pressure has been measured on nine young adults with diabetes mellitus and on eight control patients of similar age (not matched) without this condition. The diabetes mellitus patients had systolic blood pressures of 114, 120, 120, 128, 130, 135, 138, 140 and 141 mmHg. The control patients had blood pressures of 110, 112, 112, 118, 120, 122, 125 and 130 mmHg. The purpose of the study is to see if there is a relationship between blood pressure and diabetes mellitus and there is no prior conception about what the direction of this relationship may be. Also, since the sample size is small and the distribution of blood pressures may be quite skewed, it is decided that the two-sample *t* test is likely to be invalid. The most commonly used test in this situation is the *Wilcoxon two-sample rank sum test* or the entirely equivalent *Mann-Whitney U test* or *Kendall's S test*. The formulation which will be considered is that of Wilcoxon.

This test, like most non-parametric tests, is based on ranking or ordering the data. The data from the two groups are combined and ordered from lowest to highest, giving a rank of 1 to the lowest value and, in the example, 17 (the sum of the two sample sizes) to the highest observed value. The groups from which the different observations are taken must also be noted. If there are ties in the

Table 7.3 The Wilcoxon rank sum test comparing systolic blood pressures in nine diabetics (group 2) and eight controls (group 1).

Systolic blood pressures (mmHg)*	Ranks (observation numbers)	Ranks adjusted for ties*
110	1	1
112	2	$2\frac{1}{2}$
112	3	$2\frac{1}{2}$
114	4	4
118	5	5
120	6	7
120	7	7
120	8	7
122	9	9
125	10	10
128	11	11
130	12	$12\frac{1}{2}$
130	13	$12\frac{1}{2}$
135	14	14
138	15	15
140	16	16
141	17	17

* Control (group 1) values and ranks underlined.
T_1 = sum of ranks in group 1 = 49·5; T_2 = sum of ranks in group 2 = 103·5; $p < 0.05$.

data (i.e. more than one individual has the same value for a measurement), the average of the ranks that would have been given to the observations is assigned instead.

In the example, the data would be laid out as in Table 7.3, underlining the observations from (say) the control group and calling it group 1. The easiest way to assign the ranks correctly is to number the observations from lowest to highest. If there are no ties, these numbers are the ranks. If there are ties, like the two blood pressures of 112 mmHg, these are assigned a rank calculated as the average of the observation numbers. In this case the two measurements are given numbers 2 and 3, and are therefore assigned the average rank of $2\frac{1}{2}$ [(2 + 3)/2]. The three observations of 120 mmHg with numbers 6, 7 and 8 are all assigned rank 7 [(6 + 7 + 8)/3 = 7].

The Wilcoxon test is based on examining the sum of the ranks in each group. If the two populations have similar distributions, then it would be expected that the sums of the ranks in each group would be close to each other. If the distributions are different, it would be expected that the group with the lower median would have a lower sum of ranks. In the example, the sum of the ranks of the observations in group 1 (the control group) is denoted:

$$T_1 = 1 + 2\cdot5 + \ldots + 12\cdot5 = 49\cdot5$$

and the sum of the ranks in group 2 is:

$$T_2 = 4 + 7 + \ldots + 17 = 103 \cdot 5$$

This immediately suggests that the median value in group 1 might be less than that in group 2.

The actual test statistic for the Wilcoxon rank sum test is the sum of the ranks in whichever group has been called group 1.* As with all significance tests, this statistic is referred to tables of a particular distribution. The critical values for the Wilcoxon statistic are to be found in Table B.5 (Appendix B). Unfortunately, the table is rather cumbersome and spread out over 12 pages of the appendix. The table allows for sample sizes of n_1 up to 25 and n_2 up to 35. The groups can be relabelled if one has more than 25 observations. For sample sizes outside this range, a more detailed text should be consulted (see Appendix B).

Table B.5 is in three parts for values of n_1 of (a) 1–9, (b) 10–17, (c) 18–25. First, choose the appropriate part of the table depending on the value of n_1. For each range of values of n_1, there are four pages of tables, one for each of the two-sided (one-sided) significance levels of 0·10(0·05), 0·05(0·025), 0·02(0·01) and 0·01(0·005). Having chosen the required significance level, the lower (T_l) and the upper (T_u) critical values for the sample sizes in group 1 (n_1) and in group 2 (n_2) can be read from the table. If the test statistic T_1 is greater than or equal to T_u or less than or equal to T_l, a significant result can be claimed.

In the example, the controls were labelled as group 1 and $T_1 = 49 \cdot 5$. The lower and upper critical 5% two-sided values are, for $n_1 = 8$ and $n_2 = 9$, $T_l = 51$ and $T_u = 93$. The sum of ranks at 49·5 is less than T_l, so there is a significant difference between the blood pressures of the two groups. Since T_1 is less than the lower critical value, it can be concluded that the blood pressure of controls is less than that of the diabetic patients ($p < 0 \cdot 05$).

Unfortunately, however, as with many non-parametric tests, a direct measure of the magnitude of the difference between the groups is not part of the test statistic, and it is necessary to rely on the examination of group medians to determine the importance of a given result. With the t test, on the other hand, the magnitude of the difference between the two groups, $\bar{x}_1 - \bar{x}_2$, is entered directly into the calculation of the t. Although possible, the calculation of confidence limits for the difference between medians is very tedious and is not considered here.

The main assumption for the Wilcoxon test is that there is an underlying continuous distribution of the variable of interest (even if the measurements are only on an ordinal scale). In essence, the test compares the two distributions in their entirety on the assumption that the entire distribution is shifted in one of the groups, so it is a valid test for the comparison of means or medians. It is nearly as powerful as the parametric t test, even when all the assumptions for

---

* It does not matter which group is called group 1 (here it is the controls), but for the correct use of the tables it is T_2 that is the test statistic.

that test are valid, and, when the assumptions do not hold, it is always to be preferred. There are some slight problems if there are many ties in the data, but the test as outlined should be adequate for most practical situations. The application of the test is summarized in Appendix C, Section C.8.

7.8 Comparison of paired means

7.8.1 The paired *t* test for means

When data have been collected on pairs of individuals and each member of one of the groups has a match or pair in the other group, the independent *t* test cannot be used. The statistical analysis must take account of how the data were collected. Suppose that a study on the effect of a particular drug on pulse rate is performed on eight volunteers; their pulses are measured before and after the administration of the drug, giving the data shown in Table 7.4. The mean pulse rate prior to drug administration is 67·0 beats per minute and afterwards it has increased to 70·375 beats per minute. One point to note is that, in any paired situation such as this, the sample sizes in the two groups must necessarily be the same.

The approach to hypothesis testing in a paired situation is to take advantage of the fact that observations in the groups come in pairs. If, under the null hypothesis, the means of the two populations (pulse rates before and after administration of the drug) are the same, then the mean of the differences calculated on a sample of pairs of individuals should be close to 0. Column 4 of Table 7.4 shows the differences (d) in the pulse rates calculated by subtracting the 'before' reading from the 'after' reading. The mean of these differences, denoted $\bar{d}$, is 3·375, which is the same as the difference between the means of the original two groups, 67·0 and 70·375 beats per minute. This is a general result—that the mean of the differences is the same as the difference of the means.

Table 7.4 The paired *t* test. Pulse rates in eight subjects before and after administration of a drug.

Subject (pair)	Pulse rate (beats/min)		After minus before (d)
	Before drug	After drug	
1	58	66	8
2	65	69	4
3	68	75	7
4	70	68	−2
5	66	73	7
6	75	75	0
7	62	68	6
8	72	69	−3
Mean	67·0	70·375	3·375 ($\bar{d}$)

$t = 2·167$; d.f. = 7; NS.
95% CI for difference: −0·31 to 7·06.

For the analysis of a paired experiment, attention should be focused on the column of differences, essentially reducing the situation to a single sample of differences. The null hypothesis states that the population mean difference should be 0 and so, using an adaptation of the one-sample test (Eqn. 5.6), an appropriate test statistic for the paired situation is:

$$t = \frac{\bar{d} - 0}{S_d / \sqrt{n}} \qquad (7.15)$$

on $n - 1$ degrees of freedom. $\bar{d}$ is the observed mean of the differences, and the 0 in the formula is the hypothesized value for the mean population difference. S_d is nothing more than the standard deviation of the differences calculated in the usual manner. Note, though, that, if any of the differences have a minus sign, this must be taken into account and also that zero differences should be included. n is the number of pairs in the entire study, which, of course, is the number of calculated differences. There are $n - 1$ degrees of freedom, since, essentially, the paired data have been reduced to a one-sample situation, with n observations of differences.

The mean of the figures in column 4 of Table 7.4 is $\bar{d} = 3\cdot375$ and the standard deviation can be calculated as $S_d = 4\cdot406$. With n equal to 8:

$$t = \frac{3\cdot375}{4\cdot406 / \sqrt{8}} = 2\cdot167$$

There are 7 degrees of freedom and it will be assumed that a two-sided test at a 5% level of significance is to be performed. The critical 5% value for a two-sided t test on 7 degrees of freedom is $2\cdot365$ (Table B.3) and, since the calculated t of $2\cdot167$ does not exceed this value, a statistically significant result cannot be claimed. Although the drug increased the mean pulse rate by over 3 beats per minute in the subjects studied, this could be a spurious result due to sampling variation.

7.8.2 Confidence intervals for a difference in paired means

A confidence interval for the mean difference between the pulse rates can be calculated using:

$$\bar{d} \pm t_c \, S_d / \sqrt{n} \qquad (7.16)$$

where $S_d / \sqrt{n}$ is the standard error of the mean difference and t_c is the appropriate two-sided critical value of the t distribution. In the example the 95% confidence interval turns out to be:

$$3\cdot375 \pm 2\cdot365 \, (1\cdot558)$$

This gives confidence limits of $-0\cdot31$ and $7\cdot06$ beats per minute; thus, the confidence interval includes the null value of 0, as might have been expected from the result of the significance test.

The approach to this analysis of paired quantitative data is to reduce the two sets of observations to one set of differences, and the assumption underlying the use of the paired t test is that the distribution of differences in the population is not markedly skewed. The assumption required for the independent t test of equal population variances is not required, since there is now only one population of differences. Section C.9 (Appendix C) summarizes these calculations.

7.9 Comparison of paired medians

7.9.1 The sign test for paired medians

An alternative to the parametric paired t test is the non-parametric *sign test*. Essentially, this examines the null hypothesis that the medians in the two populations are the same, and it is an exceptionally easy test to perform. As with the Wilcoxon rank sum test for independent medians, the data may be quantitative or ordinal, but an underlying continuous distribution is assumed.

Suppose that the reactions of 10 patients to two different analgesics (A and B) have been studied, with the patients rating the effectiveness of each preparation on a scale from 0 to 9, a high score denoting a beneficial effect. On the basis of these scores, it is required to determine which analgesic might be judged to be more effective. The results of this study are laid out in Table 7.5. It can be seen immediately that analgesic A is superior to B according to eight of the persons studied. They are scored equally by one person, and another person judges B to be superior to A. If the median effects of the two analgesics were the same, it would be expected that, on average, half the persons would prefer A and the other half would prefer B; the sign test is, in fact, based on the number of preferences for one drug over the other, the superior drug being likely to have more preferences.

A preference (or superiority of one drug over the other) can be detected by the sign of the difference between the measured scores, a plus sign, say,

Table 7.5 The sign test (paired data). Scores assigned by 10 patients to two analgesics, A and B.

Patient (pair)	Analgesic A	Analgesic B	Sign of A − B
1	2	2	0
2	4	3	+
3	7	4	+
4	3	0	+
5	0	1	−
6	3	2	+
7	6	4	+
8	4	2	+
9	5	4	+
10	8	6	+

n_+ = number of '+' signs = 8; n = number of untied pairs = 9; $p < 0.05$.

representing a preference for A and a minus sign a preference for B. Tied results (e.g. subject number 1 who scored both drugs with a 2) must be ignored, and the number of preferences or 'pluses', denoted by n_+, should be recorded. In this case $n_+ = 8$, out of nine untied pairs. This number of preferences can be referred to critical values for the sign test, which depend on the number of untied pairs (n) and, as usual, on the significance level for the chosen one- or two-sided test. Table B.6 in Appendix B gives the lower (S_l) and upper (S_u) critical values. For $n = 9$, the two-sided 5% critical values are 1 and 8, and in this example n_+ at 8 is equal to the upper critical value. Thus, it can be concluded that there are more preferences for analgesic A in this study than could reasonably have arisen by chance, and a significant result can be claimed at the 5% level.

Note that this test does not, by its nature, take any account of the magnitude of the differences between the groups. The example shows, however, that small differences in a consistent direction, even with a small sample size, can lead to significant results. For instance, a useful rule of thumb (see Table B.6) is that six preferences in one direction and none in the other are significant at a two-sided 5% level, while an eight-to-one split gives a similar result. Section C.10 of Appendix C summarizes the application of the sign test.

7.9.2 The Wilcoxon signed rank test for paired medians

The non-parametric sign test for paired data described above took account only of the sign of the differences between the observations in the two groups, and took no cognizance of the magnitude of these differences. The test described below is more powerful than the sign test, in that the magnitude of the differences contributes to the test statistic.

The *Wilcoxon signed rank test* will be illustrated on the same data employed for the paired t test—the difference in pulse rates before and after administration of a drug (see Table 7.4). As with the paired t test (Section 7.8.1), the first step is to calculate the difference between the values for each pair ('after minus before' values). The next step is to rank these differences from smallest to largest, ignoring the sign of the difference. This is done in Table 7.6. As usual, tied ranks are given the average of the ranks that would have been given if the values were not tied. Note that the zero difference on subject 6 is not included for the purpose of ranking. (In the paired t test, this zero difference did contribute to the test statistic.) Thus, the observed difference of −2 is given rank 1 and the difference of −3 is given rank 2. The difference 4 is the next largest, and is given the rank of 3. The remainder of the ranks are assigned similarly. Once the ranks have been calculated in this manner, the sign of the difference is given back to each rank, to form the signed ranks, as shown in the last column of Table 7.6. The test statistic is then taken as the sum of the positive ranks, which is denoted T_+ and is in this example 25 ($3 + 4 + 5 \cdot 5 + 5 \cdot 5 + 7$).

Again, this test statistic is intuitively reasonable. The null hypothesis states

Table 7.6 The Wilcoxon signed rank test (paired data). Differences between pulse rates before and after administration of a drug (see Table 7.4).

Subject (pair)	Difference* in pulse rates (after − before) beats/min (d)	Rank	Signed rank
6	0	–	–
4	–2	1	–1
8	–3	2	–2
2	4	3	3
7	6	4	4
3	7	5·5	5·5
5	7	5·5	5·5
1	8	7	7

* Ordered by magnitude.
T_+ = sum of positive ranks = 25; n = number of untied pairs = 7; NS.

that the distribution from which the two sets of observations are sampled are identical and thus that the means and/or medians are the same. If this were the case, the differences (d) should be symmetrical about 0; that is, there should be as many negative differences as positive differences. Also, the sum of the positive ranks (T_+) should be close in value to the sum of the negative ranks—the sum of the ranks with the minus sign. If, however, the population mean (or median) of the 'after' group were greater than that of the 'before' group, there would be more positive differences, and thus T_+ would tend to be larger than expected under the null hypothesis. Similarly, if the differences were in the other direction, T_+ would be smaller than expected. Table B.7 in Appendix B gives the lower (T_l) and upper (T_u) critical values of T_+ for different numbers of non-zero differences, since obviously these critical values will depend on the total number of differences that were ranked. In the example, there are seven untied pairs and T_+ is equal to 25. The critical values for a 5% two-sided test are, from the table, 2 and 26; thus, T_+ does not lie in the critical region and, as with the paired t test, it must be concluded that the difference between the pulse rates before and after treatment with this particular drug is non-significant and could be ascribed to chance.

As with many of the non-parametric tests considered so far, it is necessary to assume an underlying continuous distribution for the variable, and there should not be too many ties among the differences. The calculation of confidence limits is again not considered. Section C.11 in Appendix C summarizes the use of the signed rank test.

7.10 Comparison of two independent proportions or risks (2 × 2 tables)

In many medical investigations, the variable of interest is binary and takes on two values only. Thus, one might want to compare the proportions or percentages alive or dead in two groups. In this and the following sections, techniques for the comparison of proportions in two groups are described. Since risks and proportions are synonymous, the techniques are particularly suited to the analysis of risk in cohort studies or clinical trials. A fixed follow-up is assumed (see Section 6.4). The analysis of the case–control study is also considered in terms of odds ratios. This section deals with the comparison of proportions in two independent samples. As with the one-sample situation, the analysis here is in terms of proportions and, if working with percentages is preferred, translation back to this measure at the end of the analysis is suggested.

7.10.1 The z test for two independent proportions

As an example, take the clinical trial discussed in Section 3.4.1, where the 5-year survival expressed as a proportion of the two treated groups, each of 25 subjects, was found to be 0·68 in those on drug A and 0·48 in those on drug B. Table 7.7 presents these data in a 2×2 *contingency table* (see Section 3.2.2). The test to be described for use in this type of situation is approximate, in so far as the normal distribution is being used to approximate the binomial distribution (see Section 5.9). For this reason, the applicability of the test is in doubt with small sample sizes. The test, however, is non-parametric, in that it makes no assumptions in relation to the distribution of the variables being examined.*

As with the two-sample test for means, the test statistic for the comparison of the two proportions is in the form:

$$\frac{\text{Difference between the proportions}}{\text{SE (difference)}}$$

The standard error of the difference between the two proportions depends on the value for the proportions specified by the null hypothesis. The null hypothesis specifies that the proportions in the two populations from which the samples were taken are the same. If, in the example quoted, survival is being

	5-year outcome			Table 7.7 Results of a clinical trial comparing survival in two drug-treated groups (proportions given in parentheses).
	Alive	Dead	Total	
Drug A	17 (0·68)	8 (0·32)	25 (1·0)	
Drug B	12 (0·48)	13 (0·52)	25 (1·0)	
Total	29 (0·58)	21 (0·42)	50 (1·0)	

$z = 1·433$; NS.
Survival difference $= 20\%$ (95% CI: $-6·9\%$ to $46·9\%$).

* Some prefer not to include this test under the category of 'non-parametric', reserving the term for the various 'rank tests', which can be applied to quantitative data.

analysed, then, letting π_1 and π_2 represent the population proportion of survivors in the drug A and drug B treated groups, respectively,

$$H_0: \pi_1 - \pi_2 = 0$$

or:

$$H_0: \pi_1 = \pi_2$$

If this common value for the proportion of survivors as specified by the null hypothesis is denoted π, then it can be shown that:

$$SE(p_1 - p_2) = \sqrt{\pi(1-\pi)\left(\frac{1}{n_1} + \frac{1}{n_2}\right)} \qquad (7.17)$$

where p_1 and p_2 are the observed proportions of survivors in samples size n_1 and n_2 taken from the two populations of interest, and SE $(p_1 - p_2)$ is the standard error of the difference between these two proportions. In practice, of course, this common value of π in the populations is not known and the best estimate of the quantity is the proportion of survivors observed in the two treated groups combined. In the example, there were 29 survivors in the two groups out of a total of 50 patients studied (see Table 7.7), so that the overall proportion of survivors is 29/50 or 0·58. This pooled estimate of the proportion of survivors is also obtained as a weighted average of p_1 and p_2:

$$p = \frac{n_1 p_1 + n_2 p_2}{n_1 + n_2} \qquad (7.18)$$

where the weights are the respective sample sizes, and p denotes the pooled value. Substituting this into Eqn. 7.17:

$$SE(p_1 - p_2) = \sqrt{pq\left(\frac{1}{n_1} + \frac{1}{n_2}\right)} \qquad (7.19)$$

where q is defined as $1 - p$.

Combining these results, the following test statistic is appropriate for testing the difference between proportions in independent samples.

$$z = \frac{p_1 - p_2}{\sqrt{pq\left(\frac{1}{n_1} + \frac{1}{n_2}\right)}} \qquad (7.20)$$

This should be referred to tables of the standard normal distribution (Table B.2).

Substituting in the results of the clinical trial example, this equation becomes:

$$z = \frac{0·68 - 0·48}{\sqrt{0·58(0·42)\left(\frac{1}{25} + \frac{1}{25}\right)}} = 1·433$$

For a two-sided test at a 5% level of significance, the critical z value is 1·96 and, since the calculated value of 1·433 is not greater than this, it must be concluded that the difference between the drug effects is not statistically significant. In fact, examining the table of the standard normal distribution, it can be seen that the p value is just greater than 10%. The z test for independent proportions is summarized in Section C.12 of Appendix C.

7.10.2 Confidence intervals for a difference in independent proportions (attributable or excess risk)

In some texts, the estimate of the standard error of the difference between two proportions may be given as

$$SE(p_1 - p_2) = \sqrt{\frac{p_1 q_1}{n_1} + \frac{p_2 q_2}{n_2}} \tag{7.21}$$

This is an acceptable approximation, so long as n_1 and n_2 are nearly equal and p_1 and p_2 do not differ substantially. This formula for the standard error results in a figure of 0·137 for the example, as opposed to a value of 0·140 obtained with the more exact expression given by Eqn. 7.19. The standard-error formula given by Eqn. 7.21 should, however, be used for estimating confidence intervals for the difference between two proportions, and 95% or 99% confidence intervals are given by:

$$(p_1 - p_2) \pm z_c \sqrt{\frac{p_1 q_1}{n_1} + \frac{p_2 q_2}{n_2}} \tag{7.22}$$

where z_c is the 5% or 1% critical value for the normal distribution. For example, the 95% confidence interval for the difference between the proportions alive on drug A and drug B is:

$$0·2 \pm 1·96 \,(0·137)$$

or from −0·069 to 0·469.

Translating this back to percentages, there is a 20% survival advantage for the treated group with a 95% confidence interval from −6·9% to 46·9%. The data are actually compatible with anything from an adverse effect of treatment (decreasing survival by 6·9%) to a beneficial effect of a 46·9% survival advantage. The confidence interval overlaps the null value of a 0% difference, thus confirming the non-significance of the result noted above. Note that, because of the difference in the formulation of their standard-error formulae (Eqns. 7.19 and 7.21), significance as inferred from the confidence interval may not always tally with the direct application of the significance test. This only happens in cases of borderline significance, however, and is a consequence of the approximation of the approaches.

The generally accepted conditions under which the normal distribution can be used as an approximation to the binomial are that the total sample size be greater than 20 and that the quantities $n_1 p$, $n_2 p$, $n_1 q$ and $n_2 q$ all be greater than 5 for sample sizes between 20 and 40. The approximation should be quite valid for (total) sample sizes above 40. These criteria may be too strict, however (see next section), but they are satisfied in the present example. The approach above and more exact methods for confidence interval analysis of a difference between proportions are reviewed by Newcombe (1998b).

Note that the entire discussion, which has been in the context of comparing survival proportions, could just as easily have been in terms of mortality proportions. An absolute difference in survival percentages is identical to (except for the sign) the difference in mortality percentages or risks. The standard-error term is also the same. Thus the method is suitable for the analysis of the risk difference (excess or attributable risk) also (see Section 6.5.2).

The estimation of confidence intervals for differences in proportions is summarized in Section C.12 of Appendix C.

7.10.3 The χ^2 test for two independent proportions

A more common alternative to the z test discussed in the last section is a χ^2 test to compare differences between two independent proportions. This test is easier to apply, but the computational approach, though mathematically equivalent, is quite different (see Section 5.10 for a short discussion of the χ^2 distribution).

Observed and expected numbers

The data are laid out in a 2 × 2 table, and the test statistic is based on the observed and expected (under the null hypothesis) frequencies in each of the four cells of the table. It is essential, however, that the actual numbers in the cells are used, rather than the percentages or proportions. Table 7.8 shows the results obtained when cigarette smoking in a group of 150 patients with an upper respiratory-tract infection (URTI) is compared with that of a control group of 140 patients without URTI. The aim is to determine if smoking is associated with URTI or, equivalently, if there is a difference in the proportion of smokers amongst the population of URTI patients and the comparison population. As in previous examples, it will be assumed that the comparison is valid and that the design of the study has been adequate. It is important, however, that the two samples should have been independently chosen. The null hypothesis then states that the proportion of smokers in each group is the same.

The first step in applying the test being considered is to calculate the numbers of people expected to be observed in the four cells of the table if, in fact, the null hypothesis were true. If there really is no difference between the groups, it would be expected that the proportion of smokers observed in the total sample, 165/290 = 0·5690, would be seen in each of the groups; thus, out of 150 cases of URTI, it would be expected that $0·5690 \times 150 = 85·345$ individuals would be smokers. Similarly, in the controls, $0·5690 \times 140 = 79·655$ persons would be expected to be smokers. Now, the overall proportion of non-smokers in the two groups combined is 125/290 =

Table 7.8 The χ^2 test. Smoking status in 150 patients with upper respiratory-tract infection (URTI) compared with 140 controls.

(a) Observed numbers

	URTI	Controls	Total
Smokers	95 (63·3%)	70 (50·0%)	165 (56·9%)
Non-smokers	55 (36·7%)	70 (50·0%)	125 (43·1%)
Total	150 (100·0%)	140 (100·0%)	290 (100·0%)

(b) Expected numbers

	URTI	Controls	Total
Smokers	85·345	79·655	165
Non-smokers	64·655	60·345	125
Total	150	140	290

(c) Calculation

Observed (O)	Expected (E)	O − E	(O − E)²	(O − E)²/E
95	85·345	9·655	93·219	1·092
55	64·655	−9·655	93·219	1·442
70	79·655	9·655	93·219	1·170
70	60·345	−9·655	93·219	1·545
Total				5·249

$\chi^2 = 5\cdot249$; d.f. $= 1$; $p < 0\cdot05$.

0·4310, so that in 150 cases of URTI $0\cdot4310 \times 150 = 64\cdot655$ non-smokers are expected and a similar calculation leads to 60·345 expected non-smokers in the control group.

The middle of Table 7.8 shows these expected numbers filled into the corresponding cells of a 2 × 2 table. Note that, when these expected numbers are added up across the rows and columns, the same total numbers of cases and controls and smokers and non-smokers as were in the original table are obtained. This is an important property of the expected numbers, and it can be seen that, in fact, for such a table only one of the expected numbers need be calculated and that all the others may be obtained by subtracting from the totals at the edge of the table (the marginal totals). In practice, it is advisable to calculate all the expected values and to check the calculation by ensuring that they do add up to the original totals. It is usually sufficient to keep to three decimal places in the calculation.

The test statistic

Once the expected numbers have been calculated in this way, the significance test is fairly straightforward. Obviously, the greater the difference between the observed and the expected figures, the more evidence there is to reject the null hypothesis. The test statistic is based on this observation, and also includes a factor to allow for the relative magnitude of these differences (e.g. a difference of 10 is much more striking if it arises from values of 30 and 20 than from values of 310 and 300). The test statistic used is:

$$\chi^2 = \sum \frac{(O - E)^2}{E} \tag{7.23}$$

where the O values are the four observed numbers in the body of the table and the E values are the four expected numbers. Summation is over the four cells of the table. The bottom of Table 7.8 illustrates the calculation of this sum, which turns out to be 5·249. Note that the magnitude of the $O - E$ quantities is the same for each cell of the table in the 2 × 2 case, but this is not so for larger tables. (The sum of the $O - E$ quantities is always 0, however.) Section A.3 in Appendix A gives an alternative short-cut formula for calculating χ^2 in a 2 × 2 table.

The sum 5·249 is then referred to tables of the χ^2 distribution on 1 degree of freedom (Table B.4). (For a 2 × 2 table, there is only 1 degree of freedom. If the marginal totals are fixed, the number of observations in only one of the four cells of the table is free to vary. This is because, given one, the other three can be obtained by subtraction.) Note that the chi-square test statistic as calculated must always have a positive sign and, unlike the other tests considered so far, it does not indicate which of the groups has the larger proportion. The critical values given in the χ^2 table must be *exceeded* for a significant result.[*] The two-sided critical value for χ^2 with 1 degree of freedom is 3·841 for a 5% level of significance and, since the calculated value of 5·249 is greater than this, it can be concluded that there is a significant difference in the proportion of smokers among the URTI cases and controls. The exact same result would have been obtained if the methods of the last section, using the z test, had been employed. Which test to use is quite arbitrary, though the χ^2 test is by far the most popular.[†] Although it does not enable confidence intervals to be calculated, it has the great advantage, as will be seen later, that the method extends to tables larger than 2 × 2.

Assumptions

The applicability of the χ^2 test for 2 × 2 tables depends on the same criteria as those used in the z test, which can be restated in terms of the expected values. For total sample sizes less than 20, the usual wisdom is that a more exact test

---

[*] The χ^2 table gives both one- and two-sided critical values for various significance levels. The one-sided critical values, however, do not refer to areas in one tail of the χ^2 distribution, but the interpretation of a one-sided test is as described before. The one-sided test is only valid for the 2 × 2 tables being considered in this section and in most cases is recommended anyway (see Section 5.5).
[†] It is beyond the scope of this book to prove the equivalence of the z and χ^2 tests.

should be used (see next section). For sample sizes between 20 and 40, the test is quite valid as long as none of the expected frequencies falls below 5. Some suggest, however, that, within this range of sample size, a slightly different χ^2 formula should be used, incorporating what is called Yates' correction. This is not considered here. For sample sizes greater than 40, there should be no problem with the use of the χ^2 test. Some work, however, suggests that the 2×2 table χ^2 should be used even if the sample size is smaller than noted above, as Fisher's test (in the next section) may be too conservative (D'Agostino *et al.*, 1988). This is probably the best option to take, using the χ^2 formulation above in all cases, irrespective of sample size. The application of the χ^2 test is summarized in Appendix C, Section C.13.

7.10.4 Fisher's exact test for two independent proportions [!]

As has been pointed out, the χ^2 test is considered by some not to be valid whenever the expected frequency in any of the cells in a 2×2 table falls below 5. In this case, an exact test is available called *Fisher's exact test*. Unlike all the other significance tests so far described, this test involves the calculation of the p value directly, without the use of a particular test statistic. Of all the tests encountered so far, Fisher's exact test is, without any doubt, the most difficult to calculate. Nonetheless, it is useful in many situations, and the computational method is outlined below. (Many statistical computer packages will also perform the test for you.)

Assumptions

The χ^2 test for a 2×2 table has been described as a test for the comparison of proportions in two independent samples. In such a situation, the numbers of individuals in each sample are determined by the investigator, and thus, depending on the layout of the table, the column totals are fixed, while the row totals are free to vary according to the results of the study.

The χ^2 test, however, may also be used where one sample is classified by two binary variables; thus, the numbers of smokers and non-smokers in males and females in a single sample from a population might be examined. This is still a two-group comparison, though based on a single sample. In this case, both the row totals and the column totals are free to vary; they are determined by the sex and smoking distributions in the sample and are not fixed in advance of the study. The only quantity fixed is the total sample size. The χ^2 test is also appropriate for 2×2 tables arising in this manner. It is also possible that in a 2×2 table both the row and column totals are fixed beforehand by the investigator. This type of situation rarely arises in medical applications, but again the χ^2 test is appropriate.

Now Fisher's exact test is in fact based on fixed row and column totals and so, theoretically, is not applicable to 2×2 tables arising from either the two-sample or one-sample situations described above. However, the test is often used in these cases also, with the proviso that it is conditional on (i.e. assumes) fixed row and column totals (fixed marginals), thus the test is not 'exact' in the situations in which it is often applied.

Table probabilities

Underlying the approach to all hypothesis tests is the distribution of a specific test statistic and the calculation of the area (areas)—corresponding to probabilities—in the tail(s) of the distribution cut off by the test statistic actually calculated on the basis of the observed results. In Fisher's exact test, the distribution of all possible 2 × 2 tables with the same fixed column and row totals as the one observed in the study are examined. The probability of obtaining each of these tables if there is no relationship in the population between the two factors being studied can be calculated. For a general 2 × 2 table laid out as shown in Table 7.9, this probability is:

$$P = \frac{r_1! \, r_2! \, s_1! \, s_2!}{n! \, a! \, b! \, c! \, d!} \tag{7.24}$$

The letters r and s with the subscripts refer to the row and column totals, and a, b, c and d are the numbers in each of the cells; n is the total sample size. The exclamation mark denotes 'factorial' and means successive multiplication of the integers in descending order, thus $5! = 5 \times 4 \times 3 \times 2 \times 1 = 120$. $0!$ is defined as equal to 1.

Now, to calculate a p value for Fisher's exact test, it is necessary to add up the probabilities of the observed table and any even more unlikely ones in the tail of the distribution of all possible tables. This will give a one-sided test if the only tables included are those which (a) show a more extreme result than that actually obtained and (b) at the same time also suggests the same direction of difference in the result. A two-sided test is obtained by doubling the one-sided p value.

Calculating the p value

Suppose that 16 elderly insulin-dependent patients with diabetes mellitus were studied and that six of these were classified as having had poor diabetic

Table 7.9 Fisher's exact test: general layout for a 2 × 2 table and its exact probability (p).

a	b	r_1
c	d	r_2
s_1	s_2	n

$$p = \frac{r_1! \, r_2! \, s_1! \, s_2!}{n! \, a! \, b! \, c! \, d!}$$

control during their illness. The patients were also examined to determine if they suffered any of the long-term complications of diabetes, such as deteriorating eyesight or circulatory problems. Table 7.10a displays these results in a 2×2 table. The aim is to determine if good control of diabetes is associated with a lower rate of complications. Among the seven patients with complications, four or 57·1% had poor control, while, among the nine patients without complications, only two or 22·2% could be so classified. Thus, on the basis of the sample results, there seems to be an association between the two factors, but is it statistically significant? Fisher's exact test will be illustrated on these data, even though current opinion would also accept a χ^2 test (see Section 7.10.3).

The easiest way to apply Fisher's exact test is firstly to rearrange the observed 2×2 table so that the number in the top left cell is the smallest of the observed cell frequencies. In this example, the smallest cell frequency is 2 and the rearranged table is shown in Table 7.10b. Labelling the table by the number in the top left cell, this is called set 2. The tables with more extreme results are then obtained by successively reducing the top left figure by 1, with the remainder of the table determined by the fact that the row and column totals are fixed. This process is repeated until a table with a top left cell having a 0 entry is obtained. In the example, set 1, with a 1 in the top left cell, has 5, 8 and 2 in the other three cells determined by the fixed rows and columns (Table

Table 7.10 Fisher's exact test: diabetic control and complications in 16 patients.

(a) Original table

Diabetic control	Diabetic complications		Total
	Present	Absent	
Good	3 (42·9%)	7 (77·8%)	10 (62·5%)
Poor	4 (57·1%)	2 (22·2%)	6 (37·5%)
Total	7 (100·0%)	9 (100·0%)	16 (100·0%)

(b) Rearranged table (set 2)

Diabetic control	Diabetic complications		Total
	Absent	Present	
Poor	2	4	6
Good	7	3	10
Total	9	7	16

(c) Set 1

1	5	6
8	2	10
9	7	16

(d) Set 0

0	6	6
9	1	10
9	7	16

7.10c). This table has more extreme results in the same direction as the original, in that only 1/9 (11·1%) of those with no complications had poor diabetic control, compared with 22·2% in the original table. The final set in the example, set 0 with a zero in the top left, has again even more extreme results.

The one-sided p value for the test is now obtained by summing the probabilities of these three sets of tables. In general, the number of such tables will be one more than the smallest frequency observed in any cell of the original. The probability of set 0 is calculated first. Using Eqn. 7.24:

$$P = \frac{6! \; 10! \; 9! \; 7!}{16! \; 0! \; 6! \; 9! \; 1!}$$

and cancelling this reduces to (using the subscript 0 to denote the set):

$$P_0 = \frac{10! \; 7!}{16! \; 1!}$$

This probability can be computed directly by cancelling a little more, noting that $10!/16! = 1/(16 \times 15 \times 14 \times 13 \times 12 \times 11)$. Calculated in this manner, $P_0 = 0·0008741$.* If some of the numbers are fairly large, tables of log factorials may be employed. Table B.8 gives the logarithms of all the factorials from 0 to 99. From this table, $\log P_0 = \log 10! + \log 7! - \log 16! - \log 1! = 6·55976 + 3·70243 - 13·32062 - 0·0 = -3·05843$. The decimal part of this log value must be positive to get the antilog from a table, so that $\log P_0 = \bar{4}·94157$ ($-4·0 + 0·94157$). The 0·94157 must now be looked up in an antilog table[†] (Table B.9), where its antilog is found to be 8·742. Thus, the antilog of $\bar{4}·94157$ is 0·0008742, which is almost identical to the value previously obtained for P_0.[‡]

Once P_0 (the probability of set 0) is calculated, the probabilities for the remaining sets (if any) are easily obtained. If the four entries in the body of set i, where i is any number, are denoted as a_i, b_i, c_i and d_i, then:

$$P_{i+1} = P_i \times \frac{b_i \times c_i}{a_{i+1} \times d_{i+1}} \tag{7.25}$$

That is, to obtain the probability of a set it is necessary to multiply the probability of the previous set by b and c from that set and divide by a and d from the new set. Thus:

$$P_1 = P_0 \times \frac{6 \times 9}{1 \times 2} = 0·0236007$$

$$P_2 = P_1 \times \frac{8 \times 5}{2 \times 3} = 0·157338$$

---

* Many calculators now have a factorial key, which can make this calculation even easier.
† Looking up 0·9416.
‡ These log calculation could also be performed on a calculator.

In this case, $P_0 + P_1 + P_2 = 0.1818$. Under the assumption of fixed rows and columns and the independence of the two factors being studied, this is the probability that the result, or one even more extreme, is spurious. This, of course, defines the one-sided p value and the two-sided value is obtained by doubling this figure (0.3636). Thus, in this example, diabetic complications are not significantly associated with poor control (Fisher's exact test; two-sided; $p = 0.36$).

As can be seen, Fisher's exact test is quite complex to perform, but a little practice does help. Section C.14 in Appendix C summarizes the steps involved.

Mid-p values [!]

It was pointed out in Section 7.10.3 that Fisher's exact test is considered conservative in that the p value it gives might be too large. The mid-p value has been proposed as a solution to this, and is the same as Fisher's p value described above except only *half* the probability of the observed table is included. Thus the one-sided p value for the example is:

$$P_0 + P_1 + \frac{1}{2}P_2$$

which is 0.103. The two-sided mid-p value is double this, or 0.21.

Mid-p values can be used in a number of situations and are always smaller in magnitude than the conventional p value. Confidence limits can also be based on mid-p values and they are *narrower* than conventional ones. There is controversy over the usefulness of mid-p approaches and they are not adopted in this test (see Rothman and Greenland, 1998).

7.10.5 Confidence intervals for relative risk type measures in independent 2×2 tables

When dealing with unmatched data in a 2×2 table, whether derived from a cross-sectional, a cohort or a case–control study, the appropriate significance test is the usual chi-square test of Section 7.10.3 (equivalent to the z test of Section 7.10.1). The choice of a comparative measure for the table depends on the study design or the precise point one wishes to make.

This present section considers confidence intervals in the situation when relative risks or odds ratios are chosen as the comparative measure. Confidence intervals for the risk difference (attributable risk or excess risk) were considered in Section 7.10.2. Various approaches have been suggested for calculating confidence intervals for relative risk measures and only one will be described here. The method, first suggested by Miettinen (1976), has the advantage that it can be applied to relative risks and odds ratios derived from either pair-matched or independent data. The derivation is briefly described below, but the next few paragraphs can be omitted if the reader does not wish to understand how the formulae arise and just wishes to be able to perform the calculations.

Derivation of the test-based limits [!]

In general, for any statistic that has a normal sampling distribution (such as the difference between means or proportions, for example), a 95% confidence interval is given by:

$$\text{Statistic} \pm 1.96\ \text{SE (statistic)} \qquad (4.11)$$

where SE (statistic) refers to the standard error of the statistic. Now the relative risk (RR) does not have a normal sampling distribution, but the natural logarithm of the relative risk — ln RR — does have.* Thus, if the standard error of ln RR could be found, it would be possible to obtain a 95% confidence interval for ln RR and, by taking the exponential of these limits, the confidence limits for the relative risk itself would result. This is a good example of data transformation to remove skewness and obtain a symmetric, perhaps more normal, distribution (see Section 1.6.7).

Although an exact formula for the standard error of ln RR is not available, an approximation can be obtained from the chi-square value on the 2 × 2 table on which the relative risk was calculated. First, one must remember that for a statistic with a normal sampling distribution a significance test can be formulated as:

$$z = \frac{\text{Sample statistic} - \text{null value}}{\text{SE (statistic)}} \qquad (5.5)$$

where z has a standard normal distribution. For a two-sided 5% level of significance, z must be greater than 1·96 or less than −1·96. As has been said above, the usual significance test for a 2 × 2 table is the chi-square test on 1 degree of freedom, and it so happens that the square root of a 1 d.f. χ^2 is in fact the corresponding z value from the normal distribution. For instance, the 5% (two-sided) critical χ^2 value is 3·841 and its square root is 1·96 — the 5% critical value of the standard normal distribution. Similarly, the χ^2 value of 6·635 corresponds to the z value of 2·576 (the 1% two-sided critical value).

Now, in the context of a mortality study in groups exposed and not exposed to a risk factor, a lack of association between mortality and the risk factor implies a relative risk (RR) of 1·0. Thus, for a significance test of a

---

* The 'ln' denotes the natural logarithm based on the constant e = 2·71828 . . . Usually logarithms are to the base 10, and log 100 = 2 because 10^2 = 100 (see Section 1.6.7). However, since the original derivation employed them, natural logs are also used here. Natural logs are based on powers of e and, since e^2 = 7·39 (referred to as the exponential of 2 and often written exp (2)), the natural log of 7·39 (ln 7·39) = 2. Most good calculators allow for easy calculation of e to any given power or of the ln of any quantity.

relative risk the null value would be 1·0, and for a test of ln RR the null value would be zero (the natural log of 1·0 is zero). Equation 5.5 could then be applied to the statistic ln RR, giving:

$$\chi = \ln RR/SE\ (\ln RR) \tag{7.26}$$

where χ is the square root of the chi-square for the particular table, which is equated with the z of a hypothetical significance test for ln RR. This gives an expression for SE (ln RR) based on the chi-square value:

$$SE\ (\ln RR) = (\ln RR)/\chi \tag{7.27}$$

Substituting this into Eqn. 4.11 gives the 95% confidence interval for ln RR as:

$$\ln RR \pm 1\cdot96\ (\ln RR)/\chi \tag{7.28}$$

If the exponential of this is taken to transform the confidence limits for ln RR to limits for RR, the confidence interval for the relative risk becomes:

$$e^{[\ln RR \pm 1\cdot96\ (\ln RR)/\chi]} \tag{7.29}$$

which simplifies to:

$$RR^{(1\pm1\cdot96/\chi)} \tag{7.30}$$

These confidence limits are called 'test-based limits', since they use the value of the χ^2 test statistic to derive the standard error. Limits obtained with this approach are reasonably good approximations to the exact limits, especially for relative risks not too far from unity.

Limits for the relative risk and odds ratio

An exactly similar argument applies for the odds ratio (OR), so that confidence intervals for the relative risk and odds ratio are given by:

$$RR^{(1\pm z_c/\chi)} \tag{7.31}$$

$$OR^{(1\pm z_c/\chi)} \tag{7.32}$$

where χ is the square root of the appropriate chi-square for the 2×2 table from which the measures were calculated and z_c is the critical value from the normal distribution corresponding to the confidence level chosen. To find these limits, it is necessary to have a calculator that calculates a number to a fractional power. Most scientific instruments now available can do this.

In the prognosis study of smoking following a heart attack (Section 6.5.2, Table 6.1), the relative risk of death for a continued versus stopped smoker was RR = 1·76, and a simple calculation gives χ^2 = 3·03 on 1 degree of freedom. This, of course, is non-significant at a two-sided 5% level. The 95% confidence interval for RR is then given by:

$$1.76^{(1\pm1.96/1.74)} = 1.76^{(1\pm1.13)}$$

or from $1.76^{-0.13}$ to $1.76^{2.13}$, which is from 0.93 to 3.33. Note that this interval overlaps the null value of 1.0, since the association is non-significant.

Note that, if the relative risk is greater than unity, the plus sign in Eqns. 7.31 and 7.32 gives the upper limit of the confidence interval and the minus sign gives the lower limit. If the relative risk is less than unity, the opposite holds. If the relative risk or odds ratio actually equals unity, the χ^2 value will be zero and the limits cannot be calculated using this method.

For the case–control study of head and neck cancer, the odds ratio for a smoker compared with a non-smoker was OR = 2.21 (Section 6.8.1, Table 6.4). The χ^2 for this table is 8.61 on 1 d.f. and therefore the 95% confidence interval is given by:

$$2.21^{(1\pm1.96/2.98)} = 2.21^{(1\pm0.66)}$$

which is from 1.31 to 3.73.

These confidence interval methods are summarized in Section C.13 of Appendix C.

7.11 Comparison of two independent sets of proportions

In Section 7.10.3, the use of the χ^2 test for analysing independent data laid out in a 2×2 table was described. In many cases, however, data will be laid out in a larger table than a 2×2. Either a qualitative variable with perhaps more than two categories is to be compared in two (or more) independent samples, or the relationship between two qualitative variables is being examined in one sample. (The discussion in Section 7.10.4 on Fisher's exact test drew attention to such situations in a 2×2 context.) The χ^2 test is the appropriate test to employ for such tables larger than 2×2 also.

7.11.1 The χ^2 test for tables larger than 2×2

The use of the χ^2 test for a 3×2 table with three rows and two columns will be illustrated. Table 3.2 gave the smoking status of males and females in a study of 2724 persons, and is reproduced in Table 7.11. The null hypothesis in this case would be that the distribution of smoking category is the same in males and females. The data can be equivalently interpreted as a comparison of the proportion of males (or females) between the three smoking categories, in which case the null hypothesis is that the proportion of males (females) is the same in each category.

Expected numbers

The figures in the table suggest a definite difference between males and

Table 7.11 The χ^2 test. Smoking status by sex in 2724 persons (see Table 3·2) (from O'Connor & Daly, 1983, with permission).

(a) Observed numbers

	Male	Female	Total
Current smoker	669 (49·4%)	499 (36·4%)	1168 (42·9%)
Ex-smoker	328 (24·2%)	215 (15·7%)	543 (19·9%)
Never smoker	356 (26·3%)	657 (47·9%)	1013 (37·2%)
	1353 (100·0%)	1371 (100·0%)	2724 (100·0%)

(b) Expected numbers

	Male	Female	Total
Current smoker	580·14	587·86	1168
Ex-smoker	269·71	273·29	543
Never smoker	503·15	509·85	1013
	1353	1371	2724

(c) Calculation

Observed (O)	Expected (E)	O − E	(O − E)²	(O − E)²/E
669	580·14	88·86	7896·100	13·611
328	269·71	58·29	3397·724	12·598
356	503·15	−147·15	21653·123	43·035
499	587·86	−88·86	7896·100	13·432
215	273·29	−58·29	3397·724	12·433
657	509·85	147·15	21653·123	42·470
Total				137·579

$\chi^2 = 137·579$; d.f. = 2; $p < 0·001$.

females and, with such a large sample size, it could be presumed that the observed result actually does reflect a population difference between males and females. For illustrative purposes, however, a χ^2 test will be performed on these data. The approach is identical to that used in the 2 × 2 table. Firstly, the expected numbers (E) under the null hypothesis are calculated. For instance, since there were *in toto* 1168 current smokers from a total of 2724 persons (42·9%), this percentage of males would be expected to be current smokers; 42·9% of 1353 males is 580·14, which is the expected number of male smokers. All the other expected numbers may be calculated in a similar manner and are also given in Table 7.11. In general, to calculate the expected number in any cell, multiply the corresponding row total by the corresponding column total and divide by the total sample size. Thus, the expected number of male smokers can be obtained from 1168 × 1353/2724 = 580·14. Note that, in this example, once two of the expected numbers in a particular column are calculated, the remainder follow by subtraction from the row and column totals, which remain fixed as usual.* It is suggested, however, that each expected number be calculated directly as above, and that a check on the calculations be made by confirming that they do add up to the correct row and column totals.

Once the expected numbers are calculated, the quantities $(O - E)^2/E$ are determined as before for each cell of the table, where O represents the observed numbers in the cells. (Note again that the $O - E$ quantities should sum to zero, apart from rounding errors.) The test statistic is then:

$$\chi^2 = \sum \frac{(O - E)^2}{E}$$

(7.23)

as in the 2×2 table, but with 2 degrees of freedom in this example. In general, for a table with I rows and J columns, there are $(I - 1)(J - 1)$ degrees of freedom, which, with $I = 3$ and $J = 2$, gives 2 degrees of freedom here and, of course, 1 degree of freedom for a 2×2 table. In the smoking example, an extremely large value for χ^2 of 137·579 is obtained, which, when referred to Table B.4 on 2 degrees of freedom, is seen to be highly significant. Unless the sample size is very large, χ^2 values of this magnitude are most unusual. Note that, for tables larger than 2×2, a one-sided χ^2 test is not applicable, since it is impossible to specify beforehand, or indeed interpret, a one-sided alternative hypothesis.

Assumptions

The usual advice proffered is that the χ^2 test can be employed so long as not more than 20% of the expected numbers in the cells are less than 5, with no cell having an expected frequency of less than 1. In the 2×2 situation, of course, this requires that all the expected numbers are greater than 5. As discussed previously in Section 7.10.3, this criterion is perhaps too stringent for the 2×2 table. For larger tables, the criteria are acceptable and adjacent categories can be combined together (collapsed) to satisfy the assumptions. Note that it is the expected numbers in the cells, not the observed numbers, that are relevant.

As has been said, this example could be interpreted as a three-group comparison of the proportion of males, without any change of interpretation. As will be discussed in Section 9.3.1, the χ^2 test easily extends to any size table (3×3, 4×3, etc.) and has applicability in many situations. It is the most widely used test in medical research and one of the most useful tests to know. Its application is summarized in Section C.15 of Appendix C.

---

* In the light of the discussion of the 2×2 table in Section 7.10.3, it can be said that a 3×2 table has 2 degrees of freedom.

7.12 Comparison of paired proportions

7.12.1 The McNemar test for paired (correlated) proportions

The tests for proportions in the previous sections assume that the groups being compared are independent. In this section, a simple test for use with paired samples, where the variable under examination is binary, is described. The test is sometimes called a test for correlated proportions.

Suppose that 18 patients on two different antihypertensive drugs were studied in a crossover trial (see Section 6.13.2). Each patient was given either drug A or drug B for a 1-month period, and a drop in systolic blood pressure of more than 15 mmHg was considered a success and a lesser drop or rise a treatment failure. After a wash-out period, the treatments were switched around so that those previously on drug A were now given drug B and vice versa. The same criteria were again used to assess the effectiveness of the treatment. Essentially, then, there exists a paired sample with each of the 18 patients on each of the two treatments, with the effectiveness of the drugs determined on a qualitative binary scale as either a success or failure.

Paired data like these are often incorrectly analysed. The tendency is to create a 2×2 table for the results, as shown in Table 7.12a, and perform the usual chi-square test on it. Unfortunately, however, this is incorrect; the two groups (drug A and drug B) are not independent and the analysis must take this into account. The table, although suitable for the presentation of results, cannot be used for significance testing, since the 18 persons on each treatment are the same. The analysis must be performed in terms of the 18 pairs of observations—the result on drug A and the result on drug B for each individual.

(a) Summary of results

	Drug A	Drug B	Total
Success	10 (55·6%)	4 (22·2%)	14
Failure	8 (44·4%)	14 (77·8%)	22
Total	18 (100·0%)	18 (100·0%)	36

(b) Layout for test

	Drug A		
Drug B	Success	Failure	Total
Success	1	3	4
Failure	9	5	14
Total	10	8	18

Table 7.12 The McNemar test. Outcome of a paired experiment on 18 paients.

McNemar's χ^2 on 1 d.f. $= \dfrac{(9-3)^2}{9+3} = 3.0$; NS.

Table 7.13 The McNemar test: general layout.

	Group 1	
Group 2	+	–
+	a	b
–	c	d

McNemar's χ^2 on 1 d.f.; $\dfrac{(c-b)^2}{b+c}$

This requires more information than is contained in Table 7.12a and a table must be formed for analysis purposes as shown in Table 7.12b. Note that the data required for this table are *not* derivable from Table 7.12a. The original study data are required. The entry in the top left cell of 1 means that one person (one of the pairs) had a success with both treatments. The entry of 3 means that three persons were treated successfully with drug B but unsuccessfully with drug A. Nine persons, on the other hand, had a successful outcome on drug A and not on drug B. In five persons, neither drug worked. When analysing correlated or paired proportions, the data must be laid out in this way. Table 7.13 shows this general layout. The plus and minus signs can refer to whatever the binary outcome is in the particular data being analysed. For instance, in a pair matched case–control study (see Section 6.7.2), group 1 might signify a case, group 2 a control and the plus sign would correspond to exposure (compare Table 6.5). McNemar's test for this type of data is truly one of the few tests that can be done in one's head. A χ^2 on 1 degree of freedom is calculated as:

$$\chi^2 = \frac{(c-b)^2}{b+c} \tag{7.33}$$

In the example, $\chi^2 = 6^2/12 = 3\cdot0$. For a two-sided 5% significance level, the critical χ^2 value is $3\cdot841$ (Table B.4), so that no significant difference can be claimed between the effects of the drugs.

Note that only the untied observations contribute to this test statistic. The persons (pairs) on whom the effects of the two drugs were the same (two successes or two failures) do not enter into the calculation. These are called tied pairs; only the untied pairs are used. This test is summarized in Section C.16 of Appendix C.

7.12.2 An exact test (the sign test) for paired (correlated) proportions

For small sample sizes, an exact test statistic can be used. The number of pairs with a preference for one drug rather than the other one can be referred to the table for the sign test (Table B.6) entered at *n* equal to the *total number of untied pairs*. Thus, in the example, the test statistic could be 9 (the number of pairs denoting a preference for drug A). For a 5% two-sided significance test for 12 untied pairs, the lower and upper critical values are 2 and 10. The test statistic falls within the acceptance region and theref0ore the results are non-significant. The use of this exact test is advisable when the sample sizes in the statistical table are adequate, even though the χ^2 approach is much easier to perform. See Section C.16 in Appendix C for a summary.

7.12.3 Confidence intervals for a difference in paired proportions

It may seem strange that the significance test only uses the untied pairs, *a* and *b*, and takes no account of the total sample size. This is because it is only the untied pairs that contribute information relating to the existence of a difference. However, in estimating the magnitude of the difference between the paired proportions, all data are used.

The difference between the success rate on drug A and drug B is (from Table 7.12) $0 \cdot 556 - 0 \cdot 222 = 0 \cdot 334$ (expressed as a proportion). Denoting these proportions by p_1 and p_2, it can be shown that:

$$SE(p_1 - p_2) = \frac{1}{N}\sqrt{c + b - \frac{(c-b)^2}{N}}, \qquad (7.34)$$

where c and b are the untied pairs in Table 7.13, and N in this case is the *total number of pairs*, rather than the total number of untied pairs.* The 95% confidence interval for the difference between paired proportions is then given by the usual formula:

$$(p_1 - p_2) \pm 1 \cdot 96 \ SE \ (p_1 - p_2) \qquad (7.35)$$

In the example, this is:

$$(0 \cdot 556 - 0 \cdot 222) \pm 1 \cdot 96\sqrt{12 - (36/18)}/18$$

which is $0 \cdot 334 \pm 0 \cdot 344$ or from $-0 \cdot 010$ to $0 \cdot 678$. Thus, at a 95% level of confidence, drug A could be from $1 \cdot 0\%$ worse than drug B or up to $67 \cdot 8\%$ better. Section C.16 in Appendix C summarizes the analysis of paired proportions. This and other, more exact, formulations are reviewed by Newcombe (1998c).

7.12.4 Confidence intervals for an odds ratio in paired data

For pair-matched data in a case–control study, the odds ratio is estimated from Eqn. 6.14:

$$OR = c/b \qquad (7.36)$$

where c is the number of pairs with the case exposed to the risk factor but the control not exposed, and b is the number of pairs with the control exposed but

---

* Some texts give the standard-error formula as $(1/N) \sqrt{(b + c)}$. Equation 7.34, however, is more accurate.

the case not exposed (see Table 6.5 in Section 6.8.2). The appropriate chi-square for such a matched study is McNemar's chi-square (Section 7.12.1), and test-based confidence limits, based on Eqn. 7.32, can be used for the paired odds ratio estimate if the square root of this chi-square is used in the formula. Section C.16 summarizes confidence interval estimation for the paired odds ratio.

7.12.5 Sequential analysis

The sequential clinical trial was described in Section 6.13.1. The trial is essentially based on entering and evaluating pairs of patients, with an analysis performed as each pair's outcome is determined. Suppose it is wished to compare the effects of treatments A and B. As pairs of patients, suitably matched,* become available, one of the pair receives (at random) treatment A and the other treatment B. For each pair of patients, four outcomes are possible: both treatments a success; both treatments a failure; treatment A a success and treatment B a failure; treatment A a failure and treatment B a success. For the purpose of the sequential trial, the first two outcomes are described as 'tied pairs' and are discarded from the analysis. Only the 'untied pairs' are used in the comparison of the two treatments. This is exactly the same situation as the one that arises with the tests for correlated (paired) proportions (Sections 7.12.1 and 7.12.2), but here the analysis is performed sequentially.

Now, suppose a score of +1 is given to an outcome in which treatment A is a success and treatment B a failure, and a score of −1 to an outcome in which B is a success and A is a failure. As the trial proceeds, a cumulative score is kept. It is evident that, if treatment A is markedly superior to treatment B, an increasing positive score will be cumulated, whilst an increasing negative score will cumulate in the reverse case. If there is no marked difference between A and B, then scores of +1 and −1 will occur in a random fashion, so that the total score will oscillate around zero. These three possible outcomes are then used to make a decision about the relative efficacy of the two treatments.

The application of sequential analysis makes use of a *sequential analysis chart*, and such a chart is shown in Fig. 7.1. This chart was used in the analysis of a clinical trial set up to determine if the occurrence of a particular complication of a disease was increased when a particular therapy was employed. The end-point of the trial was, unusually enough, an unwanted treatment effect. The study was performed on premature infants with the respiratory distress syndrome. Diuretic treatment of such infants to reduce fluid retention and help alleviate their symptoms is often used. It had been suggested that a particular diuretic, furosemide—which shall be called treatment A—seemed

* On the basis of prognostic variables, or using each two consecutive eligible patients to form a pair.

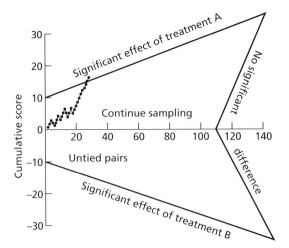

Fig. 7.1 Sequential analysis chart for comparing the effect of furosemide (A) and chlorothiazide (B) on a heart score in premature infants (from Green *et al.*, 1983, with permission).

to increase the incidence of a particular heart condition (patent ductus arteriosus), a complication in premature infants with the respiratory distress syndrome. It was decided to compare the heart functions of infants under treatment and infants on an alternative diuretic (chlorothiazide), which, for simplicity, shall be called treatment B. One of each member of consecutively admitted pairs of infants was assigned randomly to treatment A and the other to treatment B. After a specified period, a heart score, ranging from 0 to 6 (6 being a severe grading), was determined blindly on each infant and each pair was classified as 'favouring' treatment A or B (if not tied), according to which infant had the highest score. Whenever a pair of infants did not have an identical score (untied pairs), the results were entered into the chart in Fig. 7.1. The horizontal axis on the sequential analysis chart records the number of untied pairs included in the trial. The vertical axis records the cumulative score as the trial proceeds (a positive score indicating, in the example, that the treatment A infant had a higher heart score than the treatment B infant). In the figure, the cumulative score is shown by the zigzag line. The meaning of the four 'boundary lines' marked on the chart can now be explained. A trial may be terminated as soon as the score line reaches one of the boundary lines. If the score line crosses the upper boundary line, this is interpreted to mean that treatment A resulted in a significantly higher heart score than treatment B. The opposite interpretation applies if the score line crosses the lower boundary line. Of course, the score line will not cross either boundary line unless a relatively high score has accumulated in favour of one or other of the treatments. If, on the other hand, the score line crosses either of the end boundary lines, this is interpreted to mean that there appears to be no difference between the two methods of treatment; the score is not high enough in relation to the number of untied pairs tested to indicate a statistically significant advantage of one treatment over the other.

The trial continues until the score line reaches one of the boundary lines, at which point a decision can be reached, at a predetermined level of significance and power, about the relative advantages of the two methods of treatment. In the example, the score line reached the upper boundary line after 28 untied pairs had been recorded. When the heart score was higher on an infant on treatment B, the score line would move downwards. When the score was higher in a treatment A infant, it moved upwards. Twenty-two of the untied pairs favoured treatment A, six favoured B and, eventually, the cumulative score of 16 in favour of A was reached. This was sufficient to cause a rejection of the null hypothesis that there was no difference in treatment effects and to declare that treatment A significantly increased the heart score in these infants. It can be seen that once the boundary lines have been fixed, plotting and analysing the results of the trial as they become available are quite simple. The complexity of the technique lies in fixing the boundary lines for the particular experiment being conducted, and details of this are not given here. The chart is set up, however, based on the same criteria for determining a fixed sample size in the more usual type of experiment (this topic is considered in detail in Chapter 8). The chart in the trial discussed was based on a β error of 0·05 in detecting a twofold preference for one of the treatments at a two-sided significance level, α, of 0·05 (see Section 5.7.2).

7.13 Comparison of two counts

If two counts are to be compared directly, then the counts must be based on the same time period or same underlying distribution in space or time. If this is not the case, then the counts must be converted to rates to correct for the different periods of observation and it is the rates that must be compared (see Section 7.14). As discussed in Section 5.11, the sampling distribution of a count is Poisson and some of the methods below rely on a normal approximation to the Poisson distribution. Therefore, for the methods described in this section, the two counts should be greater than 10.

7.13.1 The z test for two counts

Suppose that two cultures of bacteria were prepared in equal volumes and incubated on nutrient media. The number of colonies eventually growing on the two plates is 11 and 27. Is there evidence of different bacterial concentrations? The significance test for this is rather simple. If x_1 and x_2 are the observed counts, then a test using the normal approximation to the Poisson is:

$$z = \frac{x_1 - x_2}{\sqrt{(x_1 + x_2)}}$$

(7.37)

where:

$$\text{SE}(x_1 - x_2) = \sqrt{(x_1 + x_2)} \qquad (7.38)$$

is the standard error of the difference between the counts. For this example, the z statistic is $(27 - 11)/\sqrt{(27 + 11)}$, which is $2 \cdot 60$, showing a significant difference between the counts and thus between the bacterial concentrations (5% two-sided test).

7.13.2 Confidence intervals for the difference in two counts

A 95% confidence interval for the difference between the two counts is given by:

$$(x_1 - x_2) \pm 1 \cdot 96\sqrt{(x_1 + x_2)} \qquad (7.39)$$

Note that the same standard-error estimator is employed for both the confidence interval and the hypothesis test. In this case, the confidence interval for the difference between the counts is $16 \pm 1 \cdot 96\sqrt{(38)}$ or from $3 \cdot 9$ to $28 \cdot 1$; the difference measure is not directly interpretable in the example, however, whereas the ratio of the counts would estimate the ratio of the concentrations. A confidence interval for the ratio of two Poisson variables will be considered in Section 7.14.3, when the more general ratio of two rates will be discussed. The significance test and confidence interval formulae for comparing two counts are summarized in Section C.17 in Appendix C.

7.14 Comparison of two rates

In medical applications, there are two main sources of rates for analysis. The first is in the vital-statistics area, where mortality or morbidity are expressed as events per 100, 1000, 100000 or whatever of a population (usually per year). Essentially, the rates are derived from a count of relevant cases (deaths, new cases of a cancer) over a period and the denominator is based on a census population count (usually a mid-period average). In this application, the population can be thought of in terms of a number of person-years of observation. For instance, a rate based on 2 years' worth of cases in a population with an average size of n would be calculated with $2n$ person-years of observation.

The second application where the person-year approach is useful is for cohort studies, particularly when a variable follow-up is involved. In this situation, as an alternative to life table approaches, which will be discussed in Section 7.15, the rate can be expressed with the denominator based on the total person-years of follow-up in the study. For both these scenarios, the usual statistical analysis makes the assumption that the denominator is measured without sampling variation and that the number of cases or deaths follows a Poisson distribution.

7.14.1 The z test for two rates

Suppose that the 32·10 per million population annual death rate from acute lymphatic leukaemia, discussed in Section 5.11, was to be compared with a rate of 22·41 per million in a second region. The first figure arose from 11 deaths in 0·3427 million person-years and suppose the second figure is based on 17 deaths in 0·7586 million person-years. (Remember that the person-years at risk must be expressed in the same units as the rates themselves.) Table 7.14 illustrates the data.

Using similar arguments to those in Section 7.10.1 for the comparison of two proportions, letting θ be the common rate in the two regions under the null hypothesis and using Eqn. 4.21 for the standard error of a rate:

$$SE\,(r_1 - r_2) = \sqrt{\frac{\theta}{PYRS_1} + \frac{\theta}{PYRS_2}} \tag{7.40}$$

The best estimate of this common rate θ is the total number of deaths divided by the total person-years at risk. This is equivalent to a weighted average of the two observed rates weighted by the person-years. This pooled estimate of θ is:

$$r = \frac{PYRS_1(r_1) + PYRS_2(r_2)}{PYRS_1 + PYRS_2} \tag{7.41}$$

giving as an estimate of the standard error under the null hypothesis:

$$SE\,(r_1 - r_2) = \sqrt{\frac{r}{PYRS_1} + \frac{r}{PYRS_2}} \tag{7.42}$$

where r, the pooled rate, is given by Eqn. 7.41. The significance test for comparing two rates is then formulated as:

$$z = \frac{r_1 - r_2}{\sqrt{\dfrac{r}{PYRS_1} + \dfrac{r}{PYRS_2}}} \tag{7.43}$$

Table 7.14 Childhood deaths from acute lymphatic leukaemia in two regions.

Group i	Region 1	Region 2
No. of deaths (x_i)	11	17
Person-years at risk ($\times 10^6$) ($PYRS_i$)	0·3427	0·7586
Annual rate per 10^6 (r_i)	32·10	22·41

$z = 0·93$; NS.
Rate difference: 9·69 per 10^6 (95% CI: −12·07 to 31·45).
Rate ratio: 1·43 (95% CI: 0·61 to 3·24).

This is referred to tables of the normal distribution. In the example, the pooled value of the rate (r) is 25·42 and:

$$z = \frac{32{\cdot}10 - 22{\cdot}41}{\sqrt{\dfrac{25{\cdot}42}{0{\cdot}3427} + \dfrac{25{\cdot}42}{0{\cdot}7586}}} = \frac{9{\cdot}69}{10{\cdot}38} = 0{\cdot}93$$

This does not reach the two-sided critical value of 1·96, so that a significant difference between the regions is not demonstrated at a 5% two-sided level.

7.14.2 Confidence intervals for the difference in two rates

For confidence intervals, the standard error of the difference between two rates is not based on a pooled estimate of the rates, but rather on:

$$\text{SE}\,(r_1 - r_2) = \sqrt{\frac{r_1}{PYRS_1} + \frac{r_2}{PYRS_2}} \tag{7.44}$$

which, for the example, is 11·10, compared with 10·38 based on Eqn. 7.42. The formula for the confidence interval is then:

$$(r_1 - r_2) \pm z_c \text{SE}\,(r_1 - r_2) \tag{7.45}$$

where, as usual, z_c is the appropriate value from the normal distribution. The 95% confidence interval for the rate difference in the example is:

$$9{\cdot}69 \pm 1{\cdot}96\,(11{\cdot}10)$$

which is from −12·07 to +31·45. At a 95% level of confidence, region 1 could have an annual childhood mortality rate from leukaemia ranging from a figure of 12·07 per million lower than region 2 to 31·45 per million higher. The significance test and confidence interval formulae for the difference in two rates are summarized in Section C.17, Appendix C.

7.14.3 Confidence intervals for the ratio of two rates

If it is required to put confidence limits on the ratio of two rates (as opposed to their difference), an approach can be used which does not use the results of the significance test. The same example as above will be taken, comparing childhood death rates in two regions (Table 7.14).

The ratio of the two death rates is 32·10/22·41 = 1·43, showing that the rate in region 1 is nearly one-and-a-half times as high as that in region 2. To calculate confidence limits for this, note that the rate ratio (which will be denoted RR)* can be expressed as

$$RR = (x_1/x_2)(PYRS_2/PYRS_1) \tag{7.46}$$

---

* RR was used previously to denote a relative risk as determined from a 2×2 table. The rate ratio is obviously a similar concept, though derived from a different data structure.

where x_1/x_2 is the ratio of two Poisson variables—the numbers of deaths in regions 1 and 2. The problem then reduces to determining a confidence interval for this ratio, since the person-years can be considered fixed.

Unusually enough, use is made of the binomial distribution for this calculation (Ederer & Mantel, 1974). The argument goes as follows. Out of a total of $x_1 + x_2$ events (deaths), x_1 were observed in region 1. Thus:

$$p = \frac{x_1}{x_1 + x_2} \tag{7.47}$$

can be considered as a single (binomial) proportion calculated on a sample size of $x_1 + x_2$. With the methods of Section 4.4, using either the exact method (Table B.11) or the normal approximation (Eqn. 4.5), confidence limits for the population value of p can be calculated. Let p_l and p_u denote these lower and upper binomial limits. Noting that:

$$\frac{x_1}{x_2} = \frac{p}{1-p} \tag{7.48}$$

the binomial confidence limits can be substituted into this equation to give lower and upper confidence limits for the ratio of the Poisson events as, respectively:

$$\frac{p_l}{1-p_l} \quad \text{and} \quad \frac{p_u}{1-p_u} \tag{7.49}$$

Using Eqn. 7.46, the lower and upper confidence limits for the rate ratio (RR_l and RR_u) are:

$$RR_l = \frac{p_l}{1-p_l} \frac{PYRS_2}{PYRS_1} \tag{7.50}$$

$$RR_u = \frac{p_u}{1-p_u} \frac{PYRS_2}{PYRS_1} \tag{7.51}$$

where p_l and p_u are the lower and upper binomial confidence limits for the population value of $x_1/(x_1 + x_2)$.

In the example, the relevant binomial proportion is 11/28 and, from Table B.11 (see also Section 4.4), the lower and upper 95% confidence limits for this are 0·2150 and 0·5942. When these are substituted into Eqns. 7.50 and 7.51, the confidence limits for the rate ratio of 1·43 are:

$$RR_l = \frac{(0·2150)(0·7586)}{(1-0·2150)(0·3427)} = 0·61$$

and:

$$RR_u = \frac{(0·5942)(0·7586)}{(1-0·5942)(0·3427)} = 3·24$$

Thus, the 95% confidence interval for the ratio of death rates in regions 1 and 2 is from 0·61 to 3·24. This procedure is summarized in Section C.17 of Appendix C.

7.15 Comparison of two life tables [!]

This section considers the analysis of mortality in the variable-time follow-up situation arising in cohort studies or clinical trials. (The reader should refer back to Section 6.6, where the topic is introduced without calculational detail.) The methods are not confined to mortality as an end-point but can be used to analyse any non-recurrent end-point, such as the first manifestation of a particular condition. The central point is that the analysis does not concentrate on data available at a fixed follow-up time (such as 5 years) but takes account of the entire pattern of mortality over a time period. It is possible to analyse such data using a person-years denominator, but this requires the assumption that mortality remains constant over the entire period of follow-up. The topic is illustrated using a simple example and initial concentration is on the concepts underlying a life table calculation for a single group. The comparison of two life tables is then considered.

7.15.1 Variable-time follow-up

Figure 7.2 shows, schematically, the follow-up of 14 male patients entered into a cohort study between 1990 and 1999. The study is being analysed in the year 2000 and no data after 1 January in that year are available. The left-hand side of the figure shows the 'lifespan' of each of the patients (labelled from A to N) in calendar time. Patient A, for instance, entered into the study in 1990 and died near the end of 1993 (between 3 and 4 years from study entry). Patient C

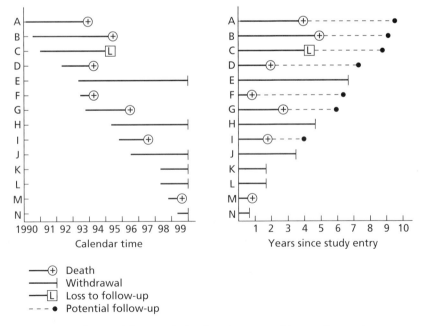

Fig. 7.2 Diagram showing follow-up of 14 male patients entered into a cohort study.

was lost track of during 1995 but was known to be alive just over 4 years after study entry (a loss to follow-up). Patient E entered the study in mid-1993 and was alive at the end of 1999 (more than 6 years after entry into the study). Similarly, patients H, J, K, L and N were all alive at the time the study was being analysed and are considered as withdrawals. The right-hand side of Fig. 7.2 shows the patient histories plotted from study entry, rather than in calendar time. The dashed lines refer to the potential periods of follow-up, had the patients not died or been lost to follow-up. Suppose now that one wanted to calculate the 4-year mortality from time of entry into the study. Some of the incorrect methods already referred to in Section 6.6.2 will be illustrated first. Using the definition of number dead within 4 years divided by the total number of patients, the figure of 6 (patients A, D, F, G, I and M) divided by 14 = 42·9% would be obtained. This, however, is unduly optimistic, because it assumes that patients J, K, L and N, the withdrawals, who were not actually followed for as long as 4 years, would in fact have remained alive until the end of the 4 years. This is an untenable assumption. Alternatively, a 4-year survival rate might have been defined, putting the number alive at 4 years over the total number in the study. This gives 4 (patients B, C, E and H) divided by 14, or 28·6%, which corresponds to a 4-year mortality of 71·4%. This is an unduly pessimistic figure, since its calculation assumes that the four withdrawals in the denominator would not have survived the full 4 years. In fact, the only unbiased estimator of a 4-year mortality rate is obtained by confining the analysis to only those patients actually followed for 4 years, or those who could have been followed if they had not died. This reduces the study cohort from the original 14 to nine patients only (A to I) and gives a 4-year mortality of 5/9 = 55·5%.* Because of the variable length of follow-up, the alternative to biased estimates of the mortality rate seems to require sacrificing much of the available information. It will now be seen how the clinical life table approach avoids this problem and yet provides an unbiased estimate of mortality.

7.15.2 Structure of the clinical life table

As was said in Section 6.6.4, this approach requires a division of the total follow-up period into intervals. Supposing the 10 years of the study are now divided into 10 intervals of 1 year each; the data required for calculating a mortality rate using the clinical life table approach are then the total number alive at the start of the study and the numbers of deaths, withdrawals alive and losses to follow-up observed in each interval.

The method is based on the law of combining conditional probabilities,

---

* It may seem strange that patient M, who died within the 4 years, is not included with A to I. It is necessary, however, to take account of the potential period of follow-up or otherwise, for later years in the study, only deaths would be included, without the possibility of any further survivors being added on (since they could not have the required potential years of follow-up). This would essentially give an over-pessimistic mortality figure.

Time (years)	0		1		2
Interval no.		1		2	
No. alive	100		45		30
No. dying		55		15	

Table 7.15 Simple example of conditional probabilities. *P* (event) means the probability of the event.

$P_1 = P$ (survival 0–1) = 45/100 = 0·45
$P_2 = P$ (survival 0–2) = 30/100 = 0·3
$p_2 = P$ (survival 1–2, given alive at 1) = 30/45 = 0·6667
$P_2 = p_2 P_1$

discussed in Chapter 2 (Eqn. 2.3). To take a simple analogy, conditional probabilities combine like stages in a journey. To fly from Paris to New York via London, one must first get to London; when in London, one has then to fly to New York. Take an example of this principle in terms of survival rates or probabilities. Table 7.15 displays a simple mortality study. One hundred persons enter the study at time zero. Fifty-five die in the first year (leaving 45 alive) and 15 persons die in the second year, leaving 30 survivors at the end of 2 years. The 2-year survival is then 30/100 = 0·3, expressed as the probability of surviving 2 years. Now the 1-year survival probability is, obviously, given by 45/100 = 0·45. Of these 45 persons who survived the first year, 15 die in the succeeding year and 30 survive, so that the survival from the start of year 2 to the end of year 2, conditional on being alive at the start, is 30/45 = 0·6667. Note, however, that 0·45 × 0·6667 = 0·3. This is an example of the application of Eqn. 2.3. To survive two intervals of time, it is necessary to survive the first interval and, given that, then to survive the second interval. If the probability of surviving from time 0 (study commencement) to time *i* (the end of the *i*th interval or year) is denoted by P_i and the conditional probability of surviving the *i*th interval (from time $i - 1$ to *i*) by p_i, then the generalization of this is:

$$P_i = p_i P_{i-1} \qquad (7.52)$$

where P_0 is the probability of surviving to time 0, the start of the study, which must be 1. The P_i are called cumulative or unconditional survival probabilities.

The clinical life table utilizes this relationship by calculating the conditional probability of surviving each interval defined for the study, and then calculating the unconditional (cumulative) probabilities of survival from study commencement to the end of each interval. The cumulative mortality probabilities are obtained by subtracting the survival probabilities from 1 and can then be converted to percentages.

How, then, can the conditional probability of surviving each interval be calculated? First, some notation must be introduced. The intervals in the study are numbered from 1 to *i*, where 1 denotes the first interval, running from time

0 to time 1 (years or months). Table 7.16 displays the notation adopted. It has already been mentioned that the life table calculation requires that n_1, the number entering the study (and therefore the first interval), and d_i and w_i, the deaths and withdrawals/losses in each defined interval, are known. No distinction is made between withdrawals due to study termination and losses to follow-up. It will now be shown how, starting with these data, an unbiased estimate of the 4-year mortality in the example discussed above can be calculated. Table 7.17 lays out the data. Fourteen persons entered the study, and in the first interval there were two deaths (patients F and M—see Fig. 7.2) and one withdrawal (patient N). If there were no withdrawals, the probability of dying in the first interval would be just 2/14, but the single withdrawal must somehow be taken into account. If it can be assumed that any withdrawals occurred on average halfway into the interval, it could be argued that each withdrawal only contributes a 'half-person' to the number at risk, and that the

Table 7.16 Clinical life table notation.

Meaning	Symbol
Interval	i
End-points of interval i	$i-1\ i$
Numbers entering interval i	n_i
Numbers dying in interval i	d_i
Numbers withdrawn or lost to follow-up in interval i	w_i
Adjusted number at risk at the start of interval i	n'_i
Conditional probability of death in interval i	q_i
Conditional probability of surviving interval i	p_i
Unconditional probability of surviving from time 0 to the end of interval i (i.e. to time i)	P_i
Unconditional probability of dying by the end of interval i (i.e. by time i)	Q_i

Table 7.17 Clinical life table for data of Fig. 7.2 (males).

(1) Interval $i\,(i-1)$ to i	(2) Numbers entering interval n_i	(3) Numbers withdrawn/ lost during interval w_i	(4) Adjusted number at risk n'_i	(5) Deaths during interval d_i	(6) Probability of death during interval q_i	(7) Probability of survival during interval p_i	(8) Cumulative probability of survival to end of interval P_i	(9) Cumulative probability of death by end of interval Q_i
1	14	1	13·5	2	0·1481	0·8519	0·8519	0·1481
2	11	2	10·0	2	0·2000	0·8000	0·6815	0·3185
3	7	0	7·0	1	0·1429	0·8571	0·5841	0·4159
4	6	1	5·5	1	0·1818	0·8182	0·4779	0·5221
5	4	2	3·0	1	0·3333	0·6667	0·3186	0·6814
6	1	1	–					

denominator of the probability of death should be reduced accordingly. Instead of 14 persons being at risk of death in the interval, there would be only 13·5 persons and the probability of death would be calculated as $2/13\cdot5 = 0\cdot1481$. This is the total number of deaths in the interval, divided by what is called the adjusted number at risk. This is a central feature of the life table, that each withdrawal alive due to study termination or loss to follow-up in an interval only contributes one-half to the number at risk required to calculate a mortality probability in the interval. This is not the only assumption that can be made. Since it is similar to an assumption made to calculate life tables in vital statistics (see Section 11.5.5), it is called the actuarial assumption and the corresponding life table is called an *actuarial life table*. The adjusted number at risk is denoted n'_i (in the ith interval) and:

$$n'_i = n_i - 0\cdot5w_i \qquad (7.53)$$

$$q_i = d_i/n'_i \qquad (7.54)$$

where q_i is the estimated probability of death in the interval. The (conditional) probability of surviving the interval is then:

$$p_i = 1 - q_i \qquad (7.55)$$

which is given in column 7 of Table 7.17 as 0·8519 for the first interval. Equation 7.52 is now used to calculate the cumulative probability of survival from the start of the study (time 0) to the end of interval 1. This is, of course, the same as the conditional probability for the first interval, so $P_1 = p_1 = 0\cdot8519$. The cumulative probability of death is then obtained by subtracting this from 1:

$$Q_i = 1 - P_i \qquad (7.56)$$

which is 0·1481 or 14·81% for $i=1$.

Now move to the second row of Table 7.17 to calculate the same quantities for the second interval. The number entering the interval is given by the number entering the previous interval, less the withdrawals and deaths in that interval:

$$n_i = n_{i-1} - (w_{i-1} + d_{i-1}) \qquad (7.57)$$

which gives a total of 11. Check this with Fig. 7.2. The calculations proceed as before. Since there were two withdrawals in this interval, the adjusted number at risk is $11\cdot0 - 1 = 10\cdot0$, and the conditional probability of surviving the interval is 0·8000. The cumulative probability of surviving to the end of the interval is again obtained using Eqn. 7.52, multiplying this conditional probability of 0·8000 by the cumulative probability of surviving to the end of the previous interval (0·8519). This gives $P_2 = 0\cdot6815$ and a cumulative probability of death by the end of the second interval at 2 years as $1 - 0\cdot6815 = 0\cdot3185$ or 31·9%. This process is continued for the next three intervals, as shown in Table 7.17. The 4-year mortality calculated in this way turns out to be 0·5221 or 52·21%. This is the best estimate of 4-year mortality available from the data. The final life table estimates the probability of death by the start of each interval to the end of the study. Usually, the cumulative probabilities of survival or death would be displayed graphically, as already illustrated in Fig. 6.2 on a real example.

The main assumption underlying the clinical life table is that withdrawals due to study termination would have subsequently experienced a similar mortality rate to those actually followed for a longer period. Thus, the method does not allow for any secular changes in mortality and requires that all study participants, irrespective of when they entered the study in calendar time, are exposed to the same risks of death. It has been mentioned that losses to follow-up are treated in the same way as withdrawals, so it is also assumed that persons lost to follow-up are similar to persons with whom contact was maintained. This is unlikely to be so and the number of losses must be kept to a minimum.

7.15.3 Confidence intervals for cumulative life table survival (mortality)

A confidence interval for the cumulative proportion surviving to the end of interval i (P_i) is easily obtained. If there were no losses to follow-up or withdrawals, then the usual method using the normal approximation (Eqn. 4.5) could be applied, giving for the 95% interval:

$$P_i \pm 1 \cdot 96 \; \text{SE} \; (P_i) \tag{7.58}$$

where:

$$\text{SE} \; (P_i) = \sqrt{\frac{P_i(1 - P_i)}{n_1}} \quad \text{(no losses or withdrawals)} \tag{7.59}$$

with n_1 as the total number alive *at the start of the study*. (Note that the subscript i here refers to the time period in the life table and does not denote a particular group of patients.)

The problem is that n_1 is too large a figure for this standard error, since the estimation of P_i is based on a smaller sample size, due to withdrawals and losses to follow-up. To correct for this, n_1 is replaced by an 'effective sample size' (denoted $n_{(\text{eff})}$) for the entire study at the end of interval i. (This effective sample size should not be confused with the adjusted number at risk at the start of any particular interval; see Eqn. 7.53).

Now, at the end of interval i, the actual number of persons alive is n_{i+1} and, in the absence of withdrawals or losses this, as a proportion of the total entering the study (n_1), would represent the cumulative survival proportion P_i of the entire study group. Thus:

$$n_{i+1} = P_i n_1 \quad \text{(no losses or withdrawals)} \tag{7.60}$$

or:

$$n_1 = n_{i+1}/P_i \tag{7.61}$$

With losses and withdrawals, however, an effective total study size which would have given rise to the same number alive at the end of the interval can be defined using Eqn. 7.61, giving:

$$n_{(eff)} = n_{i+1}/P_i \tag{7.62}$$

Note that $n_{(eff)}$ is dependent on the interval for which it is calculated, but this is not explicit in the notation. This figure is then used in Eqn. 7.59 instead of n_1 to give a standard error for P_i that allows for losses and withdrawals:

$$SE\,(P_i) = \sqrt{\frac{P_i(1-P_i)}{n_{(eff)}}} \tag{7.63}$$

When this is substituted in Eqn. 7.58, the 95% confidence interval formula for the cumulative proportion surviving to the end of interval i in the actuarial life table is:

$$P_i \pm 1.96\sqrt{\frac{P_i(1-P_i)}{n_{(eff)}}} \tag{7.64}$$

The exact same formula can be used for confidence intervals for the cumulative proportion dead by the end of an interval (Q_i). Equation 7.64 is a fairly good approximation, though it tends to give somewhat conservative values. It is possible, too, with quite small numbers, that one of the confidence limits obtained may fall outside the range 0 to 1 and be essentially uninterpretable. In such an event the upper or lower limit, as the case may be, should be set at 1 or 0. It is important to note that, as for all calculations in this book, the proportions should be expressed in decimal rather than percentage form for correct use of the formulae.

Applying this method to the 4-year cumulative survival probability of 0.4779 (47.8%) obtained in Table 7.17, the effective sample size is, with $n_5 = 4$:

$$n_{(eff)} = 4/0.4779 = 8.37$$

which is less than the actual sample size of 14. The 95% confidence interval is:

$$0.4779 \pm 1.96\sqrt{[(0.4779)(0.5221)/8.37]}$$

which is 0.4779 ± 0.3384 or from 14.0% to 81.6%.

7.15.4 The Kaplan–Meier life table

The actuarial method of calculating the life table described in Section 7.15.2 is quite easy to do with the aid of a calculator. An alternative method, which requires a computer for large sample sizes, is called the *product-limit* or

Kaplan–Meier life table (Kaplan & Meier, 1958). Essentially, this approach does not predefine the interval in terms of months or years, but instead chooses the interval on the basis of the observed data. Interval end-points are chosen at the times of each death or withdrawal, so that the intervals are as narrow as possible, given the data. The logic behind the method is similar to that described above, but the somewhat arbitrary choice of interval widths is avoided. Because of the inherent accuracy of the method and because of its availability in many computer packages, the Kaplan–Meier life table is the most commonly used in clinical research.

7.15.5 Confidence intervals for a cumulative life table survival (mortality) difference

When two life tables are being compared, the difference between the cumulative proportions surviving to the end of a particular interval (or equivalently dying before the interval end) can be calculated, together with a confidence interval for the difference. Suppose that, in addition to the 14 male patients analysed in the last section, follow-up of 20 females was also undertaken. Table 7.18 gives the life table for these patients. The 4-year survival in males is $P_4 = 0.4779$ (47·8%) and is 0·2183 (21·8%) in the females. To calculate a confidence interval for the 0·2596 (26·0%) survival advantage of males,[*] the approach of Section 7.10.2 can be used, substituting the effective sample sizes in the appropriate formula. Using obvious notation (and dropping the subscript 4 denoting the end of the fourth interval), Eqn. 7.22 gives, for the 95% confidence interval:

$$(P_M - P_F) \pm 1.96 \text{ SE } (P_M - P_F) \tag{7.65}$$

where:

$$\text{SE } (P_M - P_F) = \sqrt{\frac{P_M(1 - P_M)}{n_{M(eff)}} + \frac{P_F(1 - P_F)}{n_{F(eff)}}} \tag{7.66}$$

and $n_{M(eff)}$ and $n_{F(eff)}$ are the effective sample sizes in the males and females, respectively, at the end of year 4. Using Eqn. 7.62, these are 8·37 and 9·16, respectively. The confidence interval for the difference between male and female 4-year survival is thus:

$$0.2596 \pm 1.96 \sqrt{\frac{(0.4779)(0.5221)}{8.37} + \frac{(0.2183)(0.7817)}{9.16}}$$

which is 0·2596 ± 1·96 (0·2201) = 0·2596 ± 0·4314. The 95% confidence interval for the survival advantage of males at 4 years is from −17·2% to 69·1%.

---

[*] This is the same as the mortality excess (risk difference) in females.

Table 7.18 Clinical life table for 20 females.

(1) Interval i $(i-1)$ to i	(2) Numbers entering interval n_i	(3) Numbers withdrawn/ lost during interval w_i	(4) Adjusted number at risk n'_i	(5) Deaths during interval d_i	(6) Probability of death during interval q_i	(7) Probability of survival during interval p_i	(8) Cumulative probability of survival to end of interval P_i
1	20	2	19·0	4	0·2105	0·7895	0·7895
2	14	2	13·0	3	0·2308	0·7692	0·6073
3	9	1	8·5	3	0·3529	0·6471	0·3930
4	5	1	4·5	2	0·4444	0·5556	0·2183
5	2	0	2·0	1	0·5000	0·5000	0·1092
6	1	1		–			

Obviously it is also possible to derive a significance test to compare the cumulative life table survivals (or equivalently mortalities) at a fixed point in time, but in general it is preferable to look at the life table curves in their entirety. Sometimes, life table curves for two different groups may cross over each other, suggesting a survival advantage for one group at one point in time and a disadvantage at a second time point. In such a case, also, it is useful to have an overall comparison which in some sense might compare the average experience over time.

7.15.6 The logrank test for two life tables

The logrank test (Peto & Peto, 1972) (also referred to as the Mantel–Haenzel test; see Section 11.3.1) and its related summary measure are the most commonly employed. Usually, this method is applied to the Kaplan–Meier life table (Section 7.15.4), but, to illustrate the test, an adaptation suitable for the comparison of two actuarial life tables is described below. Essentially, the logrank test involves the comparison of the observed number of deaths in each group with the number of deaths that would be expected if the groups had similar mortalities. These observed and expected deaths are calculated in each interval for each life table and summed over all the intervals. Table 7.19 details the necessary calculations for the comparison of the male and female life tables given in Tables 7.17 and 7.18.

All calculations are based on the adjusted numbers at risk (see Eqn. 7.53) and the observed deaths for each interval. The expected number of deaths in each interval is obtained in the usual manner, under the hypothesis that the mortalities in the groups being compared are the same. In the first interval, for instance, there was a total of six observed deaths in 32·5 persons at risk. Of these 32·5, 13·5 were male, so that one would expect:

Table 7.19 Layout for the logrank test comparing male and female life tables.

Interval i	Adjusted numbers at risk			Observed deaths (O)			Expected deaths (E)	
	Male	Female	Total	Male	Female	Total	Male	Female
1	13·5	19·0	32·5	2	4	6	2·4923	3·5077
2	10·0	13·0	23·0	2	3	5	2·1739	2·8261
3	7·0	8·5	15·5	1	3	4	1·8065	2·1935
4	5·5	4·5	10·0	1	2	3	1·6500	1·3500
5	3·0	2·0	5·0	1	1	2	1·2000	0·8000
Total				7	13	20	9·3227	10·6773

$$\frac{6}{32.5} \times 13.5 = 2.4923$$

deaths among the males. Similarly, or by subtraction from the total of six deaths, one obtains 3·5077 expected deaths among the females in the first interval. Expected deaths in the remaining intervals are calculated in the same way and are summed to obtain the total expected deaths in males and females $(E_M$ and $E_F)$:*

$$E_M = 9.3227; \quad E_F = 10.6773$$

Letting O_M and O_F represent the total observed deaths in the two groups:

$$O_M = 7; \quad O_F = 13$$

The ratio of O/E in a particular group (called the relative death rate) represents the death rate, averaged over time, in that group relative to both groups combined. For the data above:

$$O_M/E_M = 7/9.3227 = 0.75$$

$$O_F/E_F = 13/10.6773 = 1.22$$

Thus, males have a death rate 75% that of the entire group and females have a death rate 22% greater. The ratio of these two quantities estimates the death rate of one group relative to the other and thus is essentially a relative risk type measure. For this example:

$$RR = \frac{O_F/E_F}{O_M/E_M} = \frac{1.22}{0.75} = 1.63 \tag{7.67}$$

showing that, averaging in some sense over the entire period of follow-up, the females have a 1·63 times higher mortality than males. The method used to

---

* Although the term 'expected deaths' is most often used, some statisticians prefer the term 'extent of exposure to risk of death', since in some situations these 'expected' numbers may actually exceed the total number of persons in the group.

calculate this gives a greater weight to mortality differences early in follow-up than differences towards the end of the life table.

The so called logrank test statistic, which tests the null hypothesis of no group difference in mortality, has a chi-square distribution with 1 degree of freedom (for a two-group comparison) and is given by:

$$\chi^2 = \frac{(O_M - E_M)^2}{E_M} + \frac{(O_F - E_F)^2}{E_F} \tag{7.68}$$

In this case:

$$\chi^2 = \frac{(7 - 9{\cdot}3227)^2}{9{\cdot}3227} + \frac{(13 - 10{\cdot}6773)^2}{10{\cdot}6773} = 1{\cdot}084$$

which on 1 degree of freedom is non-significant.

7.15.7 Confidence intervals for a life table relative risk

Although other methods are available, a confidence interval for the ratio of the death rates in the two groups (the ratios of the two O/E values) is most easily obtained with test-based limits, as described in Section 7.10.5, using the above chi-square value. Confidence limits of 95% for the RR of Eqn. 7.67 are then:

$$RR^{(1 \pm 1{\cdot}96/\chi)} \tag{7.69}$$

where χ is the square root of the chi-square of Eqn. 7.68. In this case, $\chi = 1{\cdot}04$ and the 95% confidence limits are:

$$1{\cdot}63^{(1 \pm 1{\cdot}88)}$$

giving an interval from 0·65 to 4·08.

Life table analysis is the most popular technique for mortality (or survival) comparisons in cohort studies and is used extensively in the analysis of clinical trials. Extensions of the approach to the comparison of more than two life tables are discussed in Section 9.4 and to allow for confounder correction in Section 11.3.3. A large advantage of the approach is that it makes no assumptions about the shapes of the mortality curves in the groups being compared. Mortality analysis can in fact also be performed by fitting the data to a parametric model, in which a particular functional form is assumed to hold for the mortality curve. Estimated parameters of the model are then compared with one another.

7.16 Significance testing versus confidence intervals

It is worth while commenting at this stage on the two different approaches to statistical inference—significance testing and confidence intervals. This chapter has illustrated how each of the methods can be used in the comparison of two groups and how statistical significance can be inferred from a confidence interval for an appropriate parameter (Section 7.5). Until a few years ago, most statistical analyses in medical research were via significance tests, but the majority of medical journals now insist on a reduced emphasis on p values with an increased use of confidence intervals.

It goes without saying that the results are the most important part of any research endeavour. As much effort should go into examination of the data as into its collection. As discussed throughout the book, this should include evaluation of possible biases related to study design and execution and to the influence of confounding factors, such as age and sex. This teasing out of the results is vital to determine the medical importance or relevance of a particular finding and is, in one sense, far more important than a formal statistical analysis. The purpose of a statistical analysis is purely to determine the extent to which sampling variation could explain the observed results and whether they can be validly extended to the population(s) from which the study sample(s) were drawn.

Too often, however, results have been sacrificed to the gods of significance tests and p values. A statistically significant difference between two groups does not guarantee medical importance; it just indicates that the result is unlikely to be due to chance or, more formally, that one can reject the null hypothesis of no group difference. With a large enough sample size, even the smallest and most unimportant difference can be made statistically significant.

At the other end of the scale, a non-significant difference between two groups is not synonymous with no difference. A non-significant difference means that there is not enough evidence to reject the null hypothesis. Chance may be an explanation of the observed result, but the possibility of a real difference cannot be excluded either. In many situations, medically important results can be statistically non-significant, due to an inadequate sample size. Again, it is the magnitude of the result that is critical to its interpretation, rather than its statistical significance.

The confidence interval approach to statistical analysis, on the other hand, rather than concentrating on the decision reject/do not reject, draws attention to the results actually obtained. It gives a range of values, which, at a given probability level, are likely to contain the true population value for the measure of association employed. The confidence interval at the same time presents the result and conveys the inherent variability in the estimate of that result. In addition, as discussed, statistical significance can generally be inferred by observing whether the null value of the hypothesis test falls inside or outside the confidence interval. Confidence intervals, however, do not require the prespecification of a null value, which explains why the two approaches are not completely equivalent.

The confidence interval can be particularly illuminating for the presentation of non-significant results. If the sample size is too small, the width of the confidence interval shows clearly the large range of values compatible with the observed result and thus allows one to see the possibly important effects that would be glossed over by giving only the negative result of the significance test. For non-significant results, the sample size should be sufficiently large so that the range covered by the confidence interval should be narrow enough to exclude the possibility of medically important effects.

The advantages of using confidence intervals in statistical analysis are many, and there is no doubt that their use will expand. Hypothesis testing, however, has served medical research well in the past, and a mixture of both approaches will no doubt be present for some time to come.

7.17 Summary

In this chapter, an overview was given of the confidence interval and hypothesis testing approaches for the comparison of two groups. It was shown how the sampling procedure, in terms of whether or not the groups were matched, and the level of measurement of the data both determine the specific method to employ. A point that must be made is that one cannot apply all possible valid tests to a given set of data and then choose, for presentation purposes, the one that gives a significant result. The most appropriate test must be chosen beforehand and its results accepted.

Computational details were given for the common two-group parametric and non-parametric tests and confidence interval estimates were explained. The summary boxes below review the methods discussed. Separate boxes are presented for the significance tests and for confidence intervals relating to simple comparisons (difference and ratio). The construction of life tables, with their comparative methods, is also considered separately.

It is hoped that this chapter will prove useful to researchers who wish to analyse their own data. Appendix C outlines, in step-by-step form, the computational details for all the procedures (except the life table), and Appendix B provides a useful set of statistical tables. Beware, however: different texts may give the statistical tables in a different format, and the actual test statistics for a given test, particularly for one of the non-parametric ones, although equivalent, can differ from book to book. For this reason, it is advisable to become familiar with one particular set of tables and the associated test statistics.

The next chapter considers how appropriate sample sizes are chosen for two-group studies, and the following chapter moves on to consider the comparison of more than two groups.

Comparison of	Hypothesis test		Eqn. no.
Independent means	(*t* test)*	$t = \dfrac{\bar{x}_1 - \bar{x}_2}{\sqrt{\dfrac{S_p^2}{n_1} + \dfrac{S_p^2}{n_2}}}$	(7.5)
		$S_p^2 = \dfrac{(n_1 - 1)S_1^2 + (n_2 - 1)S_2^2}{n_1 + n_2 - 2}$ d.f. $= n_1 + n_2 - 2$	(7.4)
Paired means	(paired *t* test)	$t = \dfrac{\bar{d}}{S_d/\sqrt{n}}$ d.f. $= n - 1$	(7.15)
Independent proportions	(*z* test)	$z = \dfrac{p_1 - p_2}{\sqrt{\dfrac{pq}{n_1} + \dfrac{pq}{n_2}}}$	(7.20)
		$p = \dfrac{n_1 p_1 + n_2 p_2}{n_1 + n_2}$	(7.18)
	(χ^2 test)	$\chi^2 = \sum \dfrac{(O - E)^2}{E}$	(7.23)
	(Fisher's exact test)	–	
Paired proportions	(McNemar test)	$\chi^2 = \dfrac{(c - b)^2}{b + c}$	(7.33)
Independent counts	(*z* test)	$z = \dfrac{x_1 - x_2}{\sqrt{x_1 + x_2}}$	(7.37)
Independent rates	(*z* test)	$z = \dfrac{r_1 - r_2}{\sqrt{\dfrac{r}{PYRS_1} + \dfrac{r}{PYRS_2}}}$	(7.43)
		$r = \dfrac{PYRS_1(r_1) + PYRS_2(r_2)}{PYRS_1 + PYRS_2}$	(7.41)
Independent medians	(Wilcoxon rank sum test)	$T_1 =$ sum of ranks in group 1	
Paired medians	(sign test) (Wilcoxon signed-rank test)	$n_+ \approx$ no. of preferences $T_+ =$ sum of positive ranks	

* Can be applied to transformed data also.

Difference between two	Confidence interval	Eqn. no.
Independent means	$(\bar{x}_1 - \bar{x}_2) \pm t_c \sqrt{\dfrac{S_p^2}{n_1} + \dfrac{S_p^2}{n_2}}$	(7.8)
	$S_p^2 = \dfrac{(n_1 - 1)S_1^2 + (n_2 - 1)S_2^2}{n_1 + n_2 - 2}$	(7.4)
	$\text{d.f.} = n_1 + n_2 - 2$	
Paired means	$\bar{d} \pm t_c S_d / \sqrt{n}$	(7.16)
	$\text{d.f.} = n - 1$	
Independent proportions	$(p_1 - p_2) \pm z_c \sqrt{\dfrac{p_1 q_1}{n_1} + \dfrac{p_2 q_2}{n_2}}$	(7.22)
Paired proportions	$(p_1 - p_2) \pm z_c \dfrac{1}{N} \sqrt{c + b - \dfrac{(c - b)^2}{N}}$	(7.34/7.35)
Independent counts	$(x_1 - x_2) \pm z_c \sqrt{x_1 + x_2}$	(7.39)
Independent rates	$(r_1 - r_2) \pm z_c \sqrt{\dfrac{r_1}{PYRS_1} + \dfrac{r_2}{PYRS_2}}$	(7.44/7.45)

Ratio of two	Formula/data layout	Confidence interval	Eqn. nos.
Independent geometric means	$$\frac{GM(x_1)}{GM(x_2)} = 10^{\bar{x}'_1 - \bar{x}'_2}$$	$$10^{(\bar{x}'_1 - \bar{x}'_2) \pm t_c \sqrt{\frac{S'^2_p}{n_1} + \frac{S'^2_p}{n_2}}}$$	(7.13/7.14)
		$$S'^2_p = \frac{(n_1 - 1)S'^2_1 + (n_2 - 1)S'^2_2}{n_1 + n_2 - 2}$$ d.f. $= n_1 + n_2 - 2$ where $\bar{x}'$ and S'^2 are all calculated on log-transformed values (to base 10)	(7.4)

Independent proportions (relative risk)

	Disease	
Exposure	Yes	No
Yes	a	b
No	c	d

Ratio of two	Formula/data layout	Confidence interval	Eqn. nos.
	$$RR = \frac{a/(a+b)}{c/(c+d)}$$	$$RR^{1 \pm z_c/\chi}$$	(6.7/7.31)
Independent odds (odds ratio)	$$OR = \frac{a/b}{c/d}$$	$$OR^{1 \pm z_c/\chi}$$	(6.11/7.32)

Paired odds (odds ratio)

	Cases	
Controls	E+	E−
E+	a	b
E−	c	d

E+, exposed; E−, not exposed.

Ratio of two	Formula/data layout	Confidence interval	Eqn. nos.
	$OR = c/b$	$$OR^{1 \pm z_c/\chi}$$	(6.14/7.32/7.36)
Independent rates	$$\frac{x_1/PYRS_1}{x_2/PYRS_2}$$	$$\frac{p_l}{1 - p_l} \frac{PYRS_2}{PYRS_1} \text{ to } \frac{p_u}{1 - p_u} \frac{PYRS_2}{PYRS_1}$$	(7.46/7.50/7.51)
		where p_l and p_u are binomial limits for proportion of total cases in group 1 $(x_1/(x_1 + x_2))$	

Formulae for life tables	Eqn. nos.
Basic calculations	
$$n_i = n_{i-1} - (w_{i-1} + d_{i-1})$$	(7.57)
$$n'_i = n_i - 0 \cdot 5 w_i$$	(7.53)
$$q_i = d_i / n'_i$$	(7.54)
$$p_i = 1 - q_i$$	(7.55)
$$P_i = p_i P_{i-1}$$	(7.52)
$$Q_i = 1 - P_i$$	(7.56)
Confidence interval for cumulative survival	
$$P_i \pm z_c \sqrt{\frac{P_i(1 - P_i)}{n_{(\text{eff})}}}$$	(7.64)
$$n_{(\text{eff})} = n_{i+1}/P_i$$	(7.62)
Confidence interval for difference between two cumulative survivals (at end interval i)	
$$(P_A - P_B) \pm z_c \sqrt{\frac{P_A(1 - P_A)}{n_{A(\text{eff})}} + \frac{P_B(1 - P_B)}{n_{B(\text{eff})}}}$$	(7.65/7.66)
Logrank test	
$$\chi^2 = \frac{(O_A - E_A)^2}{E_A} + \frac{(O_B - E_B)^2}{E_B}$$	(7.68)
d.f. = 1	
Overall relative risk and confidence interval	
$$RR = \frac{O_A/E_A}{O_B/E_B}$$	(7.67)
$$RR^{(1 \pm z_c/\chi)}$$	(7.69)

8 Sample Size Determination

8.1 Introduction

When planning any investigation, one of the most common problems is determining what sample size is required. Unfortunately, the question 'How many people should I study?', though simple, does not have an easy and quick answer. This surprises many people, but the question, in itself, is quite ambiguous and needs a context. It is as if someone were to ask, 'How much money should I bring on my holidays?' To answer that question, one would need to know how long the person was going for, where he was going, whether he liked to stay in a first-class hotel or to camp and all the myriad factors that could affect the amount of money he might spend. Similarly, with a question concerning sample size, a lot more information is required before a sensible answer can be provided.

This chapter describes some of the methods used to determine the best sample size for single-group descriptive studies and for two-group comparative studies and gives some simple tables that might help the investigator. An understanding of the concepts of power and significance in hypothesis tests and the ideas underlying estimation with confidence intervals are prerequisites for the material that follows.

8.2 Factors affecting the approach to sample size estimation

8.2.1 Study design and objectives

The approach taken to sample size estimation depends on the design of the investigation and its basic objectives. A major difference exists between the sample size estimation methods that should be used for comparative studies and those that should be used for descriptive studies. In medical research, the vast majority of studies involve the comparison of two or more groups. The case–control study, the two-group randomized controlled trial and a cohort study comparing individuals exposed to a factor with those not exposed all fit into the category of two-group studies. The aim of such studies is to compare the groups and determine if a difference between them exists that is not explicable by confounding or sampling variation. The statistical analysis of such studies can be performed by means of a two-sample hypothesis test, with the test used depending on whether the study comprises independent or matched samples and the type of variable (qualitative or quantitative) involved. The precise formula used for sample size estimation in a comparative study also depends on these factors, but the same underlying approach is used for all comparative investigations.

Sample size formulae are given in this chapter for both paired–matched and independent group comparative studies. If frequency matching (Section 6.7.2) or stratified randomization (Section 6.11.5) is planned, the independent sample size formulae should suffice and in fact they will give a greater sample size requirement than strictly necessary. If cluster randomization is to be used (Section 6.13.4), more advanced texts should be consulted for sample size estimation (Machin *et al.*, 1997).

For randomized controlled trials, the sample size formulae presented assume that there will be no interim analyses and that the trial will continue until the required number of patients has been recruited and evaluated. Any plans for interim analyses will require an increase in the numbers studied (see Section 6.13.1).

Some medical studies can be considered purely descriptive. The objective of the investigation is simply to estimate some parameter in a population by means of a sample. Thus, a study to determine the prevalence of smoking in a community or the mean blood pressure in that community could be considered descriptive. If a study can be considered purely descriptive, then a particular approach to sample size estimation can be used which is easier to understand than that required for a comparative study. However, the method is not appropriate if any important comparisons are to be made and should only be used if comparisons are a secondary objective of the research, and even then with care. Purely descriptive studies are, in fact, fairly rare and internal comparisons (between males and females, for example) would often be considered an integral part of the analysis of such an investigation. If comparisons are involved, then sample size estimation should reflect that fact and the methods used for single-group descriptive studies should not be used.

An assumption made in this chapter is that the populations from which the samples arise are infinite in size. For all intents and purposes, this means very large in comparison with the sample size, and the assumption underlies all of the analytic techniques discussed in this book. It should be noted that, in this situation, the size of the population makes no difference to the sample size required. Thus, studies of the same sample size could be used to draw similar inferences about the population of Ireland (about $3\frac{1}{2}$ million persons) and about the population of China (about 1000 million persons).

8.2.2 Critical variables

A sample size estimation is based on a single variable measured in one group (a descriptive study) or two groups (a comparative study). In practice, of course, many variables are examined in a study and a practical problem arises as to which variable should underpin the sample size calculation. One solution to this is to choose the 'most important' variable under consideration and to base any calculations on that variable only. A more realistic approach might be to choose a number of important variables and perform a separate sample size calculation for each, accepting the largest of the sample sizes so determined. The final sample size to be used should then be adjusted upwards to allow for non-response and, typically, calculated sample sizes should be inflated by 10–20%.*

8.2.3 Finances and resources

Sometimes, an investigator can be surprised by the large numbers that are needed for a particular study and, in practice, resources and finances have a major influence on the final sample size chosen. Even if resources are limited, sample size calculations are still relevant, since they can, at the very least, alert the investigator to the consequences of a particular choice. A required sample size, however, only gives an indicator of the number of people to study and it is foolish to believe that any calculated figure is exact. A sample size calculation may indicate that, for example, around 500 persons are required rather than 400, but would be unable to distinguish between, say, requirements of 500 and 510.

The formulae presented in this chapter allow estimation of a required sample size directly. It happens fairly often, however, that so little is known about the likely results of a study or what variables are involved that the investigator has no idea of the value of some of the parameters that are needed for the formulae. On the other hand, the possible size of the investigation in terms of available time or resource is often known. In such situations, it might be

---

* To allow for an 80% response rate, divide the calculated sample size by 0·8.

best to start, not by calculating a required sample size, but by working back-wards, starting with a sample size that is practicable and looking at the conse-quences of using that sample size.

Throughout this chapter, tables are provided showing what might be achieved with a (limited) range of different commonly used sample sizes for different types of investigations.* In that sense, the tables are fairly general and could be used to determine the order of magnitude of the sample size required. They might also be suitable for a study protocol or grant application to justify a particular sample size when a range of different variables is to be examined.

> Sample size determination depends on
> • study structure: descriptive or comparative
> • study design: paired or independent samples
> • the type of variable being analysed
> • (resources and finances available)

8.3 Sample sizes for single-group studies

8.3.1 Sample sizes based on precision

If the objective of a study is simply the estimation of the value of some para-meter in terms of, say, a percentage, a rate or a mean, then an appropriate sample size can be determined on the basis of the precision of the sample esti-mate or, in other words, on the width of its confidence interval.† Again, it must be stressed that the following approach is only suitable if no comparisons are involved.

In Chapter 4, confidence intervals for various parameters in the one-sample situation were discussed and it was shown that the standard error of a statistic decreases with increases in sample size. This provides a technique for calculat-ing the number of persons to include in an investigation. The essence of the approach is that, before the study, a decision is made as to the degree of preci-sion required of the estimate or, in other words, one sets a 'plus or minus' error limit on the sample result for a given level of confidence. Setting this precision is a matter of clinical judgement as to what would be acceptable to the scien-tific community. Very wide confidence intervals give very little information.

---

* Most sample size tables are designed for direct estimation of a required sample size and are based on the same or similar formulae to those presented here. Extensive sample size tables of this type are to be found in many books (Cohen, 1988; Machin *et al.*, 1997). The tables in this text start with the sample size and work backwards.
† In this book, the term precision, when used in the context of a confidence interval, refers to the quantity defined by the standard error (SE), multiplied by the appropriate *t* or *z* critical value. For a 95% confidence interval and a normal sampling distribution, this would be 1·96 SE. Thus the precision, which depends on the confidence level, is half the confidence interval width. Some authors use the term precision for the standard error alone.

> Precision-based sample sizes are based on
> - the confidence level
> - the required width of the confidence interval

8.3.2 Estimating a single mean

Equation 4.9 gave a 95% confidence interval for a mean as:

$$\bar{x} \pm 1 \cdot 96 \frac{\sigma}{\sqrt{n}} \qquad (4.9)$$

where n is the sample size and σ is the population standard deviation. If the '±' part of the 95% confidence interval is required to be ±δ, then the sample size needed is easily seen to be:

$$n \geq \left(1 \cdot 96 \frac{\sigma}{\delta}\right)^2 \qquad (8.1)$$

The largest whole number greater than the expression is taken. For a 99% confidence interval, 1·96 is replaced by 2·576 (see Table B.2). Of course, it is necessary to have an estimate of the population standard deviation σ, but this can be based on a pilot study or on prior investigations with the variable in question.*

  Suppose that it was required to estimate diastolic blood pressure in a population to within ±2 mmHg (using a 95% confidence interval) and the standard deviation of diastolic blood pressure was known to be 15 mmHg. Using Eqn. 8.1, the required sample size:

$$n \geq \left(1 \cdot 96 \frac{15}{2}\right)^2 = 216 \cdot 09$$

The next highest integer is taken, giving a requirement of 217 subjects. Allowing for a 10% non-response (90% response), the final required sample size is 217/0·9 or (again rounding up) 242 persons. Usually, the final sample size used in a protocol is chosen as a nice round number, so that this study would probably, given these specifications, end up with a sample size of 250.

  When dealing with quantitative data, it is convenient to express the required precision, δ, as a proportion of the standard deviation. Thus, in the example above, the precision of ±2 mmHg could be expressed as ±2/15 or ±0·13 standard deviations. Table 8.1 shows the precision achieved as a multiple of the standard deviation (i.e. δ/σ is presented) for different sample sizes and 95% and 99% confidence intervals (CI). This should give the reader a feel for how precision is affected by sample size and also may give a rough initial guide as to the broad range a required sample size should be in. For instance, a sample size of 500 gives a 95% confidence interval of ±0·088 standard

---

* The fact that the final confidence interval in the analysis of a study is based on the sample standard deviation and a t distribution does not invalidate this approach.

	$\pm\delta/\sigma$		Table 8.1 Precision (as a multiple of the standard deviation) of 95% and 99% confidence intervals for a mean ($\overline{x}$) related to sample size (n). The body of the table contains δ/σ where the confidence interval is given by $\overline{x} \pm \delta$.
Sample size (n)	95% CI	99% CI	
50	$\pm0{\cdot}277$	$\pm0{\cdot}364$	
100	$\pm0{\cdot}196$	$\pm0{\cdot}258$	
500	$\pm0{\cdot}088$	$\pm0{\cdot}115$	
1000	$\pm0{\cdot}062$	$\pm0{\cdot}081$	

deviations or $\pm8{\cdot}8\%$ of the standard deviation. Increasing the sample size up to 1000 gives a precision of $\pm6{\cdot}2\%$ of the standard deviation. A precision between these figures requires a sample size somewhere between 500 and 1000.

8.3.3 Estimating a single proportion or percentage

An identical approach is used for determining sample size to estimate a proportion with a pre-specified degree of precision. From Eqn. 4.5, the 95% confidence interval for a proportion (p) is:

$$p \pm 1{\cdot}96\sqrt{\frac{p(1-p)}{n}} \tag{4.5}$$

Pre-specification of a precision of $\pm\delta$ at a 95% confidence level gives the sample size:

$$n \geq (1{\cdot}96)^2\frac{p(1-p)}{\delta^2} \tag{8.2}$$

For a 99% interval, the 1·96 would be replaced by 2·576. Notice that, unlike the situation with estimating a mean, no prior estimate of a standard deviation is required. The precision is instead affected by the observed proportion and thus the sample size depends only on the likely result and the desired precision. Suppose it is thought that there are about 28% smokers in the population and it is required to estimate the percentage of smokers to within $\pm3\%$ (in absolute terms), using a 95% confidence interval. Converting everything to proportions and using Eqn. 8.2:

$$n \geq (1{\cdot}96)^2\,\frac{0{\cdot}28(1-0{\cdot}28)}{(0{\cdot}03)^2} = 860{\cdot}5$$

so that a survey of 861 persons is required, even before non-response is allowed for.

Table 8.2 shows the precision achieved in absolute terms by 95% and 99% confidence intervals for detecting various proportions up to 0·5, for a range of sample sizes. For detection of proportions above 0·5, the complementary figure can be used, since the precision is the same. Thus, the precision for a proportion of 0·4 is the same as that for $1{\cdot}0 - 0{\cdot}4 = 0{\cdot}6$. Again, a glance at Table 8.2 should provide a quick guide to the sample size required or, alter-

Table 8.2 Precision of 95% and 99% confidence intervals for a proportion (p), related to sample size (n) and the magnitude of the observed proportion. The body of the table contains δ, where the confidence interval is given by p ± δ.

95% CI

Sample size (n)	±δ				
	$p = 0·10$	$p = 0·20$	$p = 0·30$	$p = 0·40$	$p = 0·50$
50	±0·083	±0·111	±0·127	±0·136	±0·139
100	±0·059	±0·078	±0·090	±0·096	±0·098
500	±0·026	±0·035	±0·040	±0·043	±0·044
1000	±0·019	±0·025	±0·028	±0·030	±0·031

99% CI

Sample size (n)	±δ				
	$p = 0·10$	$p = 0·20$	$p = 0·30$	$p = 0·40$	$p = 0·50$
50	±0·109	±0·146	±0·167	±0·178	±0·182
100	±0·077	±0·103	±0·118	±0·126	±0·129
500	±0·035	±0·046	±0·053	±0·056	±0·058
1000	±0·024	±0·033	±0·037	±0·040	±0·041

natively, show the consequences of a particular sample size choice. From the table, a sample size of 500 estimates, at a 95% level of confidence, a proportion of 0·4 to within ±0·043, which corresponds to a percentage of 40% with a precision of ±4·3%.

8.3.3 Estimating a single rate

The confidence interval for a rate based on a person-years or census denominator is given by Eqn. 4.22 as:

$$r \pm 1·96 \frac{r}{\sqrt{x}} \qquad (4.22)$$

where r is the rate (expressed per 1000, 10000 or whatever is appropriate) and x is the observed number of cases.

The precision is affected by both the observed rate and the observed number of events (deaths, births or whatever the rate is being calculated for), and this latter quantity can take the place of sample size in rate determination. In other words, the number of events needed is estimated, rather than the size of the population (the person-years) giving rise to the events. If the precision is expressed in the same units as the rate, then the total number of observed cases, x, required for a 95% confidence interval precision of $r \pm \delta$ is:

$$x \geq \left(1·96 \frac{r}{\delta}\right)^2 \qquad (8.3)$$

	±δ/r	
Number of cases (x)	95% CI	99% CI
5	±0·877	±1·152
10	±0·620	±0·815
50	±0·277	±0·364
100	±0·196	±0·258
500	±0·088	±0·115

Table 8.3 Precision (as a multiple of the rate) of 95% and 99% confidence intervals for a rate (r), related to the number of observed cases (x). The body of the table contains δ/r, where the confidence interval is given by r ± δ.

Suppose that a rate is expected to be around 25 per million (per year) and it is required to estimate it with a 95% confidence interval to within ±5 per million. The number of cases required to achieve this level of precision is:

$$x \geq \left(1{\cdot}96\frac{25}{5}\right)^2 = 96{\cdot}04$$

which means that 97 cases would have to be observed. If it is wished to determine the sample size in terms of required person-years of observation, the calculation is easily performed using the relationship:

$$PYRS = \frac{x}{r} \tag{8.4}$$

PYRS is given in whatever units the rate is measured in. In the present example, to observe 96·04 cases with a rate of 25 per million (per year) would require 96·04/25 = 3·8 million person-years of observation.

Table 8.3 gives the precision of a rate estimate, expressed as a multiple of the rate (i.e. δ/r is presented), for 95% and 99% confidence intervals and selected observed number of cases. If 100 cases are observed, the relevant rate can be estimated with a 95% confidence interval to just below ±0·196 of the rate or nearly ±20% of the rate. (Note that a ±20% relative precision was required in the example above, which gave a requirement for 97 cases.) With only 50 cases, the rate can be estimated to within a little less than ±30% of the observed figure at a 95% level of confidence.

8.4 Sample size specifications for two-group comparisons

When interest lies in the comparison of two groups, it is not sufficient to base sample sizes on the precision of any estimates. The arguments underlying this are presented in Section 8.8, but for the moment the correct approach is outlined. Usually, a two-group study is designed to detect if there is a real difference between the populations from which the groups were sampled.* This real

---

* The word difference is used here qualitatively, in that it expresses the fact that the two groups are not the same. The word difference is also used quantitatively, however, when it refers to the subtraction of the value of a parameter in one group from that in another group (e.g. the difference between two means). Because measures other than difference measures can be used to quan-

difference should be distinguished from any difference that might be actually observed in a study based on samples from the populations. In the remainder of the chapter, this difference is variously referred to as the true difference, the real difference or the difference in the population. A null hypothesis of no group difference in the population is postulated and, after study completion, a significance test is performed to indicate how the observed (sample) difference between the groups should be interpreted. Either the observed result is likely to reflect a real difference between the populations and the null hypothesis is rejected—a statistically significant result—or the result is explicable by sampling variation and the null hypothesis is not rejected—a nonsignificant result. The sample size in a comparative study should be large enough for the study to be capable of detecting important (real) differences between the groups by finding them statistically significant. The next subsections discuss the input needed for a sample size estimation in a two-group comparative study.

f## 8.4.1 The significance level

In Section 5.7, it was emphasized that the chances of obtaining a statistically significant result (at a given significance level) depend on the magnitude of the real difference between the groups (in the population) and on the sample size. If there is a real difference, the investigator hopes for a significant result and, if there is no real difference, a non-significant result is required. Obviously, however, if the sample size is too small, a non-significant result may be obtained in either situation and the study may be unable to distinguish between a possible real effect and sampling variation.

The investigator protects herself against falsely deciding there is a difference (making a type I error) by setting an appropriate significance level for the test. Typically, the investigator accepts a 5% chance that she might wrongly reject the null hypothesis (when it is true) and conclude that a real difference exists, when in fact there is none. Thus the significance level of the test is also referred to as the chance of making a type I error.

8.4.2 The minimum difference to be detected

The investigator must also guard against missing a real difference if it exists by falsely declaring a non-significant result. This is called a type II error. From a clinical perspective, however, if the real difference between the groups is very small, it is probably not worth knowing about in the first place and a non-significant result would not matter. For instance, it is unlikely that there would be much interest in a blood pressure treatment which (in the population)

tify a 'lack of sameness' (e.g. the ratio of two means), use of the word difference often includes such measures also. Sometimes, the term 'effect' is used instead of difference when group differences might be due to some exposure.

reduced systolic blood pressure by only 1 mmHg. Such an effect would probably be considered too small to warrant the use of a new intervention and no
one is likely to mind that a study examining this question missed such a small
effect. Technically, the null hypothesis is false, but committing a type II error
and failing to reject it is not problematic. On the other hand, a treatment that
produced a blood pressure reduction of 15 mmHg would have to be considered worth knowing about.

This is perhaps the most difficult part of sample size determination.
The investigator must decide what size of difference she wants to be able
to detect.* This is variously called 'the minimum worthwhile difference' or
'the minimum difference to be detected'. It is chosen, not on any statistical grounds, but on the basis of clinical importance. What is often done
in practice is that two extreme differences are taken and some figure in
between is eventually chosen as the value to be detected. If the true difference (in the population) is this large or larger, the study must be big enough
to detect it (with a statistically significant result). If the true difference is
smaller than this value, it is accepted that the study might miss it (with a
non-significant result). In the blood pressure example above, the difference
worth detecting would probably be set somewhere between 1 mmHg and
15 mmHg.

8.4.3 The power of the study

Of course, one can never guarantee that a study will detect a particular real
difference between groups. All that can be done is to set a level of probability
that this difference will be detected. This is called the power of the study — the
chances of detecting a particular real difference, if it exists. Power is the com-
plement of the type II error. If the power to detect a real difference is set at
80%, then there is a 20% chance that this real difference could be missed (see
Section 5.7). To calculate a required sample size, the investigator must specify
the power she wants to have to detect this minimum worthwhile difference. If
the true difference is greater than that specified, the chances of detecting it are
greater than the chosen power; if the true difference is smaller than that specified, the power to detect it is lower. This is acceptable, since it is the *minimum*
difference to be detected that is specified.

While 5% and 1% levels of significance have become standard in medical
research, there is less universal agreement on what levels of power to choose.
Generally, power levels of 80%, 90% or 95% are used, with a useful rule of
thumb that the size of the type II error should be around four times that of the
(two-sided) significance level chosen. Thus, 80% power and 5% significance is
the most common combination in sample size determination, while 95%
power is often paired with 1% significance.

---

* Not necessarily quantified with a difference measure!

Sample sizes for two-group comparative studies are based on
- the significance level
- the minimum difference to be detected at this significance level
- the power to detect this difference

The remainder of this chapter considers sample size estimation for two-group comparative studies only. More complex approaches are necessary if comparing more than two groups. Methods are described for the comparison of means, proportions (percentages) and rates (based on person-years) in independent groups. The methods described are not suitable, however, if a variable-time follow-up is involved (see Sections 6.6 and 7.15). Methods are described for the comparison of means in a paired study, but, apart from this, no account is taken of the effect of adjusting for confounders. The sample size methods described below all assume simple random sampling or non-stratified randomization but are often used for frequency-matched studies or for trials with stratified randomization. In such cases, the calculated sample size tends to be an overestimate—which should not be a serious problem. However, the methods described give *underestimates* of the sample size if any form of cluster sampling is used to create the groups.

8.5 Derivation of a formula for two-group comparisons [!]

A simplified approach to the derivation of the required sample size is described below. It builds on the discussion of power and significance in Section 5.7. Suppose that a study is planned to compare a blood pressure-reducing medication with a placebo in a parallel two-group randomized controlled trial. Treatment efficacy is to be determined by examining the difference in mean systolic blood pressures between the treatment and placebo groups.* On the assumption that the distribution of blood pressures is not too skew, that the population standard deviation of blood pressure, σ, is the same in each group and is known and that the sample size (n) is the same in the two groups, the standard error of the sampling distribution of the difference between means $(\bar{x}_1 - \bar{x}_2)$ is given by (see Eqn. 7.3):

$$\text{SE}(\bar{x}_1 - \bar{x}_2) = \sqrt{\frac{2\sigma^2}{n}} \tag{8.5}$$

Suppose now that the sample size must be large enough to have an 80% power to detect a minimum difference of 10 mmHg at a two-sided 5% significance level. Figure 8.1, which is similar to Fig. 5.5, shows the sampling distributions of the difference between the means (a) for the situation where the null hypothesis is true and the real difference between blood pressures (in the population) is zero and (b) for the situation where the real difference is actually

---

* Initial blood pressures are taken to be similar.

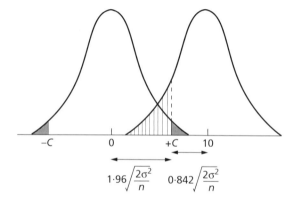

Fig. 8.1 Sampling distribution of the difference between means (a) where the null hypothesis is true — true difference is zero — and (b) where the true difference is 10 mmHg. Point C cuts off 2·5% of the area in the upper tail of the sampling distribution in the null case (heavily shaded area) and 20% in the bottom tail of the distribution obtaining if the real difference is 10 mmHg. (lightly shaded area).

10 mmHg. Each distribution is centred at the population value of the difference (0 or 10 mmHg). The distributions overlap and point C cuts off 2·5% of the area in the upper tail of the sampling distribution in the null case and 20% in the bottom tail of the distribution obtaining if the real difference is 10 mmHg.

If the difference obtained in the study were less than −C or greater than +C, the difference would be declared significant and the null hypothesis would be rejected (assuming a two-sided test). On the other hand, a non-significant result would be declared if the observed difference lay between −C and +C.

If the null hypothesis were true, the observed difference would come from the distribution on the left. The null hypothesis would be wrongly rejected 5% of the time — the probability of a type I error (the significance level) — corresponding to the heavily shaded area in the figure. If the true difference in the population were actually equal to 10 mmHg, the observed difference would arise from the sampling distribution on the right. Because 80% of the area of this distribution is above C, the observed difference would be expected to be above C 80% of the time.* This, then, is the chance that a significant result is obtained with the null hypothesis correctly rejected — the power of the study to detect a 10 mmHg difference in means.

The difference between the centres of the two distributions is determined by the value of the minimum difference to be detected. The spreads of the distributions (and thus their degree of overlap) are determined by the sample size through the standard error of Eqn. 8.5. This is the standard deviation of each of the two sampling distributions under consideration. From the properties of the normal distribution, the point C cutting off 2·5% in the top tail of the null sampling distribution is given by (see Fig. 8.1):

$$0 + 1·96\sqrt{\frac{2\sigma^2}{n}}$$

---

* The minuscule part of the overlap of the distribution on the right with the area below −C is not considered.

Now, it so happens that ±0·842 cuts off 20% in each tail of the standard normal distribution.* Thus, the value of C which cuts off 20% in the bottom tail of the second distribution is also given by:

$$10 - 0.842\sqrt{\frac{2\sigma^2}{n}}$$

If these two expressions are equated and terms are rearranged, an expression for n is obtained:

$$n = \frac{(1.96 + 0.842)^2 \, 2\sigma^2}{(10)^2}$$

The only figure that has not been given so far is σ. Assuming that this is known to be 20 mmHg, n can be calculated from the above formula to be 62·8. This is the sample size required in each of the groups to be 80% sure of detecting a blood pressure difference of at least 10 mmHg at a 5% two-sided significance level. Obviously, the value for n is rounded up to the next whole number and this gives the total sample size required for this trial as 126 (63 × 2) subjects.

Note that the power and significance levels contribute to the sample size through the term $(1.96 + 0.842)^2 = 7.8$ and that the square of the minimum difference to be detected appears as a denominator. Thus, increasing the significance level (reducing the p value), increasing the power and/or decreasing the minimum difference to be detected all increase the sample size required.

8.6 Sample sizes for the comparison of two independent groups

The sample size required for a two-group comparative study depends essentially on the significance level, the minimum difference to be detected and the power to detect this difference. In the formulae that follow, the influence of power and significance is encapsulated in the constant K given in Table 8.4. This approach makes many of the formulae simpler. The value of K should be chosen to match the significance level (one- or two-sided) and power. As has already been pointed out, the commonest choices are for two-sided tests with either 5% significance and 80% power or 1% significance and 95% power.

The formula for the comparison of two independent means is derived in the previous section (which can be omitted at first reading), and the other formulae, which are not derived explicitly, can be derived similarly. As in the sections on sample size determination through precision, tables are given which give a rough guide to the type of effects that can be detected with a few selected sample sizes. Tables are presented for 80% power and a 5% two-sided significance level only, since these are the most usual choices. Note that, in all formulae, n is the sample size required in each group and that $2n$ subjects are required altogether.

---

* This figure is not given in Table B.2, since it is not explicitly used anywhere else in this book. It can of course be found in more detailed tables of the normal distribution.

	One-sided level		Two-sided level		Table 8.4 Multiplying factor K for sample size formulae.
Power	5%	1%	5%	1%	
95%	10·8	15·8	13·0	17·8	
90%	8·6	13·0	10·5	14·9	
80%	6·2	10·0	7·8	11·7	

8.6.1 Comparing two means

For the comparison of means in two independent samples:

$$n \geq \frac{2K\sigma^2}{\Delta^2} \tag{8.6}$$

where n is the sample size required in each of the groups. K is the constant tabulated above, which depends on the chosen significance level and power for the comparison, and σ^2 is the variance in the groups being compared. This is assumed to be the same in each group and usually only a rough estimate of it is available. Δ is the minimum difference in the means that the study is required to detect at the chosen power and significance level. Note that this difference is squared.

It can be seen that Eqn. 8.6 is nothing more than a generalization of the formula derived in the previous section, and use of the equation is illustrated on the same data as that used in the derivation. Suppose a sample size is required for a randomized trial to compare two different treatments for blood pressure reduction. The researchers want to have a large chance of detecting, as statistically significant, a real (population) difference between the mean systolic blood pressures in the two groups of 10 mmHg or greater. A non-stratified randomization is to be used, so that the two groups can be considered independent. The researchers decide on a two-sided significance test at a 5% level and on a power to detect the treatment effect of 80%. An estimate of the standard deviation of systolic blood pressure is 20 mmHg.

The appropriate K for this investigation is read from Table 8.4 as 7.8, $\sigma^2 = 400$ and $\Delta^2 = 100$. Substituting these into Eqn. 8.6 gives a value for n of 62·8. This is the sample size required in each group and should be rounded up. Thus a total sample size of 126 is required for the study — 63 in each group.

In order to generalize, it is convenient to present sample size tables in terms of the difference to be detected as a multiple of the standard deviation. Table 8.5 gives the minimum difference that could be detected at a 5% two-sided significance level and 80% power for a small number of sample sizes in two-group comparisons. With a sample size of 100 persons in each group, for instance, a difference between means of 0·395 times their standard deviation is detectable.

Table 8.5 Minimum difference in means ($\Delta = \bar{x}_1 - \bar{x}_2$) that can be detected (with 80% power at a 5% two-sided significance level) between two independent groups with n subjects in each. The difference is expressed as a multiple of the standard deviation, which is assumed to be the same in the two groups (Δ/σ).

Sample size in each group (n)	Minimum difference to be detected (as multiple of standard deviation) Δ/σ
20	0·883
50	0·559
100	0·395
500	0·177

8.6.2 Comparing two proportions or percentages

For the comparison of proportions in two independent groups:

$$n \geq \frac{K[\pi_1(1-\pi_1) + \pi_2(1-\pi_2)]}{\Delta^2} \qquad (8.7)$$

where n is the number of individuals required in each group, π_1 and π_2 are the proportions in the two groups which define the minimum difference to be detected ($\Delta = \pi_1 - \pi_2$) and K is determined by the power and significance level chosen for the study. Note that, in this case, no estimate of a standard deviation from previous work is required, but that the actual proportions in the two populations must be specified, as well as their difference. As in other situations, it is easiest to work with proportions, rather than percentages. Note that the formula is somewhat inaccurate with small n, particularly if the smallest of π_1, π_2, $1 - \pi_1$ and $1 - \pi_2$ multiplied by n is less than 5.

Application to a case–control study

As an example, the sample size for a case–control study is taken. The required numbers are estimated on the assumption that no matching is to take place and that essentially independent groups of cases and controls are being compared for exposure to some risk factor. While estimates for a pair-matched study could employ the methods of Section 8.7 below, the method for independent groups is adequate for frequency matching, since it gives an overestimate of the numbers required. Though the sample size could be estimated directly from a formula based on specifying a minimum odds ratio that it was required to detect,* it is easier to use Eqn. 8.7 and base the sample size on the differences between the proportions exposed to the risk factor in both cases and controls.

Usually, the researcher has a good idea of what proportion of the controls (π_1) are exposed (it should be the same as in the population), and the minimum difference to be detected can be set in terms of detecting a particular propor-

---

* The odds ratio would be the usual measure employed in the analysis and presentation of the results of a case–control study.

tion exposed in the cases (π_2).* Suppose that the proportion exposed in controls is expected to be 25% or 0·25 and that it is decided that the study must be large enough to have an 80% chance of detecting an exposure rate of 35% in the cases, using a 5% two-sided level of significance. From Table 8.4, $K = 7·8$ and the other quantities are $\pi_1 = 0·25$, $\pi_2 = 0·35$ and $\Delta = 0·25 - 0·35 = -0·10$, which makes $\Delta^2 = 0·01$. Equation 8.7 then gives the required sample size as $n = 323·7$ in each of the groups. Thus 648 subjects should be studied.

Table 8.6 gives various values for proportions in two groups such that their differences have an 80% chance of detection at a 5% two-sided level.† The tabulation is repeated for a number of sample sizes, giving a general picture for each choice, even though the proportions that will actually arise in the study are not known. The table is laid out so that one can start with a number of different proportions, which form a baseline (π_1) in one of the groups, and see what proportion (π_2 either less than or greater than this baseline) in the other group is detectable. As mentioned above, Eqn. 8.7 is not exact for small sample sizes and therefore the table is not exact either. It does, however, give an indicative idea of what is detectable. For instance, with a sample size of 100 in each group and a baseline proportion in the first group of 0·10 (10%), a study could detect a proportion of either less than 0·01 (1·0%) or greater than 0·25 (25%) in the second group. These detectable proportions correspond to minimum detectable differences of 0·09 (9%) or 0·15 (15%), depending on whether the second group proportion is less than or greater than the baseline.

8.6.3 Comparing two rates

When comparing two rates, the sample size calculation gives the number of observations required in each group in terms of person-years. Care must be taken that all quantities are expressed in the same units. Thus, if rates are per million, the calculation gives how many person-years are required in units of a million (i.e. the actual numerical answer has to be multiplied by 1 million).

As for the proportion in the last section, the calculation requires pre-specification of the rates in each of the groups being compared. These rates define the minimum difference required to be detected. If r_1 and r_2 are the rates in the two groups then $\Delta = r_1 - r_2$ and, as usual, K, taken from Table 8.4, is based on the chosen significance level and power.‡ The required number of person-years of observation in each group is then given by:

---

* If it is wished to base the estimate on the odds ratio, a simple calculation allows conversion to the proportion exposed in cases if the proportion exposed in the controls is also given. Equation 8.7 thus has general applicability. If π_1 and π_2 are the proportions exposed in the controls and cases respectively and the minimum odds ratio to be detected is expressed (using Eqns. 6.11 and 6.13) as OR $= \pi_2(1 - \pi_2)/\pi_1(1 - \pi_2)$, the minimum proportion exposed in the cases to be detected is:

$$\pi_2 = \frac{OR\pi_1/(1 - \pi_1)}{1 + [OR\pi_1/(1 - \pi_1)]} \tag{8.8}$$

† The table is derivable from Eqn. 8.7, but requires a degree of effort!
‡ Ideally, the symbols for the rates should be in Greek script, because they represent rates in the population. This is not usually done, however.

$$PYRS > \frac{K(r_1 + r_2)}{\Delta^2} \qquad (8.9)$$

If the application is to a cohort study, then the person-years can be increased by either increasing the number of people studied or having a longer period of follow-up. Quite often, however, rate comparisons are based on observing two different geographical regions with rates based on a vital-statistics denominator of the population size and a count of the annual number of deaths. The size of the population is fixed and in a single year represents the

Table 8.6 Minimum difference in proportions ($\Delta = \pi_1 - \pi_2$) that can be detected (with 80% power at a 5% two-sided significance level) between two independent groups with n subjects in each. The proportions in each group are presented with one (π_1) as baseline and two values for the second proportion for $\pi_2 < \pi_1$ and $\pi_2 > \pi_1$.

Sample size in each group (n)	Proportion in group with lower value (π_2)	Proportion in baseline group (π_1)	Proportion in group with higher value (π_2)
20	–*	0·05	0·38
	–	0·10	0·46
	–	0·25	0·65
	0·06	0·40	0·80
	0·13	0·50	0·87
	0·20	0·60	0·94
	0·35	0·75	–
	0·54	0·90	–
	0·62	0·95	–
50	–	0·05	0·24
	–	0·10	0·32
	0·06	0·25	0·51
	0·16	0·40	0·67
	0·24	0·50	0·76
	0·33	0·60	0·84
	0·49	0·75	0·94
	0·68	0·90	–
	0·76	0·95	–
100	–	0·05	0·17
	0·01	0·10	0·25
	0·10	0·25	0·43
	0·22	0·40	0·59
	0·31	0·50	0·69
	0·41	0·60	0·78
	0·57	0·75	0·90
	0·75	0·90	0·99
	0·83	0·95	–
500	0·02	0·05	0·10
	0·05	0·10	0·16
	0·18	0·25	0·33
	0·32	0·40	0·49
	0·41	0·50	0·59
	0·51	0·60	0·68
	0·67	0·75	0·82
	0·84	0·90	0·95
	0·90	0·95	0·98

* – means that no value is compatible with the theoretical detectable difference.

person-years of observation. The only way to increase the number of person-years is to take data over a longer period than a year. All else being equal, 2 years' observation should supply twice the observed number of cases and twice the person-years, with the overall rate remaining the same. It may be difficult in practice to ensure that the person-years of observation are the same in each of the regions and adjustments, described in the next section, may be required to allow for an imbalance in the region populations. Initially, however, the calculations are illustrated on a simplified example.

Suppose it is required to compare two regions in terms of their rate of births affected by neural-tube defects. It is decided that the study should be able to detect a difference between rates of 2·5 per 1000 births in one region and 1·0 per 1000 births in the other. A 5% two-sided significance level of significance is to be used with a power of 80%. The relevant quantities for substitution into Eqn. 8.9 are: $K = 7·8$, $r_1 = 2·5$, $r_2 = 1·0$ and $\Delta = 2·5 - 1·0 = 1·5$, with the rates and difference expressed per 1000 births. On the basis of these, the required number of births (corresponding to person-years in this application)—in multiples of 1000—is 12·133, so that, multiplying by 1000, 12 133 births are required in each region.

To show what happens if the denominator of the rate is changed—say, from 'per 1000 births' to 'per 10 000 births'—the analysis above is repeated with the new figures. This time $r_1 = 25$, $r_2 = 10$ and $\Delta = 25 - 10 = 15$ (all per 10 000 births). Using Eqn. 8.8, with $K = 7·8$, gives $PYRS = 1·2133$. This is in units of 10 000, so that $1·2133 \times 10 000 = 12 133$ births are required in each region—as was obtained before.

Table 8.7 shows rates that can be detected as different for various sample sizes, again for 5% two-sided significance and 80% power. The sample sizes are given in person-years in the same units as the rates themselves. The layout is similar to that of Table 8.7. For a given $PYRS$ in each region, a range of baseline rates (r_1) is given and the rates detectable $(r_2$ less than or greater than the baseline) are given in two columns on either side of the baseline. To use the table, the study rates should be adjusted so that there are two digits before the decimal place. Thus a rate of 3 per 1000 should be treated as a rate of 30 per 10 000 and the $PYRS$ is then given in multiples of 10 000.

Suppose there are 5000 persons in each of two regions and that a baseline rate of 40 per 1000 (per year) is assumed for one of the regions. For a single year's observation, $PYRS$ is 5. Table 8.6 shows that this sample size gives an 80% power of detecting (at a 5% two-sided level of significance) rates of less than 30 per 1000 (corresponding to $\Delta = 10$ per 1000) in the second region if the rate there is less than baseline. Alternatively, rates in the second region greater than 52 per 1000 ($\Delta = 12$ per 1000) could also be detected.

8.6.4 Adjustment for unequal sample sizes [!]

The sample size calculations described above (Eqns. 8.6, 8.7 and 8.9) assume that the two groups being compared are of the same size. This is the most

Table 8.7 Minimum difference in rates ($\Delta = r_1 - r_2$) that can be detected (with 80% power at a 5% two-sided significance level) between two independent groups with person-years of observation (*PYRS*) in each. The rates in each group are presented, with one (r_1) as baseline and two values for the second rate for $r_2 < r_1$ and $r_2 > r_1$. (*PYRS* are in the same units as the rates.)

Person-years in each group (*PYRS*)	Rate in group with lower value (r_2)	Rate in baseline group (r_1)	Rate in group with higher value (r_2)
2	3	10	21
	13	25	41
	24	40	60
	32	50	72
	40	60	84
	53	75	101
	65	90	119
5	5	10	16
	17	25	35
	30	40	52
	38	50	63
	47	60	74
	60	75	91
	74	90	108
10	6	10	14
	19	25	32
	32	40	48
	42	50	59
	51	60	70
	65	75	86
	79	90	102
50	8	10	12
	22	25	28
	37	40	44
	46	50	54
	56	60	64
	70	75	80
	85	90	95

efficient situation from the statistical point of view, in that maximum power is achieved when groups being compared have the same number of subjects. Sometimes, however, situations arise when equal-sized groups are not possible or desirable. Availability of patients may dictate that the maximum number of subjects in one group is fixed, or cost considerations might dictate that more subjects should be studied in one group rather than the other. If comparisons are to be made between groups in a survey, it is unlikely that the groups will be the same size, and estimates of the total sample size should take account of that. Likewise, analyses of vital-statistics rates are rarely based on equal numbers in regions being compared.

Even if the studied groups are not going to be the same size, the numbers required for an equal-sized group comparison are estimated first. Subsequently, adjustments are made to the estimate to determine the sample size with unequal numbers in the two groups. Suppose that a sample size of n is required in each of two groups. Equation 8.10 below can be used to find (unequal) n_1 and n_2, so that a study with these numbers is equivalent to a study with equal sample size n, in terms of power, minimum difference to be detected and the significance level. The precise approach used depends on the reason for the unequal sample sizes.

$$n = \frac{2n_1 n_2}{n_1 + n_2} \tag{8.10}$$

Fixed number in one group

If the sample size in one of the groups is fixed, n_2, say, then from Eqn. 8.9, the sample size in the other group must be:

$$n_1 = \frac{n n_2}{2n_2 - n} \tag{8.11}$$

Suppose a sample size of 70 persons in each of two groups was required on the basis of power and significance criteria, but that only 50 persons were available for one of the groups (say group 2). Equation 8.11 shows that:

$$n_1 = \frac{70 \times 50}{(2 \times 50) - 70} = 116 \cdot 6$$

so that 117 persons are now needed in group 1 to give the same power and significance in detecting a given difference. This would mean a total sample size of $117 + 50 = 167$, rather than the 140 required for two equal-sized groups. Note that, if the fixed size of the smallest group is less than half the required equal sample size, a suitable study is impossible. In this case, the numbers in the smaller group are insufficient and increasing numbers in the other group cannot make up the deficit.

Sample size ratios other than 1 : 1

If the ratio of the sample size in group 1 to group 2 is fixed at $R = n_1/n_2$, then from Eqn. 8.10:

$$n_1 = \frac{n(R + 1)}{2} \tag{8.12}$$

and

$$n_2 = \frac{n_1}{R} \tag{8.13}$$

Suppose that a cross-sectional survey is to be carried out and that a comparison of blood pressures is to be made between smokers and non-smokers. The power, significance and minimum difference to be detected suggest that a sample size of 150 in each group (smokers and non-smokers) is required. Stratified sampling is not being used, however, and it is known that about 30% of the population are smokers. What effect does this have on sample size? Letting non-smokers be designated as group 1, the ratio of the sample size in group 1 to group 2 (the smokers) is $R = 70/30 = 2.33$. From Eqns. 8.12 and 8.13, the required sample sizes are:

$$n_1 = \frac{150(2.33 + 1)}{2} = 249.75$$

which can be taken as 250, and:

$$n_2 = 250/2.33 = 107$$

Thus the total survey size should be $250 + 107 = 357$, rather than the 300 required if there were the same number of smokers and non-smokers. In this survey, the percentage of smokers would, of course, be $107/357 = 30\%$.

Multiple controls per case [!]

Often, with a case–control study, multiple controls per case are taken (see Section 6.7.2). The previous subsection showed how to calculate a sample size in this situation, when R would then be the number of controls per case. There is, however, a limit to the number of controls per case in terms of efficiency or increase in power. Efficiency can be determined by comparing studies with a given fixed number of cases and different numbers of controls per case on the basis of the equivalent equal sample size situations. Letting n_1 be the number of controls and n_2 the number of cases, it is easily shown from Eqns. 8.12 and 8.13 that:

$$n = n_2 \left(\frac{2R}{R + 1} \right) \tag{8.14}$$

where n is the sample size in each group of an equivalent equal sample size study. Equivalence here means that the study has the same power to detect a minimum difference at a given significance level to the study with $R = n_1/n_2$ controls per case. Thus, the equivalent equal sample size can be used to compare the effect of increasing the number of controls per case.

With one control per case, the power of the study is that of one with (obviously) a sample size of n_2 in each group. If there are two controls per case, the study is equivalent to an equal-sized study with $(4/3)n_2$ in each group, which is 1.33 times larger than the one control per case situation. With three controls per case, this becomes $(6/4)n_2 = 1.5n_2$, which is equivalent to a study with a sample size $1.5/1.33 = 1.125$ times greater than with two controls per case. Four controls per case gives a study equivalent to an equal-sample sized one of $(8/5)n_2 = 1.6n_2$, which is $1.6/1.5 = 1.07$ times the equivalent sample size of the previous case. Thus, changing to four controls per case (adding an extra n_2 controls) is equivalent to adding only $0.07n_2$ persons to each group of the equivalent three controls per case study. Five controls per case add hardly any extra equivalent sample size. Thus, when multiple controls per case are required, any increase on three or maybe four controls per case is a complete waste of resources and gives no real increase in power.

8.7 Sample sizes for the comparison of paired means

It is generally felt that sample size calculations for pair-matched studies are difficult—particularly because the pre-specifications are either hard to understand or almost impossible to determine. The case of paired proportions, which does not often arise in practice, is not considered in this book, but a novel method for use when comparing means is described.

8.7.1 The standard approach

The usual formula given for comparing means in a paired situation is:

$$n \geq \frac{K\sigma_d^2}{\Delta^2} \tag{8.15}$$

where n is the number of pairs, Δ is the minimum difference in means to be detected, K is based on the power and significance levels chosen (Table 8.4) and σ_d is the standard deviation of the paired differences. In determining the sample size for comparing two independent means, an estimate of the standard deviation of the variable is needed and this is fairly easy to obtain from a pilot study or published data. The standard deviation of the differences, however, is difficult to determine from published data (unless in the rare case of a similar investigation), and it is equally difficult to perform a pilot study without a full dry run of the study that is being planned. 'Informed' guesses are also likely to be quite inaccurate. Thus, the formula in Eqn. 8.15, though given in most textbooks, is not likely to be very useful in practice.

A solution which was recently formulated* proposes that, rather than pre-specifying a minimum difference in means to be detected together with its standard deviation, one should specify the study requirements in terms of the percentage of differences in a particular direction.

8.7.2 Derivation of the 'percentage of differences' approach [!]

Figure 8.2 shows the distribution of differences in a population where the mean difference is Δ and the standard deviation of the differences is σ_d. Note that this distribution is likely to be much closer to normality than the original distribution of the variables (because of the central-limit theorem—see Section 4.5.1) and that the diagram shows the distribution of the actual differences in the population, not the sampling distribution of the differences.

Assuming a normal distribution, there is a known relationship between the percentage of differences above zero and the mean and standard deviation. For example, if it so happened that 95% of the differences were above zero then the distance between zero and Δ would be simply $1\cdot645\sigma_d$ (see Table B.2). Since any area cut-off in the normal distribution can be related to its mean and standard deviation through a multiplying factor, the specification of the per-

---

* By Ronan Conroy in the Royal College of Surgeons in Ireland.

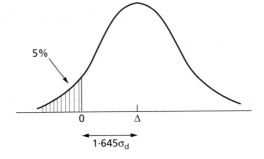

Fig. 8.2 The population distribution of differences between two quantitative measurements in a paired study with a mean difference of Δ and a standard deviation of the differences of σ_d.

Table 8.8 Conversion between percentage of differences above zero and the square of the ratio of the standard deviation (σ_d) to the mean of the differences (Δ).

% of differences above zero	$\dfrac{\sigma_d^2}{\Delta^2}$
55	63·289
60	15·586
65	6·736
70	3·636
75	2·198
80	1·412
85	0·931
90	0·609
95	0·370

centage of differences above zero can predetermine the relative sizes of the mean and standard deviation.

In the example, with 95% of differences above zero:

$$\Delta - 0 = 1.645\sigma_d$$

so that:

$$\frac{\Delta}{\sigma_d} = 1.645$$

or equivalently:

$$\frac{\sigma_d^2}{\Delta^2} = 0.370$$

This is the quantity that is required for sample size calculations for paired quantitative data in Eqn. 8.15. Though extensive tables of the normal distribution are not given in this text, Table 8.8 gives the correspondence between the percentage of differences above zero and this quantity over a range of useful values.

8.7.3 Specifying the percentage of differences

Using this approach, the investigator, instead of setting a minimum difference to be detected (with its standard deviation), sets what percentage of differences above zero (in the population) he or she would like to be able to detect. Suppose a crossover trial of two antihypertensive agents is being planned, with the end-point being systolic blood pressure. The investigator might

Table 8.9 Minimum difference in means ($\Delta = \bar{x}_1 - \bar{x}_2$) that can be detected (with 80% power at a 5% two-sided significance level) between two paired groups with n pairs. The difference is expressed as a multiple of the standard deviation of the differences (Δ/σ_d). Also given in the equivalent percentage of differences above zero (see text).

Number of pairs (n)	Minimum difference to be detected (as multiple of standard deviation of the differences) Δ/σ_d	Percentage of the differences above zero that can be detected
20	0·624	73
50	0·395	65
100	0·279	61
500	0·125	55

decide that it was sufficient to detect if one treatment had 65% of subjects (pairs) showing a lower blood pressure, with 35% showing an advantage for the other treatment. Using Table 8.8, setting a criterion to detect an effect with 65% of the differences in favour of one treatment means equivalently that $\sigma_d^2/\Delta^2 = 6\cdot736$. Substituting this into Eqn. 8.15 and assuming 80% power and 5% two-sided significance, gives the required number of pairs as $n > 52\cdot5$. Thus 53 pairs are needed, or in this case 53 subjects in the crossover trial.

Though the sample size specification was made in terms of the percentage of subjects showing a preference, the analysis should be performed using the paired t test. This is because the percentage specification was purely to obtain an estimate of the variability of the differences and the sample size equation used is based on using a t test in the analysis of the pairs.

Table 8.9 gives the minimum difference in population means that can be detected (80% power and 5% two-sided significance) in a paired comparison with different sample sizes. The difference is expressed as a multiple of the standard deviation of the differences. The equivalent percentage of differences above zero is also given.

8.8 Confidence intervals and sample sizes for comparative studies

8.8.1 Sample size based on precision

A number of sample size estimation methods for comparative studies have been proposed in recent years as alternatives to the more traditional methods based on hypothesis testing, which have been described above. These methods, similar to those described in Section 8.3 for parameters of a single group, are based on the confidence interval width or, equivalently, precision of an appropriate comparative measure. All else being equal, the larger the sample size is in a study, the narrower is the width of the confidence interval and the more precise is the sample result. Once precision has been pre-specified at a given confidence level, the sample size determination only requires a measure of the variability of the comparative measure. These specifications are clinically understandable and the difficult concepts of power, null values and minimum difference to be detected seem to be avoided altogether.

From the point of view of data analysis, hypothesis testing and confidence intervals are complementary and result in essentially similar interpretations and conclusions. However, the suggested sample size estimations based on confidence intervals tend to give much lower sample sizes than those obtained with the older, more established methods. Although the precision of any measure is very important, estimates of sample size based on confidence-interval precision alone can be misleading *in comparative studies*.

8.8.2 Explanation of the problem [!]

A correspondence is usually made between the precision of the confidence interval and the smallest difference to be detected. In Section 8.6.1, the sample size requirements for a randomized trial to compare two treatments for blood pressure reduction were discussed. A total sample of 126 patients (63 in each group) was required to give 80% power to detect, at a 5% two-sided level of significance, a (true) difference of 10 mmHg or greater between the two treatment groups. Using a confidence interval approach, it would seem that a 95% confidence interval precision for the difference in mean blood pressure of ±10 mmHg would be sufficient to distinguish a mean difference of 10 mmHg from that of a zero difference. If the confidence interval were centred around the observed difference, the expected interval of 10 ± 10 mmHg (that is, from 0 to 20 mmHg) would just exclude the null value—corresponding to a statistically significant result. In particular, using Eqn. 8.5 for the standard error of the difference between means (compare with Eqn. 7.8, which uses a critical t value and a pooled sample standard deviation), the 95% confidence interval is:

$$(\bar{x}_1 - \bar{x}_2) \pm 1{\cdot}96\sqrt{\frac{2\sigma^2}{n}}$$

where n is the sample size in each group. If this precision is set at $\pm\delta$, n can be found from the formula:

$$n \geq \frac{(1{\cdot}96)^2 2\sigma^2}{\delta^2} \qquad (8.16)$$

Substituting 10 mmHg for δ and 20 mmHg for σ, the required n is 30·7, resulting in a total sample size of 62 patients. This is less than the 126 patients required using the standard approach of specifying power to detect a minimum difference.

There are two reasons for this apparent anomaly. Assume that the real population blood pressure difference was in fact 10 mmHg and that, based on a pre-specified 95% confidence interval precision of ±10 mmHg, a sample size of 31 was used in each group. First, this width is only an expected or average width. The actual precision achieved from real data from the study would be above its expected value about 50% of the time. Thus, if centred around 10 mmHg, the confidence interval would have a 50% chance of including zero. This would correspond to a non-significant difference between the blood pressures at a 5% two-sided level. The second problem is that the sample value of the blood pressure difference calculated on the study results would be as likely to be above the population value of 10 mmHg as below it. There would thus be a 50% chance that the sample difference would lie below 10 mmHg. If the sample difference were, for instance, 9 mmHg, then a confidence interval with the expected precision of ±10 mmHg would run from −1 mmHg to +19 mmHg and would include zero difference as a possible true value.

Essentially, this means that the sample size estimated on the basis of confidence interval precision has only a power of 50% to detect the difference being sought. The fact that the power is 50% can also be seen by comparing Eqn. 8.16 (for a 95% confidence interval with precision +δ) with Eqn. 8.6 (for 80% power to detect a difference Δ at a 5% two-sided level of significance), where the full value of K has been substituted from Section 8.4.

$$n \geq \frac{(1.96 + 0.842)^2 2\sigma^2}{\Delta^2}$$

In the precision of the confidence interval (δ) and the minimum difference to be detected (Δ) are the same, the only difference between the formulae is the factor of 0.842. This is the value in the standard normal distribution that cuts off 20% in one tail—the probability of the type II error—where the power is given by 100% − 20% = 80%. The value that cuts off 50% in each tail (corresponding to a power of 50%) is the centre of the distribution, or zero, and thus the confidence interval formulation gives only 50% power to detect the specified difference.

8.8.3 Consequences

Specification of the expected precision of a confidence interval does not consider the possible true value of the difference or the power to detect it (with a confidence interval excluding the null value of zero), nor does it consider what precision might actually be achieved. In essence, the specification gives only a 50% chance that the confidence interval calculated from the data would exclude the null value of zero. Thus, in hypothesis-testing terms, the specification gives only a 50% power to detect the minimum worthwhile difference used to define the precision of the interval. The approach can therefore lead to unacceptably small sample sizes with too low a power to detect the required effect. For this reason, sample sizes based on confidence interval precision are not appropriate for comparative studies. Unfortunately, many researchers employ these methods, since they prefer a confidence interval approach to data analysis and wish their sample size estimations to fit in with that philosophy. However, it is in fact possible to employ the standard sample size equations based on hypothesis tests and use them in a confidence interval framework with only a small change in the wording of the specifications (Daly, 1991b).

8.9 Summary

In this chapter, two basic methods for sample size estimation were described. The first, suitable for single-group studies, is based on a pre-specification of confidence interval precision. The second method, which should always be employed in comparative studies, requires setting a minimum difference to be detected, together with the power to detect that difference at a given significance level. Sample size estimating formulae were described for the estimation of single means, proportions (percentages) and rates. Formulae were also provided for comparing these statistics in two independent groups and for comparing means in the paired situation. Adjustments for groups with unequal sample sizes were considered.

The next chapter of the book returns to statistical analysis and looks at the comparison of more than two groups.

Sample sizes for a single group based on precision

Estimation of	Sample size in group	Eqn. no.
A mean	$n \geq \left(z_c \dfrac{\sigma}{\delta} \right)^2$	(8.1)
A proportion	$n \geq z_c^2 \dfrac{p(1-p)}{\delta^2}$	(8.2)
A rate	$x \geq \left(z_c \dfrac{r}{\delta} \right)^2$	(8.3)
	$PYRS = \dfrac{x}{r}$	(8.4)

Sample sizes for two-group independent comparisons based on power to detect differences

Comparison of	Sample size in each group	Eqn. no.
Means	$n \geq \dfrac{2K\sigma^2}{\Delta^2}$	(8.6)
Proportions	$n \geq \dfrac{K[\pi_1(1-\pi_1) + \pi_2(1-\pi_2)]}{\Delta^2}$	(8.7)
Rates	$PYRS > \dfrac{K(r_1 + r_2)}{\Delta^2}$	(8.9)

Sample sizes for paired comparisons based on power to detect differences

Comparison of	Number of pairs	Eqn. no.
Means	$n \geq \dfrac{K\sigma_d^2}{\Delta^2}$	(8.14)

9 Comparison of More than Two Independent Groups [!]

9.1 Introduction

Chapter 7 considered in detail the comparison of two groups using hypothesis tests and confidence intervals. Here the analysis of more than two groups is considered. The major part of what follows deals with a technique called analysis of variance, which, despite its name, is actually used for the comparison of means. The logic behind the approach is explained, together with computational details in simple examples. It is hoped that this will provide the reader with enough detail to appreciate the very general applications of this methodology. The comparison of proportions in more than two groups using a simple extension of the chi-square test is also examined, and a test for a trend in proportions is introduced. The techniques discussed are for the comparison of more than two independent groups only. Comparison of individually matched data in more than two groups is relatively uncommon. The analysis of stratified or frequency-matched data is considered in Chapter 11 in the context of controlling for confounders.

There is a vast body of analytical techniques for multigroup analysis and the material in this chapter can only be considered a brief foray into this area. As has been pointed out previously, however, two-group comparisons are much more common in medical applications, and in many cases problems may be reduced to the two-group case by appropriate grouping of categories. The contents of this chapter are somewhat difficult and require the reader to be conversant with much of the material covered so far in this text.

9.2.1 Multiple comparisons with *t* tests

When analysing means in more than two groups that are not paired or matched, it would seem tempting to employ the usual independent *t* test and compare the groups in pairs. Thus, for three groups, A, B and C, one might compare A with B, A with C and finally B with C. With more than three groups, the number of comparisons increases quite quickly. Such a procedure is not to be recommended, however, for two basic reasons. The first is that *in the one analysis* many *t* tests would be used and, overall, the chances are greater than 5% that any single one of them might give a statistically significant result, even if the groups being compared had the same population means (see Section 9.2.6 also). The second reason is that the correct approach uses the data from all groups to estimate standard errors, and this can increase the power of the analysis considerably.

The correct technique for comparing means in three or more groups is called *analysis of variance* or ANOVA for short. When there is only one qualitative variable which defines the groups, a *one-way* ANOVA is performed. ANOVA is a very powerful method and can be extended to quite complex data structures. (A two-way ANOVA is used when groups are defined by two qualitative variables. See Chapter 11 for a fuller discussion.) Despite its misleading name, the analysis of variance is a technique for the comparison of means, which happens to use estimates of variability in the data to achieve this.

(One-way) analysis of variance
• a technique for comparing independent means in more than two groups

---

9.2.2 Between-groups and within-groups variation

The logic behind an analysis of variance is quite different from anything encountered so far in this text. Supposing blood pressures in three groups are being compared. Figure 9.1 shows the distribution of the blood pressures in two possible situations. In Fig. 9.1a, the blood pressures in the three groups are fairly tightly spread about their respective means and it is easy enough to see that there is a difference between the means in the three groups. In Fig. 9.1b, the three groups have the same means as previously but the individual blood pressure distributions are much more spread out and it is quite difficult to see that the means are in fact different.

On this basis, one could say, more formally, that to distinguish between the groups, the variability *between* or among the groups must be greater than the variability of, or *within*, the groups. If the within-groups variability is large compared with the between-groups variability, any differences between the

(a)

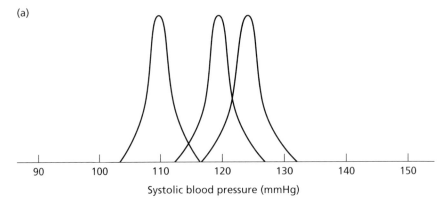

(b)

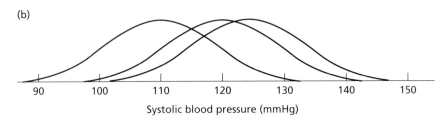

Fig. 9.1 Distribution of blood pressure in three groups: (a) with low variance, (b) with high variance.

groups are difficult to detect. Thus, the determination of whether or not group means are significantly different can be achieved by a comparison of between-groups and within-groups variability, both of which are measured by the variance. (Remember that the variance is the square of the standard deviation and is a measure of variability or spread in the data.)

A simple example comparing three groups should suffice to explain the basic concepts involved. In general, the number of groups will be denoted by k, and here $k = 3$. Suppose that systolic blood pressure is to be compared between current, ex- and non-cigarette-smokers and that there are four persons in each group. (The sample size in each group will be denoted n for the equal sample size situation considered in this section.) The null hypothesis for this example is that the mean (population) systolic blood pressure is the same in the three smoking categories. Table 9.1 shows the data, with the means and variances in the three groups separately. ($\bar{x}_i$ and S_i^2 represent the mean and variance in the ith group. $\bar{x}$ without a subscript represents the mean of all the observations, called the grand mean, and N is the total sample size — $3n$, or 12 in this example.)

Within-groups mean square

One of the assumptions of the analysis of variance is that the (population) variances in the groups being compared are all equal. From an examination of the data in the table, this seems to be a reasonable assumption and is the same

Table 9.1 Data for one-way analysis of variance in three equal-sized groups.

Group (i)	Smokers (1)	Ex-smokers (2)	Never smokers (3)	$k = 3$
Systolic	125	110	95	
blood	135	125	100	
pressure	145	125	105	
	155	140	120	
n	4	4	4	$N = 12$
$\bar{x}_i$	140·00	125·00	105·00	$\bar{x} = 123·33$
S_i^2	166·67	150·00	116·67	

as that made for the independent t test also (see Section 7.4.3). Under this assumption, the three sample variances within current, ex- and never smokers all estimate this common value, which will be denoted σ^2. In this case of equal sample sizes, the best estimate of the common population variance from the within-sample values is the average of the three of them. This estimate is called the *within-groups variance* or, more commonly, the *within-groups mean square* or the *error mean square*, and is denoted S_W^2 (the use of the latter two terms will be explained later):

$$S_W^2 = \sum S_i^2 / k \quad \text{(equal sample sizes)} \tag{9.1}$$

which in this case is:

$$S_W^2 = (166·67 + 150·00 + 116·67)/3 = 144·45$$

Note that the summation is over the k ($i = 1, 2, 3 \ldots k$) values of S_i^2. Since equal population variances have been assumed, this estimate of the population variance, derived from the separate within-groups estimates, is valid whether the null hypothesis (that the three means are the same) holds or not.

Between-groups mean square

If the null hypothesis were true, the three groups could be considered three random samples, each of size n, from the same population, and the three sample means would be three observations from the same sampling distribution of the mean. Now, the sampling distribution of the mean has variance σ^2/n (the square of the standard error, where n, the sample size, is in this case equal to 4 and σ^2 is the population variance — see Section 4.5) and this gives a method for obtaining a second estimate of the population variance. The variance of the sample means is obtained directly from the usual formula for a variance (cf. Eqn. 1.6), where, in this case, the three sample means ($\bar{x}_i$) replace the observations and the grand mean ($\bar{x}$) is the figure subtracted from each value. In general, the summation is over the k groups and the divisor is $k - 1$:

$$\frac{\sum (\bar{x}_i - \bar{x})^2}{k - 1}$$

If this is equated with σ^2/n (the theoretical value for the variance of the sampling distribution of the mean), then the between-groups estimate of the population variance, denoted S_B^2, is:

$$S_B^2 = \frac{n\sum(\bar{x}_i - \bar{x})^2}{k-1} \qquad \text{(equal sample sizes)} \qquad (9.2)$$

This quantity, which is calculated from the between-groups variance, is called the *between-groups mean square*. If the null hypothesis is true, then it is a second estimate of the population variance. However, if the population means of the groups are not all equal, S_B^2 should be greater than the population variance. On this basis, a comparison of S_B^2 and S_W^2 (which always estimates the population variance) should indicate if the null hypothesis is likely to be true. If S_B^2 is much greater than S_W^2, there is more variability between the groups than would be expected given the variability within the groups, and the null hypothesis might be suspect. In the example, the between-groups mean square is:

$$S_B^2 = \frac{4\left[(140 - 123\cdot33)^2 + (125 - 123\cdot33)^2 + (105 - 123\cdot33)^2\right]}{3-1}$$

which is equal to 1233·33. Now this is considerably larger than S_W^2 which was calculated as 144·45 so that one might doubt the null hypothesis in this case.

> The within-groups mean square
> - is the average of the variances in each group
> - estimates the population variance
> - is also called the error mean square
>
> The between-groups mean square
> - is calculated from the variance between the groups
> - estimates the population variance, if the null hypothesis is true

9.2.3 The F distribution and the F test

The question is, of course, how much larger than S_W^2 must S_B^2 be before the null hypothesis can be rejected formally at a particular level of significance. Now, there is a significance test available that will test the hypothesis that two variances are equal. It is based on the ratio of the two variances and is called the *F* test:

$$F = S_B^2 / S_W^2 \qquad (9.3)$$

In the example, $F = 1233\cdot33/144\cdot45 = 8\cdot54$. If F is sufficiently larger than unity, one can reject the hypothesis that the two variances are equal, which, in the situation considered here, translates to a rejection of the null hypothesis that the means of the groups being compared are equal. This is how an analysis of variance allows for a comparison of group means. As for the z, t and χ^2 distributions, tables of the F distribution are available. The validity of the F test is based on a requirement that the populations from which the variances were taken are normal, but, as usual, approximate normality will suffice.

Note that the critical value, F_c, for the F distribution must be equalled or exceeded for a significant result and, in the analysis of variance, a one-sided F test must be employed. This is because no interpretation can be attached to the ratio $F = S_B^2/S_W^2$ if it is less than 1. An F value of less than 1 must be a chance occurrence and it is only when F exceeds 1 that the null hypothesis can be rejected. Note that rejection of the null hypothesis just means that the population means do not all have the same value. A significant result does not indicate which means are different from which.

An unusual property of the F distribution is that, unlike the t and χ^2 distributions, it has a *pair* of degrees of freedom. These are based on the degrees of freedom for the two variances in the F ratio. Looking at Eqn. 9.1, S_W^2 is based on the sum of k variances, each with $n - 1$ degrees of freedom, so that its degrees of freedom are $k\,(n-1)$. Now since k (the number of groups) multiplied by n (the sample size in each group) is equal to N (the total sample size), this gives a total of $N - k$ degrees of freedom for S_W^2. From Eqn. 9.2, S_B^2 obviously has $k - 1$ degrees of freedom. For a one-way analysis of variance, $F = S_B^2/S_W^2$ has then $k - 1$ and $N - k$ degrees of freedom, the first member of the pair taken from the numerator of the F ratio and the second from the denominator.

Table B.14 in the Appendix gives tables of the F distribution. Separate pages are provided for *one-sided p* values of 0·05 and 0·01. (As stated above, two-sided tests are inappropriate for the analysis of variance.) Degrees of freedom for the numerator run from 1 to 10 along the top of the table, allowing for comparison of up to 11 groups. The degrees of freedom for the denominator are given in the table from 1 to 20 with all values, up to 100 in jumps of 10 and up to 500 in jumps of 100. If the value of the degrees of freedom for a particular analysis is not given, then the next lowest should be taken and used.

In the example, the F ratio was 8·54 on 2 and 9 degrees of freedom (d.f.). From the table, the critical 5% (one-sided) value is 4·26 and the 1% value is 8·02. Thus the F value is sufficiently large to enable rejection of the null hypothesis at a 1% level of significance. The mean blood pressures are not the same in the three smoking categories ($F = 8\cdot54$; d.f. $= 2, 9$; $p < 0\cdot01$). The question of which mean is significantly different from which will be discussed below.

The F test
- is the appropriate hypothesis test for the comparison of more than two means
- is based on the ratio of the between-groups sum of squares to the within-groups sum of squares

Table 9.2 Data for one-way analysis of variance in three unequal sized groups.

Group (*i*)	Smokers (1)	Ex-smokers (2)	Never smokers (3)	$k = 3$
Systolic	125	115	95	
blood	135	125	100	
pressure	140	135	105	
	145		120	
	155			
n_i	5	3	4	$N = 12$
$\bar{x}_i$	140·00	125·00	105·00	$\bar{x} = 124·58$
S_i^2	125·00	100·00	116·67	

9.2.4 Unequal sample sizes [!]

The discussion above and the formulae for the two estimates of the population variance were for equal sample sizes in the three groups. Although it is somewhat easier to understand the logic with equal sample sizes, extension to unequal sample sizes is not difficult. Table 9.2 shows almost identical data relating to blood pressure by smoking status, but this time, rather than four persons in each group, there are five smokers, three ex-smokers and four never smokers. The sample size in group *i* will be denoted n_i. Note that, while the overall mean $\bar{x} = 124·58$ is the mean of the 12 blood pressure observations, it is not equal to a simple (unweighted) average of the three group means. It is in fact a weighted average of the group means, with the weights equal to the sample sizes in the groups.

As before, there are three separate estimates of the population variance within the three groups, but they are based on different sample sizes. With equal sample sizes, the average of the three was taken, but now a weighted average of the variances is required. Remember that, in the independent *t* test, a weighted average of the two variances was taken to get what was called the pooled variance (see Eqn. 7.4 in Section 7.4). A similar procedure is followed here and each variance is weighted by its degrees of freedom ($n_i - 1$):

$$S_W^2 = \frac{(n_1 - 1)S_1^2 + (n_2 - 1)S_2^2 + (n_3 - 1)S_3^2}{(n_1 - 1) + (n_2 - 1) + (n_3 - 1)}$$

This, of course, reduces to an unweighted average when the sample sizes are all equal. For the smoking example:

$$S_W^2 = \frac{4(125) + 2(100) + 3(116·67)}{4 + 2 + 3} = \frac{1050}{9} = 116·67$$

This generalizes to:

$$S_W^2 = \frac{\sum(n_i - 1)S_i^2}{N - k} \quad \text{(unequal sample sizes)} \qquad (9.4)$$

The extension of the formula for S_B^2 is slightly more difficult to justify. The usual result for the sampling distribution of the mean under the null hypothesis cannot be invoked, because the sample size is not the same in each group. However, it can be taken on faith that, instead of Eqn. 9.2:

$$S_B^2 = \frac{n\sum(\bar{x}_i - \bar{x})^2}{k-1} \quad \text{(equal sample sizes)} \quad (9.2)$$

the correct expression with unequal sample sizes is:

$$S_B^2 = \frac{\sum n_i(\bar{x}_i - \bar{x})^2}{k-1} \quad \text{(unequal sample sizes)} \quad (9.5)$$

This is, in the example:

$$S_B^2 = \frac{5(140 - 124 \cdot 58)^2 + 3(125 - 124 \cdot 58)^2 + 4(105 - 124 \cdot 58)^2}{3-1}$$

$$= 2722 \cdot 9/2 = 1361 \cdot 45$$

Again, the significance test is performed by calculating the F ratio, $F = S_B^2/S_W^2 = 1361 \cdot 45/116 \cdot 67 = 11 \cdot 67$, with 2 and 9 degrees of freedom, as before. The 1% critical value is $8 \cdot 02$ and, again, in this example the null hypothesis of no group differences in means is rejected at this level of significance.

It should be noted that, if the one-way ANOVA is used for the comparison of two groups only, the analysis is exactly and mathematically equivalent to the use of the independent t test of Section 7.4.1. The one-way ANOVA, like the independent t test, requires that the groups under comparison are independent. Adaptations of the method must be employed for 'paired' or frequency-matched data. It is important also to remember the assumptions underlying an analysis of variance. In the situation of a straightforward comparison between groups, the distribution of the variable must be near-normal in each group, with the same underlying variance. If, on examination of the data, these assumptions appear suspect, a transformation of the variable may alleviate the problem (see Sections 7.4.4 and 1.6.7) Section C.18 of Appendix C summarizes calculations for the one-way ANOVA.

9.2.5 Sums of squares, mean squares and degrees of freedom [!]

It is hoped that the above description of the analysis of variance is sufficient to allow an understanding of the basic ideas behind the technique. Usually, however, the approach is explained and carried out from a slightly different perspective. This section can be omitted without any loss of understanding of the technique.

So far in this text, the Greek capital sigma sign (Σ) has been used in a fairly straightforward manner to denote summation and it has been obvious what exactly is being summed up. For this section, a slight extension of the use of Σ and the general notation must be made. Instead of using x on its own to denote one of the observations in a group, x_{ij} will explicitly refer to the jth observation in the ith group. j can thus have values ranging from one up to n_i (the sample size in the ith group). The summation sign will also have an explicit subscript to indicate what is being summed. Σ_i will mean summation over the k groups, Σ_j will mean summation over the observations in a group, and $\Sigma_i\Sigma_j$ will mean summation over all observations. To give an example, the mean and variance in the ith group would be expressed as:

$$\bar{x}_i = \frac{\Sigma_j x_{ij}}{n_i} \tag{9.6}$$

$$S_i^2 = \frac{\Sigma_j (x_{ij} - \bar{x}_i)^2}{n_i - 1} \tag{9.7}$$

where the summations are over the n_i observations in the ith group.

Now, the deviation of any individual observation (x_{ij}) from the grand mean $(\bar{x})$ can be expressed:

$$(x_{ij} - \bar{x}) = (x_{ij} - \bar{x}_i) + (\bar{x}_i - \bar{x}) \tag{9.8}$$

This states simply that the deviation of any observation from the grand mean can be split into two components, a deviation of the observation from *its own* group mean and the deviation of the group mean from the grand mean. It can be shown that, if each of these deviations is squared and summed over all observations, the following equality also holds:

$$\Sigma_i \Sigma_j (x_{ij} - \bar{x})^2 = \Sigma_i \Sigma_j (x_{ij} - \bar{x}_i)^2 + \Sigma_i \Sigma_j (\bar{x}_i - \bar{x})^2 \tag{9.9}$$

Each of these is referred to as a *sum of squares*. The expression on the left is called the total sum of squares and the two components on the right are called the within-groups and between-groups sums of squares, respectively. Letting 'SSq' denote sum of squares:

$$\text{Total SSq} = \text{Within-groups SSq} + \text{Between-groups SSq} \tag{9.10}$$

In some sense the sums of squares are measures of the variability observed in the data. The total SSq measures the total variability independently of group membership, the within-groups SSq measures the variability within the groups only (irrespective of how the group means differ) and, finally, the between-groups SSq measures the variability between the groups with no contribution from the variability within.

As well as partitioning the total sum of squares into components within and between groups, the total degrees of freedom can be similarly partitioned. Remember that degrees of freedom refer to how many of the components of an expression are free to vary. Using the same arguments of Section 1.8.2, the total SSq has $N - 1$ degrees of freedom, because there is a total of N observations and the grand mean is included in the SSq. The within-groups SSq has $N - k$ degrees of freedom, because all observations are included in its calculation, in addition to the k group means. Note that the between-groups SSq can be expressed as:

$$\sum_i \sum_j (\bar{x}_i - \bar{x})^2 = \sum_i n_i (\bar{x}_i - \bar{x})^2 \qquad (9.11)$$

since the Σ_j just repeats the summation n_i times in each group. With this formulation, it is clear that the between-groups SSq has $k - 1$ degrees of freedom:

$$\text{Total d.f.} = \text{Within-groups d.f.} + \text{Between-groups d.f.}$$
$$N - 1 \quad = \quad N - k \quad + \quad k - 1 \qquad (9.12)$$

When a sum of squares is divided by its degrees of freedom, the result is called a mean square (MSq for short). Comparing Eqns. 9.11 and 9.5, it is obvious that:

$$S_B^2 = \text{Between-groups MSq}$$

Also, by substituting the value for S_i^2 from Eqn. 9.7 into Eqn. 9.4 for S_W^2 and comparing with Eqn. 9.9:

$$S_W^2 = \text{Within-groups MSq}$$

The analysis of variance F test can thus be expressed in terms of MSq as:

$$F = \text{Between-groups MSq/Within-groups MSq} \qquad (9.13)$$

on $k - 1$ and $N - k$ degrees of freedom (see Eqn. 9.3).

Note that the total mean square (total SSq/total d.f.) is nothing more than an estimate of the variance of all the observations, taking no account of group membership. It is often given the symbol S_T^2:

$$S_T^2 = \frac{\sum_i \sum_j (x_{ij} - \bar{x})^2}{N - 1}$$

The actual magnitude of this quantity is not very important in an analysis of variance, however.

For the unequal sample size example in the last section, the total SSq can be calculated as 3772·9. From earlier calculations in the same example, the values for the other two sums of squares are seen to be:

$$\text{Within-group SSq} = 1050 \cdot 0$$
$$\text{Between-groups SSq} = 2722 \cdot 9$$

which add to the total SSq. Most computer printouts and presentations of the analysis of variance are in terms of the sums of squares, giving rise to what is called an ANOVA table, and analyses of variance for more complex situations (see Chapter 11) are all based on an appropriate partitioning of both the total SSq and the degrees of freedom. Short-cut formulae for calculating sums of squares are given in Appendix A. The ANOVA table for the second example, with unequal sample sizes, is given in Table 9.3.

The between-groups SSq is sometimes referred to as the *model sum of squares* and the within-groups figure is often called the *residual sum of squares* (what is left over when the between-groups variation is taken out) or the *error sum of squares* (the variation that cannot be explained by anything else).

Source of variation	d.f.	SSq	MSq	F ratio
Between groups	2	2722·9	1361·45	11·67
Within groups	9	1050·0	116·67	(p < 0·01)
Total	11	3772·9		

Table 9.3 ANOVA table for the study of blood pressure and smoking (unequal-sample size example).

9.2.6 Multiple comparisons and the interpretation of a significant *F* test

It has already been pointed out that, when means in more than two groups are being compared, use of many independent *t* tests on pairs of groups is not valid, because of the possibility of misinterpretation of a significant result. For *k* groups, there are $k(k-1)/2$ pairs of means which could be compared, and for seven groups there would be 21 *t* tests. One of these would be likely to be significant at a 5% level (1/20), even if the null hypothesis were true and there were no real differences between the groups. Multiple *t* tests are, then, not appropriate.

When an *F* test is significant, the correct conclusion is that the population means in the groups are not all the same. There is a difference among the means somewhere, but it is not clear where. Perhaps the most straightforward solution is just to examine the data and note which means are different from which, without further formal statistical analysis. If, however, the design of the study was specifically to compare certain *pre-specified* means, then the approach below is quite acceptable, as long as the comparisons were chosen before examination of the data. If the data are examined just to see what significant comparisons turn up, more complex *multiple comparison* techniques must be used. These essentially adjust the *p* value for the large number of comparisons that must be made and allow an appropriately interpretable significance test to be performed. Multiple comparison tests are not considered in this text.

If certain specific comparisons were chosen beforehand, then the equivalent of an independent *t* test can be used on the relevant means. The general wisdom is, however, that this should only be done if the overall *F* test is itself significant. Essentially an independent *t* test (Eqn. 7.5) is used:

$$t = \frac{\overline{x}_1 - \overline{x}_2}{\text{SE}(\overline{x}_1 - \overline{x}_2)} \quad (9.14)$$

where, without loss of generality, the comparison is assumed to be between groups 1 and 2. However, for the standard-error term, the estimate of the population variance based on all groups in the analysis (S_W^2 from Eqn. 9.4) replaces the usual pooled estimate based on the specific two groups being compared (Eqn. 7.3):

$$\text{SE}(\overline{x}_1 - \overline{x}_2) = \sqrt{\frac{S_W^2}{n_1} + \frac{S_W^2}{n_2}} \quad (9.15)$$

Note that the divisors in the standard-error term are n_1 and n_2, but the degrees of freedom for the test are $N - k$ (rather than $n_1 + n_2 - 2$, used in the usual t test). These are the degrees of freedom that the variance estimate is based on. Remember that one of the assumptions of the analysis of variance was that the variances in the groups were the same, so that S_W^2 estimates the variance of each of the groups. This is a far more accurate estimate than that based on two groups, but it is the increase in the number of degrees of freedom for the t test that increases the efficiency of the analysis. For small sample sizes, this is quite important, since the increased degrees of freedom mean that the critical t value for the test will be smaller and more easily exceeded.

Assume that in the smoking/blood pressure (unequal sample size) example that prior interest had been on the comparison of blood pressures between current smokers and each of the other two groups. For the comparison of (current) smokers and never smokers the t test gives:

$$t = \frac{140 - 105}{\sqrt{\dfrac{116 \cdot 67}{5} + \dfrac{116 \cdot 67}{4}}} = 35/7 \cdot 25 = 4 \cdot 83$$

on 9 degrees of freedom. The critical 1% (two-sided) t value is $3 \cdot 25$, so there is a highly significant difference between the blood pressures of current smokers and never smokers. For the comparison between current smokers and ex-smokers the t can be calculated:

$$t = \frac{140 - 125}{\sqrt{\dfrac{116 \cdot 67}{5} + \dfrac{116 \cdot 67}{3}}} = 15/7 \cdot 89 = 1 \cdot 90$$

again on 9 degrees of freedom. The critical two-sided 5% value is $2 \cdot 262$, so that the smokers and ex-smokers do not have significantly different blood pressures. The significant differences between the groups determined by the omnibus F test seems to be due to differences between current smokers and never smokers.

9.2.7 Confidence intervals

Confidence intervals for individual means or for the difference between two means are based on the usual approaches described in Sections 4.6.4 and 7.4.2, except that the within-groups mean square S_W^2 is used as the estimate for the population variance in the standard errors and the degrees of freedom are $N - k$ (total sample size in all groups less the number of groups). The confidence interval for the mean in a single group (group i) is given by:

$$\bar{x}_i \pm t_c \frac{S_W}{\sqrt{n_i}} \tag{9.16}$$

where S_W is the square root of S_W^2 and there are $N - k$, rather than $n_i - 1$, degrees of freedom for the t statistic (cf. Eqn. 4.14). The 95% confidence interval for the mean systolic blood pressure in current smokers (unequal-sample size example) is therefore:

$$140 \pm 2.262\sqrt{(116.67/5)} \quad \text{or} \quad 140 \pm 10.93$$

which is from 129.07 to 150.93 mmHg. Note that the critical value of the t distribution for 9 degrees of freedom (2.262) was used, rather than the value for 4 degrees.

Similarly, the confidence interval for the difference between the means in groups 1 and 2 is given by:

$$(\bar{x}_1 - \bar{x}_2) \pm t_c\sqrt{\frac{S_W^2}{n_1} + \frac{S_W^2}{n_2}} \tag{9.17}$$

Again, there are $N - k$ degrees of freedom (cf. Eqn. 7.8). For the difference between the blood pressures of current smokers and never smokers, the 95% confidence interval is:

$$(140 - 105) \pm 2.262\sqrt{\frac{116.67}{5} + \frac{116.67}{4}}$$

which is 35 ± 16.40.

Confidence interval calculations for ANOVA are summarized in Section C.18 of Appendix C.

Comparing means	Formulae	Eqn. nos.
Overall comparison between means (F test)	$F = S_B^2/S_W^2$ d.f. $= k - 1$ and $N - k$	(9.3)
	$S_B^2 = \dfrac{\sum n_i(\bar{x}_i - \bar{x})^2}{k - 1}$	(9.5)
	$S_W^2 = \dfrac{\sum (n_i - 1)S_i^2}{N - k}$	(9.4)
Comparison between two means (t test)	$t = \dfrac{\bar{x}_1 - \bar{x}_2}{\sqrt{\dfrac{S_W^2}{n_1} + \dfrac{S_W^2}{n_2}}}$ d.f. $= N - k$	(9.14/9.15)
Confidence interval for a single mean	$\bar{x}_i \pm t_c \dfrac{S_W}{\sqrt{n_i}}$ d.f. $= N - k$	(9.16)
Confidence interval for difference between two means	$(\bar{x}_1 - \bar{x}_2) \pm t_c\sqrt{\dfrac{S_W^2}{n_1} + \dfrac{S_W^2}{n_2}}$ d.f. $= N - k$	(9.17)

9.3.1 Extension of χ^2 to $2 \times k$ tables

Section 7.11 considered the chi-square (χ^2) test for comparing many proportions in two groups, using an example of the association of smoking status (current, ex- and never smokers) in males and females. Equivalently this example could have been considered a comparison of the proportion of males in the three groups defined by smoking status. Thus, the usual chi-square test is appropriate for multigroup comparisons. In fact, the test is applicable to tables of any dimension (3×3, for instance), as long as the groups in the table are independent. The expected numbers in each cell (E) are calculated in the usual manner and the observed (O) and expected (E) numbers are entered into the standard formula:

$$\chi^2 = \sum \frac{(O - E)^2}{E} \tag{7.23}$$

As mentioned in Section 7.11, the degrees of freedom for the test are $(I - 1)$ $(J - 1)$, where I and J are the number of rows and columns. It is usually suggested that, for valid application of the test, not more than 20% of the cells should have expected numbers less than 5 and no cell should have an expected frequency less than 1. If these conditions are not met, then adjacent categories should be combined and the chi-square recalculated.

When comparing proportions in, say, k groups, the analysis is that of a $2 \times k$ contingency table. As an example, Table 9.4 examines in-hospital mortality after coronary artery bypass surgery in groups defined by increasing severity of angina, using the New York Heart Association classification.

The proportions being compared are denoted p_i in the table, and the usual chi-square can be calculated from Eqn. 7.23. In the special case of a $2 \times k$ table, however, there is a short-cut computational formula, which is entirely equivalent. Firstly, the deaths (or whatever the proportion is being calculated on) in each group are squared and divided by the total number in the group.

Table 9.4 In-hospital mortality after coronary artery bypass surgery, by severity of angina.

Classification of angina:		I	II	III	IV	
Group:	i	1	2	3	4	Row totals
Dead	d_i	2	12	11	22	$D = 47$
Alive	$n_i - d_i$	160	545	403	559	$N - D = 1667$
Total	n_i	162	557	414	581	$N = 1714$
Proportion dead	$p_i = d_i/n_i$	0·0123	0·0215	0·0266	0·0379	
For χ^2 calculation:	d_i^2	4	144	121	484	
	d_i^2/n_i	0·0247	0·2585	0·2923	0·8330	$\mathcal{A} = 1·4085$

This quantity is then summed over all k groups and denoted $\mathscr{A}$. The chi-square, on $k - 1$ degrees of freedom, is then:

$$\chi^2 = \frac{N(N\mathscr{A} - D^2)}{D(N - D)} \tag{9.18}$$

where N is the total sample size, D is the total number of deaths and:

$$\mathscr{A} = \sum (d_i^2 / n_i)$$

In the example:

$$\chi^2 = \frac{1714\left[1714\,(1 \cdot 4085) - (47)^2\right]}{47(1714 - 47)} = 4 \cdot 49$$

The reader should verify that this is exactly the same answer that would have been obtained if Eqn. 7.23 had been employed instead. The critical 5% chi-square on 3 ($k - 1$) degrees of freedom is 7·815, so that, on the basis of the usual chi-square test, the differences between the proportions of deaths in the four anginal categories is non-significant.

If a chi-square test comparing more than two groups is significant, the question is often asked, as with the comparison of means, which groups are significantly different from which. Formal, more advanced, methods are available to help answer this, but it is often sufficient just to examine the data and draw conclusions from a visual inspection of the table.

Without doubt, the chi-square test is the most commonly used test in medical statistics. The fact that it is just as applicable to multigroup comparisons as to the comparison of two groups explains this in part. The popularity of the chi-square test, however, is mainly due to the fact that it can be used to analyse quantitative data also. All one has to do is categorize the quantitative variable (working with, for example, age-groups rather than exact age) and apply the chi-square test in the usual way. The loss of information by categorizing into four or five groups is not great and often a table with a grouped variable can be more informative than working with the mean of the (ungrouped) variable. The categories, however, must be chosen before examination of the data and should not be selected to maximize group differences. This application of the chi-square test is summarized in Section C.15 of Appendix C.

9.3.2 Testing for a trend in proportions [!]

When analysing proportions in more than two groups, it is often of interest to know if the proportions increase or decrease as one moves along the groups. Such a question can only be asked, of course, if the groups have some intrinsic order.

If *prior to the analysis* a trend in the proportions had been considered likely, then a more powerful statistical test than the usual chi-square for a $2 \times k$ table is available. Note that this test should be applied only if the trend is hypothesized prior to examination of the data. Essentially, the test is based on a null hypothesis of no group differences against an alternative hypothesis of a linear trend in proportions. If there is a real linear trend (in the population), then the test is more likely to give a significant result than the usual chi-square. On the other hand, if there are real group differences without a clear trend, the test is less powerful than the usual test.

The exact formulation of the chi-square test for trend is somewhat difficult to justify, so the formula will be given here without explanation. The method is illustrated on the data for mortality after coronary bypass related to anginal status already examined in Table 9.4 and it is assumed that the researchers involved wished to examine whether mortality increased with increasing severity of angina. For examination of a trend, a score must be assigned to each of the groups being compared. The choice of this score is arbitrary and usually it is quite adequate to assign scores of 1, 2, 3, etc. to each category. If the categories represent a grouping of a continuous variable (e.g. age-groups), then the mid-point of the group could be used instead. In the example, scores of 1 to 4 will be assigned to the four anginal groups. The data for the example, together with the quantities required for calculation of the chi-square for trend, are given in Table 9.5.

The chi-square for trend χ^2_{TR}, on 1 degree of freedom (irrespective of the number of groups, is calculated as

$$\chi^2_{TR} = \frac{N(N\mathscr{C} - D\mathscr{B})^2}{D(N - D)(N\mathscr{D} - \mathscr{B}^2)} \tag{9.19}$$

where N is the total sample size, D is the total number of deaths,

$$\mathscr{B} = \sum n_i x_i$$

$$\mathscr{C} = \sum d_i x_i$$

$$\mathscr{D} = \sum n_i x_i^2$$

Table 9.5 In-hospital mortality after coronary artery bypass surgery by severity of angina (chi-square test for trend).

Classification of angina:		I	II	III	IV	
Group:	i	1	2	3	4	Row totals
Dead	d_i	2	12	11	22	$D = 47$
Total	n_i	162	557	414	581	$N = 1714$
For χ^2 calculation:	Score x_i	1	2	3	4	
	$n_i x_i$	162	1114	1242	2324	$\mathscr{B} = 4842$
	$d_i x_i$	2	24	33	88	$\mathscr{C} = 147$
	x_i^2	1	4	9	16	
	$n_i x_i^2$	162	2228	3726	9296	$\mathscr{D} = 15412$

and x_i is the assigned score. From the table:

$$\chi^2_{TR} = \frac{1714\left[1714\,(147) - 47\,(4842)\right]^2}{47\,(1714 - 47)\left[1714\,(15412) - (4842)^2\right]} = 4\cdot38$$

This value exceeds the critical 5% value for chi-square on 1 degree of freedom, so that one can conclude that there is a significant tendency for increased mortality rates to be associated with an increased severity of angina. Note that, in the last section, the ordinary chi-square (on 3 degrees of freedom) did not achieve significance for the same data, illustrating clearly the increased power of this test to detect a trend if it exists. No matter how many groups are involved, χ^2_{TR} has 1 degree of freedom and, if significant, the null hypothesis of no group difference is rejected in favour of a trend of increasing (or decreasing) proportions with group membership.

One can also test if there is a significant departure from a linear trend. (A linear trend holds if the proportions increase at a constant rate in proportion to the score assigned to the groups.) The chi-square for this test is obtained by subtracting the trend chi-square from the total (usual) chi-square and has $k - 2$ degrees of freedom, where k is the number of groups:

$$\chi^2_{DEP} = \chi^2 - \chi^2_{TR} \tag{9.20}$$

In the example, $\chi^2_{DEP} = 4\cdot49 - 4\cdot38 = 0\cdot11$, which, on 2 degrees of freedom, is obviously non-significant. Thus, there is no evidence that the trend is not linear in this case. A significant departure from trend can arise together with a significant trend if there is an increase (decrease) in proportions that is not linear. A significant departure from trend in the absence of a significant trend is interpreted to mean that group differences exist but that there is no trend in the data.

Different formulae for the chi-square test for trend are to be found in different texts. Mostly, these are equivalent formulations of the version given above (Eqn. 9.19), but sometimes there is a factor of $N - 1$ rather than N. This makes no difference in practice. As with the ordinary chi-square test, the test for trend should not be used if more than 20% of the expected numbers in the cells of the table fall below 5 or if any fall below 1. The chi-square test for trend is summarized in Section C.19, Appendix C.

Hypothesis test comparing proportions	Formulae	Eqn. nos.
Overall test	$\chi^2 = \sum \dfrac{(O - E)^2}{E}$	(7.23)
	$= \dfrac{N(N\mathcal{A} - D^2}{D(N - D)}$	(9.18)
	d.f. $= k - 1$	
Test for linear trend	$\chi^2_{TR} = \dfrac{N(N\mathcal{C} - D\mathcal{B})^2}{D(N - D)(N\mathcal{D} - \mathcal{B}^2)}$	(9.19)
	d.f. $= 1$	

(Continued.)

Test for departure from linear trend	$\chi^2_{\text{DEP}} = \chi^2 - \chi^2_{\text{TR}}$	(9.20)

$$\text{d.f.} = k - 2$$

$$\mathscr{A} = \sum (d_i^2 / n_i)$$

$$\mathscr{B} = \sum n_i x_i$$

$$\mathscr{C} = \sum d_i x_i$$

$$\mathscr{D} = \sum n_i x_i^2$$

$$N = \sum n_i$$

$$D = \sum d_i$$

x_i is the assigned score

9.4 Comparison of other statistics in more than two groups

This chapter has concentrated on comparing means and proportions in more than two groups. A non-parametric ANOVA equivalent is available to compare medians, but is not covered in this text. The comparison of rates is usually done in the context of vital statistics and typically includes age adjustment (i.e. correction for the confounding effect of age) as part of the methodology. The topic is therefore considered in Chapter 11, which considers confounder control. Comparison of life table mortality between k groups is a simple extension of the two-group logrank test considered in Section 7.15.6. The two-term logrank χ^2 of Eqn. 7.68 now has k terms, one for each comparison group, and the statistic has $k-1$ degrees of freedom:

$$\chi^2 = \sum \frac{(O - E)^2}{E} \tag{9.21}$$

where the summation is over the O and E calculated separately in each comparison group, in a similar manner to the two-group case.

9.5 Summary

In this chapter, the comparison of independent proportions and means in more than two groups has been discussed. The analysis of variance (ANOVA) was introduced as the appropriate technique for the comparison of means and it was indicated that this is a very powerful method that can extend to complex data structures. It was also shown how the chi-square test for the comparison of two groups extends to multigroup comparisons, and the chi-square test for a trend of proportions was described. Indications of approaches available for multigroup comparisons of medians and life table mortality were also given.

The chapter only considered independent data. Individually matched data in multigroup comparisons are relatively unusual in the medical area, and frequency-matched groups are considered in Chapter 11, where stratified analyses are described in the context of confounder control. The next chapter of the book turns to the analysis of associations between two numerical variables.

10 Associations between Two Quantitative Variables: Regression and Correlation

10.1 Introduction

Chapters 7 and 9 of this book showed how one could statistically analyse differences between groups as regards quantitative variables (comparing mean or median values) and qualitative variables (comparing percentages or proportions). As already mentioned, such a comparison of two or more groups can be viewed as an examination of the association or relationship between two variables, one of which is qualitative and defined by group membership. If, for instance, the proportions of smokers in groups of individuals with and without lung cancer are being compared, essentially the relationship between two qualitative variables is being examined. These are the variable 'lung cancer' (present or absent) and the variable 'smoking category'. If blood pressure is being compared in males and females, the relationship between a quantitative variable (blood pressure) and a qualitative variable (sex) is being examined.

The third possible combination of two variables is that both are quantitative, and this chapter examines associations between two such variables. Although details of some of the simpler calculations are included, these can be omitted at first reading.

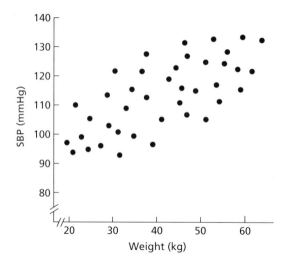

Fig. 10.1 A scattergram of systolic blood pressure (SBP) and weight in 40 10-year-olds.

10.2 Describing relationships between two quantitative variables

There are essentially two possible objectives to the analysis of the relationship between two quantitative variables. The first is to determine if an association between them exists—in other words, if the values of one variable have a tendency to either increase or decrease with values of the other. Allied to this is the requirement to quantify and describe the nature of the relationship, perhaps with a view to prediction. The second objective is that of measuring agreement between two numerical measurements, such as the results of a biochemical blood test performed by two different instruments. Agreement is not the same as association, and regression and correlation techniques are not appropriate for the analysis of agreement. The topic of agreement will be covered separately in Chapter 12.

10.2.1 Scattergrams

In Section 3.2.3, it was explained that an essential first step in the analysis of the relationship between two quantitative variables was to draw a picture of the data as either a graph or a scattergram. Without examination of this picture, it is impossible to describe or analyse any relationship that might exist. Figure 10.1, for instance, shows the relationship between systolic blood pressure (SBP) in mmHg and weight (W) in kilograms in 40 10-year-old schoolchildren.* The points on the scattergram show a trend upwards and to the right; this indicates a direct or positive relationship between the two sets of readings. High (low) values of one variable, blood pressure, are associated with high (low) values of the other, weight. In simple terms, there seems to be a tendency

---

* Adapted from Pollock *et al.* (1981) with permission. Although the regression equation and correlation coefficient (to be discussed later) are taken from this article, which is actually based on a study of 675 children, the scattergram presented here is not based on the actual data and is used for illustrative purposes only.

for blood pressure to increase with weight. A scattergram, then, gives a visual impression of what the relationship between the two variables might be.

Figure 10.2 shows a number of different types of scattergrams that could be obtained when a relationship between two variables is examined. The scattergrams labelled (a) and (b) show relationships that could be considered linear. By linear is meant that, in some average sense, a straight line could be drawn on the scattergram to summarize the relationship. In scattergram (a) the values of the two variables increase together—as in the blood pressure/weight example—and the relationship is called direct. Scattergram (b) shows an indirect or inverse relationship, where the value of one variable decreases as the value of the other increases. The idea of a linear relationship is perhaps best understood when a definite non-linear relationship is seen. In scattergram (c) it does not seem possible to summarize the relationship by means of a straight line and this relationship is called non-linear or curvilinear. Finally, there seems to be no relationship at all between the two variables shown in scattergram (d)—high or low values of one variable are not associated with high or low values of the other.

The reason it is so important to examine the relationship between two quantitative variables by means of a scattergram before any analysis is undertaken is that the techniques to be considered, those of regression and correlation, are only valid for linear relationships. If a relationship seen in a scattergram seems non-linear, then alternative approaches will have to be employed (see Section 10.6). The methods give, for a linear relationship, the line of 'best fit' to the data, a measure of the scatter of points about this best-fit line and a method of determining if the relationship could be due to chance.

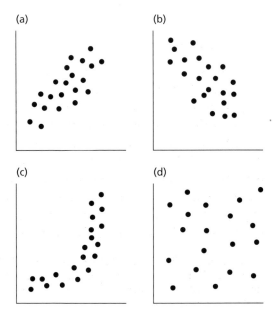

(a)   (b)

(c)   (d)

Fig. 10.2 Scattergrams showing different relationships: (a) linear (direct), (b) linear (inverse/indirect), (c) non-linear (curvilinear), (d) none.

However, just because a scattergram shows a linear relationship between two variables does not necessarily mean that regression and correlation are the correct techniques for the analysis. An important requirement is that the observations be independent. In essence, this means that each pair of observations (e.g. blood pressure and weight) comes from a different subject. If some subjects contribute more than one data point in a scattergram (e.g. blood pressure and weight measured a few years apart on the same person), the correct analysis can be quite complex. It is not considered in this text.

Regression and correlation
• analyse the association between two quantitative variables
• assume independent observations
• assume a linear relationship
• allow hypothesis testing of the relationship

Regression
• gives the 'best-fit' line to the data

Correlation
• gives a measure of scatter of data points around this line

10.2.2 Linear equations

Having identified the existence of a linear relationship between the two variables, the next step is to describe or summarize the relationship in some compact way. Equations are often used to describe relationships, for example:

$$F = 32 + (1\cdot 8 \times C)$$

describes the exact relationship between the two common scales for measurement of temperature. C is the temperature in degrees Celsius or centigrade (°C) and F is the same temperature in degrees Fahrenheit (°F). From the equation a temperature of 0°C corresponds to a temperature of 32°F and 10°C correspond to 50°F. If this relationship were to be represented graphically and a number of different points were to be plotted, the points would be seen all to lie on a straight line. Figure 10.3 shows five such plotted points and the straight line that defines the relationship between the two temperature scales.

A 'straight line' relationship such as this is called *linear*. In general, the equation of a straight line can be expressed as $y = a + bx$, where the variable y is drawn on the vertical axis and the variable x is on the horizontal axis. 'a' is the intercept of the line on the y axis (the value of y when x is zero) and 'b' is the slope of the line. The slope of the line, b, measures how much the y variable changes for every unit increase in the x variable. Thus every 1°C increase in temperature corresponds to an increase of 1·8°F. An equation always implies an exact relationship, which, in the case of two variables x and y, means that, given a value for x, a value for y can be precisely determined. When the two

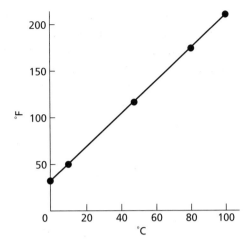

Fig. 10.3 Relationship between °F and
°C.

variables increase together, the relationship is said to be direct and the value
of *b* is positive. When the relationship is inverse or indirect, the value of *b* is
negative and, as one variable increases, the other decreases.

The equation of a straight line
- $y = a + bx$

10.2.3 The regression equation and regression coefficient

Now, let us return to the example of the relationship between weight and
blood pressure, for which the scattergram was given in Fig. 10.1. It is obvious
that there is some form of relationship between the two variables but, obviously, this relationship cannot be described exactly by means of an equation.
No line (straight or smoothly curved) could pass through all the points on
the scattergram. However, some sort of 'average' equation could summarize
the relationship, and might be obtained by drawing a smooth line through the
middle of the data points. In Fig. 10.1, a straight line would seem to be the best
choice and, although such a line could be fitted by using a ruler, there would be
a subjective element about this and different people would fit different lines.
There is, however, a mathematical technique for finding the 'best-fit' line to a
set of data points. This line is called a *regression line* and its corresponding
equation is called a *regression equation*. This text deals, for the most part,
with linear regression, which means that the relationship as seen in the scattergram should at least appear to be linear in the first place. For the moment,
also, only relationships between two variables, or what is technically referred
to as *bivariate regression*, will be considered. The regression equation, then, in
some sense, measures the average relationship between two variables. It can
be expressed in the form:

$$\hat{y} = a + bx \tag{10.1}$$

where $\hat{y}$ is the 'computed', 'expected' or 'predicted' value of y given any value of x. 'a' and 'b' are constants, to be determined on the basis of the data, as described later, by a technique called the *method of least squares*. In many situations, the '^' above the y variable will be omitted, although it should always be remembered that, in a regression equation, it is an expected value which is being calculated. In the blood pressure study, the actual regression equation calculated turns out to be:

$$SBP = 79{\cdot}7 + 0{\cdot}8\,W \qquad (10.2)$$

where SBP represents systolic blood pressure in mmHg, W represents weight in kilograms and the coefficents 79·7 and 0·8 are calculated from the data. This regression line is drawn in on the scattergram in Fig. 10.4. The line passes through the middle of the scatter points, and the regression line might reasonably be claimed to represent, approximately, the relationship between the two variables. On the basis of the regression line, it would be expected or predicted that a child weighing 40 kg, for instance, would have a systolic blood pressure of:

$$SBP = 79{\cdot}7 + 0{\cdot}8(40) = 111{\cdot}7\,mmHg$$

This result could also have been read off Fig. 10.4 using the regression line. Note, however, that there may not have been anyone in the study who actually weighed 40 kg and, even if there was, he or she need not necessarily have had a blood pressure of 111·7. The figure of 111·7 mmHg is interpreted as the average blood pressure that would be expected among a large number of children, all of whom weighed 40 kg, or, in other words, the average blood pressure associated with this weight.

The regression equation also implies that systolic blood pressure will increase by 0·8 mmHg with every 1 kg increase in weight. The coefficient 0·8 in the equation is called the *regression coefficient* and, in general, means the change in y per unit change in x. It is, in fact, the slope of the regression line. One further point may be noted; if a value of zero is substituted for weight in Eqn. 10.2, an expected systolic blood pressure of 79·7 would be calculated. It is plainly nonsensical to estimate a blood pressure for a child weighing nothing. The regression equation is derived from the observed values of the two variables, and it is only valid within the ranges actually observed for the variables. Extrapolation beyond this range may be misleading and is often totally invalid.

Another example of a regression analysis relates to indicators of prognosis after a myocardial infarction (heart attack). The left ventricular ejection fraction (LVEF) is one such indicator, but, unfortunately, is difficult to measure and also expensive. On the other hand, the taking of an electrocardiogram (ECG) is much faster and cheaper, and a particular index called the QRS score is easily derived from an ECG tracing. Twenty-eight patients had their LVEF measured 3 weeks after their heart attack. This was then compared with the patients' QRS score to evaluate the usefulness of this score in determining

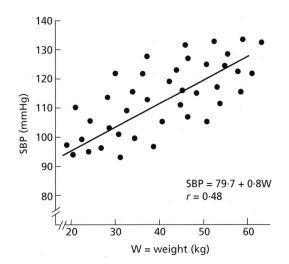

Fig. 10.4 Scattergram of systolic blood pressure (SBP) and weight (w) with the regression line drawn in.

LVEF. Figure 10.5 shows the scattergram and regression line for the relationship between these two variables. From inspection of the plot points on the diagram, it is clear that the relationship is linear but inverse. The regression equation can be calculated as:

$$LVEF = 62{\cdot}01 - 3{\cdot}44QRS \tag{10.3}$$

where the LVEF is measured as a percentage. In this case, the regression coefficient is −3·44, which means that, for every increase of 1 unit in the QRS score, the value of the LVEF decreases by 3·44%. An inverse relationship will always give rise to a negative regression coefficient.

The regression equation
- the best-fit line to the data
- has the form $y = a + bx$

The regression coefficient 'b'
- measures what the relationship between the variables is
- measures the amount of change in the y variable for a unit change in the x variable
- is positive for a direct relationship and negative for an inverse one

---

10.2.4 Dependent and explanatory (predictor or independent) variables

In both the above examples, it was meaningful to consider how one variable depended on the other. The aim was to determine, in the first case, how blood pressure depended on weight and, in the second case, how the LVEF could be determined by the QRS score. Blood pressure and the LVEF are both called *dependent* variables, while weight and the QRS score are called the explanatory, predictor or independent variables. The question of which variable in a regression analysis is explanatory and which is dependent is decided on the

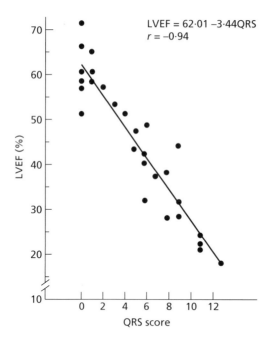

Fig. 10.5 Scattergram showing relationship between the left ventricular ejection fraction (LVEF) and the QRS score in 28 patients after a myocardial infarction (from Palmeri *et al.*, 1982, with permission).

basis of logic (a child's weight is hardly dependent on blood pressure) or on the precise question the researcher is trying to answer. (In the heart-attack example, the purpose was to predict a patient's LVEF on the basis of the QRS score.) It is important to note, however, that a regression equation only expresses a numerical association between two variables; it does not establish a causal link between the two or prove that one variable is causally dependent on the other.

In a regression equation, the dependent variable is written on the left-hand side of the equation and the explanatory variable is written on the right-hand side; it is usual to talk about the regression of the dependent variable on the explanatory. Thus, the first example is of the regression of blood pressure on weight. In the scattergram, the dependent variable is put on the y axis. It is important, in calculating regression equations, that one is clear which variable is to be considered explanatory. Without going into detail here (see Section 10.4), the regression of a variable y on a variable x does not give the same mathematical relationship as the regression of x on y, although, unless there is a large scatter of points around the regression line, the relationships are usually very close.

10.3 Correlation

10.3.1 Strength and goodness of fit

Consider the regression Eqn. 10.2. For a given value of W (body weight), a corresponding value of SBP (systolic blood pressure) can be calculated. This calculated value can be written SB̂P. SB̂P can be interpreted as the expected or average value of SBP associated with the given value of weight. Now, if all the points in the scattergram lay on the regression line, for any given value of W the expected and observed values of SBP would be identical. The regression equation would describe the relationship between systolic blood pressure and weight exactly. The variation in systolic blood pressure would be completely explained by, or be dependent upon, the variation in weight.

In practice, this is not the case. Systolic blood pressure can vary independently of variation in weight, so that two children of the same weight may have different blood pressures. Weight is not the only factor affecting systolic blood pressure. Given any particular value for weight, the expected blood pressure can be calculated. However, since blood pressures do vary independently of weight, the blood pressure associated with any particular weight cannot be predicted exactly. In this sense, the regression equation can be described as measuring the average relationship between the two variables. It does not, however, measure the *strength** or *goodness of fit* of the relationship.

In the blood pressure and weight example (Fig. 10.4), there is a fairly large dispersion of the plot points around the regression line. This suggests a fairly weak relationship between the two variables. Given a weight of 40 kg, a child's systolic blood pressure could be estimated as 111·7 mmHg, but the child's actual blood pressure could vary quite appreciably around this. A considerable amount of the variation in the dependent variable is unexplained by the variation in the explanatory variable. Although, on average, systolic blood pressure increases with weight, there are obviously many other factors that influence this variable.

In Fig. 10.5, which shows the relationship between the LVEF and the QRS score, the plot points lie close to the regression line, which suggests a strong relationship between the two variables. The observed values for LVEF do not differ markedly from the expected values represented by the regression line. This implies that most of the variation in LVEF can be 'explained' by the variation in the QRS score. Given a particular QRS score, the estimated LVEF could be predicted, and it would be fairly certain that the actual value would be quite close to this predicted one.

10.3.2. The correlation coefficient

A measure of the degree of scatter of the data points around the regression line is given by the *correlation coefficient*, denoted by '*r*'. The measure is also called the *coefficient of linear correlation* or (to distinguish it from a different correlation coefficient) *Pearson's product-moment correlation*. An analogy can be made with the position of the mean and standard deviation as descriptive statistics of the distribution of a single quantitative variable. The mean is a summary or average value and the standard deviation measures the spread of

---

* Strong in this sense means a relationship that allows good prediction of one variable from the other, or, in other words, a relationship that shows little scatter around the regression line.

the data around the mean. In the case of a relationship between two quantitative variables, the regression line summarizes or gives the average relationship and the correlation coefficient gives the degree of spread around that relationship.

Values of r can only lie between +1 and −1, the sign of r depending on whether or not there is a direct relationship between the two variables, as in Fig. 10.4, or an inverse relationship, as in Fig. 10.5. If the relationship between the two variables is perfect or exact — that is, if all the points on the scattergram lie on the regression line — r will be equal to +1 or −1. A positive sign indicates a direct relationship; a negative sign indicates an inverse one. If there is no relationship at all between the two variables, r will be 0. The greater the numerical value of r, the stronger the relationship between the two variables.

Methods for calculating the correlation coefficient are given in Section 10.4, but for the moment only the results for the two examples are given. The correlation coefficient for the relationship between blood pressure and weight in 10-year-old children is $r = 0 \cdot 48$, which is not very high. On the other hand, $r = -0 \cdot 94$ for the relationship between LVEF and the QRS score, which confirms the strength of that relationship as determined visually. (Note that r is negative for this inverse relationship.)

It has been said that r ranges from −1 to +1, but it is not immediately clear how to interpret different values of this coefficient. It happens, however, that the value of r^2 has a readily understandable interpretation in terms of the strength of a relationship. Take the example of blood pressure and weight. Blood pressures will show a fair degree of variation from child to child due to the many factors, one of which is body weight, that affect blood pressure. This can be referred to as the total variation in the variable. Prediction of the systolic blood pressure of a 10-year-old without reference to these factors would be subject to quite a degree of uncertainty. If, however, only children of a particular weight were examined, the variation in their blood pressures would be considerably less. (See Fig. 10.4, where the scatter of blood pressures for a given weight is far less than the total scatter of blood pressure in all the children studied.) Some of the total variation in blood pressure measurements can be explained by the variation in children's weights (the 'explained' variation), while the remainder of the variation must be due to other factors, which were not considered explicitly or are unknown (the 'unexplained' variation). The larger the first component is, relative to the second, the stronger is the relationship between the two variables.

It can be shown that r^2 (the square of the correlation coefficient — sometimes called the *coefficient of determination*) is equal to the proportion of the total variation in the dependent variable (SBP) that is explained by the regression line. If the relationship between the two variables is perfect, all the variation in the dependent variable is explained by the regression line, and thus r^2 equals, 1, so that r equals ±1. r is written plus or minus according to whether the relationship is direct or inverse. The more closely the points in the scattergram are dispersed around the regression line, the higher will be the proportion of variation explained by the regression line and hence the greater the value of r^2 and r. In the blood pressure example, it was said that r equals 0·48, so that r^2 equals 0·2304. Thus, the variation in the weights of the children explains just over 23% of the total variation in blood pressure. The other 77% of the variation is unexplained and must be due to many other factors, not considered in this analysis. In the LVEF example, $r^2 = (0·94)^2 = 0·8836$, which means that over 88% of the variation in LVEF is explained by the variation in the QRS score.

The correlation coefficient (r)
- measures the degree of scatter of the data points around a regression line
- measures the goodness of fit or strength of the relationship
- lies between −1 and +1

10.3.3 Correlation without regression

In most cases involving the use of regression analysis, it is advisable to include the value of the correlation coefficient or its square. There are situations, however, where determination of the exact form of a linear relationship is not relevant, or where identification of which of the variables being examined is dependent and which explanatory or predictor is not obvious. In these cases, a correlation analysis examining only the strength of a relationship may be all that is required, and the actual regression equation may be irrelevant. A regression analysis is not symmetrical in that one variable must be taken as dependent and the other as explanatory. Correlation, however, results in a measure of association that does not imply any dependence of one variable on the other.

Figure 10.6 is a case in point. This shows a scattergram for the relationship between the age at which 38 females with frequent urinary-tract infections (UTI) developed their first kidney stone and the age at which they first developed UTI. Rather than one age determining the other age, it is much more likely that another factor or factors determined the timing of each event. A regression analysis would not seem to be appropriate, but a correlation analysis examining the strength of the relationship would be. For this example, r turns out to be equal to 0·86 ($r^2 = 0·74$), showing a reasonably strong association between the age at first infection and the age at first stone. The interpretation of this particular association in terms of a causal hypothesis is much more difficult, however.

10.4 Calculation of regression and correlation coefficients [!]

In Section 10.2.3, it was pointed out that a regression line could be fitted by hand by drawing a line through the middle of the points on the scattergram.

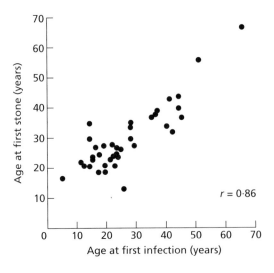

Fig. 10.6 Relation between age at first stone and age at first infection in 38 females with two or more stone-associated urinary-tract infections (see Fig. 3.4) (from Parks *et al.*, 1982, with permission).

Obviously, as was said, this is rather a haphazard way of fitting the line, and a more systemic procedure is required. The most common technique is called the *method of least squares*. Assume that the scatter of points is such that a straight line would be appropriate to describe the relationship. From the infinite number of straight lines that could be drawn, it is desirable to select that line to which the points on the scattergram are, in some sense, closest. That is, the line should be drawn in such a way as to minimize the distance between the scatter points and the line. In Fig. 10.7, a line has been fitted to minimize the sum of vertical distances between the four plot points and the line. Actually, since some of these distances will be positive (points above the line) and some will be negative (points below the line), the line is fitted to minimize the sum of squares of the vertical distance between the plot points and the line. This is why it is called the method of least squares.

When the line is fitted in this way, the overall difference between the plot points and the line is minimized. This is the line of 'best fit'. The mathematical derivation of the regression coefficients a and b in the regression line:

$$\hat{y} = a + bx \qquad (10.1)$$

are not given here, but they can be calculated from the following formulae:

$$b = \frac{\sum (x - \bar{x})(y - \bar{y})}{\sum (x - \bar{x})^2} \qquad (10.4)$$

$$= \frac{\sum (x - \bar{x})(y - \bar{y})}{(n - 1)S_x^2} \qquad (10.5)$$

$$a = \bar{y} - b\bar{x} \qquad (10.6)$$

These are the slope and intercept of the regression line, as determined by the method of least squares. The numerator in the expression for b, $\sum (x - \bar{x})(y - \bar{y})$, looks formidable and, as it stands, requires subtraction of the mean of the x

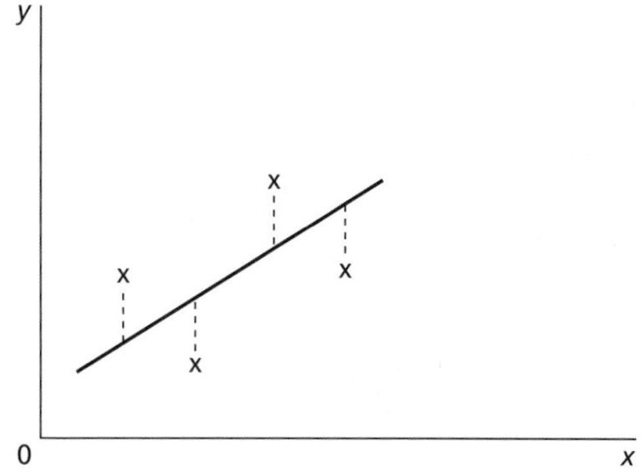

Fig. 10.7 Illustration of the 'method of least squares'.

variable from each x value, the mean of the y variable from each corresponding y value, multiplication of the two results together, and summing over all the pairs of xy values. Appendix A, however, outlines an easier computational approach. The denominator of the expression for b is identical to $(n-1)S_x^2$ where S_x^2 is the variance (square of the standard deviation) of the x values (see Eqn. 1.6). The equation for a requires only the means of both x and y, together with the calculated value of b.

Once the regression equation has been estimated, it can easily be drawn in on the scattergram. Choose two representative values for x; calculate the predicted or expected $\hat{y}$ values; plot in these points and connect with a straight line.

The formula for the correlation coefficient r is also fairly cumbersome;

$$r = \frac{\sum(x-\bar{x})(y-\bar{y})}{\sqrt{\sum(x-\bar{x})^2 \sum(y-\bar{y})^2}} \qquad (10.7)$$

$$= \frac{\sum(x-\bar{x})(y-\bar{y})}{(n-1)S_x S_y} \qquad (10.8)$$

where S_x and S_y are the standard deviations of the x and y variables, respectively. Appendix A outlines in detail the calculation of these quantities for the LVEF data of Fig. 10.5.

10.5 Statistical inference in regression and correlation

10.5.1 Populations and samples

In the examples used so far, and in general, analysis is based on a sample of the pairs of variables of interest. Thus, the data in Fig. 10.1 are based on a sample of 10-year-old children. Now, in the same way that the mean and standard deviation of a random sample are estimates of the mean and standard deviation of the population from which it is drawn, so the regression coefficient and correlation coefficient of a sample of pairs of two variables are estimates of the regression coefficient and correlation coefficient for the population of pairs of these values. Let the regression coefficient for the sample be denoted by b and the correlation coefficient by r; similarly, denote the regression coefficient for the whole population by β (beta) and the correlation coefficient by ρ (rho, the Greek letter 'r'). Then, the sample statistics b and r are estimates of the unknown population parameters β and ρ. The regression equation in the population may thus be written:

$$y = \alpha + \beta x \qquad (10.9)$$

where α and β are the regression coefficients in the population. (a and α are also called regression coefficients, although the term is more usually employed for b and β.) Note that there is no implication that all the data points in the population lie *on* the regression line. There will be a degree of scatter in the population as well.

An interesting possibility now arises; suppose, for the whole population of pairs of values, that $\beta = 0$ and $\rho = 0$. This would occur in cases where there was no relationship between the two variables.* The two variables are said to be independent of one another. An example would be pairs of values that arise in throwing two dice simultaneously. There is no relationship (or should not be!) between the number that turns up on one die and the number turning up on the other. A regression analysis between pairs of values should yield $b = 0$ and $r = 0$.

10.5.2 Confidence intervals and hypothesis tests

However, if a sample of pairs of values is analysed, it is quite possible that, just by chance, non-zero values will be obtained for b and r. In the same way that the mean ($\bar{x}$) of a single sample is unlikely to be exactly equal to a population mean (μ), the values of a regression coefficient b and a correlation coefficient r derived from a sample are unlikely to be exactly equal to the population values β and ρ. Hence, it is likely that, even if β and ρ equal 0, b and r will be non-zero. This means that the results of a regression analysis may suggest a relationship between two variables that is quite spurious. To guard against this possibility, some method is needed to make inferences about the population values of b and r (β and ρ, respectively) on the basis of the sample results. In previous chapters, it was explained how confidence intervals for and significance tests on unknown population parameters could be based on the sample statistics and their standard errors. Similarly, confidence intervals and significance tests are available for the regression and correlation coefficients (β and ρ) based on the standard errors of their sample values. Tests for the value of α (the y-intercept) are also available, although less commonly employed.

It is important to distinguish between the strength of a relationship as measured by the correlation coefficient, or its square, and its statistical significance

---

* β is a measure of the average change in one variable (y) per unit change in the other (x). If there is no relationship between x and y, an increase of 1 unit in x is equally likely to be associated with a decrease or increase in y. Hence the average change in y per unit change in x will be 0. Similarly, if no relationship can be postulated between x and y, $\rho = 0$.

for a null hypothesis of zero population correlation. A significant correlation does not mean a strong relationship; thus an *r* of 0·12 explaining only 1·4% [$(0·12)^2 = 0·0144$] of the variation in the dependent variable could be highly significant from the statistical point of view but would probably be of little consequence. On the other hand, a high value for *r* may be non-significant if based on a very small sample size. Correlation coefficients can only be interpreted if both their magnitude and significance are reported.

10.5.3 Assumptions

As with other significance tests, however, some assumptions concerning the underlying distribution of the data must be made for valid use of these inferential approaches. For inferences relating to a regression analysis, it must be assumed that the distribution of *y* for each fixed value of *x* is normal (or nearly so), that the standard deviation of this normal distribution of *y* is the same for each *x* and that the mean values of the *y* distribution are linearly related to *x*. These assumptions are explained below in the specific example of the regression of blood pressure on weight in 10-year-old children, considered earlier. The assumptions state that, for children of a given weight (40 kg, say), the distribution of systolic blood pressure is normal with a standard deviation (σ), and that, no matter which weight is chosen, children of that weight will have a normally distributed blood pressure with this standard deviation. This assumption, which is often stated in terms of variances, rather than standard deviations, is called the assumption of homoscedasticity (see Section 7.3.2). The final assumption is that the population mean systolic blood pressure for each different weight is a linear function of weight.

For inferences on the correlation coefficient, a further assumption about the distribution of the *x* variable is required. Essentially, the *x* variable must also have a normal distribution for each value of *y*, in which case *x* and *y* have what is called a bivariate normal distribution. There is no such requirement for inferences on regression and the *x* values can be fixed in the design of the investigation. For example, a number of children of pre-specified weights could have been chosen for the study of blood pressure and weight, rather than carrying out a survey of whatever children happened to be available. Some suggestions of what approach to take when the assumptions do not hold are considered in Section 10.6.

Assumptions for valid inferences in regression and correlation
- independent data
- distribution of *y* normal for each *x*
- variances the same at each *x*
- linear relationship between the mean of the *y* values and each corresponding *x*
- bivariate normal distribution (correlation only)

10.5.4 Mathematical details [!]

This section summarizes some of the formulae used in making statistical inferences for regression and correlation analyses. First, a standard error for the regression coefficient is given by:

$$SE(b) = \frac{\sigma}{\sqrt{\sum(x - \bar{x})^2}} \tag{10.10}$$

$$= \frac{\sigma}{\sqrt{(n-1)}S_x} \tag{10.11}$$

where σ is the (unknown) standard deviation of the y variable at each x value. The assumption of equality of variances is important, and more advanced techniques may have to be used if the assumption is not tenable, or perhaps a transformation of the data (see Section 10.6.2) may suffice. Note that, of course, σ is unknown and must be estimated from the data. Again, without deriving the result, it can be shown that an estimate of σ is given by:

$$S_{y,x} = \sqrt{\frac{\sum(y - \hat{y})^2}{n-2}} \tag{10.12}$$

where y represents the observed y values obtained, and $\hat{y}$ is the predicted or expected y calculated from the regression equation on the corresponding x (Eqn. 10.1). The similarity of this formula to that of the usual standard deviation should be noted. The quantity is some sort of average of the deviations of each point from its predicted value, but, as for the standard deviation, it is the squared deviations that are averaged. It can be seen, however, that $S_{y,x}$ is a reasonable estimator for σ. (An easier computational form is given in Appendix A.) $S_{y,x}$ is variously referred to as *the standard deviation from regression* or *the standard error of the estimate* or when squared as *the residual mean square*. $n - 2$ is sometimes called the residual degrees of freedom. The subscript y,x on S means that we are talking about the regression of y on x.

The standard error of b is estimated as (see Eqn. 10.11):

$$SE(b) = \frac{S_{y,x}}{\sqrt{(n-1)}S_x} \tag{10.13}$$

This standard error of b has $n - 2$ degrees of freedom, so that:

$$b \pm t_c SE(b)$$

gives a confidence interval for b where t_c is the critical value of the t distribution on $n - 2$ degrees of freedom for the required confidence level. In the LVEF example, it can be shown that (see Appendix A) $S_{y,x}$ equals 5·102 on 26 degrees of freedom, and S_x equals 4·118. It has already been seen that b equals −3·438 (to three decimal places), so that a 95% confidence interval for β is given by:

$$-3{\cdot}438 \pm 2{\cdot}056\,(0{\cdot}238)$$

where $SE(b) = 0{\cdot}238$ from Eqn. 10.13, and $t_c = 2{\cdot}056$ is the critical t value on 26 degrees of freedom, corresponding to 5% of the area in both tails. The lower and upper confidence limits are thus $-3{\cdot}927$ and $-2{\cdot}949$.

To recap: usually, a calculated regression equation is determined on a sample of values, so that, in particular, the regression coefficient b is a sample estimate of the regression coefficient (β) in the population. As with sample means and proportions, it is possible (given certain assumptions) to calculate the standard error of the regression coefficient and thus give a confidence interval estimate for the unknown value of β. A hypothesis test for β is also easily derived. If the null hypothesis specifies a particular value β_0 for the regression coefficient in the population, the test statistic is:

$$t = \frac{b - \beta_0}{SE(b)} \tag{10.14}$$

where b is the sample value of the regression coefficient, β_0 is the hypothesized vale and $SE(b)$ is given by Eqn. 10.13. This provides a t test on $n - 2$ degrees of freedom. The usual null hypothesis specifies a value of $\beta = 0$, so that the test is of the existence of any relationship in the first place, and Eqn. 10.14 becomes, when Eqn. 10.13 is used for $SE(b)$:

$$t = \frac{b S_x \sqrt{n-1}}{S_{y,x}} \tag{10.15}$$

If t is greater than the appropriate (usually two-sided) critical value, then the existence of a real relationship in the population can be accepted. For the LVEF data, $t = -14{\cdot}42$, d.f. $= 26$, $p < 0{\cdot}01$. Thus, the value of b is significantly different from zero. This, of course, is consistent with the confidence interval for β calculated above, which did not include zero as a possible value.

Although formulae are not given in this text, it is also possible to derive standard errors for a predicted $\hat{y}$ value, given a particular value for x, or for the population mean y value for that x. Confidence intervals can then be obtained.

The null hypothesis of zero population correlation $(\rho = 0)$ uses the test statistic:

$$t = r\sqrt{\frac{n-2}{1-r^2}} \tag{10.16}$$

on $n - 2$ degrees of freedom. For the LVEF data, $t = -14{\cdot}42$ on 26 degrees of freedom. This is numerically the same as that obtained using the t test of zero regression coefficient mentioned above (Eqn. 10.15). This is not an accident; it can be shown that the two tests are mathematically equivalent. Confidence intervals for ρ and tests of hypotheses for population values other than $\rho = 0$ are more complex and are not considered here.

Section C.20 of Appendix C summarizes the statistical calculations of this section.

10.6 When the assumptions do not hold [!]

10.6.1 Residual analysis

The assumptions underlying the regression techniques discussed in this chapter are important. These are, essentially, a linear relationship, equality of variances and normality of the data. One method of checking on the assumptions is to perform what is called an analysis of residuals. The residual is the difference between the observed value y and the predicted value $\hat{y}$ obtained by applying the regression equation to the corresponding x value for the dependent variable. Plots of the residuals against x or $\hat{y}$ can provide insights into how well the assumptions hold and can aid greatly in choosing the correct approach. A more advanced text should be consulted for details on this topic.

10.6.2 Data transformations

In previous sections, it was shown how suitable transformation of the data might reduce skewness (Section 1.6.7) or decrease differences between group variances (Section 7.4.4). Data transformations may also linearize a curved relationship. Figure 10.8 shows some curvilinear relationships and the transformations that could be applied to either the y or the x variable to linearize the relationship. One common cause of non-linearity is a skew in the distribution of one or both of the variables, and the transformations to reduce skewness can be used. If a transformation succeeds, then a linear regression analysis can be carried out on the transformed data. In practice, some experimentation may be necessary with different transformations of either the x or y variable to produce the best result.

10.6.3 Polynomial regression

Another approach to curvilinear regression is to run a *polynomial regression* on the data, where, without transformations, a dependent variable y might be related to an independent or predictor variable x with a polynomial equation of the following form:

$$Y = a + bx + cx^2 \tag{10.17}$$

with terms in x^3 and x^4, etc., if necessary. With such an approach, more than one regression coefficient must be estimated (e.g. b and c above). Often, curvilinear relationships can be expressed in such a polynomial form and the analysis is very similar to that of *multiple regression*, to be discussed in the following chapter.

10.6.4 Rank correlation

When other assumptions underlying linear regression do not hold, non-parametric alternatives are available, and rank correlation is such a procedure

Form of non-linear relationship	Cause of non-linearity

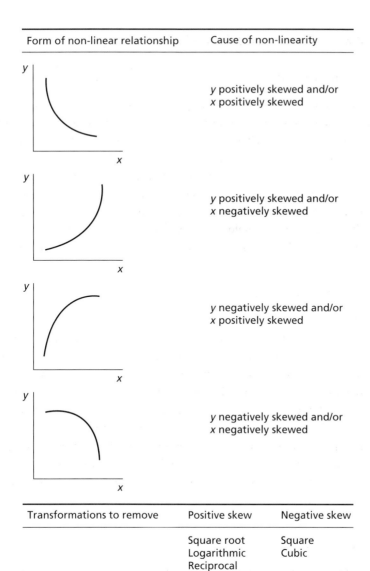

y positively skewed and/or
x positively skewed

y positively skewed and/or
x negatively skewed

y negatively skewed and/or
x positively skewed

y negatively skewed and/or
x negatively skewed

Transformations to remove	Positive skew	Negative skew
	Square root	Square
	Logarithmic	Cubic
	Reciprocal	

Fig. 10.8 Data transformations to linearize relationships.

for calculating a correlation coefficient. As such, it does not require the assumptions made for the usual approach when Pearson's product-moment correlation coefficient is employed. There are two common rank procedures which will be encountered in the medical literature. The first is called *Kendall's rank correlation coefficient* or *Kendall's tau* (tau is the Greek letter 't'). The calculations can be complex and are not given in this text. An alternative rank-correlation method, due to Spearman, is given instead, which results in the calculation of *Spearman's rank correlation coefficient*. When in doubt about the underlying assumptions required for an ordinary correlation analysis, when a transformation of the data will not work or when perhaps only a ranking of the data is available, there should be recourse to this method. The first step is to rank the observations on each variable. Suppose 10 children are subjected to a form of intelligence test by two independent assessors. The ranks assigned to the children by each investigator are shown in Table 10.1.

The ranking order given by the two assessors, although similar, is different.* If the ranking orders were exactly the same, a coefficient of correlation of +1 would be expected. On the other hand, if the ranking order of assessor B were exactly the *reverse* of that of assessor A, the coefficient of correlation would be expected to be −1. If there is no relationship at all between the two rankings, the coefficient of correlation would be expected to be almost 0.

For each student, one calculates the differences between the ranks given by the two assessors: d = 'the rank for assessor A' minus 'the rank for assessor B'. These differences are shown in Table 10.1. They are squared and summed up to:

$$\sum d^2 = 70{\cdot}5 \qquad (10.18)$$

Spearman's rank correlation coefficient is then simply calculated as:

$$r_s = 1 - \frac{6\sum d^2}{n(n^2 - 1)} \qquad (10.19)$$

where n is the number of pairs (10 in this case). r_s in the example turns out to be 0·5727. This correlation coefficient can be interpreted in a similar manner to the parametric correlation coefficient discussed earlier. The formula given is not quite exact if there are a lot of tied ranks in the data.

A significance test can also be performed on Spearman's rank correlation coefficient. The test statistic is actually r_s itself, and Table B.10 gives the critical values for a given number of pairs. If the calculated correlation coefficient is equal to or outside the limits defined by $\pm r_c$ given in the table, a significant result can be declared. For 10 pairs and a two-sided significance level of 5%, r_s would have to lie outside $\pm$ 0·6485. The calculated r_s in the example is not outside these limits, and so it can be concluded that there is no significant difference between the ranks assigned by these two assessors. Section C.21 of Appendix C summarizes the steps required to do these calculations.

Table 10.1 Spearman's rank correlation coefficient. Rank assigned to 10 children by two assessors.

Child	1	2	3	4	5	6	7	8	9	10
Assessor A	7	6	1	2	3	8·5	8·5	10	4	5
Assessor B	6	7	3	2	1	4	9	8	10	5
d	1	−1	−2	0	2	4·5	−0·5	2	−6	0
d^2	1	1	4	0	4	20·25	0·25	4	36	0

$\sum d^2 = 70{\cdot}5; \ r_s = 1 - \dfrac{6(70{\cdot}5)}{10(99)} = 0{\cdot}5727; \ \text{NS}.$

* See Section 12.5.1 for discussion on measuring agreement.

10.7 Biases and misinterpretations in regression

10.7.1 Origins of the term 'regression'

The term 'regression' for the type of analysis that has been considered seems a bit strange and was first used by Sir Francis Galton in describing his 'law of universal regression' in 1889. 'Each peculiarity in a man is shared by his kinsman, but *on the average* in a less degree.' Thus, for example, intelligent fathers tend to have intelligent sons, but the sons are, on average, less intelligent than their fathers. There is a regression, or 'going back', of the sons' intelligence towards the average intelligence of all men. Sons of intelligent fathers will, of course, on average be more intelligent than the average in the population. Galton's 'law', which has a genetic explanation, is illustrated graphically in Fig. 10.9, which shows the scattergram and regression line for the IQs of fathers and sons (one son for each father!) in a number of families. For any parental IQ, the mean of the sons' IQ is closer to the mean IQ (about 100) than their fathers' was. From the diagram, for example, fathers who had an IQ of 110 had sons with an average IQ of 106. Similarly, sons of fathers with an IQ of 90 themselves had an average IQ of 93. Because Galton used a scattergram to illustrate his ideas, the word 'regression' is now applied to the analysis of any relationship between two numerical variables. Galton's observation on regression is not confined to genetic situations, however, and the phenomenon of *regression to the mean* can cause confusion in the interpretation of certain types of data.

10.7.2 Regression to the mean

Take a simple example. Suppose the mid-year examination results of 100 first-year medical students in statistics are obtained and the group of 25 with the

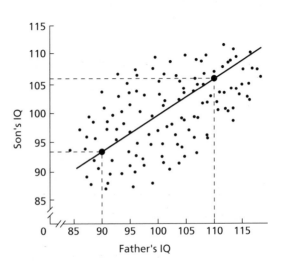

Fig. 10.9 Regression to the mean of sons' IQ.

highest marks are identified. Call these students, identified at this exam, the 'bright students' and suppose their average mark is 62% while the average mark for the whole class is 51%. Because of regression to the mean, it can be predicted that, when the end-year examination is held, the average mark of these 25 bright students will on this second occasion be less than 62%. This will occur even if the average mark for the whole group remains at 51%, with an overall similar spread of marks. Why this happens is not very hard to see. Some of the 25 bright students will have got very high marks in the mid-year examination that they are most unlikely to improve on, or not much anyway. On the other hand, some of the 25 could drop their marks appreciably in the second examination; this could be due to luck on the first examination or a bad day on the second. Essentially, some of the bright students disimprove but, because they have further to fall, this is not balanced by a similar magnitude of improvement in the bright students who improve. As a consequence, the average mark of the bright students is likely to fall, or regress downward, to the mean of the full group. If, instead, the 25 worst students on the first examination had been taken, their average mark would be likely to increase or regress upward to the mean.

Regression to the mean can occur when a variable is measured on two separate occasions, when that variable can change its value in the individual on whom it is measured and when a subgroup of the larger study group is defined on the basis of high (or low) values of the variable at the first measurement. Any subgroup so defined will have an average value for the variable that is lower (or higher) the second time it is measured.

Regression to the mean occurs when
- a group is defined by extreme values of a factor that varies within a person
- a second measurement of the factor is made
- the initial and subsequent mean levels of the factor are compared within the group

---

10.7.3 Misinterpretation of regression to the mean

It is very easy to be misled by the phenomenon of regression to the mean in clinical situations. For instance, it would seem logical to decide that a blood pressure above a certain level (say, 180 mmHg) would be an appropriate entry criterion to a trial of blood pressure reduction. Because of regression to the mean, however, the average blood pressure of this group would be lower on a repeat examination than it was at study entry. Such a decrease could be mistakenly interpreted as the effect of a particular treatment, whereas it would occur without any intervention whatsoever. Allowing for regression to the mean mathematically is not usually an easy procedure. The problem is probably best solved by ignoring the first measurement on the basis of which the individuals were categorized and to take, as a baseline, measurements taken at a subsequent examination when spuriously high (or low) levels have 'settled down'. Comparison with a control group might also allow the effect to be distinguished from the effect (if any) of treatment.

Regression to the mean can also cause problems in examining any change in a variable over time related to the initial value. Correlations suggesting larger changes in those with high initial values are often spurious. A similar problem arises when correlating two variables, one of which in some sense 'contains' the other. Regression to the mean creates spurious correlations, for instance, between total cholesterol and low-density cholesterol (which is part of the former). The user of regression and correlation techniques should always be wary of the possibility of bias due to regression to the mean.

10.7.4 Non-random sampling

Related to the problem of regression to the mean is the situation where one of the variables involved in the analysis has been used to define the group of persons actually analysed. Thus, if, for example, the blood pressure/weight study had been performed only on those who weighed over 40 kg (see Fig. 10.1), a regression analysis would not be valid. Random sampling is assumed and restricting the analysis to certain subgroups defined by values of the variables in the regression invalidates the statistical approach and the resulting regression or correlation coefficients are not easily interpreted.

10.7.5 Agreement

Often regression and/or correlation is employed in the examination of agreement between two numerical measurements. Certainly, for example, a scattergram can be used to display data relating to, say, blood glucose values as measured by two different 'pocket' glucometers on the same blood sample. It would be surprising, however, if there was not a good 'correlation' between the readings on the two machines, but correlation is not the same as agreement and the techniques described in this chapter are generally not suited to the analysis of such data. Rank correlation methods (Section 10.6.4) may be used however. The topic will be discussed in detail in Chapter 12, to which the reader is referred.

10.7.6 Spurious correlations

It is tempting, when faced with a regression equation, to make certain assumptions about what it means in reality. As has been mentioned, extrapolation is always dangerous and a regression equation should not be assumed to apply outside the range of the original data used in its derivation. When interpreting regression results (as, indeed, any statistical results), one should also be careful not to assume causal effects. Changing the value of the predictor variable in an individual will not necessarily result in that individual achieving the predicted value of the dependent variable—even on average. The direction of causality may be wrong or, indeed, the relationship may be due to confounding by one or more other variables (see Section 3.5).

Often, correlations will be found between factors measured over time and it is easy to be misled by such relationships. For instance, correlations are often quoted between the divorce rate in a country and the number of television sets per 1000 of the population, or between two biochemical measurements in an individual measured over time. Correct analysis and interpretation of such time-series data is quite complex. Many variables show correlations over time without being in any way causally related.

10.8 Summary

In this chapter, it has been explained how the relationship between two quantitative variables may be described by means of regression equations and how the strength of the relationship between the variables may be measured. It has been shown, also, how the significance of statistics such as the regression coefficient and the correlation coefficient may be tested. The calculations are summarized in Sections C.20 and C.21 in Appendix C.

Summary of formulae for regression (see Appendix A for computational formulae)		
Application	Formulae	Eqn. nos.
Regression equation	$\hat{y} = a + bx$	(10.1)
	$b = \dfrac{\sum(x - \bar{x})(y - \bar{y})}{(n-1)S_x^2}$	(10.5)
	$a = \bar{y} - b\bar{x}$	(10.6)
Correlation coefficient	$r = \dfrac{\sum(x - \bar{x})(y - \bar{y})}{(n-1)S_x S_y}$	(10.8)
Hypothesis test ($\beta = 0$)	$t = \dfrac{bS_x\sqrt{n-1}}{S_{y,x}}$	(10.15)
	d.f. $= n - 2$	
Confidence interval for β	$b \pm t_c \dfrac{S_{y,x}}{\sqrt{(n-1)}S_x}$	(10.13)
	d.f. $= n - 2$	
Hypothesis test ($\rho = 0$)	$t = r\sqrt{\dfrac{n-2}{1-r^2}}$	(10.16)
	d.f. $= n - 2$	
Spearman's rank correlation coefficient	$r_s = 1 - \dfrac{6\sum d^2}{n(n^2 - 1)}$	(10.19)

11 Multivariate Analysis and the Control of Confounding[!]

11.1 Introduction

So far in this book, the statistical methods have concentrated on the analysis of the association between two variables only. For two quantitative variables, the association is displayed by means of a scattergram, with simple regression techniques to perform the statistical analysis (e.g. blood pressure and age). For a quantitative and a qualitative variable, the association can be examined by looking at the mean level of one variable in groups defined by categories of the other (e.g. mean blood pressure in males and females). The statistical techniques in this situation include t tests and analysis of variance. The final case of two qualitative variables is dealt with by contingency-table analysis, using one of the chi-square tests.

As has been pointed out, medical research is, to a large extent, aimed at determining associations between two variables, but, in most cases, account has to be taken of other variables, which may act as confounders of an observed association (see Chapter 3). This chapter considers techniques that will correct for the existence of confounders and provide a valid statistical inference of confounded relationships. Confounding can be controlled for analytically, using either stratified analyses or employing multiple regression techniques. A stratified analysis essentially performs separate analyses at each level of the confounder. Multiple regression, on the other hand, is an extension to simple regression that allows for more than one explanatory (independent) variable, including the confounding variable as one of these. With both approaches, there is a single dependent variable, which is related to the other variables considered. The chapter considers quantitative and qualitative dependent variables separately and takes, for the most part, fixed follow-up mortality as an example of a dependent qualitative variable. In fact, the analysis of mortality in the context of cohort studies is discussed in some detail and some methods for mortality analysis, used mainly in vital statistics, are also introduced.

Although control of confounders at the analysis stage of a study is important, it must be remembered that confounding can also be controlled at the design stage. Thus, matching for potential confounders or restriction, can be used in case–control studies, and stratified randomization is employed in clinical trials. Control of confounding in study design is preferable to control with a statistical technique and should be done where feasible. However, it is never possible to exclude all confounders at the design stage and the analysis of any data must include the search for and control of nuisance variables for which adjustment has not been made.

If some form of matching (frequency or paired) or stratification has been used in the study design to control for confounders, the statistical analysis should also take account of this. In Chapter 7, the analysis of paired data was discussed, while some of the methods in this present chapter are suitable for the analysis of frequency-matched or stratified data. Failure to take account of frequency matching will result in a reduction of power, although the analysis will not be biased.

Some of the multivariate methods (particularly the regression approaches) considered in this chapter are also used when one wishes to examine the relationship between one variable (the dependent variable) and a number of other explanatory variables considered simultaneously.

11.2 Quantitative dependent variable

11.2.1 Quantitative explanatory variables: multiple regression

Bivariate correlations

In Chapter 10, simple regression and correlation were used in the examination of the association between two quantitative variables. Analysis that involves more than two quantitative variables can be approached in two ways. Using the first approach, the relationship between pairs of variables may be examined independently of the other variables. Thus, if there are three variables, say x_1, x_2 and x_3, the relationship between the pairs can be examined: x_1 and x_2, x_1 and x_3, and x_2 and x_3, in each case ignoring the third variable. An example of this kind of analysis is shown in Table 11.1. There are four variables in this example: cigarette and dairy product consumption in 1973, and male and female coronary heart disease (CHD) mortality in 1974, determined in 14 countries. The figures in the table are the values of the correlation coefficient between any pair of variables. Thus, in the first line, the correlation between cigarette consumption in 1973 and dairy product consumption in 1973 is negative, with a value of $r = -0.36$. The correlation between cigarette

Table 11.1 Zero-order correlation coefficients between cigarette consumption (1973), dairy product consumption (1973) and male and female coronary heart disease (CHD) mortality (1974) in 14 countries (adapted and abbreviated from Salonen & Vohlonen, 1982, with permission).

	Cigarettes in 1973	Dairy products in 1973	Male CHD in 1974	Female CHD in 1974
Cigarettes in 1973	1·0	−0·36	0·17	0·33
Dairy products in 1973		1·0	0·78*	0·70*
Male CHD in 1974			1·0	0·96*
Female CHD in 1974				1·0

* $p < 0.05$.

consumption in 1973 and male CHD mortality in 1974 is 0·17 and so on. In the second line, the correlation between dairy product consumption and cigarette consumption in 1973 is omitted, since it already appears in the first line. The correlation between any variable and itself is necessarily unity, as shown in the diagonal of the table.

Each correlation coefficient is calculated between two variables quite independently of the other two variables. The table therefore consists of a number of separate bivariate correlation coefficients, calculated by the method described in Section 10.3 and interpreted in the same way. Each correlation coefficient has been tested for significance, and those coefficients that are significantly different from zero at the 5% level are marked with an asterisk. A table of this kind, sometimes referred to as a matrix of bivariate correlation coefficients, is a useful method of summarizing the independent relationships between a number of variables and of showing which relationships are significant. In Table 11.1, there are three significant relationships; the remaining correlations can be ignored. This example shows some of the problems in the interpretation of bivariate correlation coefficients. The relationships between dairy product consumption and male and female CHD deaths could possibly be attributed to a causal connection between the factors, while the association between male and female deaths is of little relevance in developing a causal hypothesis. This latter relationship is likely to be due, almost totally, to the influence of dairy product consumption (and other factors) on the CHD deaths in both sexes.

Multiple regression equations

The second approach to analysing relationships between more than two quantitative variables is quite different, involving the simultaneous analysis of the variables. This is called *multiple regression analysis*, as distinct from simple regression analysis, which deals with only two variables.

In Chapter 10, the relationship of systolic blood pressure (SBP) to weight in 10-year-old children was summarized by the simple linear regression equation:

$$SBP = 79 \cdot 7 + 0 \cdot 8 \, W$$

where SBP was the systolic blood pressure in mmHg and W was the weight in kilograms. In this study, many other variables besides weight were examined for their influence on systolic blood pressure. The authors also presented a multiple regression equation, again with SBP as the dependent variable, but with diastolic blood pressure (DBP) and the time of day at which the measurement was taken as two extra variables, in addition to weight. Such variables are often called independent variables, to distinguish them from the dependent variable. Due to the fact, however, that some of these 'independent' variables may be highly correlated with each other, it is preferable to refer to them as explanatory or predictor variables. Some of these variables may also play the role of confounders.

Multiple regression is essentially a technique that examines the relationship between a single quantitative dependent variable and many quantitative explanatory variables. (The extension to qualitative explanatory variables is considered in the next section.) In the blood pressure study, the authors presented the following multiple regression equation:

$$SBP = 39 \cdot 6 + 0 \cdot 45 \, W + 0 \cdot 69 \, DBP + 0 \cdot 45 \, T$$

where SBP and DBP are systolic and diastolic blood pressures in mmHg, W is weight in kilograms and T is the time of day, measured in number of completed hours. In this multiple regression equation, SBP is the dependent variable and DBP, W and T are the explanatory variables.

The coefficients 0·45, 0·69 and 0·45 are called *partial regression coefficients*. For example, for *any* given values of W and T, the equation shows that an increase in DBP of 1 mmHg results in an increase of 0·69 mmHg in SBP. This is true no matter what values are chosen for W or T; the partial regression coefficient of 0·69 thus summarizes the relationship between systolic and diastolic blood pressure when weight and time of day are kept constant, or, in other words, independently of these other two variables. This, of course, is equivalent to adjusting for any confounding effect of weight or time of day. Similarly, the coefficient 0·45 is the partial regression coefficient for weight, which shows the relationship of systolic blood pressure and weight when diastolic blood pressure and time of day are held constant. The coefficient for T is also 0·45 and measures the relationship between systolic blood pressure and time of day when the other two factors are held constant. Note that the partial regression coefficient for weight (0·45) is much less than the simple regression coefficient of 0·8 obtained when weight was the only explanatory variable included in the analysis. Thus, the relationship of systolic blood pressure with weight is not as marked when diastolic blood pressure and time of day are taken into account. For a fixed time of day and fixed diastolic blood pressure, systolic blood pressure will increase by 0·45 mmHg for every 1 kg increase of weight, compared with 0·8 mmHg when the other variables are not allowed for. Multiple regression can thus control for the confounding effects of other variables on any bivariate relationship. Note that, with a multiple regression, any of the explanatory variables can be considered as potential confounders.

Coefficients of multiple correlation

The strength of the relationship between the dependent variable and the explanatory variables may also be estimated by calculating the *coefficient of multiple correlation (r)*. This is analogous to the simple correlation coefficient and, as before, its square measures the proportion of the total variation in the dependent variable that can be 'explained' by variations in the explanatory variables. The 'unexplained' variation may be due, of course, to other variables that have not been included in the regression equation. If these variables can be identified, then a new multiple regression equation can be calculated with these additional variables included. The value of r^2 will be increased, since the proportion of 'explained' variation in the dependent variable will be higher. The value of r^2 for the multiple regression equation above is 0.53, compared with the value of 0.23 in the simple regression equation with only weight included. More of the variation in systolic blood pressure is explained by inclusion of the extra variables. Moreover, by calculating what are called *partial correlation coefficients*, the strength of the relationship between the dependent variable and any *one* of the explanatory variables may be calculated, assuming the other explanatory variables are held constant. These partial correlation coefficients differ from the simple bivariate (or zero-order) correlation coefficients described earlier. In the former, the simultaneous influence of other variables is taken into account; in the latter, the correlation between two variables is calculated without any explicit attempt to remove the possible confounding effect of other factors.

Usually, multiple regression analysis is performed on a computer, as the calculations are, to say the least, fairly tedious. Computational details will not be given in this text. A multiple regression package will give as part of its output the constant term and the partial regression coefficients. As with simple regression, confidence intervals can be calculated for these coefficients (the coefficient ± 1.96 times its standard error for a 95% interval) and significance tests can be performed for the null hypothesis that the coefficient is zero (i.e. no association with the dependent variable).

Stepwise methods

When performing a multiple regression, there is a limit to the number of explanatory variables that can be included and this limit is related to the sample size. From a practical point of view, also, the number of variables should be kept to a manageable level. The choice of which variables to include is dictated by many factors. If one is controlling for confounders, then variables should be retained in the equation if their inclusion materially alters the value of the regression coefficient of the principal variable of interest, even if they are not statistically significant. If one is looking for factors that best explain the variation in the dependent variable, then there are a number of techniques available to choose the 'best' subset of the explanatory variables. *Forward (stepwise) inclusion* methods search through all the possible variables not already in the equation and add in, at each step, the variable that increases the coefficient of multiple correlation to the greatest extent. The process continues until either the increase in the coefficient is non-significant or a pre-specified number of variables has been included. *Backward elimination*, on the other hand, starts with all possible variables in the regression equation and deletes them one by one to eventually obtain the 'best' set of explanatory variables. Variations on both these techniques are also available, but most methods, depending on the criteria used for inclusion or exclusion, tend to give the same set of predictors.

When a number of explanatory variables are highly correlated with each other, the effect of one of them on the dependent variable will often totally mask the effect of the others, resulting in some of these variables having small and non-significant partial regression coefficients. Usually, only one of a set of such variables will be included in the final equation, because it will act as a proxy for the remainder. Variables excluded in this way may, however, be important predictors of the dependent variable, and dealing with such *multicollinearity* can be a problem.

It must be stressed, however, that multiple regression techniques should not be used blindly to solve all problems with more than two quantitative variables. In essence, a multiple regression analysis imposes a particular type of linear additive model on the interrelationships between the dependent and explanatory variables. The appropriateness of this model should be determined on theoretical grounds, if possible, and it should not be glibly assumed that nature obeys such constructs. (See Section 11.2.3 for methods that do not assume linear effects and Section 11.4 for methods to examine interaction or effect modification, which is also discussed in Section 6.5.4.) The use of automated stepwise selection methods has also been criticized. Some suggest that variable selection should be based on a knowledge of biological or epidemiological relationships rather than on purely statistical criteria.

Multiple regression
- single quantitative dependent variable
- many quantitative explanatory variables, some of which can be confounding

Partial regression coefficient for an explanatory variable
- relationship between dependent variable and the explanatory variable adjusted for the other confounding explanatory variables
- amount of change in dependent variable for unit change in explanatory variable with other variables held constant

Table 11.2 Mean serum cholesterol (mg/100 ml) by exercise level and sex (hypothetical data).

	Male		Female		Total	
Exercise	(*n*)	Cholesterol	(*n*)	Cholesterol	(*n*)	Cholesterol
Heavy	(50)	220	(25)	215	(75)	218·3
Light	(50)	240	(75)	235	(125)	237·0
Total	(100)	230	(100)	230	(200)	230

11.2.2 Qualitative explanatory variables: analysis of variance

Section 9.2 explained how a one-way analysis of variance (ANOVA) could be used to compare the mean of one variable between more than two groups. The term 'one-way' was used because means were examined for their association with one qualitative variable only. ANOVA easily extends to the examination of the association of a quantitative variable with more than one qualitative variable.

Table 11.2 shows the results of a hypothetical study of serum cholesterol related to two qualitative variables—exercise (heavy or light) and sex. Note that in the total study group of 100 males and 100 females the mean cholesterols are the same in each sex. However, in both the heavy and light exercisers separately, cholesterol in males is 5 mg/100 ml greater than in females. The cholesterol relationship with sex is confounded by exercise. If exercise had not been examined in this situation, one might conclude that cholesterols were identical in the two sexes. The further breakdown by exercise level shows that males really have higher levels of serum cholesterol than females, but, because they exercise more (50% heavy exercisers compared with 25% in females), this association does not appear in the crude data. In this example, the confounding effect of exercise masks the sex difference because exercise is related both to sex and to serum cholesterol. Remember that a confounding variable can either mask a real relationship (as in this example) or create an apparent association where none exists.

Note too that the exercise effect is only marginally confounded by sex—the difference between heavy and light exercisers in males and females combined is 18·67 mg/100 ml compared with 20 mg/100 ml in each sex group. Thus, when associations are being examined, the degree of confounding is not a symmetrical property. The fact that the sex relationship with cholesterol is strongly confounded by exercise does not necessarily imply that the exercise relationship with cholesterol is strongly confounded by sex.

To test the sex/cholesterol association for statistical significance while allowing for the influence of exercise, the usual technique would be a *two-way analysis of variance*, 'two-way' referring to the fact that cholesterol is classified by two qualitative variables—sex and exercise. The analysis is complicated by the fact that the data are what is referred to as 'unbalanced'—there are unequal numbers in each of the four sex/exercise categories. It was this, of course, that gave rise to the confounding in the first place. The computations for the analysis of variance in this case are quite complex and would usually be performed on a computer. The logic of the method involves comparisons of various estimates of variance, as in the one-way case (see Section 9.2), but the output of any computer program requires careful interpretation and the advice of a statistician should be sought. (Note, too, that some computer programs do not handle unbalanced data.)

In this example, an analysis of variance would include significance tests comparing cholesterols between males and females, taking account of the differences within each category of the confounder (exercise), and would also allow the calculation of confidence intervals for the corrected or adjusted cholesterol differences. The estimate of the (corrected) mean cholesterol difference between males and females would be 5 mg/100 ml—the figure seen in each of the exercise groups. In general, the corrected difference is some form of average of the differences in each category of the confounder. Analysis of variance is essentially performing a stratified analysis and should also be used when the data have been frequency matched. It is the usual approach for the comparison of means between groups formed through frequency matching (Section 6.7.2) or stratified randomization (Section 6.11.5).

The analysis of variance can, of course, handle qualitative variables with more than two categories and can be applied to quite complex data structures with more than two qualitative variables involved. The technique is much easier to apply when the data are balanced (usually meaning equal numbers in the various cells) and is a most powerful method for the analysis of experimental data, particularly in animal and laboratory experiments, when balance can and should be achieved. The techniques, however, are too advanced for this text.

What happens when the effect of a quantitative variable is also to be allowed for—e.g. age in the above example? One possibility is to create age-groups and treat age as a qualitative variable. The alternative is to use what is called an *analysis of covariance*, which allows for the influence of both qualitative and quantitative variables. Thus, an analysis of covariance would handle the relationship between the dependent variable serum cholesterol and the explanatory variables age (quantitative), exercise and sex (both qualitative).

Analysis of variance (ANOVA)
- single quantitative dependent variable
- many qualitative explanatory variables, some of which can be confounding or stratifying
- relationship between the dependent variable and groups defined by one of the explanatory variables adjusted for the other (confounding) variables

---

11.2.3 Quantitative and qualitative explanatory variables: analysis of covariance

Analysis of covariance lies between multiple regression, where all the explanatory variables are quantitative, and analysis of variance, where they are all qualitative. In fact, although the approaches seem quite different, the three techniques are very closely allied and both the analysis of variance and the analysis of covariance can be formulated in a multiple regression framework with identical numerical results. The trick is to include qualitative variables in the multiple regression. This is done by means of 'dummy variables'. If the qualitative variable is binary (two categories only), then the use of this method is very straightforward. A binary variable is numerically coded for entry into a multiple regression, using the value 1 for one category and 0 for the other. If the variable called MALE is coded 1 for a male and 0 for a female, and EXER-CISE is coded 1 for heavy and 0 for light, the multiple regression equation formulation of the analysis of covariance discussed above would be:

$$\text{CHOL} = a + b_1 \text{ AGE} + b_2 \text{ MALE} + b_3 \text{ EXERCISE}$$

Here b_1, b_2 and b_3 are the partial regression coefficients and a is the constant term. b_1 gives the change in cholesterol for a year's change in age, corrected for sex and exercise. b_2 can be interpreted as the difference in cholesterol between males and females corrected for the other factors. This is because the predicted cholesterol for a male (MALE = 1) is b_2 higher than the value for a female of similar age and exercise level. (With MALE equal to 0, the b_2 sex term disappears.) Similarly, the b_3 term is the corrected difference in cholesterol between heavy and light exercisers. If there were only a single explanatory 0/1 coded binary variable (say, MALE) in the above regression, the analysis would be fully equivalent to an independent t test (Section 7.4.1) and the regression coefficient would be just the (unadjusted) sex difference in cholesterol.

If the qualitative variable to be included has more than two categories, the dummy coding scheme becomes more complicated. Suppose cigarette smoking status with three categories of current, ex- and never smokers were to be included in the above equation. Two dummy variables (CURR and EX) would be created, as shown in Table 11.3, and both would be entered into the regression equation, instead of the original three-category variable.

Arbitrarily, one of the categories of the original smoking status variable is considered as reference—in this case, the never smokers. The regression equation, including smoking status via the two dummy variables, would now read:

$$\text{CHOL} = a + b_1 \text{ AGE} + b_2 \text{ MALE} + b_3 \text{ EXERCISE} + b_4 \text{ CURR} + b_5 \text{ EX}$$

Note, of course, that the a, b_1, b_2 and b_3 coefficients would be unlikely to have

Table 11.3 Dummy coding.

Smoking status	Dummy variable coding	
	CURR	EX
Current	1	0
Ex-smoker	0	1
Never smoker	0	0

the same values as in the previous equation, because of the addition of the smoking variables. Using a similar argument as above in the case of binary variables, b_4 is the corrected difference in cholesterols between current smokers and never smokers, while b_5 is the corrected difference between ex-smokers and never smokers. Both coefficients measure the difference from the reference category. The difference between the cholesterols of current and ex-smokers would be given by $b_4 - b_5$. In general, the number of dummy variables that have to be created to allow a qualitative variable to enter into a multiple regression is one less than the number of categories of the variable.

It was pointed out in Section 11.2.1 that a multiple regression approach to data analysis imposed a linear relationship between the dependent and explanatory variables. If the relationship is not linear, the regression analysis may give misleading results. One way of examining if the dependent variable increases or decreases linearly with a particular quantitative explanatory variable is to categorize the latter (e.g. age into age-groups) and enter it into the regression equation as a set of dummy variables. The partial regression coefficients for these dummy variables show immediately if a trend is present. If a linear trend is apparent, it is quite legitimate to employ the original quantitative variable in the regression equation. If a non-linear trend is apparent, transformation of the original variable (see Section 10.6.2) may linearize it, and the transformed quantitative variable could be retained in the equation. Alternatively, the dummy variables could be used in the regression, rather than the original quantitative one.

Although calculational details are not given here for either multiple regression or analysis of variance/covariance, it is hoped that the discussion above will guide the researcher as to what is possible with these techniques. The choice between a multiple regression or an analysis of covariance in a particular situation often depends on the computer software available, but it can be argued strongly that the interpretation of the former is much more tractable, which is why it has been covered in more detail.

Analysis of covariance
- equivalent to multiple regression with dummy variables
- single quantitative dependent variable
- many qualitative and/or quantitative explanatory variables, some of which can be confounding or (qualitative only) stratifying

---

11.3 Qualitative dependent variable: (i) case–control and cohort studies

The distinction between fixed-time and variable-time follow-up in a cohort study was emphasized in Section 6.6. In a fixed-time follow-up study, the survival status of each individual is known at a fixed time (for instance, 5 years) after study commencement and the analysis is of the 5-year mortality or survival risks. When there are no confounders, the data are in the form of a $2 \times n$

table with mortality (two categories) compared between n exposure groups. For 2×2 tables, the summary measures of association include the excess (attributable) risk, the relative risk and the odds ratio.

349

*Section 11.3
Qualitative
dependent
variable:
case–control
cohort studies*

Significance tests and confidence interval calculations for these measures are discussed in Section 7.10. The techniques discussed in the present section extend these approaches to account for confounding variables or variables used to stratify or match in the formation of the comparison groups. For categorical confounders, the Mantel–Haenzel methods are employed and logistic regression extends the ideas of multiple regression to encompass a qualitative binary dependent variable and qualitative or quantitative confounders. Though this discussion is almost entirely in terms of analysing mortality as an end-point in a cohort study (or clinical trial), the methods can be used for examining any binary variable. In particular, the methods can be used for analysing case–control data.

For variable-time follow-up, the techniques for group comparisons of mortality without confounders are considered in Sections 7.15 and 9.4. A brief indication of the extensions to allow for confounders or stratifying variables is also given below.

11.3.1 Qualitative explanatory variables: the Mantel–Haenzel techniques

This section discusses the problem of confounding when the dependent variable and the explanatory variables are all qualitative. In this case control of confounding can be achieved with contingency-table analysis. Emphasis will be placed entirely, in what follows, on confounding in the analysis of two binary variables. As seen in Chapter 6 on medical studies and the clinical trial, the 2×2 table with two binary variables is the starting-point for many analyses, with the relative risk or the odds ratio as the usual measure of the association.

Computational details are included in this section because it is feasible to carry out the calculations without the use of a computer and, even if a computer package is used to generate the relevant tables, the output often does not include the statistics required and the actual statistical analysis may have to be performed by hand.

Table 11.4 shows the basic data from a cohort study to examine reasons for females having a higher 24-hour mortality after coronary artery bypass surgery (CABS) than males. It is clear from this table that females have a significantly higher 24-hour mortality. The odds ratio (OR) is 1·96 and the relative risk (RR) is 1·93.* Using the usual chi-square test, this result is statistically significant at the 5% level ($\chi^2 = 5\cdot24$; degrees of freedom (d.f.) = 1). The confidence intervals (CI) are based on the methods of Section 7.10.5. This example is going to consider both the relative risk and the odds ratio as measures of the association between mortality and sex, though the former would be

---

* The calculations in this section are based on the numbers in the tables and not the rounded percentages.

Table 11.4 Twenty-four-hour mortality after coronary artery bypass surgery, by sex. (Unpublished data from the Irish Cardiac Surgery Register, with permission.)

| Sex | Total | At 24 hours | | OR (95% CI) | RR (95% CI) |
		Dead	% Dead		
Female	544	15	2·8	1·96	1·93
Male	3366	48	1·4	(1·10–3·50)	(1·09–3·39)
Total	3910	63	1·6		

Table 11.5 Twenty-four-hour mortality after coronary artery bypass surgery by body surface area (BSA). (Unpublished data from the Irish Cardiac Surgery Register, with permission.)

| | Total | At 24 hours | | OR (95% CI) | RR (95% CI) |
		Dead	% Dead		
Low BSA	1250	35	2·8	2·71	2·66
High BSA	2660	28	1·1	(1·68–4·37)	(1·66–4·25)
Total	3910	63	1·6		

more likely to be used in practice, since this is a cohort study. If the data had arisen from a case–control study, then the odds ratio would be the only possible measure of the two.

One possible confounder examined was body surface area (BSA). BSA can be taken as a proxy for body size and it has been suggested that bypass surgery may be more difficult in persons of small stature, due to smaller coronary vessels. BSA was categorized into thirds on the basis of the tertiles in all 3910 persons; those in the lowest third were designated 'low BSA' and those in the top two thirds were designated 'high BSA'. As might be expected, a much larger proportion of the females, 483/544 (88·8%), had a low BSA, compared with 767/3366 (22·8%) of the males. Table 11.5 shows that BSA (in both sexes combined) also related very strongly to 24-hour mortality, those with low BSA faring much worse ($\chi^2 = 16\cdot38$; d.f. = 1; $p < 0\cdot01$). It would thus seem that the sex relationship with mortality might be confounded by BSA. The fact that low BSA is associated with a higher mortality and that females tend to have a low BSA could explain the higher mortality in females. Table 11.6 shows that this is so.

In the low-BSA group, males and females fared almost identically (OR: 1·06; RR: 1·06). In the high-BSA group, though females did have a higher mortality than males (OR: 1·59; RR: 1·58), this was non-significant and a smaller difference than seen in the unadjusted analysis (OR: 1·96; RR: 1·93). Given this, it would seem legitimate to conclude that, *within BSA categories*, females do not fare worse than males and that the lower BSA of females explains their observed higher mortality.

351

*Section 11.3
Qualitative
dependent
variable:
case–control
cohort studies*

Table 11.6 Twenty-four-hour mortality after coronary artery bypass surgery by sex within each BSA category. (Unpublished data from the Irish Cardiac Surgery Register, with permission.)

Sex	Total	At 24 hours Dead	At 24 hours % Dead	OR (95% CI)	RR (95% CI)
Low BSA					
Female	483	14	2·9	1·06	1·06
Male	767	21	2·7	(0·54–2·10)	(0·54–2·10)
High BSA					
Female	61	1	1·6	1·59	1·58
Male	2599	27	1·0	(0·21–11·79)	(0·22–11·40)

Table 11.7 Layout of the *i*th 2 × 2 table in a series of 2 × 2 tables.

Exposure	Disease Yes	Disease No
Yes	a_i	b_i
No	c_i	d_i

$n_i = a_i + b_i + c_i + d_i$ (total sample size for the table).

The Mantel–Haenzel χ^2

As was done Section 11.2 for means, it would be useful to be able to adjust for BSA and to estimate an adjusted odds ratio or relative risk for females versus males, together with an appropriate significance test and confidence intervals. The first step is to perform a significance test, and the appropriate test is called the Mantel–Haenzel chi-square (Mantel & Haenzel, 1959). It is used to test the null hypothesis of no overall relationship in a series of 2 × 2 tables derived either from a cohort or a case–control study. (In the CABS example, there are only two tables in the series, defined by the low and high BSA categories.) A series of tables could also be created for the categories of a factor employed in frequency matching—and this is the preferred method for the analysis of frequency matched data.

For a single table, the usual chi-square would apply and the Mantel–Haenzel chi-square is a type of combination or average of the individual chi-squares for each table in the series. Suppose there are s 2 × 2 tables in the series and the *i*th table is laid out like Table 11.7 (note that the layout allows for either case–control or cohort data). The quantities required in each of these tables for the Mantel–Haenzel chi-square are the number with disease and exposed, a_i, the expected value of a_i, $E(a_i)$, and the variance (standard-error squared) of a_i, $V(a_i)$. The expected value of a_i is obtained, as for the usual chi-square, by multiplying the totals in the appropriate margins and dividing by the total sample size for the table (n_i):

$$E(a_i) = \frac{(a_i + b_i)(a_i + c_i)}{n_i} \tag{11.1}$$

The variance of a_i is given by the following formula:

$$V(a_i) = \frac{(a_i + b_i)(c_i + d_i)(a_i + c_i)(b_i + d_i)}{n_i^2(n_i - 1)} \qquad (11.2)$$

It so happens that the quantity:

$$\frac{[a_i - E(a_i)]^2}{V(a_i)} = \frac{(n_i - 1)}{n_i}\chi^2 \qquad (11.3)$$

where χ^2 is the usual 2×2 table chi-square. For large enough n_i, the difference between the two expressions is negligible. It may seem strange that the chi-square can be obtained by looking at the entry in one cell of the table only, but, of course, once the value in one cell of a 2×2 table is known, the others are predetermined and can be obtained by subtraction.

Now, once the three quantities, a_i, $E(a_i)$ and $V(a_i)$, have been calculated from each of the 2×2 tables in the series, the Mantel–Haenzel chi-square (which has 1 degree of freedom, no matter how many tables are in the series) is obtained by the following formula, which sums up the individual components of the individual table chi-squares:

$$\chi^2_{MH} = \frac{[\sum a_i - \sum E(a_i)]^2}{\sum V(a_i)} \qquad (11.4)$$

The calculation of this chi-square for the example is detailed in Table 11.8 below. In this case, the a_i cell refers to female deaths, with disease corresponding to death and exposure corresponding to being a female. $\chi^2_{MH} = 0.08$ on 1 degree of freedom and this non-significant result suggests that, when allowance is made for BSA, there is no real relationship of sex to 24-hour mortality in the post-CABS patient.

Table 11.8 Calculation of Mantel–Haenzel chi-square.

Sex	Dead			a_i	$E(a_i)$	$V(a_i)$
	Yes	No	Total			
Low BSA						
Female	14	469	483			
Male	21	746	767			
Total	35	1215	1250	14	13·524	8·072
High BSA						
Female	1	60	61			
Male	27	2572	2599			
Total	28	2632	2660	1	0·642	0·621
Summation:				15	14·166	8·693

$$\chi^2_{MH} = \frac{(15 - 14 \cdot 166)^2}{8 \cdot 693} = 0.0800$$

353

*Section 11.3
Qualitative
dependent
variable:
case–control
cohort studies*

As with the usual chi-square, however, there are some rules relating to when it is legitimate to apply the Mantel–Haenzel test. Essentially, the criterion is that the sum over each table of the minimum and maximum possible values that the numbers in the a_i cell could take, assuming fixed margins, must be at least 5 away from the actual Σa_i. Taking the low BSA figures in Table 11.8, the minimum number that could have died among the females is zero (assigning all the 35 deaths to the males) and the maximum that could have died is 35 (assigning all deaths to females). In the high BSA table, the corresponding minimum and maximum are 0 and 28. The two relevant sums are, then, 0 and 63, which are both more than 5 away from the observed sum of 15, showing the validity of the Mantel–Haenzel chi-square for this example. Usually, the calculation of the maximum and minimum values is straightforward, as in this example, but, in some situations, care must be taken when the minimum might not be zero. The maximum is always the smaller of the first column total and the first row total (i.e. the smaller of 483 and 35 in the low BSA table and of 61 and 28 in the high BSA table).

The Mantel–Haenzel chi-square essentially tests for a consistent association in the series of 2×2 tables examined. A non-significant chi-square means that there is no overall association or that there is no consistent association that predominates in the tables. Thus, if some of the tables suggest an association in one direction and others suggest the reverse of this association, the Mantel–Haenzel chi-square may end up non-significant. Such a case involves an interaction between the factors, and a summary analysis should probably not be attempted. This will be discussed further below.

The Mantel–Haenzel method can also be used with two or more qualitative confounders by forming a single composite variable and adjusting for that (e.g. age/sex groups from the single variables defined by age-group and sex). It is interesting to note also that the logrank test for the comparison of two life tables (see Section 7.15.6) is in fact an adaptation of the Mantel–Haenzel chi-square.

The Mantel–Haenzel summary measures

Having described the significance test for overall association, an overall summary measure of association is now required. A summary measure of association must, in some sense, average the measure of association in each of the individual tables. In the CABS example, the relative risks for female versus male mortality were 1·06 and 1·58 in the low- and high-BSA groups, respectively, and any summary measure of relative risk would be expected to lie somewhere between these two estimates. Remember, the crude relative risk was 1·93 and was excessively inflated due to the confounding effect of BSA. The summary or adjusted measure should correct for such confounding.

There are a number of different methods to calculate summary measures for relative risks and odds ratios in a series of 2×2 tables, but only one will be considered here. The measures to be discussed below are referred to as the

Table 11.9 Definition of quantifies involved in calculation of the Mantel–Haenzel summary
odds ratio and relative risk.

SINGLE TABLE

Exposure	Disease		Odds ratio (OR)	Relative risk (RR)
	Yes	No		
Yes	a	b	ad/bc	$a(c + d)/c\,(a + b)$
No	c	d		

$n = a + b + c + d$

SERIES OF TABLES

Exposure	Disease		OR	RR
	Yes	No		
First table				
Yes	a_1	b_1	$\dfrac{a_1 d_1}{n_1} \Big/ \dfrac{b_1 c_1}{n_1}$	$\dfrac{a_1(c_1 + d_1)}{n_1} \Big/ \dfrac{c_1(a_1 + b_1)}{n_1}$
No	c_1	d_1		

$n_1 = a_1 + b_1 + c_1 + d_1$

Exposure	Disease		OR	RR
	Yes	No		
ith table				
Yes	a_i	b_i	$\dfrac{a_i d_i}{n_i} \Big/ \dfrac{b_i c_i}{n_i}$	$\dfrac{a_i(c_i + d_i)}{n_i} \Big/ \dfrac{c_i(a_i + b_i)}{n_i}$
No	c_i	d_i		

$n_i = a_i + b_i + c_i + d_i$

MANTEL–HAENZEL SUMMARY MEASURES

OR_A	RR_A
$\sum \dfrac{a_i d_i}{n_i} \Big/ \sum \dfrac{b_i c_i}{n_i}$	$\sum \dfrac{a_i(c_i + d_i)}{n_i} \Big/ \sum \dfrac{c_i(a_i + b_i)}{n_i}$

Mantel–Haenzel estimates. Essentially, they are a type of average of the component measures in each of the constituent 2×2 tables.

Table 11.9 shows the layout of a series of tables for which a summary measure is to be estimated. The first part shows the standard layout for a single 2×2 table with the usual formulae for the odds ratio and relative risk. The first and *i*th 2×2 tables in the series are then shown with the odds ratios and relative risks again given. However, the table totals have been included in both the numerator and denominator of each expression. (This does not affect the calculated value.) The final section shows how the Mantel–Haenzel summary measures, OR_A and RR_A, are formed by summing the numerator and denominators of the individual table measures

355

*Section 11.3
Qualitative
dependent
variable:
case–control
cohort studies*

Table 11.10 Calculation of Mantel–Haenzel adjusted measures.

Exposure	Disease Yes	No	Total	Odds ratio (OR)	Relative risk (RR)
Low BSA					
Female	14	469	483	8·3552/7·8792 = 1·06	8·5904/8·1144 = 1·06
Male	21	746	767		
Total	35	1215	1250		
High BSA					
Female	1	60	61	0·9669/0·6090 = 1·59	0·9771/0·6192 = 1·58
Male	27	2572	2599		
Total	28	2632	2660		
Summation = adjusted measure				9·3221/8·4882 = 1·1	9·5675/8·7336 = 1·1

$$\text{OR}_A = \sum \frac{a_i d_i}{n_i} \Big/ \sum \frac{b_i c_i}{n_i} \tag{11.5}$$

$$\text{RR}_A = \sum \frac{a_i(c_i + d_i)}{n_i} \Big/ \sum \frac{c_i(a_i + b_i)}{n_i} \tag{11.6}$$

The calculations for the CABS study are shown in Table 11.10, in which the data from the two component tables are summed.

Thus, we see that the Mantel–Haenzel adjusted odds ratio in this case is 1·1, as an average of the two component odds ratios of 1·06 and 1·59. Greater weight is given to the risk of 1·06, since it is based on much larger numbers of deaths. The conclusion of this analysis, then, is that 1·1 is the best summary estimate of the odds ratio between females and males within the low- and high-BSA categories. The crude odds ratio of 1·96 seen in the total group is due to the fact that females tend to have a much lower BSA. The relationship of sex and mortality was confounded by BSA. Males and females with similar BSA, in fact, have almost identical mortalities after CABS. Working with the relative risks instead of the odds ratios gives an identical conclusion.

It is also possible to put confidence limits on the Mantel–Haenzel adjusted odds ratios and relative risks. This is done with the 'test-based limit' method that was employed in Section 7.10.5 to obtain confidence intervals for the crude measures. The Mantel–Haenzel chi-square is used in the confidence-interval formula for both the odds ratio and the relative risk. The 95% confidence limits are given by:

$$\text{OR}_A^{[1\pm(1·96/\chi)]} \tag{11.7}$$

$$\text{RR}_A^{[1\pm(1·96/\chi)]} \tag{11.8}$$

where χ is the square root of the Mantel–Haenzel chi-square and RR_A and OR_A are the adjusted relative risks and odds ratios.

The Mantel–Haenzel chi-square was 0·08 so that $1 - (1·96/\chi)$ is $-5·93$ and $1 + (1·96/\chi)$ is 7·93. This gives the 95% confidence interval for the corrected odds ratio of 1·1 as 0·57 to 2·13. The confidence interval for the corrected relative risk of 1·1 is obviously the same.

Mantel–Haenzel χ^2
- analysis of more than two qualitative variables
- single qualitative dependent variable (e.g. mortality)
- one qualitative binary explanatory variable and one qualitative confounding or stratifying variable
- suitable for cohort or case–control data

Mantel–Haenzel relative risk or odds ratio
- relative risk or odds ratio adjusted for a qualitative confounder

---

Mantel–Haenzel techniques

*i*th table in series of 2×2 tables	Formulae	Eqn. nos.

Disease

Exposure	Yes	No	$n_i = a_i + b_i + c_i + d_i$	
Yes	a_i	b_i	$E(a_i) = \dfrac{(a_i + b_i)(a_i + c_i)}{n_i}$	(11.1)
No	c_i	d_i	$V(a_i) = \dfrac{(a_i + b_i)(c_i + d_i)(a_i + c_i)(b_i + d_i)}{n_i^2(n_i - 1)}$	(11.2)

Mantel–Haenzel chi-square

$$\chi^2_{\text{MH}} = \frac{[\sum a_i - \sum E(a_i)]^2}{\sum V(a_i)}$$

d.f. $= 1$ (11.4)

Mantel–Haenzel summary measures

$$OR_A = \sum \frac{a_i d_i}{n_i} \bigg/ \sum \frac{b_i c_i}{n_i} \qquad (11.5)$$

$$RR_A = \sum \frac{a_i(c_i + d_i)}{n_i} \bigg/ \sum \frac{c_i(a_i + b_i)}{n_i} \qquad (11.6)$$

Confidence intervals

$$OR_A^{(1 \pm z_c/\chi)} \qquad (11.7)$$

$$RR_A^{(1 \pm z_c/\chi)} \qquad (11.8)$$

357

*Section 11.3
Qualitative
dependent
variable:
case–control
cohort studies*

11.3.2 Quantitative and qualitative explanatory variables: logistic regression

It was seen in Section 11.2 how multiple regression allowed for the analysis of the relationship between a quantitative dependent variable and both qualitative and quantitative explanatory variables. Multiple regression can be used both to determine the joint effect of the explanatory variables on the dependent variable and to determine the association between the dependent variable and a single explanatory variable corrected for the (confounding) effects of the remaining factors. Is there any way that multiple regression could be extended to cover the case of a qualitative dependent variable? Suppose, for example, that an analysis was to be performed relating the explanatory variables blood glucose level (G), age (A), systolic blood pressure (SBP), relative weight (W), cholesterol (C) and number of cigarettes per day (NC) to a qualitative dependent variable, measuring the presence or absence of major abnormalities on an electrocardiograms (ECGs). It is possible to imagine a multiple regression analysis with the presence or absence of an ECG abnormality as a dependent variable, obtaining an equation such as:

$$P = a + b_1G + b_2A + b_3SBP + \ldots$$

where b_1, b_2, etc. are the partial regression coefficients for the corresponding variables, and P has a value of 1 for the presence of the abnormality and 0 otherwise. The problem about this approach is that the predicted values for P from the equation, for given values of the explanatory variables, could quite easily be less than 0 or greater than 1 and would thus be totally uninterpretable. If P could be constrained to lie between 0 and 1, it could be interpreted as the probability of an ECG abnormality given the set of values for the explanatory variables. In a fixed-time follow-up cohort study, P would be the probability or risk of the end-point over the period of follow-up.

The logistic regression equation

This is precisely the situation that was faced in trying to analyse the Framingham cohort study of coronary disease in the 1960s (Section 6.4.1), and a technique called *logistic regression* was developed to deal with binary dependent variables. Basically, one works with a transformed dependent variable, running a multiple regression on the transformed variable:

$$Y = \ln \frac{P}{1-P} \qquad (11.9)$$

obtaining a regression equation (for the current example) like this:

$$Y = \ln \frac{P}{1-P} = a + b_1G + b_2A + b_3SBP \ldots \qquad (11.10)$$

where P is interpreted as the probability of an ECG abnormality. Given the form of this equation, P is constrained to lie between 0 and 1, and so has the required properties of a probability. If P is the probability of an event, then $P/(1-P)$ is the odds of that event, so that Eqn. 11.10 is a type of multiple regression equation, with the dependent variable transformed to be the ln of the odds* (see Section 7.10.5 for a discussion of the natural log and exponential functions). Obviously:

$$P/(1-P) = e^Y \qquad (11.11)$$

The ln of the odds can also be converted back to a probability, giving a direct relationship between the probability of disease and the explanatory variables:

$$P = \frac{e^{\hat{Y}}}{1+e^{\hat{Y}}} \qquad (11.12)$$

where:

$$\hat{Y} = a + b_1 G + b_2 A + b_3 SBP \ldots \qquad (11.13)$$

is the predicted value of Y for a given set of values for the explanatory variables. Table 11.11 shows the multiple logistic regression coefficients obtained for a study on ECG abnormalities, using the variables already discussed. Coefficients significantly different from 0 are marked with an asterisk; relative weight was defined as the percentage of desirable weight based on standard weight tables. To show how the results of such an analysis might be employed, the equation will be used to predict the probability of an ECG abnormality for a male aged 50 years, with a blood glucose level of 98·2 mg/dL, a systolic blood pressure of 140 mmHg, a relative weight of 115% and a cholesterol level of 230 mg/dL and who smokes 25 cigarettes per day. The predicted $\hat{Y}$ value for this individual, using the values of the coefficients in Table 8.2, is:

$$\begin{aligned}
\hat{Y} = &-12{\cdot}1041 + 0{\cdot}0009(98{\cdot}2) + 0{\cdot}1339(50) + 0{\cdot}0178(140)\\
&-0{\cdot}0079(115) + 0{\cdot}0034(230) + 0{\cdot}0075(25)\\
= &-2{\cdot}768
\end{aligned}$$

When this value is substituted into Eqn. 11.12, the value for P is found to be 0·059. (This P is not to be confused with p denoting significance level.) Thus,

Variable	Logistic regression coefficients (b)
Constant	−12·1041
Age	0·1339*
Glucose	0·0009
SBP	0·0178*
Relative weight	−0·0079
Cholesterol	0·0034
No. of cigarettes	0·0075

* $p < 0{\cdot}05$.

Table 11.11 Multiple logistic regression coefficients for the relationship between six variables and ECG abnormalities in 3357 men aged 40–54 (abbreviated from Hickey *et al.*, 1979, with permission).

* It should be noted, however, that logistic regression cannot be performed using a standard least-squares multiple regression package on a computer. A special program is needed.

on the basis of this study, an individual with the listed characteristics would have a 5·9% chance of having an ECG abnormality. The magnitude of the logistic regression coefficients gives some idea of the relative importance of various factors in producing the probability of an abnormality.

The coefficient for a particular factor can be interpreted as giving the amount of change in the ln(odds) for a unit change in that factor, holding all other explanatory variables constant. A multiple logistic regression coefficient for a variable expresses its relationship with the dependent variable, corrected for the confounding effects of the other explanatory variables.

359

Section 11.3
Qualitative
dependent
variable:
case–control
cohort studies

Logistic regression coefficients and the odds ratio

When, however, there is a qualitative explanatory variable with 0/1 coding, the interpretation of its regression coefficient is particularly appealing. For instance, a logistic regression analysis on the CABS data of Section 11.3.1 gives the following equation for the odds of death:

$$\frac{P}{1-P} = e^{[-4\cdot236+0\cdot673(\text{FEMALE})]}$$

where P is the probability of a 24-hour death and FEMALE is a binary variable coded 1 for a female and 0 for a male. From this, the odds of death for a female are:

$$e^{(-4\cdot236 + 0\cdot673)}$$

and the odds for a male are:

$$e^{(-4\cdot236)}$$

The odds ratio for females compared with males is simply the first of these quantities divided by the second, which, using the properties of exponents, gives:

$$\text{OR} = e^{(-0\cdot673)} = 1\cdot96$$

where the constant term cancels out. Thus, the exponential of the logistic regression coefficient gives the odds ratio for that factor. The same value for the odds ratio has already been calculated directly from the 2×2 table of sex by mortality in Table 11.4. This is a general result if there is only one explanatory variable. The logistic regression equation for the CABS example with two explanatory variables, FEMALE and LOWBSA, is:

$$\frac{P}{1-P} = e^{[-4\cdot546+0\cdot095(\text{FEMALE})+0\cdot961(\text{LOWBSA})]}$$

where LOWBSA is a variable taking on a value of 1 for those with low BSA and 0 otherwise. Note first that the logistic regression coefficient for FEMALE is quite reduced compared with the situation when LOWBSA was not in the model—confirming the confounding effect of that variable. Using similar arguments to those above, the exponential of 0·095 can be interpreted as the odds ratio for females compared with males, in those with high BSA *and* also in those with low BSA. Thus the estimate corrects or adjusts for BSA:

$$OR_A = e^{(-0.095)} = 1.1$$

This is the same as the Mantel–Haenzel corrected estimate of Table 11.10, but strict equality may not always hold between the two approaches when a confounder is present.

In general terms, the odds ratio for a binary 0/1 coded explanatory variable is given by:

$$OR = e^b \qquad (11.14)$$

where b is the logistic regression coefficient for the variable. If there are a number of other explanatory variables in the regression, this odds ratio is adjusted for their confounding effect.

Logistic regression thus provides an alternative method for the control of confounding in 2×2 tables. With all binary variables in a logistic regression, the numerical results for the adjusted odds ratios are usually quite close to the Mantel–Haenzel estimates. Ninety-five per cent confidence intervals for the odds ratio can be obtained by taking the regression coefficient plus or minus 1.96 times its standard error (given by most computer outputs) and taking the exponential of the result.

Applications for logistic regression

Logistic regression, of course, entails using the odds ratio as the measure of association and the above method can thus also be used for case–control data. Note, however, that the constant term in the regression has no interpretation in the case–control situation, even though the computer package is likely to calculate it. In the case–control study, the odds of disease cannot be calculated from the logistic regression equation, but the odds ratio for a factor can be obtained from its logistic regression coefficient, using Eqn. 11.14.

Logistic regression is a very powerful technique and, though not as easy to use as the Mantle–Haenzel approach, has a number of advantages in the analysis of a binary dependent variable. First, it can deal with a large number of variables when the Mantel–Haenzel adjustment may fail to work because of very small numbers in the component 2×2 tables. Logistic regression, too, can account for quantitative confounders without having to categorize them, and can examine effect modification (interaction) easily (see Section 11.4). Being a regression technique, it examines many variables simultaneously, whereas the Mantel–Haenzel technique is specifically for the control of confounding on one particular association.

Logistic regression is often used for the analysis of mortality, though it must be stressed that it can only analyse mortality determined at a fixed time point from study commencement. The dependent binary variable alive/dead must be

defined for each subject at this specific time point and withdrawals or losses to
follow-up cannot be accounted for.

361
*Section 11.4
Confounding
vs. interaction*

> Logistic regression
> - single qualitative dependent variable (e.g. mortality)
> - many qualitative or quantitative explanatory variables, some of which can be confounding or stratifying
>
> Logistic regression coefficient for a binary exposure
> - its exponential is the odds ratio for exposure if it is coded 0/1

11.3.3 Variable follow-up

Confounding effects can, of course, also arise in the analysis of mortality in a variable follow-up situation. The logrank test of Section 7.15.6, however, can be extended to allow control of the confounding effect of other qualitative variables in life table comparisons, in addition to its extension to com-pare more than two groups (see Section 9.4). An alternative to this approach is to use *Cox's life table regression* model or, as it is sometimes called, the *proportional hazards* model (Cox, 1972). Essentially, this is a multiple regression approach to the analysis of censored data. Remember that logistic regression, discussed in Section 11.3.2, can only be used for the analysis of survival or mortality when the status of all subjects is known at a fixed time point, and Cox's regression is to the life table what logistic regression is to the ordinary 2×2 table. An advanced text should be consulted for details of this regression method.

11.4 Confounding versus effect modification or interaction [!]

Note that, when performing a stratified analysis to summarize a measure of association in any set of tables, the associations in the individual tables must be examined first. Otherwise, if the associations are in different directions or are of very different magnitude or no one pattern predominates, a summary significance test or a summary measure may not validly describe the situation.

In the CABS example, taking age as a potential confounder, suppose that in young patients females had a higher mortality than males, but that in older patients females had a lower mortality. A summary measure in this case might suggest that females had a similar mortality to that of males, totally obscuring the important fact that age modifies the sex relationship with mortality. In this case, age would be referred to as an *effect modifier* of the relationship between sex and mortality. The concept of effect modification is the same as that of synergy or antagonism, as described in Section 6.5.4. Effect modification is also referred to as *interaction*.

It is important to distinguish between an effect modifier and a confounder, though a variable may at the same time act as both. Effect modification relates essentially to differences between the measure of association at different levels of the effect modifier. The crude (unadjusted) measure of association obtained when the data are analysed ignoring the effect modifier is irrelevant to the concept of effect modification. Of course, the measure of association is in practice likely to vary between different tables in any breakdown and it is, to some extent, a matter of judgement whether there is effect modification or not. Statistical tests are available to determine whether the measure of association varies significantly between the tables, and these tests for homogeneity of the association can act as a guide to the presence of effect modification. When effect modification is present, no summary or adjusted measure can adequately summarize the association found in categories of the effect modifier.

Confounding, on the other hand, means, essentially, that the crude or unadjusted measure of association does not reflect the measure in each of the component tables or does not average it in some reasonable way. When a variable acts as a confounder (and not as an effect modifier), the measure of association at each level of the confounder should be, to a certain extent, consistent and an adjusted measure is said to summarize the underlying association.

It is possible for a variable to act simultaneously as both a confounder and an effect modifier. Table 11.12 presents some hypothetical examples of different series of relative risks (the chosen measure of association) in three categories of a confounder/effect modifier (referred to as a control or stratifying variable).

In Example A, the crude relative risk of 2·5 does not reflect the underlying risks in the three categories or strata of the control variable and is in fact larger than each of them. Thus confounding is present. The three risks, however, are not too dissimilar, so that the control variable, though a confounder, is not an effect modifier. In Example B, the control variable is still not an effect modifier but could not be considered a confounder either, since the crude relative risk is, in a broad sense, representative of the three risks in the three categories. In Examples C and D, the control variable would be considered an effect modifier, since the relative risks are not consistent across the three categories. In fact, the heterogeneity is quite extreme, in that the risk in the third category is in the opposite direction to that in the other two categories. When effect modification is present, the question of confounding becomes somewhat aca-

Table 11.12 Examples of confounding and effect modification.

| Level of control variable: | Relative risk (exposed vs. non-exposed) | | | | Control variable is | |
	1st stratum	2nd stratum	3rd stratum	Total (crude)	Confounder	Effect modifier
Example A	1·4	1·8	1·3	2·5	Yes	No
Example B	1·4	1·8	1·3	1·5	No	No
Example C	1·4	1·8	0·2	1·5	(No)	Yes
Example D	1·4	1·8	0·2	2·5	(Yes)	Yes

demic, since no single measure can *adequately* summarize the three component relative risks. However, in Example C, the crude risk of 1·5 might be said to be an average of the three risks and thus the result could be considered not to be confounded. In Example D, the crude value cannot in any sense be considered representative of the three category values and thus confounding could be considered present in addition to effect modification.

It must be stressed again, however, that the whole concept of confounding or effect modification of an association depends on the precise measure used to quantify the association. Concentration here has been on the relative-risk-type measures, but, of course, in follow-up studies the attributable risk (risk difference or excess risk) might also be employed. A variable may be an effect modifier or confounder of the relative risk, for example, but not of the excess risk. Generally, in epidemiological analysis, concentration tends to be on relative risk type rather than difference measures.

Effect modification can, of course, also be present when relationships between quantitative variables are in question, and one can determine the existence of effect modification with a regression approach also. This is done by introducing an *interaction term* into the regression equation. Suppose it were suspected that age was an effect modifier of the association of exercise with serum cholesterol in the example of Section 11.2.3. An interaction term for exercise and age would involve creating a new variable AGE × EXERCISE, which would have the value of the individual's age if they were heavy exercisers and zero otherwise. (Note that this is just the multiplication of the values of the component variables AGE and EXERCISE, which is the general formulation of an interaction term.) The multiple regression equation might then be:

$$\text{CHOL} = a + b_1\,\text{AGE} + b_2\,\text{MALE} + b_3\,\text{EXERCISE} + b_4\,\text{AGE} \times \text{EXERCISE}$$

If the b_1 coefficient were significant or large enough, it might be kept in the equation, showing the effect-modifying action of age on the exercise/cholesterol relationship. A change in exercise level from low to high would result in a change in cholesterol of $b_3 + b_4\,\text{AGE}$. The effect of a change in exercise depends on age and, if b_4 were positive in the example, the older the subject, the greater the cholesterol change with exercise would be. If effect modification is suspected or to be looked for, then it is necessary to include the relevant interaction terms in a multiple regression analysis. Three-way interaction terms are also possible, though their interpretation becomes somewhat difficult. Again, either judgement or the results of significance tests will have to be employed to determine if such terms should be retained in the final model. It is worth while noting, too, that interaction or effect modification is symmetrical, in that in the above example, for instance, one could talk about age modifying the effect of exercise on cholesterol or exercise modifying the effect of age. The degree of effect modification relative to the main effect will, of course, depend on the magnitude of the partial regression coefficients b_1 and b_3.

With a qualitative (binary) dependent variable logistic regression approaches can be used to examine the presence of interaction or effect modification on an odds-ratio measure of effect.

11.5 Qualitative dependent variable: (ii) vital statistics approaches

A branch of statistics that is of particular interest to medical and social scientists is that concerned with the study of human populations, usually described as *demography*. Demographic studies involve *vital statistics*, such as death rates and birth rates.

Vital statistics measures are commonly expressed in the form of *rates* (see Section 6.51). This section considers the comparison of mortality rates between different populations as usually implemented in vital statistics applications. Typically, such comparisons adjust for the confounding effect of other variables—notably age, which is dealt with as a grouped and therefore a stratifying variable.

11.5.1 Crude and age-specific rates

The simplest measure of mortality is the crude death rate, defined as the number of deaths in a particular time period (usually a year) per thousand population. The annual crude death rate can be expressed as:

$$\frac{\text{Annual number of deaths}}{\text{Mean population during the year}} \times 1000 \qquad (11.15)$$

Note that, since, typically, the population varies slightly during the year, the denominator is an estimate of the 'mid-year' population (often, however, this is difficult to estimate accurately, unless there are regular and up-to-date population census data available; see Section 6.5.1).

Separate crude death rates can be calculated for males and females, for particular areas of a country and for other subgroups in the total population, including particular age-groups, to which reference is made below. The denominator would then refer to the mean population of the particular subgroup or area of interest.

For analytical purposes, crude death rates are of limited usefulness and may be misleading if used for comparisons. For example, country A may have a higher crude death rate than country B simply because, at the time of the comparison, the former had a higher proportion of elderly people. The death rate at every age may be lower and the expectation of life higher in A, and it would therefore be misleading to conclude, on the basis of a comparison of crude death rates, that country B's population is healthier or enjoys a higher level of medical care than that of country A. Comparisons must take into account the age distribution of the population. In addition, the overall crude death rate is also affected by the sex ratio in the population, since females generally have a longer expectation of life than males, and, usually, separate death rates for females and males are calculated.

365

*Section 11.5
Qualitative
dependent
variable: vital
statistics*

A way of neutralizing the effect of age distribution on the crude death rate is to calculate separate death rates for each age-group in the population. These are called *age-specific death rates*, defined as:

$$\frac{\text{Number of deaths in a specific age group}}{\text{Mean population of that age group}} \times 1000. \qquad (11.16)$$

(Deaths and mean population relate to a specific calendar period, usually a year, although some rates are calculated at quarterly or even monthly intervals.)

Corresponding age-specific death rates for different populations can then be compared. An overall test for any significant difference in the mortality experience of two populations, allowing for differences in age structure, can be carried out using the Mantel–Haenzel χ^2 test (see Section 11.3.1). The comparability of these rates is also affected by the age distribution *within* each age-group, but, provided that the age-group class intervals are fairly narrow, the influence of the within-group age distribution can be considered negligible. Five-year and 10-year age-group intervals are commonly used.

Although age-specific death rates provide an appropriate basis for comparing the mortality experience of different populations, it is useful to have a single overall measure of mortality which, unlike the crude death rate, allows for the effects of age distribution (assume throughout that males and females are considered separately). This is achieved by the calculation of one or more of a number of *standardized* mortality measures, the best known of which will be described in the following sections.

11.5.2 Direct standardization

As noted above, crude death rates for different populations cannot be properly compared because of the confounding effect of age. One particular method for age adjustment in vital statistics is called the *direct method*. Rather than giving an example comparing geographical populations, the method will be illustrated on a comparison of the mortality of travellers* in Ireland in 1986 with that of the entire population. The traveller population is called the study population. Table 11.13 shows the relevant data for the travellers and the full Irish population. For simplicity of presentation, wider than normal age-groups are used for the age-specific mortality rates, and the data refer to males and females taken together. Capital letters are used to denote the full Irish population and lower-case letters are used for the study population of travellers. Letters with a subscript denote age-specific quantities and letters without a subscript refer to crude or total figures.

---

* Travellers are a subgroup of the population with a unique cultural identity. Their lifestyle tends to be nomadic.

Table 11.13 Mortality experience of the Irish traveller population, 1986 (data aggregated and rounded; from Barry & Daly, 1988, and Barry *et al.*, 1989, with permission).

Age-group	Population ('000)	Deaths	Age-specific death rate (per 1000)
General Irish population	(N_i)	(D_i)	(R_i)
0–24	1640	1200	0·7317
25–44	920	1300	1·4130
45–64	590	5500	9·3220
65+	390	26000	66·6667
All ages (crude rate)	3540	34000	9·6045
Irish traveller population	(n_i)	(d_i)	(r_i)
0–24	11·7	22	1·8803
25–44	2·8	10	3·5714
45–64	1·1	24	21·8182
65+	0·3	28	93·3333
All ages (crude rate)	15·9	84	5·2830

The crude mortality rate in the Irish population (expressed per 1000) is:

$$R = \frac{D}{N} = \frac{34000}{3540} = 9\cdot60 \; per \; 1000 \tag{11.17}$$

Similarly, the crude rate in the travellers is 5·28 per 1000. Thus, on the basis of the crude rates, the travellers would seem to have a lower mortality than in the general population. However, looking at the age-specific rates in Table 11.13, it is clear that, within each age-group, the travellers have a higher mortality. The crude death rate for travellers is lower because that population contains a much higher proportion of people in the youngest age-group (in which age-specific mortality is lowest) and a lower proportion of people in the oldest age-group (in which age-specific mortality is highest). Age is acting as a confounder.

Expected number of deaths

The direct method of age standardization requires initial selection of a *standard population*. This is a population with a known age distribution and its choice will be considered below. The age-specific death rates of the populations to be compared are applied to this standard to get an expected number of deaths (in the standard population). Mortality comparisons between different populations can then be based on this expected or standardized number of deaths.

Table 11.14 shows the calculation of the expected deaths for the traveller population, using the national population as the standard. The expected number of deaths is given by:

$$E_{direct} = \Sigma r_i \times N_i \tag{11.18}$$

367

Section 11.5
Qualitative
dependent
variable: vital
statistics

Table 11.14 Direct age standardization of traveller mortality.

Age-group	Age distribution of standard population ('000) (N_i)	Age-specific death rates in study (traveller) population (per 1000) (r_i)	Expected deaths ($r_i \times N_i$)
0–24	1640	1·8803	3 083·7
25–44	920	3·5714	3 285·7
45–64	590	21·8182	12 872·7
65+	390	93·3333	36 400·0
Total	3540	–	55 642·1

Directly standardized rate

$$R_{direct} = \frac{E_{direct}}{N} = \frac{55\,642.1}{3\,540} = 15.72 \text{ per 1000.}$$

where the r_i are the age-specific rates in the study population and the N_i are the number of persons in each age-group in the standard population. In the example, this is calculated as 55 642·1 deaths. This is the number of deaths that would be expected to occur among the travellers if they had this (standard) age distribution; or, alternatively, it is the number of deaths that would be expected in the standard (national) population if it experienced the same age-specific death rates as the travellers.

Directly standardized rates

The directly age-standardized death rate is obtained by dividing the expected number of deaths by the size of the standard population—in this case, 3540 (thousands). The directly standardized mortality rate for travellers is then:

$$R_{direct} = \frac{\sum N_i \times r_i}{\sum N_i} = \frac{E_{direct}}{N} = \frac{55\,642·1}{3\,540} \qquad (11.19)$$

which is 15·72 per thousand. Like the expected number of deaths, it is the rate that would be observed if the traveller age-specific rates applied in the standard population or if the travellers had the standard age distribution. Note that the directly standardized rate is a weighted average of the age-specific rates in the study population, with weights defined by the standard-population age distribution.

The expected number of deaths and the directly standardized rate are both fictitious figures and do not represent the mortality experience of any actual population. The value of the measures, however, is that they can be compared with similarly calculated figures from a different population to give an age-standardized, or age-adjusted, comparison, correcting for the confounding effect of age.

The standard population

Obviously, the choice of the standard population influences the numerical value for the expected number of deaths and the standardized mortality rate. Often, the standard population, as in the present example, is one of the populations to be compared, but any standard can be used, as long as it represents a 'reasonable' population. When different regions, occupations or socio-economic groups are being compared, a common practice is to select as standard the national population of which the study populations form a part. For comparisons over time, however, there is a choice of standard populations, and the numerical values of the standardized figures will vary, depending on which year is selected as the population standard. If the age structure of the standard population remains relatively stable over time, which year is chosen as standard will not make a great deal of difference. In any case, it is usually the relative sizes of the standardized measures that are of relevance. There are advantages if different researchers use the same standard population (which would allow comparability between researchers), but this is difficult to achieve.

Comparative mortality figure (CMF)

The expected number of deaths and the directly standardized rate are descriptive figures that apply to the study population for which they are calculated. The *comparative mortality figure* (CMF) is a relative risk type measure that gives an age-adjusted comparison of the study population with the standard population or with a second study population. The CMF comparing the study population with the standard population is obtained from either of the following ratios:

$$\text{CMF} = \frac{\text{Expected deaths in standard population}}{\text{Observed deaths in standard population}} \times 100$$

$$= \frac{E_{direct}}{D} \times 100 \tag{11.20}$$

$$\text{CMF} = \frac{\text{Directly age-standardized rate in study population}}{\text{Crude rate in standard population}} \times 100$$

$$= \frac{R_{direct}}{R} \times 100 = \frac{E_{direct}/N}{D/N} \times 100 \tag{11.21}$$

The equivalence of the two formulations is clear and, for the travellers compared with the national population, the CMF is 163·7. A CMF of over 100 means that the study population has a higher mortality than the standard; one less than 100 means that mortality is lower. Here, the CMF shows clearly that, once age is taken into account, the mortality in travellers is considerably higher than in the national population, even though the crude rates showed the exact opposite.

Though the CMF as defined above is a figure that compares the study population with the standard, it can also be used to compare two study populations directly. The ratio of two CMFs gives an age-adjusted comparison between two study populations directly as (in the formulation of Eqn. 11.21) the crude rate in the standard population cancels out. The ratio of two CMFs is simply the ratio of the directly age-standardized rates in the two respective populations:

369

Section 11.5
Qualitative
dependent
variable: vital
statistics

$$\frac{\text{CMF}_{Population\ A}}{\text{CMF}_{Population\ B}} = \frac{(R_{direct(PopulationA)}/R) \times 100}{(R_{direct(PopulationB)}/R) \times 100} = \frac{R_{direct(PopulationA)}}{R_{direct(PopulationB)}} \quad (11.22)$$

A feature of direct standardization that can cause problems, however, arises when the population of interest (the study population) contains small numbers in particular age-groups. In these circumstances, the chance occurrence of one or two extra individual deaths in a particular age-group may give rise to a much greater than normal age-specific mortality rate and hence distort the CMF. The converse (i.e. an atypically low mortality rate in a particular age-group) may also occur.

Direct age standardization

Requirements
- age distribution of a standard population
- age-specific mortality rates in the study population

Method
- apply age-specific mortality rates in study population to the standard population, giving expected deaths in the standard population
- directly standardized rate $= \dfrac{\text{Expected deaths in standard population}}{\text{Standard population total}}$
- $\text{CMF} = \dfrac{\text{Directly standardized rate}}{\text{Crude rate in standard}}$

11.5.3 Indirect age standardization

Expected deaths

Indirect standardization overcomes the problem of small-sized study populations and unstable age-specific rates. In the indirect method of standardization, age-specific rates in a standard population are applied to the age distribution of the study population to give expected deaths in the study population. (Expected deaths in the *standard* population were calculated in direct standardization.) The standard population is usually taken as a relevant national population, which defines the age-specific rates with a good degree of precision. These expected deaths are the deaths that would be observed in the study population if the standard rates had applied to it. Table 11.15 shows the calculation of the expected deaths in the traveller population, using the age-specific rates of the national population as standard (see Table 11.13).

$$E_{indirect} = \Sigma R_i \times n_i \quad (11.23)$$

Table 11.15 Indirect age standardization of traveller mortality.

Age-groups	Age-specific death rates in standard population (per 1000) (R_i)	Age distribution of study (traveller) population ('000) (n_i)	Expected deaths $(R_i \times n_i)$
0–24	0·7315	11·7	8·56
25–44	1·4130	2·8	3·96
45–64	9·3220	1·1	10·25
65+	66·6667	0·3	20·00
Total	–	–	42·77

Observed deaths in study population $O = 84$
Expected deaths in study population $E = 42·77$

$$\text{SMR} = \frac{O}{E} = \frac{84}{42.77} = 196.4$$

The standardized mortality ratio (SMR)

In indirect standardization, a relative-risk-type index comparing the study and standard populations is calculated immediately and is called the *standardized mortality ratio* (SMR). It is the ratio (multiplied by 100) of the actual number of deaths observed in the study population to the expected number of deaths (on the basis of the standard age-specific rates applying, rather than the study rates). The observed number of deaths in indirect standardization is usually given the symbol O and therefore

$$\text{SMR} = \frac{\text{Observed deaths in study population}}{\text{Expected deaths in study population}} \times 100$$

$$= \frac{O}{E} \times 100 \tag{11.24}$$

To be consistent with notation used so far in these sections, however, Eqn. 11.24 should read:

$$\text{SMR} = \frac{d}{E_{indirect}} \times 100 \tag{11.25}$$

where the *d* represents the total observed number of deaths and the numerator is given by Eqn. 11.23.

    Like the CMF, the SMR is based on a comparison of observed and expected deaths and is similarly interpreted. The former compares observed deaths in the standard population with the number that would have occurred if that population had been subject to the age-specific mortality rates of the subgroup of interest. The latter compares the observed deaths in a particular subgroup with the number that would have occurred if that subgroup had been subject to the age-specific mortality rates of the standard population. For both measures, values over 100 suggest a higher mortality in the study population and values under 100 suggest lower mortality. From Table 11.15, the expected number of deaths among the travellers is 42·77, while the observed number is 84. The SMR for travellers is therefore 196·4, again highlighting the much higher (age-adjusted) mortality experienced by this group.

371

*Section 11.5
Qualitative
dependent
variable: vital
statistics*

Indirectly standardized rates

As with direct standardization, indirect standardization also permits the calculation of an overall age-standardized death rate. In analogy with Eqn. 11.21, this is obtained as the product of the SMR (defined as a ratio rather than a percentage) and the crude death rate in the standard population:

$$R_{indirect} = SMR \times R \qquad (11.26)$$

Thus, in the travellers example, the indirectly age-standardized death rate for travellers is $1·964 \times 9·6045 = 18·86$ per 1000.

Unlike the CMF, SMRs are in theory not directly comparable. The SMR compares each study population with the standard, but the ratio of two SMRs does not compare the two component populations correctly. However, comparisons between different groups are often made using the SMR and, usually, little bias is involved.

In many applications, the CMF and the SMR will actually be very close in value, but this is by no means always the case. In the travellers example, for instance, the CMF and the SMR are quite different, because the age distributions of the two populations are so different, but both measures point to the same conclusion. Like the CMF, the SMR has a number of limitations, but it requires less information to calculate. In particular, it is not necessary to know the age distribution of deaths in the subgroups of interest. SMRs are commonly used in analysis of mortality in different socio-economic or occupational groups.

Indirect age standardization

Requirements
- age distribution of the study population
- number of deaths in study population
- age-specific mortality rates in a standard population

Method
- apply age-specific mortality rates from the standard population to the study population, giving expected deaths in the study population
- $SMR = \dfrac{\text{Observed deaths in study population}}{\text{Expected deaths in study population}} \times 100$
- indirectly standardized rate = SMR × crude rate in standard

11.5.4 Confidence intervals for standardized measures

Directly standardized rates

Confidence intervals for age-specific rates and crude rates can be estimated using the methods of Section 4.9.2, assuming a Poisson distribution for the number of deaths. Now, the directly standardized rate is defined by:

$$R_{direct} = \frac{\sum N_i r_i}{\sum N_i} \tag{11.27}$$

where i represents the age-group, N_i is the standard population in age-group i and r_i is the age-specific rate in the study population. For example, in Table 11.13 for the first age-group 0–24, $N_i = 1640$ (thousands) and $r_i = 1\cdot8803$ (per 1000). The directly standardized rate was 15·72 per 1000. The standard error of a directly standardized rate is given by:

$$SE(R_{direct}) = \frac{\sqrt{\sum N_i^2 \, r_i/n_i}}{\sum N_i} \tag{11.28}$$

where n_i is the number in the study population on which the age-specific rate (r_i) is based. Note that n_i and r_i must both be expressed in the same form (e.g. in thousands and per 1000, respectively). The N_i may be expressed in any convenient unit and, in this example, it is in thousands. Using the data on travellers in Table 11.4:

$$SE(R_{direct}) = \frac{\sqrt{(1640)^2 \, 1\cdot8803/11\cdot7 + (920)^2 \, 3\cdot5714/2\cdot8 + \ldots}}{1640 + 920 + \ldots}$$

which turns out to be 2·11 (per 1000). A 95% confidence interval for the standardized rate is then (using a normal approximation):

$$R_{direct} \pm 1\cdot96 \; SE \, (R_{direct}) \tag{11.29}$$

which is:

$$15\cdot72 \pm 1\cdot96 \, (2\cdot11)$$

or from 11·58 to 19·86. Note that this interval does not include the death rate of 9·60 per 1000 for the (standard) population of Ireland, so that the travellers can be said to have a significantly higher (age-adjusted) mortality.

Confidence intervals are available for the CMF, which directly compares the travellers with the Irish population, but are not considered here. It is also possible, when there are two populations, to calculate a standardized rate for each and compare these rates. This can be done using a difference or ratio measure. The ratio measure is essentially the ratio of two CMFs. Confidence intervals (and significance tests) are available for such comparisons, but confidence intervals for the SMR and ratios of SMRs will be given instead.

Standardized mortality ratios

373
Section 11.5
Qualitative
dependent
variable: vital
statistics

Because, for reasons which will not be gone into, the SMR has a lower standard error than the CMF, it is often preferable to work with indirect rather than direct standardization. The SMR is simply a ratio of observed to expected deaths (multiplied by 100), and the observed deaths can be considered to have a Poisson distribution. The methods of Section 4.9.1 can be used to obtain a confidence interval based on the observed deaths and, if these limits are divided by the expected deaths and multiplied by 100, the confidence interval for the SMR results. The limits are:

$$100 \ (x_l/E) \text{ and } 100 \ (x_u/E) \tag{11.30}$$

where x_l and x_u are the lower and upper limits, respectively, for the observed number of deaths (O). In the travellers example:

$$SMR = 100 \ (O/E) = 100 \times (84/42 \cdot 77) = 196 \cdot 4$$

From Table B.13, the 95% confidence interval based on a count of 84 is from $67 \cdot 00$ to $104 \cdot 00$, so that the 95% limits for the SMR are from $6700/42 \cdot 77$ to $10400/42 \cdot 77$ or from $156 \cdot 7$ to $243 \cdot 2$.

Ratio of two SMRs

Although, as briefly mentioned in Section 11.6.3, one must be careful in comparing SMRs for different groups, comparisons are frequently made and are acceptable provided that the groups being compared are broadly similar in age distribution. For instance, relative mortality in two groups, A and B, may be expressed as:

$$SMR_A/SMR_B = \frac{O_A}{E_A} \bigg/ \frac{O_B}{E_B} = \frac{O_A}{O_B} \bigg/ \frac{E_A}{E_B} \tag{11.31}$$

This is seen to be very similar to Eqn. 7.46, used to compare two (unadjusted) rates, and, in fact, the approach to the calculation of a confidence interval for the ratio of two rates can be used for the ratio of two SMRs. Section 7.14.3 explains the method, which treats O_A as a binomial proportion on a sample size of $O_A + O_B$. Confidence limits for this proportion are obtained as p_l and p_u and the lower and upper limits for the ratio of the two SMRs are, respectively:

$$(SMR_A/SMR_B)_l = \frac{p_l}{1-p_l} \frac{E_B}{E_A} \tag{11.32}$$

$$(SMR_A/SMR_B)_u = \frac{p_u}{1-p_u} \frac{E_B}{E_A} \tag{11.33}$$

11.5.5 Population life tables

The clinical life table was discussed in Section 7.15 as a method for analysing variable-time follow-up data from a cohort study. The essence was the display of cumulative mortality over time from the start of the study. Two methods for calculating such life tables were described—the actuarial method and the Kaplan–Meier method.

The cohort or generation life table

A slightly different type of life table is based on 'following' a group of persons from birth to death. This life table, often called a *population life table*, is distinguished from the clinical life table in that it starts with birth and everyone is followed to death. Unfortunately, the terminology is not universally agreed and the term 'population' as applied to a life table can refer to two separate situations. The first, *the generation or cohort life table*, arises when an actual real population is followed up. Since many individuals survive to over 100 years, such a life table can only be constructed for groups of births in the distant past.

The central measure obtained from a population life table is the expectation of life or the average number of years a person can be expected to live. Though the mathematical manipulations to actually calculate this figure may seem somewhat convoluted, the concept is simplicity itself. Suppose that a follow-up study had been carried out on 100 persons born in the year 1900 and that all are now dead. Suppose, too, that the age at death (the lifespan) of each of these is known. The average lifespan of these 100 persons would be calculated by adding up the 100 individual lifespans and dividing by 100. This is the expectation of life at birth. It is calculated by adding up the person-years lived by each individual (to death) and dividing by the number of individuals.

The current or period life table

There is another form of population life table called the *period or current life table*. This is the best-known type of life table and it allows for a comparison of mortality between two populations, adjusted for age. As pointed out, a cohort life table can only be calculated for persons born 100 years or more ago. The current life table, on the other hand, is based, not on actual follow-up of real individuals, but on the experience of a hypothetical cohort. The approach is to take a cohort of 100 000 births. Instead of actually following them, however, the *current* age-specific mortality rates are applied to the cohort to see how it would fare if these current rates continued to apply over the next 100 or more years. The resulting expectation of life is the figure that would be obtained if the age-specific mortality rates observed now were to remain constant over the next 100 years. Though this is not a tenable assumption in reality, the expectation of life from the current life table is a good and easily understood summary of a population's current mortality experience.

	Age x	I_x	d_x	L_x	T_x	e_x^0
	0	100 000	818	99 310	7 229 754	72·30
	1	99 182	66	99 149	7 130 444	71·89
	2	99 116	53	99 090	7 031 295	70·94
	3	99 064	31	99 048	6 932 205	69·98
	4	99 033	30	99 018	6 833 156	69·00

Table 11.16 Part of Irish life table no. 12, 1990–92, males (supplied by the Central Statistics Office, Ireland).

The life table is also called a *period life table* since, usually, the current mortality rates used are calculated over a short period of 2–3 years.

Construction of the current life table [!]

Table 11.16 shows part of the Irish life table for males 1990–92 and the construction of a current life table will be described in relation to this. The life table starts with the cohort of 100 000 births in the second column headed I_x. A number of these will die during their first year of life, and the number is estimated by means of the current infant mortality rate. In the period 1990–92, the average infant mortality rate in Ireland was 8·18 per 1000 (per year), so that out of 100 000 male births the 'expected' number of deaths can be estimated as 818. Thus, of the original cohort, 99 182 may be expected to survive to age 1. These figures are shown in the columns headed I_x and d_x in the table.*

How many of the hypothetical cohort will survive to age 2? This can be estimated by using the actual (1990–92) specific mortality rates for Ireland for the age-group 1 and under 2 years of age. Thus, it is estimated that 66 of the cohort will die between the ages of 1 and 2, leaving 99 116 to survive until age 2.

The general procedure will now be clear. At each age, the cohort is subjected to the specific mortality rates for that age-group. Eventually, of course, the cohort will 'die off'. The number who die at each age is determined by the age-specific mortality rates, and these are usually based on the average mortality rates for the most recent period for which accurate statistics are available.†

Consider now the column headed L_x. The figures in this column measure the estimated total number of years lived by the cohort at each age. To explain this, suppose the whole cohort had survived to age 1 (the infant mortality rate was zero). In this case, the total number of years lived by the cohort, between

---

* The infant mortality rate is defined as the number of deaths in those aged under 1 year, divided by the number of live births. Thus, the number of expected deaths is obtained directly by multiplying the cohort size by the 'rate', which, in this instance, is actually a risk and is not defined on the average population.

† Apart from infant mortality in the first year, age-specific death rates are calculated using the MID-year population as denominator (see Eqn. 11.16). The expected number of deaths, therefore, cannot be calculated by simply multiplying the number in the cohort alive at a particular age by the rate. A small adjustment must be made to change the rate to a risk first (see Section 6.5.1).

birth and age 1, would be 100000 — each member of the cohort would have lived for 1 year.

However, it is estimated that only 99182 of the cohort live for a year, while 818 live for only part of a year. Thus, the total number of years lived by the cohort is 99182 plus some fraction of 818. The simplest assumption would be that those who die live on average 6 months each, so that the 818 of the cohort who die before reaching age 1 would live for a total of 818/2 = 409 years. This assumption is made for all age-groups *except* the age group 0–1, since most deaths in this group occur in the first month of life. The precise method of calculation used for age 0–1 will not be explained here, but it can be estimated that the total number of years lived by this cohort, between the ages of 0 and 1, is 99310.

The total number of years lived by the cohort between the ages of 1 and 2 is 99116 (the number of years lived by the survivors to age 2) plus a half of 66 (those who die before reaching the age of 2). This is 99149. The interpretation of the L_x column should now be clear.

Turning now to the T_x column, the first figure in this column is the total number of years lived by the cohort at all ages — in fact, the sum of *all* the figures in the L_x column when the complete life table for all ages is constructed. Thus, the lifespan of all the members of the cohort is estimated to account for a total of 7229754 years. Since there were originally 100000 persons in the cohort, the average number of years lived by the cohort is 7229754/100000 = 72·30 years. This average, recorded in the last column of the table, is the expectation of life at birth of an Irish male. It indicates how many years an Irish male may be expected to live — or, alternatively, the average age of an Irish male at death — subject to the current age-specific mortality rates prevailing for the next 100 years or so.

The other entries in columns T_x and e_x^0 are also of interest. For example, the second figure in the T_x column measures the total number of years lived by the cohort from the age of 1 onwards; the second figure (71·89) in the e_x^0 column is the number of years lived from age 1 onwards, divided by the cohort size at age 1 (7130444/99182), and measures the *expectation of life* at age 1. That is, a male who has survived to age 1 may expect, on average, to live a further 71·89 years. Thus, the figures in the e_x^0 column measure the expectation of life at each age.

Incidentally, although not observed in the present life table the expectation of life at 1 can exceed the expectation of life at birth, though on *a priori* reasoning it would be expected that the expectation of life would fall with increasing age. This apparently perverse result is due to the effect of a high infant mortality on the life expectancy of the cohort at birth. From age 1, however, the expectation of life invariably declines with age, as expected.

There are many other features of life tables that could be discussed, but sufficient has been explained to demonstrate their relevance in analysis of mortality, despite their limitations.

377

*Section 11.5
Qualitative
dependent
variable: vital
statistics*

Life tables can be constructed for different populations and comparisons made on the basis of life expectancy. Separate tables can be constructed for males and females, for different areas of the country (e.g. urban and rural) and for different occupations. Comparisons can be made that are independent of the effects of age and sex composition, and the expectation of life is a useful and simple concept to understand.

It must be stressed again, however, that the current life table does not reflect the likely future experience of any real birth cohort. The currently *prevailing* age-specific mortality rates are used to calculate the *expected* mortality experience of the cohort. In the example above, age-specific mortality rates for 1990–92 were used. (There was a population census in 1991, so that the population of each age-group could be ascertained with a high degree of accuracy, and this enabled firm estimates to be made of age-specific death rates.) If these are used to calculate the expected mortality experience of a cohort of 100 000 male births commencing in 1991, then for the year 2021, for example, the figure applied to the survivors of the cohort is the age-specific death rate for males aged 30 that prevailed in 1990–92. As the cohort ages, the applicability of the 1990–92 age-specific death rates becomes increasingly open to question. The actual mortality experience of a cohort of male births in 1991 (and hence their life expectancy) is not known. Thus, the expectation of life derived from a life table is a purely hypothetical measure, based upon prevailing (recent) age-specific mortality rates. It is, of course, possible to attempt to anticipate changes in mortality conditions by *predicting* changes in age-specific mortality rates, based, perhaps, on an extrapolation of past trends, but, in certain respects, this introduces a greater degree of ambiguity in the interpretation of the life table statistics.

Clinical life table
- mortality experience of a defined study cohort
- not necessarily starting at birth, and not everyone followed to death

Cohort or generation life table
- actual mortality experience of a cohort
- usually starting at birth with everyone followed to death

Current or period life table
- mortality experience of a hypothetical cohort
- starting at birth with everyone 'followed' to death
- based on current prevailing age-specific mortality rates

Expectation of life (life expectancy) at a given age
- average number of further years a person of that age can expect to live
- based on current prevailing mortality

Years of potential life lost

Standardized rates and ratios are, to a large extent, influenced by the mortality experience of the older age-groups. Deaths in younger age-groups may, however, be more relevant in comparing two populations. This gives rise to the concept of premature mortality. Underlying this is the notion that death implies a loss of potential years of life and that the younger the age at death, the greater the loss. For instance, suppose the (average) expectation of life in a particular population is 70 years. An individual who dies aged 40 can be said to 'lose' 30 years of potential life. If we know the age at death of every individual who dies in a particular calendar period, it is possible to calculate the total years of potential life lost (YPLL) for that population in the given calendar period. If we also know the cause of death, it is possible to calculate YPLL for specific causes of death (in effect, to disaggregate by cause the overall YPLL). Alternatively, if we know the occupation or socio-economic status of each decedent, YPLLs for particular occupations or socio-economic groups can be calculated.

Before commenting further on the method of calculation, the distinctive feature of the premature-mortality approach is the emphasis on mortality experience in younger age-groups. The younger the age at death, the greater the YPLL; hence, in the overall measure of YPLL, the mortality experience of the younger age-groups is given greater weight. This contrasts with more conventional measures, such as cause-specific mortality rates, which are dominated by the mortality experience of the elderly (since most deaths occur amongst the elderly). As a result, a ranking of causes of death by YPLL may be quite different from a ranking by cause-specific (crude) mortality, and this could have implications for health planning priorities. Moreover, comparisons of YPLL for different socio-economic groups may identify vulnerable or high-risk groups (e.g. ethnic minorities) to which additional health resources could be targeted.

Several different definitions and methods of calculation of premature mortality have been proposed. The most contentious issue concerns the selection of the upper end-point for the calculation of YPLL. As suggested above, one possibility is to take the average expectation of life at birth as the end-point. Thus, if the average expectation of life at birth is 70 years, the YPLL for any individual decedent is 70 minus age at death. For individuals who die at age 70 or above, the YPLL would be zero. Some suggest that age 65 should be chosen as a cut-off, since, in many countries, this marks the age of retirement and cessation of a contribution to the economy. An alternative method is to take as the end-point the expectation of life at age of death. For instance, if the average expectation of life at age 75 were 8 years, a death at age 75 would contribute 8 YPLL to the calculation, corresponding to an end-point of 83 years. Since expectation of life varies with age, this method involves the use of a range of end-points, but also ensures that every individual death, including deaths among the elderly, contributes to the calculation of the YPLL.

YPLL can be employed to compare (premature) mortality between populations and can be easily standardized by estimating the number of deaths at each age in a standard population and assigning YPLL to these expected deaths.

11.6 Multivariate analysis

The methods discussed so far in this chapter are often referred to as multivariate techniques, since they are concerned with the variability of a dependent variable related to multiple explanatory variables. Technically, however, multivariate analysis is a body of methods designed to handle simultaneous variation in a number of dependent variables. Only a brief excursion through these techniques is attempted here, and the reader should be warned that the techniques are difficult to use and can easily be misapplied. An example of a multivariate technique is *discriminant analysis*. Suppose two populations are defined by a set of characteristics, such as height, weight, serum cholesterol level, etc., and that for each characteristic the two distributions overlap, so that, for example, the distribution of heights in population A overlaps with the distribution of heights in population B. Thus, although the mean height of individuals in population A may be less than the mean height of individuals in population B, one individual picked at random from population A may be taller than an individual picked at random from population B. Consequently, if an individual were encountered and it was not known which population that individual belonged to, he could not be definitely assigned to a particular population unless, for any one of the variables concerned, the distributions were known not to overlap.

The purpose of discriminant analysis is to enable individual units to be assigned to one or other of the populations with, in some defined sense, the greatest probability of being correct (or smallest risk of error). The techniques of analysis, which are not explained here, involve the specification of a discriminant function, in which the relevant variables are assigned a weight or coefficient. If the discriminant function is linear in form, it will 'look like' a multiple regression equation. For a particular individual or case, values of the variables (height, weight, etc.) are substituted in the discriminant equation and a value for the function calculated. On the basis of this value the individual is assigned to a particular population. As an indication of the possible application of discriminant analysis, suppose it is desired to allocate individuals to a 'high risk' or 'low risk' category for a particular disease, the allocation being made on the basis of certain diagnostic variables, e.g. blood pressure and age. Coefficients of the discriminant function are estimated using sample observations of those who have and have not contracted the disease in some past period. Individuals can then be assigned to one or other category using the discriminant function as the method of allocation. Discriminant analysis has very close theoretical connections with logistic regression, but can easily be extended to the case of more than two groups.

Other multivariate techniques do not require specification of group membership prior to analysis, and can classify individuals or allocate them to groups which are distinct in some sense. These groups are defined by the data structure, and may or may not be logical or natural in themselves. *Principal-components analysis, factor analysis* and *cluster analysis* (numerical taxonomy) are different techniques used in this area. However, not many applications in the general medical literature are seen, although the techniques have, for example, been used to classify psychiatric diagnosis on the basis of patient symptoms.

11.7 Summary

This chapter has considered in detail the analytic approach to the control of confounding and the examination of multiple explanatory factors. The stratification techniques for qualitative confounders should also be used when frequency matching is employed in the design of an investigation. Some of the methods discussed are mainly used in the analysis of rates in vital statistics.

Explanatory or confounding variable(s)	Dependent variable			
	Mean	Binary proportion (risk)	Rate	Life table survival (mortality)
Qualitative only	ANOVA	Mantel–Haenzel techniques	Direct and indirect standardization Current life tables	Logrank methods
Quantitative and/or qualitative	Multiple regression Analysis of covariance	Logistic regression	–	Cox regression

12 Bias and Measurement Error

12.1 Introduction

Bias may be defined as any factor or process that tends to produce results or conclusions that differ systematically from the truth.* Any research study in a medical field is open to bias from many sources, and it is important that the researcher be aware of these biases and, in designing, executing and analysing a study, avoid them where possible. Many of the biases that can arise in the planning and execution of the study are avoidable, but a badly run study cannot be rescued by clever statistical manipulation of figures. For this reason, study design is a far more important aspect of research than pure statistical analysis.

In the body of this book, it has been indicated at various stages how bias may interfere with the eventual outcome of a study, and this chapter brings together some of these ideas and introduces some new ones. Particular forms of bias are more likely with some study designs than others, and the discussion below indicates which pitfalls are more likely in which studies.

Sackett (1979) has identified 56 sources of bias in medical research and, although all these biases are not considered individually here, the article makes for fascinating reading. This chapter considers some of the different biases that can arise in the context of the different stages of a study execution — the design stage, patient selection, data collection, data analysis

---

* This broad definition of bias thus includes errors in analytical methodology and errors of interpretation.

and interpretation of results. Particular emphasis is given to biases inherent in the measurement process, and in the interpretation of diagnostic tests.

12.2 Biases in study design

Chapter 6 outlined the four main study designs often used in medical research—the cross-sectional, the cohort and case–control observational studies and the experimental trial. The avoidance of bias in the experimental trial by the use of randomization and double-blind procedures was discussed in some detail. These arguments are not repeated here, but, instead, points relating to the design of studies in general are considered.

Perhaps the first question to ask about any study is whether a comparison or control group is required. In most cases, the answer will be yes and, indeed, many research studies are uninterpretable without a comparison group. The fact that, for example, 80% of a group of lung-cancer patients smoke does not in itself suggest a relationship between smoking and lung cancer. It is necessary to know what the percentage of smokers is in the general population (the comparison group). This fact is often overlooked. Similarly, in evaluating a preventive or therapeutic measure, there must be a comparison group against which to evaluate the results. Some studies, of course, will not require a specific comparison group. In a cohort study, for example, the comparison groups are often defined by the variables measured at the start of the study, and an explicit comparison group need not always be built into the study design. A sample survey to estimate some parameters may also fit into this category. For instance, a study to determine the factors relating to birth weight would not require a control group.

Given, however, that many studies will require an explicit control group, it is necessary to ask if, at the end of the day, confounders may be present which would bias any comparisons. If confounders can be eliminated by designing a study in a particular way, it is far better than adjusting for extraneous differences between groups at the analysis stage. Thus, in a case–control study, some form of matching may be employed or, in an experimental trial, randomization (stratified or simple) may be used.

An important source of bias in many situations relates to the number of individuals studied. This is discussed in the context of interpreting the results in Section 12.7 below, and methods for determining the appropriate sample size for an investigation are detailed in Chapter 8. Obviously, the design of a given investigation depends critically on the question to be answered and it must be ascertained whether the study as designed will answer that question.

12.3 Biases in selecting the sample

The selection of individuals or items to be included in a study is the area with the greatest potential for bias and relates, to a large extent, but not exclusively, to whether the results of a study are generalizable. As already mentioned, for example, studies based on volunteers can cause great difficulties in this area. If, however, those studied form a random sample (in the strict sense of that term) from the population of interest, then selection bias should not be a problem, as long as results are generalized only to the actual population from which the sample was taken. Studies based on hospital admissions, however, are not generalizable to all patients with a particular condition. Comparisons between admissions to different hospitals are also often biased for the same reason. The type of patient admitted to a particular hospital will depend on, among other things, the catchment population for the hospital, admission criteria, the fame of the physicians and surgeons, the facilities and diagnostic procedures available and the intensity of the diagnostic process. These, and other factors which determine admission to a particular institution or hospital, are even more important when it is remembered that many studies are based on a presenting sample of patients. Admissions to a hospital will, of necessity, exclude, for example, patients managed in the community and patients who do not survive long enough to be admitted to hospital in the first place. A further bias (Berkson's bias) can result in spurious associations between an exposure and disease in a case–control study if the admission rates to hospital differ in different disease/exposure categories (see Section 6.7.2).

A general rule relating to studies of any particular disease is to commence the study in all patients at some fixed point in the natural history of the disease. Failure to do this properly can be a further source of bias. This is why it is suggested in a case–control study, for instance, to include newly diagnosed (incident) cases only—diagnosis being usually a fixed point in a disease's history. Evidence of exposure to a particular factor may be masked if the disease is present for some time. A problem does arise, however, if some patients are diagnosed earlier than others, and the bias is often called *lead time bias*. Suppose a group of breast-cancer patients, diagnosed when they presented with a definite lump in the breast, had been studied and that it is wished to compare their subsequent survival with a group of cases diagnosed by mammography (X-ray) at a screening clinic. This latter group would enter the study at an earlier stage in the natural history of the disease (before an actual lump was detectable) than the former group and thus would be likely to have a longer survival anyway, due to this earlier diagnosis. Some correction for this lead-time bias would have to be made when analysing or interpreting the results.

Selecting patients at a fixed point in the natural history of a disease in a survival study is not achieved, however, by retrospectively determining the data of disease onset. Apart from problems in patient recall and adequacy of available records, such a process would result in a biased group with a spuriously long survival. A researcher who determined the survival of a group of cancer cases attending a clinic by measuring the time from their diagnosis (in the past) to the present would necessarily exclude patients who had died earlier and would thus load the group with those who survived the longest. Such an investigation can only be performed if the survival of *all* patients is determined from diagnosis, and requires a cohort study design.

For any study of disease, the diagnostic criteria must be clear and explicit. Different centres may label different conditions with the same name, and it is important to know precisely what patients were studied, and thus to which population results can be applied. The exclusion of cases because of concomitant disease or other factors may affect the general applicability of findings, although it is usually necessary to avoid contamination of the study groups. In addition to these selection biases, the problems raised by a large number of patients refusing to participate in a study must not be forgotten. This question of non-response bias has been discussed before, and it is best reduced by making the study as simple as possible and not in any way daunting to potential participants.

12.4 Accuracy: measurement error for a single test

Every study in medicine involves data collection or measurement and an interaction between the observer and the patient or object being observed. There are a large number of biases that can occur in this area. Some are related to the process of data gathering and recording, but some are intrinsic to the process of measurement itself.

12.4.1 Data gathering and recording

All studies should employ a predesigned data collection form with the information required, whether it be based on interview, case records or direct measurement, laid out neatly and comprehensively. If data are to be processed by computer, the form should be laid out in a manner suitable for easy transferral of the data to the computer or, indeed, the data may be entered on a computer directly. The specific problems of questionnaire and form design are not considered here, except to note that a questionnaire is much more that just a list of questions that require an answer. Streiner and Norman (1995) give an account of developing questionnaires in the health area.

Some of the biases of data collection, in the context of the case–control study and the experimental trial, have been discussed, emphasizing the necessity, where possible, of blinding the observer to the particular group (case/control, treatment/control) from which information is being collected. This is to avoid biases in the observer's elicitation and interpretation of a response. Bias can also, of course, be due to non-response and lack of complete follow-up, when missing items of information can cause very definite problems.

The problems of measurement go deeper than this, however, but unfortunately there is no standardized terminology to describe the concepts in this area. The definitions given in this text are widely, but not universally, accepted and represent an attempt to put the subject into a realistic framework. What is finally recorded on a questionnaire or record form is a number (e.g. a systolic blood pressure of '124 mmHg') or a category (e.g. 'diabetic') that is in some sense the outcome of a measurement process. This process is often called a test and in what follows the terms measurement and test, depending on context, are used interchangeably. Often the term test specifically refers to a situation where the result is not a measured quantity but rather a category, such as in a diagnostic test, but this is not general. For instance, a test for occult blood gives a category of 'blood present' or 'blood absent' in a stool sample, while a liver-function test usually gives a numerical result. In this text, a quantitative test will refer to a test or measurement that results in a number and a qualitative test will refer to a test that categorizes an individual into one of a number of distinct groups. For the most part, the remainder of this section is concerned with quantitative tests, though a number of the conceptual ideas apply to qualitative tests too.

12.4.2 Accuracy, bias and precision

Any time a test is performed on an individual, there is an underlying quantity that the test is trying to estimate. Measurement error relates to the fact that an observed test result may not reflect this underlying quantity exactly. It is assumed, however, that repeated applications of the test produce a set of results that vary around the unknown underlying quantity in some defined way.

In this chapter, an *accurate* measurement is defined as one that is *precise and unbiased*. These terms can be applied to the actual measurement or the test/instrument that gives rise to them. (For further discussion, see Section 12.4.4) Perhaps the best way to illustrate these two terms is by reference to Fig. 12.1. This shows the hits obtained on four targets by four individuals using different airguns. Mr A's shots are closely grouped around the centre of the target. From this, it might be assumed that the sight of the gun was properly aligned, so that the shots went where they were aimed and also that he was a 'good shot' and had a steady hand, because of the close grouping around the bull's-eye. Ms B, however, did not achieve a close bunching of her shots, although obviously, 'on average', she was hitting where she was aiming for. It might be assumed that the sight of her rifle was well-adjusted, but that her hand was not too steady, resulting in a wide spread of shots. Ms C, on the other hand, obviously had a steady hand, since her shots were grouped closely together, but she was consistently off target; either the sight of her gun was badly adjusted or there was, perhaps, a strong wind. Mr D is most unfortunate; not only is his hand a bit shaky, but, by looking at where his shots are grouped, it would appear also that his sight was out of alignment.

Precision relates to the scatter of shots caused by, for instance, the random shake in an individual's hand, while bias refers to whether or not the shots are hitting the target on average. A faulty sight or a crosswind causes a *systematic*

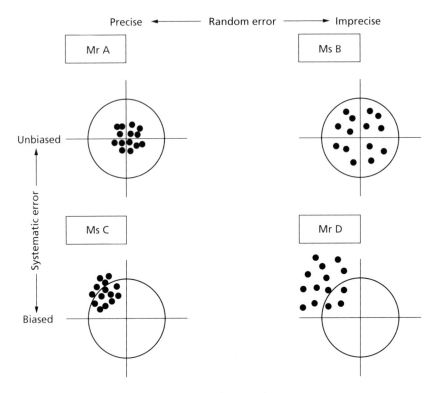

Fig. 12.1 Precision and bias: target practice in a fairground.

error in one particular direction away from the bull's-eye. In terms of a measurement, a bias tends to make the recorded measure consistently above (or below) the true value. Technically, the existence of bias or error can only be determined if the true answer is known from some external source. Relative bias, however, means that two measurements of the same thing are different, without necessarily knowing which of them, if either, is true. The term measurement error should probably only be used if the true underlying value of the measurement is known, but the terms 'measurement error' and 'measurement variation' are often used interchangeably.

The precision of a quantitative measurement relates to the amount of *random variation* about a fixed point (be it the true value or not). An imprecise measurement will sometimes be above this fixed point and sometimes below it, but will vary randomly about it.* If the error is defined as the observed reading minus the true value, then random errors have a zero mean but can have any standard deviation. They can be assumed to have a normal distribution. Random errors can also be considered independent of each other.

---

* Sometimes, the term precision is used in the sense of 'a height of 2·544 m is a more precise measurement than that of 2·5 m'. The two usages are similar, however, in that a measurement with a large amount of random variation cannot be expressed with the same degree of exactness as one with little such variation.

An accurate measurement, then, is one that varies very little (precise) around the true value (unbiased) of what is being measured. If a measurement is biased, the usual way to solve the problem is to correct for this bias by adjusting the observed value. Thus, for example, blood glucose levels determined on the basis of a small finger-prick drop of capillary blood are somewhat lower than the level of glucose in a venous blood sample. Capillary-blood glucose gives a biased estimate of venous-blood glucose and should be adjusted upwards to allow comparison with venous-blood values. A biased measurement, however, can be used to monitor change in an individual, as long as the bias is constant (that is, it is not related to the true value of the measurement). Thus, a weighing scale that consistently underestimated weight by a half a kilogram could be used to determine if a patient were losing or gaining weight. If a measurement lacks precision, repeated measurements of the same characteristic, finally using an average of all these readings, will reduce or eliminate the problem. Repeated measurements will not, of course, correct for bias.

Biased measurement
- systematic error
- on average over- or underestimates true value
- is corrected by adjustment of observed value

Imprecise measurement
- random error
- values of repeated tests vary
- is overcome by taking average of repeated measurements

Accurate measurement
- unbiased and precise

12.4.3 Sources of measurement variation

What then can affect the accuracy of a given measurement? Or, putting it another way, what factors could cause observed measurements to be different from each other and from the true underlying value of a parameter being measured? Different factors affect both precision and bias, and Fig. 12.2 displays some of these. Remember, to define bias it is necessary to know the true value of the measurement and, for the moment, it will be assumed that the factor being measured is actually the factor about which information is required. (See discussion of validity in Section 12.6.) Thus, in evaluating measurements of blood pressure, what is being evaluated is the measurement's capability of determining the pressure exerted by the artery on the cuff of the measuring device. The example of blood pressure determination will be used throughout the rest of this subsection.

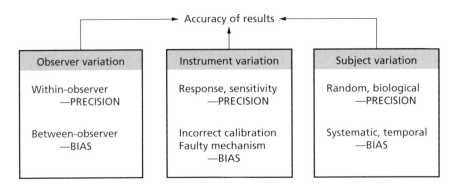

Fig. 12.2 Sources of variation in measurement results.

Observer variation

Observer variation has a major impact on measurement accuracy, and can be split into two components—*within- (intra-) observer variation and between- (inter-) observer variation*. Within-observer variation refers to the variation between different recorded measurements by one observer when the observations (on the same individual) are made on different occasions. In theory, this assumes that the true underlying value is constant and that the differences in the measurements are due only to the observer. In practice, it is impossible to distinguish such observer variation from that of subject variation (if it exists) when the same individual is tested more than once. However, if an observer is interpreting or taking a measurement from, for example, an electrocardiogram (ECG) tracing or an X-ray, 'pure' within-observer variation can be detected. Within-observer variation may be caused by factors such as misreading a dial or judging the height of a column of mercury in a sphygmomanometer at slightly different angles each time. Slight errors in diluting a sample for assay, different inflections in the voice in administering a questionnaire or just misinterpreting a result all contribute to within-observer variation. The important point is that within-observer variation does not, in itself, cause bias, but does affect precision. The variation within an observer is assumed to be random.

Between-observer variation, on the other hand, can bias results and can cause great difficulty in interpreting measurements recorded by different individuals. Between-observer variation is the variation in a recorded measurement performed by two or more different observers. The results of between-observer variation can be severe and, in any study, should be allowed for. Between-observer variation can be caused by different criteria for making a measurement (phase 4 or phase 5 in measuring diastolic blood pressure, for instance) or by different measurement techniques (blood pressure taken supine or standing).

Different methods of actually recording a measurement can also lead to between-observer variation. In blood pressure again, *digit preference* is a large problem. A blood pressure of 117/89 mmHg is rarely recorded; observers tend to have a preference for certain values, or end digits, especially 5 and 0. Thus, readings of 120/85 mmHg and similar are far more common in recorded blood pressures than would be expected on any reasonable distribution of the underlying variable. Again, whether measurements are rounded up or down to the nearest even value or to values ending in 5 or 0, for instance, affects between-observer variation. In administering questionnaires, between-observer variability can be due to different ways of asking questions and even the general demeanour of the interviewer. Between-observer variation can be reduced substantially by very careful standardization of methods and by training of observers. In any study where observations are to be made by different individuals, this must be done to avoid spurious differences between groups. This is particularly so in multicentre trials, for instance. Between-observer variation, too, is always a problem when clinical records or charts are being employed as a data source. Between-observer variation can also be due to unconscious bias on the part of the observer who knows the group in which the individual has been classified. This can be avoided, as has been discussed, by appropriate blinding. Between-observer variation, in essence, biases results, in so far as two different observers recording non-identical results cannot both be right.

Instrument variation

A second major influence on the accuracy of observed measurements is *instrument variation*. The precision of an instrument may be low, in so far as an actual reading is difficult to determine. The term instrument is used in the widest possible sense and includes physical measuring devices (weighing scales, sphygmomanometers, thermometers), questionnaires and interview schedules, and even biological assays. The precision of an instrument depends on its 'sensitivity' or response to the quantity being measured. An instrument from which a measurement is recorded by reading a pointer on a dial would be considered imprecise if the pointer hovered around but never actually stopped at a particular reading. The response or sensitivity of an instrument, however, can often not be distinguished from the effects of observer variation or, indeed (as with questionnaires, for instance), from the effect of subject variation also.

Instrument variation resulting in bias is usually the result of a faulty machine or incorrect calibration. If the scale of a mercury sphygmomanometer slips down, a blood pressure reading will be higher than its true value. Careful maintenance of equipment and testing in a situation where the true value of a measurement is known can reduce this bias enormously.

Subject variation

Subject variation also affects the accuracy of test results, but, of course, in one sense, it is often subject variation that is of interest—for example, a drop in blood pressure due to treatment in an individual patient. Random or biological subject variation relates to the fact that an individual's blood pressure, say, varies in a random way around some fixed value. This, of course, affects the precision of a blood pressure's determination and such within-subject variation is the main cause of the phenomenon known as regression to the mean (see Section 10.7.2). If there is no random within-subject variation, then the quantity being measured is said to be *stable*. Random subject variation is best controlled for, of course, by repeating measurements. This is why, in many studies, for instance, the mean of duplicate or even triplicate blood pressures is used for statistical analysis.

Systematic subject variation will cause a measurement bias. Many parameters can be affected by the subjects' mood, the conditions under which the measurements are taken, the time of day, the season and even the very fact that the subjects know that they are being observed. Such bias is, of course, intrinsically linked to observer variation, in that standardization of measurement technique can reduce some of the systematic variation in this area. Bias can also be due to the subjects' awareness of why they are being studied. *Recall bias*, for instance, can occur if subjects in a case–control study ruminate overmuch concerning exposure to possible causal factors, and thus remember more than if they were, in fact, controls without the disease. In a clinical trial, an individual's response may be affected by his knowledge that he or she is in a group on a 'new wonder drug' which he/she knows should work (the placebo effect).

An interesting bias that can affect study results in different ways is *compliance bias*. For convenience, it is mentioned under the general heading of subject variation. If, in a controlled trial, participants in a treatment group fail to comply fully with their therapy, the apparent effect of that therapy in the full group is diluted. Also, it has been noted in some clinical trials that compliers with the placebo therapy can fare better than non-compliers with this therapy—even though there is no direct effect of the placebo. This is an interesting variation of the placebo effect. If the proportion of compliers in the treatment and control groups differs, a biased comparison may result.

In the final analysis, however, knowledge of whether measurement variation is random or systematic is far more important than knowledge of its source. Systematic variation in any measurement is a problem; individuals will be wrongly classified on the basis of such measurements, which is serious in screening programmes or actual clinical practice. As mentioned, however, a measurement that is systematically biased can remain useful for comparative purposes.

Random variation, on the other hand, causes less of a problem than systematic variation or bias. For the individual, of course, random variation can cause misclassification, but it can be controlled by taking repeat measurements and averaging them. In statistical-type investigations, analysis is performed on groups and random variation will tend to cancel out. Thus, the mean blood pressure of a group of 100 individuals may represent the true situation of the group very well, while any single reading on an individual may lack precision. Random variation, in general, will tend to obscure group differences and reduce the magnitude of correlations between groups.

> Accuracy of measurements is affected by
> * observer variation
> * subject variation
> * instrument variation

12.4.4 Terminology

So far, the term precision has been used somewhat loosely for a 'measurement' or a 'test'. However, a quantitative measurement is just a number and, in itself, is not precise or imprecise. Precision is more a quality that belongs to the measurement process that gives rise to a recorded measurement. This process can include contributions by the observer, the measuring instrument, the subject and interactions between them. A determination of the amount of precision, however, can only be determined by repeating a measurement a number of times under similar conditions. Of course what exactly is meant by 'similar conditions' will determine what sources of imprecision are present.

The term *reliable* can be used instead of precision when describing a test. In this sense, a reliable test is generally defined as one that gives consistent results when administered a second, third or any number of times. Reliability measures the extent to which test results can be replicated, but how the replications are actually made determines both the interpretation of the reliability and the terminology used to describe it. The box lists a number of more or less synonymous terms, even though some authors manage to distinguish between a few of them. Context may make some terms preferable to others, but the reader should be aware that there is a lack of consistency (repeatability, reproducibility!) in the definitions used in the literature. Essentially, however, the terms all refer to the extent that repeated or replicated measures agree with each other. Obviously, the term agreement is best used when comparing results given by two observers on two different tests and, in fact, a reliability analysis of the data is inappropriate in that situation. (See Section 12.5, where the concept of agreement is considered.) The other terms seem more germane when two close time periods are being compared or when within-observer variation is being examined. In many real-life situations, differences between two test results may arise from a combination of a number of these factors; thus, with blood pressure taken on two occasions, it is impossible to distinguish the contribution of the subject from that of the observer in any difference observed. Table 12.1 indicates possible study situations, the variation detectable and the terms probably most appropriate to describe the variability or lack of it.

Table 12.1 Descriptions often applied to measurement variation studies. (The descriptions are indicative only and will not meet with universal agreement.)

Study situation	Variation detectable	Descriptive term
Same subject Same observer Different times	Within-subject variation and within-observer variation	Repeatability Reliability Reproducibility Stability Consistency
Same test material Same observer Different times	Within-observer variation	Reproducibility
Same test material Different observers	Between-observer variation	Agreement
Same test material Different tests	Between-test variation	Agreement

---

Precision
• the extent to which repeated measurements under similar conditions on the same individual or test material agree with each other

Near-synonyms for precision
• reliability
• repeatability
• stability
• consistency
• reproducibility
• (agreement)

12.4.5 Quantifying precision of a quantitative test [!]

For simplicity, the situation of just two administrations of a test or measurement is considered in deriving a measure of reliability. This certainly eases calculations but is not necessary for all the measures considered. A test can be repeated or replicated in a number of different ways. The test can be done on the same individual by the same observer at two different time points (e.g. blood pressures 5 minutes apart); the test can be done on the same test material (e.g. detecting an abnormality in a chest X-ray) by the same observer at different times or by two different observers.

Why is it important to quantify the precision of a test? There are three main reasons. Tests with low precision are unlikely to be very useful in clinical practice and, for this reason, it is important to have a measure relating to this concept. Secondly, a comparison of precision between two different tests may be important in choosing the 'best'—all else being equal (see Section 12.5 for further discussion of comparing different tests). Finally, an estimate of test precision is needed to determine whether an observed difference in test results (within an individual on different occasions—before and after treatment,

Table 12.2 Repeated readings of blood glucose levels 5 minutes apart in 10 well-controlled diabetics using a glucometer with the same observer.

Subject	Glucometer 1st reading (mmol/L)	Glucometer 2nd reading (mmol/L)	Variance of the readings within each subject
1	10·0	10·4	0·080
2	8·0	8·0	0·000
3	7·9	8·2	0·045
4	9·8	9·6	0·020
5	9·0	9·1	0·005
6	8·3	8·0	0·045
7	9·0	8·6	0·080
8	6·5	6·6	0·005
9	6·3	6·8	0·125
10	10·6	10·4	0·020
Mean	8·54	8·57	0·0425

say — or between different individuals) reflects a true difference in the underlying parameter being measured.

Table 12.2 shows early morning blood glucose levels in 10 well-controlled diabetics. Measurements were taken 5 minutes apart by a single observer, using a home glucometer on capillary blood. The purpose of the study was to examine the reliability of a home glucometer in measuring blood glucose. Within-subject variation over 5 minutes is likely to be very small, but both instrument and observer variation (due perhaps to slightly different ways of using the machine) contribute to the differences between the readings in any individual. The data are illustrative only.

There are a number of different ways that such data can be examined in terms of precision and the reader will see different approaches throughout the literature. A few methods are described below. Unfortunately, some of the methods used in published papers are not appropriate for the measurement of test reliability.

The correlation coefficient

Given the structure of these data, the first thing that many people do is to draw a scattergram, as in Fig. 12.3, and calculate a correlation coefficient (see Section 10.3). The line drawn on this scattergram is not the regression line, but is the 'line of agreement', which is the line that would be observed if the two measurements were identical within each individual. In this context, the correlation coefficient is called the 'test–retest reliability'. There are problems with this measure, however, and it should probably not be used. First, the concept of reliability or repeatability would seem to allow for an arbitrary number of observations per subject, while the correlation coefficient is only estimable when there are exactly two observations for each person. Secondly, the correlation coefficient depends on the range of the observed data. The range of blood glucose for these diabetics is fairly small (from 6·3 to 10·6 mmol/L), but, in a larger, more heterogeneous and less well-controlled group, blood glucose

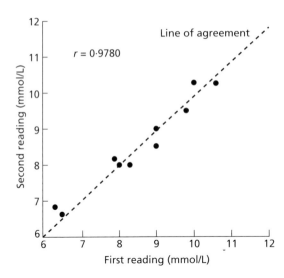

Fig. 12.3 Scattergram showing relationship between repeated blood glucose measurements using a glucometer in 10 subjects. The line of agreement is shown.

levels might vary much more between patients. In general, the larger the range of the data, the higher is the correlation coefficient, so that different correlation coefficients have to be presented for different defined populations. A third difficulty is that, theoretically, there should be no distinction between the first and second observation, since all that is being measured is the variability within each person and the order of the readings should not matter. (Order might, of course, matter if the measurement were taken after a large intake of glucose, in which case the second reading, even only 5 minutes later, would be expected to be higher than the first.) The correlation coefficient fails on this criterion too since it is the relationship between (all of) the first readings and (all of) the second readings that it measures. An *intra-class correlation coefficient* is sometimes calculated, which overcomes this problem by essentially averaging the correlations among all possible orderings of the pairs. This measure extends to more than two observations per person but is not considered here. In the blood glucose example, the correlation coefficient is $r = 0.9780$.

> Correlation coefficient between repeated measures as a measure of precision
> - not an ideal measure
> - two measures per subject only
> - is a function of the order of the measurements
> - depends on the range of the data
> - the higher the correlation coefficient, the greater the precision

Variance/standard deviation of the measurements: error limits

Essentially, precision relates to the variability of repeated measurements on the same person (ideally, taken under similar conditions with the same observer, etc.). The variance of repeated measurements would thus be a reasonable measure of precision—the smaller the variance, the greater the precision or reliability. To make any sense out of this, it is necessary to assume that this variance does not depend on the individual studied and that there is an underlying variance that is the same for everyone.* On this basis, the variance of repeated measurements within any single individual would be an estimate of this underlying variance of the measurements. Table 12.2 shows the variances of the two blood glucose measurements calculated separately for each of the 10 subjects. The variance is calculated, using Eqn. 1.6, on the sample of two observations within each subject (see also Section 12.4.6). Under the assumption of a common underlying vari-ance, an average of the 10 within-subject variances gives a direct measure of the variability due to measurement error. This average is referred to as the '(within-subject) variance of the measurements' and its square root as the '(within-subject) standard deviation of the measurements'.[†] This variance (or standard deviation) is perhaps the commonest measure of precision used for quantitative data. Though it directly measures the variability of repeated measurements, the magnitude of the variance is not easily interpretable — how high an error vari-ance is acceptable? The answer depends on the situation and there is no unique response.

The assumption that the variability of the measurement is independent of the magnitude of the observation can be informally checked by examining a plot of the standard deviation in each subject versus the mean of the two repeated readings. Since each reading gives an estimate of the same underlying quantity, the mean of the two is taken, rather than either one on its own. For reasons that will be discussed in Section 12.4.6, the standard deviation of *two* readings is proportional to their absolute difference (i.e. the difference ignor-ing its sign), and the suggested plot is given in Fig. 12.4. This plot does not suggest any consistent relationship between the variability of the blood glucose measurement and its magnitude. If a relationship is discernible, a common underlying variance does not exist and a transformation of the data is necessary to allow for this (Bland & Altman, 1996).

In the blood glucose example, the (within-subject) variance of the measure-ments (obtained by averaging the 10 variances in column 4 of Table 12.2) is:

$$S_W^2 = 0 \cdot 0425 \qquad (12.1)$$

where the W subscript stands for 'within-subject'. The standard deviation of the measurements is calculated by taking the square root of this figure as:

$$S_W = 0 \cdot 2062 \qquad (12.2)$$

---

* An exception to this assumption, whereby the variance depends on the magnitude of the measurement (usually increasing with it), can be accounted for but is not considered in this text.

[†] Note that the square root of the average of the variances is taken and not the average of the indi-vidual standard deviations. Note too that the variance and standard deviation of repeated measurements can go by a number of different names. Though the term 'within-subject variance/standard deviation of the measurements' is cumbersome, it is used here to avoid confusion. Other texts may use a different descriptor for the same quantity.

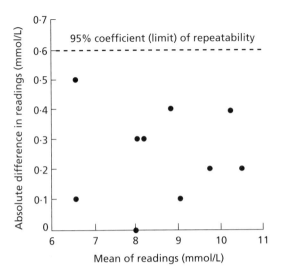

Fig. 12.4 Plot of absolute difference between repeated blood glucose measurements (using a glucometer) against their mean in 10 subjects. The absolute difference is proportional to the standard deviation of the repeated measurements in each individual. The 95% coefficient (limit) of repeatability is shown.

If the values of replicate measures of the same underlying quantity are normally distributed around the true value of that quantity and the variability is the same within each individual, 95% of the measurements in any individual should lie within plus or minus 1·96 (standard deviations) of the quantity. It could be said that, 95% of the time, the quantity is measured to a precision of:

$$\pm 1{\cdot}96\, S_W \qquad (12.3)$$

For the glucometer data, the precision is within ±0·40 mmol/L. Essentially, this means that the true underlying value is (95%) likely to be within 0·40 mmol/L of the recorded measurement. The figures obtained when this number is added to and subtracted from an observed reading are called the 95% error limits. For an observed measurement of m, these limits are:

$$m \pm 1{\cdot}96\, S_W \qquad (12.4)$$

Obviously, this approach extends easily to the case of more than two repeated measurements per person and to different numbers of replicates being available for different persons. Again, the variance within each person is taken and these are then averaged. (See Section 12.4.6 for further details and some short-cut computational methods for calculating the final estimate of the within-subject variance of the measurements.)

The within-subject standard deviation of the measurements S_W as a measure of precision
- assumed independent of the magnitude of the reading
- assumed the same for each individual
- direct measure of variation of repeated measures in an individual
- not confined to two replications per individual
- the larger its value, the lower the precision
- gives the 95% error limits for a single measurement m, as $m \pm 1{\cdot}96\, S_W$

Bland and Altman (1986) suggest that any measure of precision in the medical context should be directly relevant to the clinical use of such a measure and that the analytic approach should be able to quantify relative bias and precision separately. Since the interpretation of test differences is one of the most important aspects of clinical measurement, they propose that the emphasis should be on the variability of differences between measurements given by the test, rather than just on the variability of repeated measurements of a single test. Their method is simple, has a direct clinical interpretation and provides what is, perhaps, the measure of choice for precision in the medical context.

Table 12.3 gives the blood glucose data shown previously in Table 12.2, but this time the differences between the repeated values are also presented. In general, if two test values are being compared in clinical practice, what is needed is some guidance as to whether the observed difference reflects a real underlying difference or whether it could be explained by measurement variation. If a measurement has high precision, then observed differences between two observations are likely to reflect real differences. If the precision is low, then differences may well be explicable by the random variability introduced by the measurement process. In the example, the mean of the 10 differences (d = 1st reading minus 2nd reading), taking account of their sign, is:

$$\bar{d} = -0.03\,\text{mmol/L} \tag{12.5}$$

This mean is close to zero, as expected, since there is no physical reason for one reading to be consistently lower or higher than the other. The mean of the differences is a direct measure of relative bias between the two measurements

Table 12.3 Repeated readings of blood glucose levels 5 minutes apart in 10 well-controlled diabetics using a glucometer with the same observer.

Subject	Glucometer 1st reading (mmol/L)	Glucometer 2nd reading (mmol/L)	d 1st minus 2nd reading (mmol/L)	Mean of 1st and 2nd readings (mmol/L)
1	10·0	10·4	−0·4	10·20
2	8·0	8·0	0·0	8·00
3	7·9	8·2	−0·3	8·05
4	9·8	9·6	0·2	9·70
5	9·0	9·1	−0·1	9·05
6	8·3	8·0	0·3	8·15
7	9·0	8·6	0·4	8·80
8	6·5	6·6	−0·1	6·55
9	6·3	6·8	−0·5	6·55
10	10·6	10·4	0·2	10·50
Mean	8·54	8·57	−0·03	8·555

$\bar{d} = -0.03\,\text{mmol/L}$
$SD(d) = 0.3057\,\text{mmol/L}.$

and, if it is quite different from zero, there is a possibility of a systematic difference between the first and second readings. In such a case, the methods described for the analysis of precision are not applicable to the data and methods for analysing agreement may have to be employed instead (Section 12.5). A paired *t* test can be performed to determine if the mean difference is significantly greater than or less than zero (see Section 7.8).

In the example, the variance of the 10 differences in blood glucose is (applying Eqn. 1.6 to the differences in Table 12.3):

$$Var(d) = 0.0934 (\text{mmol}/\text{L})^2 \tag{12.6}$$

and the standard deviation is the square root of this, which is:

$$SD(d) = 0.3057 \, \text{mmol}/\text{L} \tag{12.7}$$

The population of differences between the two replicated measurements can safely be assumed to have an approximately normal distribution.* From the properties of the normal distribution, 95% of differences between any two replicated measurements should lie between:

$$0 - 1.96 \, SD(d) \quad \text{and} \quad 0 + 1.96 \, SD(d)$$

where the population of differences is assumed to have a zero mean (no relative bias) and the sample standard deviation is taken as an estimate of the standard deviation in the population. Thus, since the sign of the difference is irrelevant when repeated measures are in question, 95% of the differences (ignoring the sign) should be less than $1.96 \, SD(d)$. The value given by this quantity is called the 95% *coefficient of repeatability* or the 95% *limit of repeatability*. In the example:

$$\text{Coefficient of repeatability} = 1.96 \, SD(d)$$
$$= 1.96(0.3057)$$
$$= 0.5992 \, \text{mmol}/\text{L} \tag{12.8}$$

95% of differences between two repeated measures of fasting blood glucose on the same individual should be less than 0.60 mmol/L (rounding to two decimal places). Thus, if two observed readings are less than 0.60 mmol/L apart, the difference could be (but is not necessarily) explained by measurement error or lack of precision of the determination. On the other hand, blood glucose determinations more than 0.60 mmol/L apart are likely to reflect a real difference in blood glucose and not an artefact of measurement variability.

If there is a relationship between the size of the difference and the magnitude of the observation, the coefficient of repeatability as defined above is not

---

* The population referred to here is the population of all possible replications of a particular measurement in an individual, since it is also assumed that the variability of replicated measurements is the same for each individual. Due to the central-limit theorem (see Section 4.5.1), differences between two quantities are also more likely to have a normal distribution than the quantities themselves.

valid. If there is a relationship, it is usually that the size of the difference between replicated readings increases with the size of the readings. In this case, a transformation of the data may allow a suitable coefficient to be estimated (Bland & Altman, 1996).

A check on this assumption can be made by constructing a diagram showing the relationship between the differences and the magnitude of the readings. Since there is no interest in the direction of the difference between two readings replicated under similar conditions, the absolute value of the difference is plotted. Also, as argued in the previous subsection, the mean of the two readings is the best representation of the magnitude of the underlying quantity. Thus, the absolute difference between the readings is plotted against the mean of the two of them.* Figure 12.4 shows this plot for the replicated blood glucose readings, with the relevant figures given in Table 12.3. This is a popular method of illustrating studies of precision and usually includes a line representing the coefficient (limit) of repeatability, given by Eqn. 12.8. The diagram allows one to see what the magnitude of the measurement error actually is and whether it is related to the size of the quantity being measured. In this example, there does not seem to be any such relationship. In addition to the visual check on any relationship between the differences and the mean, the diagram is a good check for outlying observations, which may have to be investigated further.

The 95% coefficient (limit) of repeatability
- is given by $1 \cdot 96 \, SD(d)$
- is the value below which 95% of the differences between two replicated readings should lie
- is the upper limit of differences that are (95%) likely to be due to measurement error
- assumes that the size of the differences is independent of the magnitude of the observations

---

12.4.6 Computations and interrelationships between measures of precision for quantitative tests [!]

This section considers the close connections between the coefficient (limit) of repeatability and the within-subject variance of the measurements discussed above. Included are some short-cut computational methods and a description of the approach to be taken for the estimation of the coefficient of repeatability when more than two repeated measures are available per subject. This section is somewhat technical and can be omitted at first reading.

---

* It should be noted that some authors suggest that the actual values of the differences, rather than their absolute value, be plotted. See Section 12.5, where this is done for estimating agreement, as opposed to reliability.

Within-subject variance with two replicated measurements

In the case of two replicates per individual, as was considered in Section 12.4.5, the within-subject variance of the two observations in any single individual is particularly easy to calculate. From Eqn. 1.6, the variance of two observations x_1 and x_2 is:

$$Var(x_1 \text{ and } x_2) = \frac{\left(x_1 - \frac{x_1 + x_2}{2}\right)^2}{2-1} + \frac{\left(x_2 - \frac{x_1 + x_2}{2}\right)}{2-1}$$

$$= \frac{(x_1 - x_2)^2}{2} = \frac{d^2}{2} \tag{12.9}$$

where $d = x_1 - x_2$ is the difference between the readings in each individual studied.

The standard deviation of the replicated measurements (within each individual) is given by the square root of the variance in the individual as:

$$|d|/\sqrt{2} \tag{12.10}$$

where $|d|$ is the absolute value of the difference. Thus, when there are two replicates, a plot of $|d|$ against $(x_1 - x_2)/2$ is equivalent to a plot of the standard deviation against the mean (apart from the factor $\sqrt{2}$) (see Fig. 12.4). In the general situation of a variable number of replicates per subject, the actual standard deviation is plotted against the mean to check on the assumption that the measurement variation is independent of the size of the observation.

The within-subject variance of the measurements, which is the average of the subject variances given by Eqn. 12.9, is obtained by summation and division by the number of subjects (n):

$$S_W^2 = \sum (d)^2 / 2n \tag{12.11}$$

The square root of this quantity gives the common within-subject standard deviation of measurements S_W (see Eqn. 12.1).

Analysis of variation (ANOVA) and within-subject variance

As mentioned in the previous section, the within-subject variance of the measurements can be obtained from a study where there are more than two replicates and the number of replicates is different for each individual. Again, the variance within each individual is calculated and averaged over however many individuals there are. A weighted average is taken, reflecting the number of replicates in each person. The astute reader may have noticed a correspondence with analysis of variance (ANOVA) here (see Section 9.2.2). In fact, the estimation of the within-subject variance in the most general case is best performed using an ANOVA approach. Usually, an ANOVA compares groups

Table 12.4 One-way ANOVA table for the data of Table 12.2. Comparisons are between subjects.

Source of variation	Degrees of freedom	Sum of squares	Mean square
Between subjects	9	33·7445	3·7494
Within subjects	10	0·4250	0·0425
Total	19	34·1695	

with a number of subjects in each group. If, instead, the ANOVA is set up to compare subjects, with a number of observations per subject, what is called the within-group variance when comparing groups now corresponds to a within-subject variance. Table 12.4 shows the ANOVA table for the data of Table 12.2. The ANOVA estimate of within-subject variance (0·0425) is identical to that obtained by averaging the individual within-subject variances (see Eqn. 12.1). Note that the notation S_W^2 is use for both quantities.

Within-subject variance and the variance of the difference between two replicates

There is a close connection between the within-subject variance of the measurements, $S_W^2 = 0·0425$ (Eqns. 12.1 and 12.11), and the variance of the difference between two replicated measurements, $\text{Var}(d) = 0·0934$ (Eqn. 12.6). Both are measures related to precision, the former giving the variability of an individual measurement and the latter giving the variability expected in the difference between two replicated readings. In Section 7.4.1, it was mentioned that the variance of a difference is equal to the sum of the variances of the individual components, as long as the observations are independent. If S_W^2 is known, then the variance of the differences between two replicate measures can be obtained as:

$$\text{Var(differences)} = 2S_W^2 \qquad (12.12)$$

because each component of the difference has variance S_W^2. The standard deviation of the differences is then:

$$SD\text{(differences)} = \sqrt{2}S_W \qquad (12.13)$$

In the blood glucose example, this quantity was obtained directly by calculating the standard deviation of the differences between the two replicate measurements (Eqn. 12.7). Using Eqn. 12.13 is an alternative approach. The 95% coefficient (limit) of repeatability is then (from Eqn. 12.8):

$$1·96\sqrt{2}S_W = 2·77S_W \qquad (12.14)$$

This is the method that should be employed to estimate the coefficient of repeatability in the general study situation of more than two replicates per subject.

For reasons that are too technical for this text, the standard deviation of the differences obtained using Eqn. 12.13 is numerically slightly different from the figure obtained using Eqn. 12.7.* For the blood glucose data, Eqn. 12.13 gives the answer of $\sqrt{2}(0{\cdot}2062) = 0{\cdot}2916$, with S_W given by Eqn. 12.2. On the other hand, Eqn. 12.7 gives the direct answer as $0{\cdot}3057$. The difference is not large and the reader should not be over-worried about the discrepancy. He or she should be aware that either method described here can be used to estimate the standard deviation of differences between two replicated readings and, from that, the coefficient of repeatability.

12.5 Agreement: comparing two different tests or observers

The discussion in the last section of measurement error concentrated to a large extent on the idea of precision (reliability, repeatability or reproducibility) in the context of a quantitative test. The analytic approach discussed assumes that the same underlying quantity is being measured under, as far as possible, similar conditions. Thus, replicated measurements vary randomly around this quantity and the differences between two replicates are assumed to have (in the population of all measurements) a zero mean. The question of bias or relative bias does not arise. If, however, two different observers or two different tests are involved, there may be a relative bias between the measurements. Measurements made by one observer may vary randomly around one particular value, while measures (of the same underlying quantity) by a second observer may vary around a different value. When two different observers or tests are involved, the problem is whether measurements obtained by the two *agree* or not. Precision is a quality related to a single test; agreement refers to two (or more) tests, or to two (or more) observers.

The methods for measuring agreement, however, are closely connected with those for measuring precision, but there are subtle distinctions—one, of course, is that relative bias becomes an issue when examining agreement. It is important, too, that the observers or tests being compared should have a high level of precision or this will also contribute to lack of agreement.

As for measures of reliability, significance testing is not the most relevant statistical analysis for measures of agreement. The rejection of a null hypothesis of 'no agreement' is not very enlightening. The measures discussed are estimates of the true underlying parameter in the populations of all comparisons between the two tests, and confidence intervals can give the sampling error of the measures discussed. In general, formulae for confidence intervals of the measures discussed in this book are complex to calculate and a more advanced text should be consulted.

---

* The discrepancy is related to the fact that the average difference between the two replicates $\bar{d}$ is not exactly zero and to the fact that a divisor of $n-1$ is used in the definition of the variance, rather than n.

Agreement
• the extent to which two different tests or two different observers agree with each other when measuring the same subject/test material

12.5.1 Quantifying agreement between quantitative tests [!]

Table 12.5 shows the blood glucose levels determined by a glucometer on a finger-prick of blood, together with the laboratory results on a venous blood sample taken at the same time. The glucometer data are the mean of the two readings from the study of precision in Table 12.3. The point of examining agreement is to see if two instruments or observers give the same readings on essentially the same observation. If two instruments agree well, for instance, then perhaps they could be interchanged and, in the example, the glucometer might be a real alternative to a laboratory-based blood test.

There are a number of different approaches that have been used to analyse agreement data. Unfortunately, many of these methods are simply wrong, and often little thought seems to be given to the purposes of the analysis.

The first point to note from Table 12.5 is that, overall, there is a difference in the mean values given by the different tests. On average, the laboratory gives readings 0·2750 mmol/L higher than the glucometer. Thus, there is a systematic difference or relative bias between the two instruments.

Correlation and agreement

Again, the first approach that is often used with agreement data, similar to the situation for precision, is that of a correlation analysis. Figure 12.5 shows a

Table 12.5 Blood glucose levels from a glucometer (mean of replicated readings in Table 12.3) and from a blood sample taken simultaneously and analysed in a laboratory.

Subject	Laboratory reading (mmol/L)	Glucometer reading (mmol/L)	d Laboratory minus glucometer reading (mmol/L)	Mean of laboratory and glucometer readings (mmol/L)
1	10·2	10·20	0·00	10·200
2	8·2	8·00	0·20	8·100
3	8·7	8·05	0·65	8·375
4	9·6	9·70	−0·10	9·650
5	9·6	9·05	0·55	9·325
6	8·2	8·15	0·05	8·175
7	9·4	8·80	0·60	9·100
8	7·0	6·55	0·45	6·775
9	6·6	6·55	0·05	6·575
10	10·8	10·50	0·30	10·650
Mean	8·83	8·555	0·275	8·6925

$\bar{d} = 0·2750$ mmol/L
$SD(d) = 0·2741$ mmol/L.

scattergram of the glucometer and laboratory data. The correlation coefficient is $r = 0.9798$ ($p < 0.001$). Thus, there is a high, statistically significant, degree of correlation between the two instruments in measuring blood glucose. The line drawn on Fig. 12.5 is not, however, the regression line but the line of agreement, which represents perfect agreement between the two measuring instruments (see Section 12.4.5). The data points tend to fall below the line, since the laboratory gives higher readings than the glucometer.

The problem with using this diagram is that agreement and correlation are completely different concepts and, since it is agreement that is of relevance, correlation is irrelevant. Correlation measures whether there is a linear relationship, but a strong linear relationship does not necessarily mean a high level of agreement. Suppose a basic mistake had been made in the manufacture of the glucometer and it gave a reading that was twice the 'true' reading that it was estimating. Figure 12.6 shows what the data comparing this 'bad' glucometer with the laboratory might look like. (The data for the 'bad' glucometer are obtained by taking half the glucometer measurements from Table 12.5) The correlation coefficient for these data, $r = 0.9798$, is identical to that obtained in Fig. 12.5, but, of course, the two instruments do not agree at all! This serves to illustrate the difference between correlation and agreement. If two measures agree fully, they will be perfectly correlated. However, perfect correlation does not imply any agreement at all. Agreement means that the readings from the two instruments are the same; correlation examines whether or not the readings are related to each other (linearly) — quite a different concept. Unfortunately, many analyses and published papers use correlation coefficients as a measure of agreement and are wrong in so doing.*

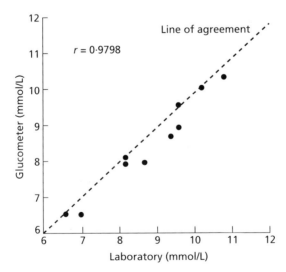

Fig. 12.5 Scattergram showing relationship between blood glucose measurements by a glucometer and a laboratory method in 10 subjects. The line of agreement is shown.

* Rank correlation coefficients (see Section 10.6.4) do not suffer from this problem but only measure agreement on the *ordering* of the different test results.

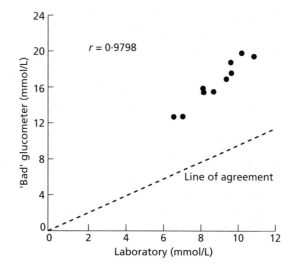

Fig. 12.6 Scattergram showing relationship between blood glucose measurements by a badly calibrated glucometer and a laboratory method in 10 subjects. The line of agreement is shown.

Of course, precision and agreement are closely allied concepts and, essentially, precision is agreement in the context of repeated readings under similar conditions with no relative bias. However, the absence of a systematic difference allows analytic methods to be used for precision, which would be quite inappropriate for analysing agreement.

> • A correlation coefficient cannot be used to measure agreement

Other approaches to analysing agreement, using regression, have been proposed. Perfect agreement implies a regression coefficient of 1·0 (the slope of the regression line—see Section 10.2.3), but, unfortunately, random measurement error always reduces the regression coefficient on observed data to below the required 1·0. If agreement is to be measured, why not do so directly?

Limits of agreement

The approach is similar to that employed for examining precision. Since the difference between readings is of interest, these are examined directly. Table 12.5 gives the difference between the laboratory and glucometer determinations (d = laboratory minus glucometer), together with their mean, on each individual studied. The mean and standard deviations of the 10 differences are:

$$\bar{d} = 0.2750\,\text{mmol/L} \qquad\qquad (12.15)$$

$$SD(d) = 0.2741\,\text{mmol/L} \qquad\qquad (12.16)$$

Figure 12.7 shows a plot of the 10 differences against their mean value to examine whether the differences between the instruments are related to the size of the measurement. The mean value of the two observations is used,

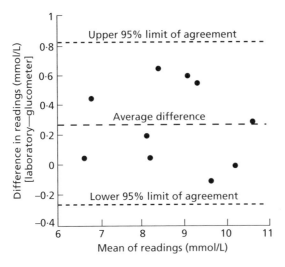

Fig. 12.7 Plot of difference between laboratory and glucometer blood glucose measurements against their mean in 10 subjects. The average difference line and the 95% limits of agreement are shown.

because of a spurious correlation that exists between the difference between two readings and any one of them. The differences are scattered on either side of the 'average difference' line and there is no tendency for the differences to increase as the magnitude of the readings increase. (Remember that the equivalent diagram in the context of precision, Fig. 12.4, plotted the absolute difference between the readings rather than their difference.)

On the further assumption that the difference between the two instruments is independent of the individual on whom the readings were made, the diagram can be examined to find out how much agreement there is. First, the average difference line, plotted at $\bar{d} = 0.2750$, shows the relative bias. As was pointed out at the beginning of this section, on average the laboratory results are higher than those based on the glucometer. Using similar arguments to those in Section 12.4.5, the distribution of the differences should be approximately normal. Therefore, 95% of the differences in readings (laboratory minus glucometer) are expected to lie between:

$$\bar{d} - 1.96\,SD(d) \quad \text{and} \quad \bar{d} + 1.96\,SD(d) \qquad (12.17)$$

where $\bar{d}$ is the average difference and $SD(d)$ is the standard deviation of the (in this case, 10) differences. These are called the 95% *limits of agreement*. The 95% limits of agreement between the laboratory and glucometer determinations of blood glucose are:

$$0.2750 \pm 1.96(0.2741)$$

or -0.2622 and 0.8122 mmol/L. Thus, while on average the glucometer measures 0.28 mmol/L lower than the laboratory, on 95% of occasions the glucometer reading could be anywhere from 0.26 mmol/L above the laboratory determination to 0.81 mmol/L below it. This is a succinct and easy-to-understand statement of how two instruments agree. Figure 12.7 shows the

95% limits of agreement also, and the diagram is a good method of presenting the results of an agreement study.

Note that one distinction between the analysis of agreement and the analysis of precision is that, for precision, the mean of the differences between replicates is assumed to be zero. There is thus a single coefficient (limit) of repeatability below which 95% of the (absolute) differences between replicated readings should lie (see Section 12.4.5). Because, however, there may be bias, there are two limits of agreement *between* which 95% of the differences between two instruments should lie.

Whether the agreement between two instruments is reasonable will depend on the clinical situation and on the degree of accuracy required in a determination. In the blood glucose example, the bias could be corrected for and, allowing for that, differences between the instruments, 95% of the time, would be between $\pm 1.96(0.2741)$ or ± 0.54 mmol/L. This is for a measurement that ranges from (in these patients) around 6.0 to 10.0 mmol/L. Often, a plot of the difference between readings versus their mean, together with the limits of agreement, highlights a major lack of agreement between two instruments that is not obvious from the scattergram or the correlation coefficient.

The limits of agreement are expressed in absolute terms in mmol/L since they are unaffected by the magnitude of the observation. If the plot of the difference versus the mean showed that the difference between the instruments increased with the magnitude of the observations, then, as for precision, a transformation of the data is necessary. In this case, the limits of agreement have to be presented as a percentage of the observed value, rather than in absolute terms (Bland & Altman, 1996).

Of course, if either of the instruments (or observers) being compared has a low precision or repeatability, agreement cannot be good. Ideally, precision should be examined first. It is possible, of course, to compare two tests, with each test performed twice. This allows examination of agreement between the tests and the precision of each test in one analysis. Bland and Altman (1986) detail the required calculations.

The 95% limits of agreement
- are given by $\bar{d} \pm 1.96 \, SD(d)$
- are used when comparing two instruments or two observers
- are limits within which are found 95% of the differences between measurements from two different instruments or observers

---

12.5.2 Quantifying agreement between qualitative tests — kappa

This section introduces a measure of agreement suitable for qualitative tests, but only considers those with a simple binary response — the presence or absence of some factor. Data relating to how two observers interpret a number

Table 12.6 Diagnosis of sight-threatening eye disease in 200 patients, on the basis of retinal photographs (a) by two different observers Dr A and Dr B and (b) by Dr A and a monkey.

(a) Observed data

Dr B's diagnosis	Dr A's diagnosis		Total
	Sight-threatening eye disease	Not sight-threatening	
Sight-threatening eye disease	50	20	70
Not sight-threatening	10	120	130
Total	60	140	200

Observed agreement $A_O = \dfrac{50 + 120}{200} = 85\%$

(b) Chance data

Monkey's diagnosis	Dr A's diagnosis		Total
	Sight-threatening eye disease	Not sight-threatening	
Sight-threatening eye disease	21	49	70
Not sight-threatening	39	91	130
Total	60	140	200

Agreement expected due to chance $A_E = \dfrac{21 + 91}{200} = 56\%$.

of retinal photographs are used to illustrate how agreement is measured. The same approach would be used to compare two different tests — for instance, diagnosis of an eye condition by retinal photograph versus direct examination by an ophthalmologist. Note that the context here is examining how well two observers or two tests agree with each other. There is no question of knowing which test gives a 'correct' result at this stage (see Section 12.6).

Table 12.6a shows the results of determining the presence of sight-threatening eye disease in a group of 200 diabetics on the basis of retinal photography.* Each of the 200 sets of photographs was examined by two observers — Dr A and Dr B — and a determination of the presence or absence of disease was made. The table shows how each observer graded each patient. Dr A made a positive diagnosis in 60/200 = 30% and Dr B's corresponding figure on the same photographs was 70/200 = 35%. There is thus some relative bias between the two observers, since Dr A tends to be less stringent overall than Dr B. In terms of how individuals were classified, however, there were only 50 patients on whom the two doctors could agree on the presence of disease and there were 120 whom they agreed were disease-free. The most obvious measure of agreement is the percentage of patients in whom an agreed diagnosis was made and, on this basis, the observed agreement is:

* Illustrative data only.

$$A_O = \frac{50+120}{200} = 85\% \qquad (12.18)$$

This figure measures agreement directly but it does not allow for the possibility that some of this agreement might be due to chance. The easiest way to understand chance agreement is to replace one of the observers, Dr B say, with a monkey, who makes the diagnosis entirely by chance—perhaps by just creating two different piles of the photographs! Table 12.6b shows a table comparing Dr A's results with that of the hypothetical monkey. The results of the monkey in this table are obtained by assuming that the monkey gives the same overall percentage of those with disease as did Dr B (70/200 = 35%) but assigns this 35% randomly with no diagnostic skill whatsoever. Thus 21 of Dr A's 60 positive patients (35%) are determined by the monkey to have the disease.* Similarly, the monkey gives a positive diagnosis to 35% of Dr A's 140 negative patients, which is 49 patients. The remaining patients are diagnosed as disease-free by the monkey and the numbers can be obtained by subtraction from the totals in the margins of the table. The numbers in Table 12.6b are, then, the numbers expected on the basis of chance alone. The same expected numbers can be obtained by replacing Dr A with a monkey and performing similar calculations to the above. The reader will note that these expected numbers are calculated in the same way as the expected numbers in the chi-square analysis of a 2×2 table (see Section 7.10.3, which discusses some of the short cuts and checks when calculating these numbers).

From Table 12.6b, Dr A and the monkey agree on $21 + 91 = 112$ diagnoses. The percentage agreement between the two observers expected due to chance is then

$$A_E = \frac{21+91}{200} = 56\% \qquad (12.19)$$

Therefore the amount of observed agreement beyond chance is

$$A_o - A_E = 85\% - 56\% = 29\% \qquad (12.20)$$

The interpretation of this 'agreement beyond chance', however, depends on how much agreement beyond chance is actually possible. The final step in creating a useful measure of agreement is to express the observed agreement beyond chance as a proportion of the total possible or potential agreement beyond chance. Figure 12.8 shows the percentages involved. Since 56% agreement in these data can be ascribed to chance, there is a potential of up to $100\% - 56\% = 44\%$ agreement beyond chance. Kappa (κ—the Greek lowercase letter 'k') is defined as the observed agreement beyond chance as a proportion of the potential agreement beyond chance:

$$\kappa = \frac{A_O - A_E}{100\% - A_E} = \frac{85\% - 56\%}{100\% - 56\%} = \frac{29\%}{44\%} = 0.66 \qquad (12.21)$$

* If this chance-expected figure ends up as a fractional number of patients, that is perfectly all right. It often does.

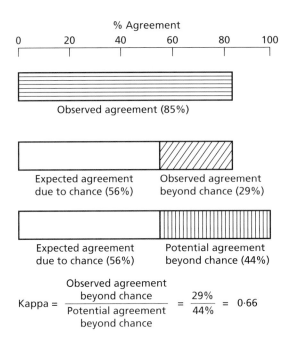

Fig. 12.8 Derivation of kappa using data from Table 12.6.

$$\text{Kappa} = \frac{\text{Observed agreement beyond chance}}{\text{Potential agreement beyond chance}} = \frac{29\%}{44\%} = 0{\cdot}66$$

Kappa	Level of agreement
$\kappa \leq 0{\cdot}2$	Poor
$0{\cdot}2 < \kappa \leq 0{\cdot}4$	Fair
$0{\cdot}4 < \kappa \leq 0{\cdot}6$	Moderate
$0{\cdot}6 < \kappa \leq 0{\cdot}8$	Good
$0{\cdot}8 < \kappa$	Excellent

Table 12.7 Level of agreement expressed by kappa.

Kappa values can range from zero, representing no agreement beyond what would be expected by chance, to a value of 1·0, representing perfect agreement. Negative kappa values are possible but unusual in practice. (Such values arise if the observed agreement is worse than expected on the basis of chance.) What constitutes an acceptable level of agreement is often hard to say, but Table 12.7 indicates ranges for kappa with some corresponding qualitative terms. It can be surprising in practice to see the low levels of agreement often achieved between observers or between purportedly similar tests. Kappa can be employed any time agreement between two qualitative tests is being sought, and its most common use is for the comparison of two different tests or two different observers.

Extensions of kappa to tests that give an ordinal response ('severe disease', 'moderate disease', 'no disease', for example) and to more than two observers/tests are possible, but a more advanced text should be consulted for details (Fleiss, 1981).

Kappa for measuring precision

Kappa can also be used for examining the precision of a qualitative test when the data are obtained by repeating the test on the same subject/test material. Essentially, the only difference between precision and agreement is the context. A qualitative test can be considered precise if the results of repeated tests agree with each other.

Kappa
- is a measure of agreement between two different tests or observers
- corrects for chance agreement
- ranges from 0 for no agreement beyond chance to 1 for perfect agreement
- is the amount of observed agreement beyond chance as a proportion of the potential agreement beyond chance
- can also be used for measuring precision

12.6 Validity: comparing a test with a gold standard

12.6.1 Criterion validity

The last sections discussed, in terms of precision and bias, problems with measurement relating to the question, 'How and why does an observed result differ from the true underlying value of the quantity being measured?' This section considers the other important question, 'Are we actually measuring what we are trying to measure?', which relates to the *validity* or correctness of a particular observation. For instance, a sphygmomanometer is said to measure blood pressure, but it does not actually measure the intra-arterial pressure exerted by the blood. This can be measured directly and the question is whether or not the indirect measurement, obtained by deflating a cuff placed on the arm and noting the height of a column of mercury at the appearance and disappearance of sounds, is a valid method of doing this. From this point of view, the validity of any procedure is only determinable if some 'gold standard' of absolute truth exists, and the results of the measurement are gauged against this. Validity based on a gold standard external criterion is called *criterion validity*.

There are a number of other types of validity that can be defined, and there is a large literature on the meaning of validity in the context of questionnaires and disease scales. The reader is referred to Streiner and Norman (1995) for a general discussion.

Sometimes, such a gold standard may not exist and the operational definition of the variable being measured itself becomes a standard. If intelligence is defined as what is measured by an IQ test, then an IQ test is a valid measure of intelligence. The validity of a test or measurement can only, in a sense, be considered in the context of an accurate test, because, obviously, problems with bias and precision will reduce a test's validity. An accurate test, however, is not necessarily a valid one.

An especially important area in which validity merits attention is in the process of making a diagnosis. The 'true' (gold standard) diagnosis is usually made on the basis of a history, clinical examination, signs, symptoms and the results of one or more biochemical, electrical, radiological or other measurement processes. Although it may be difficult to lay down exactly what the criteria are for the diagnosis of a given condition, unless perhaps autopsy reports are available and relevant, a clinical diagnosis based on all available information is, perhaps, the best available 'gold standard' for diagnosis.

12.6.2 Sensitivity and specificity

Evaluating the validity of a single diagnostic test is done by comparing the test results with the 'true' diagnosis. This is different from the situation of agreement, where what is of interest is whether two different tests agree with each other, with no test having precedence in terms of correctness or truth. Obviously, validity has important consequences in categorizing individuals. A single diagnostic test will misclassify some individuals, and this is extremely important in screening studies and in clinical practice. A *false-positive* result is a result that suggests an individual has a disease whereas, in terms of some 'gold standard', he/she does not. A *false-negative* result categorizes an individual as disease-free whereas, in reality, he/she has the disease. Table 12.8 shows the classification of 1000 individuals by whether or not a particular diagnostic test gave a positive result and by their actual disease status. In general, the entries in the cells of the table are labelled a, b, c and d, as noted. In the example, there are 180 false positives and 10 false negatives.

The *sensitivity* of a test measures its ability to detect true cases, and is defined by the number of true positives as a percentage of the total with the disease, or, in this case, $90/100 = 90\%$. The *specificity* of a test, on the other hand, measures its ability to detect disease-free individuals, and is defined as the number of true negatives divided by the total without the disease, or $720/900 = 80\%$. Ideally, a test should have high sensitivity and high specificity. One without the other is useless. For example, a test that defines bowel cancer to be present in all persons with a height above 0.25 m is 100% sensitive, in that, certainly, all cases of bowel cancer will be detected. A test that diagnosed

Test result	Disease		
	Present	Absent	Total
Positive	90 (a)	180 (b)	270 ($a + b$)
Negative	10 (c)	720 (d)	730 ($c + d$)
	100 ($a + c$)	900 ($b + d$)	1000 (n)

Table 12.8 Measures relating to the validity of test results.

Sensitivity: $a/(a + c) = 90/100 = 90\%$
Specificity: $d/(b + d) = 720/900 = 80\%$
Predictive value: $a/(a + b) = 90/270 = 33.3\%$
(False-positive rate: $b/(a + b) = 180/270 = 66.7\%$)
False-negative rate: $c/(c + d) = 10/730 = 1.4\%$.

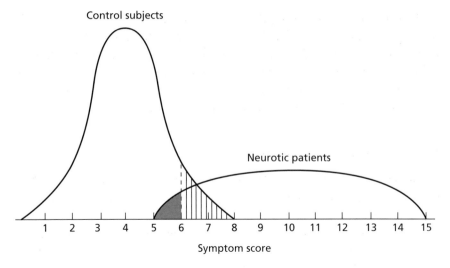

Fig. 12.9 Distribution of a symptom score in neurotic patients and normal controls.

bowel cancer as present in all persons over 2·5 m high would be 100% specific. Unfortunately, however, sensitivity and specificity are not usually independent and, in any particular test, as one increases, the other is likely to decrease.

Figure 12.9 shows the hypothetical distribution of a symptom score obtained by questionnaire in a group of psychiatric cases with a diagnosis of neurosis, compared with a normal control population. The controls have a mean score of 4 and the neurotics a mean score of 10. If a cut-off point of 6 in the symptom score were used to determine a diagnosis of neurosis, the sensitivity of the test would be fairly high, only missing neurotics with a symptom score of less than 6, as shown by the dark shaded area. The specificity of the test would not be so great, however, since it would misclassify any persons in the control population with a score of 6 or over, as denoted by the striped area in Fig. 12.9. Moving the cut-off point down to a score of 5 would give a test with a 100% sensitivity, while a test based on a score of 8 would achieve 100% specificity. Any intermediate point would result in the sensitivity and specificity indices increasing and decreasing in tandem. In a situation such as this, the best cut-off point to use can be determined only by the relative costs (to the investigator and to the patient) of the two types of misclassification. This is, obviously, a subjective judgement.

Reality is never as clear-cut as this example, however. Diseased persons may just have higher values of a particular quantitative variable in a unimodal distribution and it could be questioned whether the presence of some diseases can ever be determined as definite. The grey area of uncertain diagnoses should always be allowed for. The sensitivity and specificity of a diagnostic procedure can be altered by the inclusion of more than one test to determine disease status. A diagnosis may be made only if the results of two different tests are both positive. This is called *testing in series*, and tends to increase specificity at the expense of sensitivity. Alternatively, a diagnosis might be made if either of two tests showed a positive result. Such testing *in parallel* would increase the sensitivity of the diagnostic procedure.

In general, individual tests not having 100% specificity and sensitivity will distort any estimates of disease prevalence. For example, in Table 12.8, the true prevalence of the disease is 10% (100 per 1000), while, on the basis of the test results, the prevalence is 27% (270 per 1000). If the validity of a test is different in two population groups being compared, spurious differences between the groups may occur. A real difference may be magnified, or it may be masked. If the validity of a test is consistent across comparison groups, the effect is always to dilute or weaken any association that may be observed between the disease and a factor.

A common error, which can lead to serious bias, arises in studies where the validity of a test is incorrectly adjusted for. In many studies, the often small number of individuals with a positive test result are examined further to try to reduce the number of false positives. Unfortunately, no corresponding effort is made in those with a negative test result to reduce the number of false negatives; this will tend to result in a spuriously low prevalence estimate.

Sensitivity
- ability of a test to identify true cases of a disease
- true positives/total with disease

Specificity
- ability of a test to identify those without the disease
- true negatives/total without disease

12.6.3 Predictive values and false-positive and false-negative rates

Although sensitivity and specificity may seem adequate in determining the validity of a diagnostic test, there are two further measures, which are perhaps even more important in describing the effect of misclassification errors. Sensitivity and specificity can be determined independently by studying separate groups of diseased and non-diseased individuals. However, the usefulness of a diagnostic test also depends on the true prevalence of the condition in the population being studied. For the practising clinician or organizer of a screening programme, the *predictive value (diagnostic value)* of a test is a most important parameter. The predictive value of a test is the proportion of true cases among all those with a positive test result; in other words, it relates to what a clinician sees — those individuals with positive tests. In Table 12.8, the predictive value of the test is 90/270, or only 33·3%. Thus, although the sensitivity and specificity of the test are 90% and 80%, respectively, only one-third of the persons for whom the test results were positive actually had the disease. The usefulness of the test would be quite questionable.

The predictive value of the test can be calculated if, in addition to the test's sensitivity and specificity, the true prevalence of the disease is known, or if, as in the example, the test is performed on a sample from the population in which it is to be applied. The predictive value of a test of given sensitivity and specificity increases (decreases) as the true prevalence of the condition increases (decreases). Thus, a test with a high predictive value developed in a hospital setting (where a high prevalence of any condition is to be expected) may be quite inapplicable when applied to a general population.

The *false-positive rate* for a test is calculated as the number of false positives as a percentage of all positive test results, and is 66·7% in the example. It is, of course, 100% minus the predictive value, and is another way of looking at that parameter. The *false-negative rate* for a test is the false negatives as a percentage of the total negative test results, and has, in the example, the low value of 1·4%. Note that the false-positive and false-negative rates are calculated with, respectively, the number of positive and negative test results as denominator, *not* the total number with or without the disease.*

Although the sensitivity and specificity of a test are measures of its validity, high values for these parameters do not in themselves make for a usable test in clinical practice. The usefulness of a test depends also on the prevalence of the condition being studied and, in any evaluation of a diagnostic test, predictive values and false-negative rates should be calculated if it is to be judged adequately. If the true prevalence of the condition is unknown, these calculations could be done for a series of prevalences that might be observed in practice.

Predictive (diagnostic) value
- the proportion of those with a positive test who have the disease
- true positives/total with a positive test result
- increases as the true disease prevalence increases

False-positive rate
- false positives/total with a positive test result
- 100% minus predictive value

False-negative rate
- false negatives/total with a negative test result

12.7 Bias in statistical analysis and interpretation

If a study has been well designed and well executed, the main hurdles have been overcome. Errors in the statistical analysis and interpretation of results can, of course, still occur, but can be corrected. That such errors do occur is continually pointed out (Altman, 1994). Errors of interpretation can, of course, be on the part of the investigator or the reader of a published paper.

---

* Some sources define the false-positive and false-negative rates with denominators of all diseased and non-diseased persons, respectively. The definition given here is more generally used.

Errors related to the statistical analysis can arise in various ways, and most relate to failure to use appropriate statistical techniques. Errors of omission mean that a technique that should have been used on the data was not; errors of commission mean that a technique was applied incorrectly. Some of the more common errors are detailed below.

Failure to distinguish between independent and dependent observations causes many problems. If measurements are repeated on the same individual, they are not independent, and it is totally invalid to analyse them as if they were. For instance, if 20 diabetic patients were studied to determine pancreatic activity, and five observations were made on each patient, the data cannot be analysed for a sample size of $20 \times 5 = 100$ observations. The most important factor is the number of different individuals and, in such a case, the analysis could be performed on the 20 mean levels calculated on each individual. Analysis of variance also provides a very useful technique, which can handle replicate observations in comparative studies. Failure to distinguish between independent and dependent data often arises also in clinical trials or case–control studies, where the two groups are paired or matched. The use of the independent t test or χ^2 test, instead of the paired t test or McNemar's χ^2 test, is a common error in paired comparisons.

Many errors relate to ignoring the assumptions underlying the parametric significance tests. The assumptions of approximate normality and equality of variances in group comparisons are important in many cases and, although some tests are fairly robust (departures from some of the assumptions do not seem to matter a great deal), biased analyses can result from misapplication of tests to highly skewed data, for instance. Transformation of the data may iron out such problems. With small sample sizes in particular, however, assumptions can often not be checked and the non-parametric tests should perhaps be used more frequently.

Problems also arise with repeated use of significance tests. If a set of data is dredged for any significant relationships without reference to the purpose for which the study was set up, some relationships will appear statistically significant purely due to chance. A similar problem arises in an experimental trial with a fixed sample size, where interim analysis of results takes place before the requisite number of patients have entered. In such situations, spurious differences may appear by chance, and the p value required to declare a significant result should be decreased to allow for multiple testing. This, of course, will usually require an increase of sample size if the conventional levels of statistical significance are to be claimed.

Lack of understanding of the significance tests available and the type of data they can be applied to can result in biased analysis. This is particularly true in prospective studies of survival, where the problems of variable follow-up and losses to follow-up cause much difficulty. Clinical life table methods or, less preferably, the 'person-years at risk' concept can be used to great advantage in such situations.

In many studies, failure to adjust for confounding variables can result in a totally biased analysis. As has been said, however, controlling for the confounders at the design stage through randomization or matching is preferable to statistical adjustment, although the latter is usually necessary.

Over-interpretation of the data is a problem that can also arise. The erroneous assumption that sensitivity and specificity, on their own, are good indicators of the usefulness of a particular diagnostic test has already been discussed. The problem also occurs when appropriate denominators are not available for the calculation of rates. For example, it is not possible to estimate absolute risk in a case–control study. Also, if a study of causes of death is being performed, only proportional mortality analyses can be carried out, unless the population from which the deaths arose is known. Thus, it might be determined that 2% of all deaths under the age of 1 year were due to infectious diseases, while the proportion among deaths in those aged 1–2 years was 8%. This would not mean that the death rate (per 1000 of the population in these age-groups) from infectious diseases was greater in the older age-group. In fact, the death rate would be much higher in those under 1 year. When the number of deaths, only, is available for analysis, the large number of deaths from all causes under the age of 1 year results in the proportional mortality for any single cause being considerably reduced.

Misinterpretations of the meaning of statistical significance abound. The confusion of statistical association with causation must be avoided and the results should not be generalized to inappropriate populations. Also, a non-significant result does not mean a negative result; it means only that chance is a possible explanation of an observed association, not that chance is *the* explanation. Important results may be non-significant, due mainly to small sample sizes. On the other hand, a statistically significant result does not necessarily mean a medically important result. A trivial difference between two groups can always be made statistically significant with a large enough sample size.

12.8 Critical reading of the literature

One of the purposes of this book is to enable doctors to approach the medical literature with a critical mind. Many published studies are not all they seem to be at first reading, and it is up to the reader to judge a study's conclusions in the light of its design and analysis. Many biases can be detected if a report is approached with a logical mind and if the important question 'What else could have produced the results obtained?' is asked. Errors in statistical analysis are often difficult to spot, but flaws in design and execution are more easily detectable. It goes without saying, of course, that a report must describe the study adequately in order for a judgement to be made, and many published reports fail to give sufficient information in this respect. Sackett *et al.* (1991) give sound advice on keeping up to date with the medical literature.

A report in the medical literature is usually given the following headings: 'Introduction'; 'Materials and Methods'; 'Results'; 'Discussion' or 'Conclusions'. In the introduction, there should be a clear statement of the objectives of the study and the population to which the findings are to be related. Without this, it is difficult to see if the study design and analysis are appropriate to the question being asked. The materials and methods section, usually in small print, should give in some detail the design of the study, whether a cross-sectional case–control or cohort observational study or an experimental trial. Precise definitions of inclusion and exclusion criteria should be given, together with the description of the population from which the study group was formed. If random sampling was employed, this should be stated, as should also the procedure used for randomization. If matched groups are involved, it should be clear whether frequency or paired matching was employed. From these descriptions, it should be possible to detect any sources of selection or other biases and to see if the researchers have made any attempt to allow for them.

There should be clear definitions of all the variables studied; this is particularly important for the major end-points of the study, and details of how the measurements were made, whether from case records, interview, direct measurement or official sources, should be indicated. If necessary, comments on the accuracy and validity of the data should be included. If patient follow-up is involved, the methods of tracing patients should be stated and an indication as to whether complete follow-up was achieved should be given.

The statistical techniques employed in the analysis should be described in 'Materials and Methods', and should state, at least, which tests were performed, the significance level adopted and whether one- or two-sided tests were used. If less common techniques were used, references, or a full description, should be given. It should be asked if appropriate techniques were actually employed and if, in fact, the data were worthy of statistical analysis. This book has attempted to cover a fair proportion of the statistical techniques employed in medical research, but techniques will be encountered that have not been detailed. In such cases, the adequacy or appropriateness of an analysis may be difficult for the general reader to judge. This section of a published paper should also, ideally, give an indication as to how the study sample size was arrived at—was any attempt made to use statistical methods, or was the size of the study group decided totally on the basis of convenience?

The results section of a paper is, without any doubt, the most important. Are the results presented clearly and in a comprehensible manner? A problem with many reports is that the results section is incomprehensible, with too much detail, too many large and complex tables and a totally inadequate explanation as to how the results were actually arrived at. If a study is to be widely read and understood, simplicity of presentation is vital. This must be balanced, however, by the necessity to present sufficient detail for judging the adequacy and applicability of the results to the problem under investigation. The results of a study may have arisen from an extremely complex and comprehensive analysis; all aspects of this cannot be presented, and extensive summarizing may be necessary to present the kernel of what was found. There is a danger of swamping the reader with too much detail. The procedure adopted in some reports relegates such detailed results to an appendix, to 'mini-print' tables or to a page on the Internet. The results section should at least include a simple description of the distribution of the important variables studied in the different comparison groups, so that the reader may make a judgement about any confounding effects. Any statements made in a results section, such as 'males did better than females', should be backed up by summary statistics of the comparison. If confounders have to be adjusted for statistically, it is advisable that both adjusted and unadjusted results are given, to enable the actual effect of the confounding to be seen.

In addition to significance testing, confidence intervals should be presented for comparative measures, particularly if a study is reporting statistically non-significant results.

It is surprising how often numerical inconsistencies appear in published reports. Often there are discrepancies between figures given in tables and figures given in the text, or numbers in tables or percentages do not add up to the required totals. These should be checked by the reader, because, although such errors are easy to make (with revision of drafts, bad proofreading, etc.), they may indicate more serious deficiencies in the study.* Do the numbers in the tables and text differ because some patients with missing observations were omitted from the final report but were included originally? Inconsistency may often be due to missing data (refusals, lost records, losses to follow-up) and the paper should state clearly how these problems were dealt with.

The discussion section of a paper should highlight the main results, show how they throw light on the research question being studied and put the results in context by referring to the relevant literature.

In any study, bias may not be actually present, but the possibility of bias may put a question mark on the acceptance of final conclusions. No study can be perfect, however. The important factor is whether the results do give new information, which, of course, may be examined in a different way in a further investigation. If the authors of a paper identify possible sources of bias and discuss their potential influence on the results, any conclusions are all the more worthwhile. Finally, if you do discover inadequacies in a published study, ask yourself, 'Could I have done it better?' In many situations, it will be found that there is no feasible alternative to that of the approach adopted, and it will be concluded that an excellent piece of research has indeed been performed.

12.9 A note on research procedures

For those who may become involved in setting up a research project, or for those who are involved in analysing or writing up a study, a few simple words of advice are offered below. First, do not rush into any project. A good research project may take months of planning before any individual is actually studied. Some statistical advice should be sought at a very early stage, especially as regards an appropriate sample size and the design of data collection forms if a computer analysis is even a possibility. A good literature survey is

---

* The astute reader may discover some inconsistencies in this text!

essential, to give an idea of what has already been done in the area of interest and to provide insights into the particular problems the study might face. It must then be decided whether the study is to be observational or experimental and what design features can reasonably be included.

The sections in this book on study design and bias in research provide an overview of the areas that must be considered, but further reading will most probably be necessary. A preliminary *pilot study* on a smaller number of individuals is often very helpful, to test data collection procedures and to provide preliminary estimates on the distribution of some variables as an aid to sample size calculations.

It is often difficult in a study to decide what variables should be measured. Do not be tempted to measure everything. The literature review and knowledge of what is being studied should be a guide to the relevant variables. A good procedure to judge what variables are really needed is to plan out in a rough way what tables would, ideally, be presented in a final report, and thus to determine the variables that are most likely to be related to the study outcome; use only these. Avoid, too, taking measurements which will have missing information in a large number of subjects.

It is worthwhile considering, in the planning stages of a project, the type of statistical analysis that might be undertaken. This may also be a guide as to which variables to include in the data collection. It is advisable in any project to describe the complete study design and all ancillary information in a written *protocol*. This will greatly aid in the final write-up of a study and help ensure that the original design is strictly adhered to. Where many persons are involved in a project and for multicentre trials, this is particularly important. This protocol can then be consulted by anyone involved in the project if there are any doubts about exactly what should be done in a particular situation. A written protocol is also necessary for submission to funding agencies (if funds are required!) and most research proposals must be submitted to an ethics committee for approval before study commencement. A good research protocol should include a precise statement concerning the objectives of the study and its importance in the light of current medical knowledge. The actual design of the study should be given in great detail, with careful attention paid to the selection of study participants (including the sample size) and potential sources of bias arising therefrom. Ethical problems must also be considered. Clear and concise definitions of the variables to be measured and the measurement techniques to be employed are essential, as are considerations of the relevance, accuracy and validity of these measurements. Data-collection forms and questionnaires should be included, as should an indication of the type of statistical analysis that will be performed.

The protocol must be a practical document and should include far more than will ever appear in a published report. It should detail the manpower required for successful implementation of the study and estimate costings in terms of diagnostic tests and other procedures, stationery, printing, etc., travel, computer costs and all the administrative overheads that will accrue.

The likely duration of the study must be indicated and a timetable for completion of the various stages (e.g. planning, subject recruitment, follow-up, data collection and cleaning, analysis and report (paper) writing) should be given. How the study is to be implemented in practice, together with an outline of the responsibilities of those involved, should also be presented. Much thought should go into this area.

The execution of a study design demands careful adherence to the written protocol. All individuals involved with any of the subjects being studied should know that a special investigation is being carried out and should have read the protocol. Often, departures from the protocol may be necessary for ethical or other reasons, and careful note should be taken of such departures. Often, as a study progresses, certain decisions, especially as regards exclusion or admission criteria, may have to be made in situations not considered in the original design. These too should be noted.

Once the study data have been gathered, a statistical analysis will have to be undertaken. For a large study, this will usually require the use of a computer and professional advice may be required. Many analyses can be undertaken by computer that would be impractical by hand, but pencil-and-paper methods are no more outmoded than the wheel. The statistical methods detailed in this book should be sufficient to enable a fair proportion of the data in any reasonably sized study to be analysed with the use of nothing more than a calculator. This book also details some of the methods used for the control of confounding, which are not implemented in all statistical computer packages, and the description of multiple regression techniques may help in the interpretation of such analyses.

At the end of the study, the results must be written up for publication. Choose a journal appropriate to the subject-matter of the study and read a good number of articles in that journal to gauge the requirement in presentation. Also, pay careful attention to the 'instructions for authors', which are usually published in each journal on a regular basis. It is not easy to write up a research report, and a fair amount of time and effort is required. The previous section in this chapter, on the critical reading of the literature, should provide some guidelines as to what should be included in an article. Apart from that, it is all up to you.

12.10 Summary

The purpose of this chapter has been to bring together and expand on the subject of bias in medical research. Bias can arise in every stage of a research project, from design, subject selection and data collection to statistical analysis and interpretation. The chapter highlighted some, but not all, of the difficulties and considered in some detail the problems inherent in measurement. It is hoped that this chapter may prove useful to the reader of the medical literature and to the individual involved, for the first time, in the setting up, execution or analysis of a project.

Appendix A Computational Shortcuts

A.1 Introduction

This appendix outlines some short-cut computational formulae that will simplify some of the calculations discussed in the text. In particular, simple formulae for the standard deviation, for the χ^2 test for 2×2 tables, for regression and correlation coefficients and for analysis of variance are presented.

A.2 The standard deviation

The calculation of the standard deviation using Eqn. 1.7:

$$S = \sqrt{\frac{\sum (x - \bar{x})^2}{n - 1}}$$

is fairly cumbersome and an easier computational formula can be derived, which gives the same numerical answer.* The sum of squared deviations in the numerator can be expressed:

$$\sum (x - \bar{x})^2 = \sum x^2 - \frac{\left(\sum x\right)^2}{n} \tag{A.1}$$

so that:

$$S = \sqrt{\frac{\sum x^2 - \left(\sum x\right)^2 / n}{n - 1}} \tag{A.2}$$

This involves squaring each observation, taking their sum (Σx^2) and subtracting from this the square of the sum of all the observations ($\Sigma x)^2$ divided by the total sample size (n). This is then divided by $n - 1$ and the square root taken.

Table A.1 illustrates the layout for this calculation. Column 1 gives six observations (x) for which the standard deviation is to be calculated. The sum of the observations (Σx) is given at the foot of the column. Column 2 is the square of each value (x^2) with the sum of these squares (Σx^2) at the foot of the column. These values are then substituted into Eqn. A.1 to give the standard deviation.

It is advisable to keep as many digits in the intermediate steps as are dis-

* Many calculators perform this calculation automatically.

Table A.1 Calculation of the standard deviation.

1	2
x	x^2
530	280 900
518	268 324
572	327 184
595	354 025
527	277 729
548	300 304
3290	1 808 466

$$n = 6$$
$$\Sigma x = 3\,290$$
$$(\Sigma x)^2 = 10\,824\,100$$
$$(\Sigma x)^2/n = 1\,804\,016\cdot 7$$
$$\Sigma x^2 = 1\,808\,466$$
$$\Sigma x^2 - (\Sigma x)^2/n = 4\,449\cdot 334$$

$$\frac{\Sigma x^2 - (\Sigma x)^2/n}{n-1} = 889\cdot 8668$$

$$S = \sqrt{889\cdot 8668} = 29\cdot 83$$

played on the calculator. The final computed standard deviation, however, need only be expressed to two decimal places more than the original observations, unless it is to be used in further calculations. Most calculators display only eight digits and sometimes an intermediate computed quantity may exceed the display capacity. In such cases, the original observations can be rescaled to a size more manageable on the calculator. If the original units are too large, either a constant should be subtracted from each observation, or each observation should be divided by some constant. If the units are too small, then each observation should be multiplied by a constant. The calculations as described are carried out on the rescaled observations. If subtraction of a constant was employed in the rescaling, then the computed standard deviation needs no adjustment and is the same as would have been obtained on the original data. If multiplication (or division) was employed, the computed standard deviation must be divided by (multiplied by) the chosen constant to obtain the correct result. The example in Table A.1 is recomputed in Table A.2 using rescaled values obtained by subtracting 500 from each observation and then in a separate calculation by dividing each observation by 100. The same final standard deviations are obtained. Although rescaling was not necessary in this example, the advantages of the smaller numerical quantities at each step are clear.

If a series of observations has many repeat values or if the standard deviation of grouped data is being calculated, again there are some short-cut computational methods. In grouped data, remember that all the observations in an interval are assumed to have a value equal to the mid-point of the interval. If there are f occurrences of the value x, then the standard deviation is defined:

Table A.2 Example of rescaling in calculating standard deviations.

	Original units	−500	÷100
	530	30	5·3
	518	18	5·18
	572	72	5·72
	595	95	5·95
	527	27	5·27
	548	48	5·48
Σx	3290	290	32·90
$(\Sigma x)^2$	10824100	84100	1082·41
Σx^2	1808466	18466	180·8466
$\Sigma x^2 - (\Sigma x)^2/n$	4449·334	4449·334	0·4449334
$\sqrt{\dfrac{\Sigma x^2 - (\Sigma x)^2/n}{n-1}}$	29·8306	29·8306	0·298306
S	29·83	29·83	29·83

$$S = \sqrt{\frac{\Sigma f(x-\bar{x})^2}{\Sigma f - 1}} \qquad (A.3)$$

where the sample size is given by the sum of the frequencies in each class (Σf). A computationally easier formula is given by:

$$S = \sqrt{\frac{\Sigma fx^2 - (\Sigma fx)^2/\Sigma f}{\Sigma f - 1}} \qquad (A.4)$$

The application of this to calculate the standard deviation of the birth weight data discussed in Chapter 1 is illustrated in Table A.3. Column 1 gives the mid-points of each class interval, which correspond to the observations x. Column 2 gives the frequencies (f) observed in each class, and the sum of their values (Σf) is the total sample size. Column 3 contains the square of each x value and column 4 gives each of these x^2 values multiplied by its frequency f. The sum of this column is Σfx^2. Column 5 gives each observed value multiplied by its frequency, giving the sum Σfx. Σf, Σfx and Σfx^2 are then substituted into Eqn. A.4 to give the standard deviation. Again, the original values, x, can, if necessary, be rescaled to make the calculations more manageable on a calculator.

A.3 The χ^2 test for independent 2 × 2 tables

An alternative to the usual χ^2 formula in 2 × 2 tables (Eqn. 7.23):

$$\chi^2 = \Sigma \frac{(O-E)^2}{E}$$

which is computationally simpler, is often used. It has the disadvantage, however, that the expected values (E) are not computed, so that there is no

Table A.3 Standard deviation for grouped data (birth-weight data of Table 1.3).

1 Class mid-points x	2 No. of observations f	3 x^2	4 fx^2	5 fx
1·88	4	3·5344	14·1376	7·52
2·13	3	4·5369	13·6107	6·39
2·38	12	5·6644	67·9728	28·56
2·63	34	6·9169	235·1746	89·42
2·88	115	8·2944	953·8560	331·20
3·13	175	9·7969	1 714·4575	547·75
3·38	281	11·4244	3 210·2564	949·78
3·63	261	13·1769	3 439·1709	947·43
3·88	212	15·0544	3 191·5328	822·56
4·13	94	17·0569	1 603·3486	388·22
4·38	47	19·1844	901·6668	205·86
4·63	14	21·4369	300·1166	64·82
4·88	6	23·8144	142·8864	29·28
5·13	2	26·3169	52·6338	10·26
	1 260 (Σf)		15 840·822* (Σfx^2)	4 429·05 (Σfx)

* Eight digits accuracy.

$$S = \sqrt{\frac{\sum fx^2 - \left(\sum fx\right)^2 / \sum f}{\sum f - 1}}$$

$$= \sqrt{\frac{15840\cdot822 - (4\,429\cdot05)^2 / 1260}{1259}}$$

$$= 0\cdot4650$$

Table A.4 Short-cut χ^2 formula for independent 2×2 tables.

| | a | b | r_1 |
| $\chi^2 = \dfrac{(ad - bc)^2 n}{r_1 r_2 s_1 s_2}$ on 1 degree of freedom |
| | c | d | r_2 |
| | s_1 | s_2 | n |

direct check on whether all of these are greater than 5 (which used to be a requirement for valid application of the test).

Table A.4 shows the layout of a general 2×2 contingency table. a, b, c and d are the four observed quantities, r_1 and r_2 are the row totals and s_1 and s_2 are the column totals; n is the sample size. With this notation:

$$\chi^2 = \frac{(ad - bc)^2 n}{r_1 r_2 s_1 s_2} \qquad (A.5)$$

When using a calculator, the numerator of this expression may exceed the capacity of the display. This can usually be avoided by first calculating $(ad - bc)^2$, then dividing by r_1 and r_2, multiplying by n and finally dividing by s_1 and s_2.

A.4 Regression and correlation

The formulae for both the regression and correlation coefficients (Eqns. 10.4 and 10.7) involve the expression:

$$\sum (x - \bar{x})(y - \bar{y})$$

while the formula for the standard error of the estimate $S_{y,x}$ (Eqn. 10.12), requires the calculation of:

$$\sum (y - \hat{y})^2$$

where the y values are the observed values of the dependent variable and the $\hat{y}$ values are the predicted or expected values on the basis of the regression equation. As they stand, both these expressions are computationally awkward and alternatives are available. First:

$$\sum (x - \bar{x})(y - \bar{y}) = \sum xy - \frac{(\sum x)(\sum y)}{n} \tag{A.6}$$

where n is the number of pairs on which the regression equation or correlation coefficient is being calculated. This expression involves calculating the product of each pair of x and y variables and summing to obtain Σxy. The Σx and Σy terms are the sums of the x and y variables separately.

Table A.5 shows the original data for the regression of the left ventricular ejection fraction (LVEF) on the QRS score, discussed in Chapter 10.[*] Columns 1 and 2 give the QRS values (x) and the corresponding LVEF values (y), which, when summed, give Σx and Σy. Column 3 gives the xy values obtained by multiplying each x value by its y value, and the sum of these is Σxy. Columns 4 and 5 give the squares of the x and y values and their sums. These are the basic quantities required for regression and correlation calculations. The number of pairs, n, is 28. Table A.6 shows, explicitly, the calculations for the regression coefficients (Eqns. 10.4 and 10.6) and the correlation coefficient (Eqn. 10.7) for the LVEF data.

The computational expression for $\Sigma(y - \hat{y})^2$ is given by:

$$\sum (y - \bar{y})^2 - \frac{\left[\sum (x - \bar{x})(y - \bar{y})\right]^2}{\sum (x - \bar{x})^2} \tag{A.7}$$

All these quantities have already been calculated and Table A.7 shows the final computations for $S_{y,x}$ using Eqn. 10.12.

A.5 Sums of squares in ANOVA

Underlying all calculations in the analysis of variance are the quantities referred to as 'sums of squares' (SSq) (see Section 9.2.5). The formulae for

---

[*] These data are based on the published diagram (Palmeri *et al.*, 1982) and the resulting calculations differ slightly from those appearing in the publication.

Table A.5 Computation of basic quantities required for simple regression calculations (data from Fig. 10.5).

1 QRS score x	2 LVEF y	3 xy	4 x^2	5 y^2
0	51	0	0	2 601
0	57	0	0	3 249
0	58	0	0	3 364
0	60	0	0	3 600
0	66	0	0	4 356
0	71	0	0	5 041
1	58	58	1	3 364
1	60	60	1	3 600
1	65	65	1	4 225
2	57	114	4	3 249
3	52	156	9	2 704
4	51	204	16	2 601
5	44	220	25	1 936
5	46	230	25	2 116
6	32	192	36	1 024
6	40	240	36	1 600
6	42	252	36	1 764
6	48	288	36	2 304
7	37	259	49	1 369
8	28	224	64	784
8	38	304	64	1 444
9	28	252	81	784
9	31	279	81	961
9	43	387	81	1 849
11	21	231	121	441
11	22	242	121	484
11	24	264	121	576
13	18	234	169	324
142 (Σx)	1 248 (Σy)	4 755 (Σxy)	1 178 (Σx^2)	61 714 (Σy^2)

Table A.6 Regression calculations for LVEF/QRS data.

Quantity	Computational formula	Value	
$\Sigma(x-\bar{x})(y-\bar{y})$	$\Sigma xy - (\Sigma x)(\Sigma y)/n$	$4755 - (142)(1248)/28$	$-1574{\cdot}1429$
$\Sigma(x-\bar{x})^2$	$\Sigma x^2 - (\Sigma x)^2/n$	$1178 - (142)^2/28$	$457{\cdot}85714$
$\Sigma(y-\bar{y})^2$	$\Sigma y^2 - (\Sigma y)^2/n$	$61714 - (1248)^2/28$	$6088{\cdot}8572$
$\bar{x}$	$\Sigma x/n$	$142/28$	$5{\cdot}0714$
$\bar{y}$	$\Sigma y/n$	$1248/28$	$44{\cdot}5714$
Regression coefficient b (Eqn. 10.4)	$\Sigma(x-\bar{x})(y-\bar{y})/\Sigma(x-\bar{x})^2$	$-1574{\cdot}1429/457{\cdot}85714$	$-3{\cdot}4381$
Regression coefficient a (Eqn. 10.6)	$\bar{y} - b\bar{x}$	$44{\cdot}5714 + 3{\cdot}4381(5{\cdot}0714)$	$62{\cdot}0074$
Correlation coefficient r (Eqn. 10.7)	$\dfrac{\Sigma(x-\bar{x})(y-\bar{y})}{\sqrt{\Sigma(x-\bar{x})^2\,\Sigma(y-\bar{y})^2}}$	$\dfrac{-1574{\cdot}1429}{\sqrt{457{\cdot}85714 \times 6088{\cdot}8572}}$	$-0{\cdot}9428$

$$\sum(y-\hat{y})^2 = \sum(y-\bar{y})^2 - \frac{\left[\sum(x-\bar{x})(y-\bar{y})\right]^2}{\sum(x-\bar{x})^2}$$

$$= 6088.8572 - \frac{(-1574.1429)^2}{457.85714}$$

$$= 676.8501$$

$$S_{y.x} = \sqrt{\frac{\sum(y-\hat{y})^2}{n-2}}$$

$$= \sqrt{\frac{676.8501}{26}}$$

$$= 5.1022$$

these, as presented, are tedious to compute and a more convenient approach is
described below.

$$\text{Total SSq} = \sum_i \sum_j (x_{ij}-\bar{x})^2$$

$$\text{Within-groups SSqs} = \sum_i \sum_j (x_{ij}-\bar{x}_i)^2$$

$$\text{Between-groups SSqs} = \sum_i \sum_j (\bar{x}_i-\bar{x})^2$$

where Σ_i means summation over the number of groups being compared (k)
and Σ_j means summation over the n_i values in a group (see Eqn. 9.9).

The easiest way to compute these quantities is to first calculate the total SSq,
using the methods of Section A.1 (Eqn. A.1). Letting T be the sum of all the
observations, and S be the sum of all the observations after squaring:*

$$T = \sum_i \sum_j x_{ij} \quad \text{and} \quad S = \sum_i \sum_j x_{ij}^2$$

it is easy to see that:

$$\text{Total SSq} = S - \frac{T^2}{N} \tag{A.8}$$

where N is the total sample size in all k groups.

The within-groups SSq for a single group—group i—is:

$$\sum_j (x_{ij}-\bar{x}_i)^2 = S_i - \frac{T_i^2}{n_i}$$

where T_i and S_i denote the sums of the observations and the squared observations in group i, and n_i is the sample size in that group. The within-groups SSq
for all the groups is then:

$$\text{Within-groups SSq} = \sum_i S_i - \sum_i (T_i^2/n_i)$$

$$= S - \sum_i (T_i^2/n_i) \tag{A.9}$$

---

* S *in this section* refers to the sum of the squared observations and should not be confused with
the standard deviation, which, elsewhere in this text, is also denoted S.

The between-groups SSq can be obtained, after the total and within-group SSqs have been calculated with Eqns. A.8 and A.9, by using Eqn. 9.10:

$$\text{Between-groups SSq} = \text{Total SSq} - \text{Within-groups SSq} \qquad (A.10)$$

These calculations are illustrated in Table A.8 on the data from Section 9.2.4 (Table 9.2).

Table A.8 Illustration of sums of squares calculations on the data of Table 9.2.

Group i	Smokers (1)	Ex-smokers (2)	Non-smokers (3)	$k = 3$
Systolic blood	125	115	95	
pressures	135	125	100	
	140	135	105	
	145		120	
	155			
n_i	5	3	4	$N = 12$
T_i	700	375	420	$T = 1495$
T_i^2	490 000	140 625	176 400	
T_i^2/n_i	98 000	46 875	44 100	$\Sigma_i(T_i^2/n_i) = 188\,975$

S (obtained directly) $= 190\,025$

Total SSq	$= S - (T^2/N)$
	$= 190\,025 - (1\,495)^2/12$
	$= 3\,772{\cdot}9$

Within-groups SSq	$= S - \Sigma_i(T_i^2/n_i)$
	$= 190\,025 - 188\,975$
	$= 1\,050$

Between-groups SSq	$= 3\,772{\cdot}9 - 1\,050$
	$= 2\,722{\cdot}9$

Appendix B Statistical Tables

B.1 Introduction

This appendix gives the statistical (and other) tables necessary in the calculation of significance levels and confidence intervals for the methods described in this book. For ease of use, an attempt has been made to employ a uniform layout for these tables and the upper and lower critical values for a range of one- and two-sided significance levels are presented. Consequently, some of the tables may have a different appearance from those that are more customary, but hopefully they will prove easier to employ in practice. Note also that the tables relate to the critical values of the test statistic as described in this text, which may have a slightly different formulation (especially for the non-parametric tests) from that given in other sources. Most of the tables have been reproduced or adapted from the *Geigy Scientific Tables* (1982), which is a very useful reference work, but Tables B.11, B.12, B.13 and B.14 have been produced directly using algorithms written by one of the authors (L.D.).

Sometimes the sample size may be too large for use of the statistical tables for the non-parametric tests. In such cases, if a non-parametric test must be used, the *Geigy Scientific Tables* give formulae for approximate large-sample size significance levels. The non-parametric tests, however, tend to be used more often with small sample sizes, so this should not be a major problem in most practical applications. Note, too, that, in many of the non-parametric tests, the significance levels given in the tables are not exact, due to the discrete nature of the particular distributions.

B.2 Tables

Table B.1 Table of random numbers (abbreviated from *Geigy Scientific Tables*, 1982, with permission).

20557	43375	50914	83628	73935	72502	48174	62551	96122	22375	96488
83936	45842	78222	88481	44933	12839	20750	47116	58973	99018	22769
36077	82577	16210	76092	87730	90049	02115	37096	20505	91937	69776
78267	31568	58297	88922	50436	86135	42726	54307	29170	13045	65527
00232	98059	07255	90786	95246	15280	61692	45137	17539	31799	64780
65869	64355	91271	49295	98354	28005	69792	01480	51557	70726	35862
35454	51623	98381	11055	32951	28363	16451	67912	66404	76254	75495
99542	44247	12762	54488	74321	36224	95619	16238	25374	13653	25345
36087	32326	52225	72447	77804	57045	27552	72387	34001	83792	66764
64899	62390	68375	42921	28545	33167	85710	11035	40171	04840	69848
11994	97820	06653	27477	61364	22681	02280	53815	47479	44017	37563
02915	81553	92012	50435	73814	96290	86827	81430	45597	82296	28947
62895	09202	48494	95974	33534	94657	71126	71770	16092	03942	90111
39202	82110	82254	03669	03281	11613	36336	98297	48100	71594	52667
53252	18175	09457	83810	46392	02705	85591	33192	65127	80852	42030
17820	50756	80608	35695	72641	26306	76298	32532	22644	96853	18610
85245	12710	60264	74650	92126	08152	32147	17457	56298	48964	64733
85822	44424	88508	66190	74060	93206	92840	44833	81146	64060	62975
24804	24720	66501	74157	42246	41688	72835	87258	89384	11251	34329
31942	85419	93017	28087	78323	77109	56832	78400	24190	37978	85863
72838	10933	99964	13468	17211	48046	51122	92668	96750	11139	06275
38546	49559	71671	53603	24491	57570	90789	32932	67449	05115	45941
38051	39391	92039	71664	40219	97707	93975	66981	19556	24605	52169
28101	38543	54214	48928	32818	51963	87353	15094	29529	87305	01361
70476	44242	54227	28598	64422	29361	20359	48577	05971	92373	22765
64999	11468	74149	81386	94127	67342	38010	92522	57728	39432	27914
73641	52165	54336	89196	40042	37889	06003	58033	59082	94988	62152
67421	83093	77038	55399	67893	89597	85630	08059	35757	49479	63531
30976	66455	90708	08450	50120	17795	55604	51222	17900	55553	02980
29660	30790	65154	19582	20942	81439	83917	90452	64753	99645	19799
82747	97297	74420	18783	93471	89055	56413	77817	10655	52915	68198
46978	87390	53319	90155	03154	20301	47831	86786	11284	49160	79852
19783	82215	35810	39852	43795	21530	96315	55657	76473	08217	46810
12249	35844	63265	26451	06986	08707	99251	06260	74779	96285	31998
58785	53473	06308	56778	30474	57277	23425	27092	47759	18422	56074
69373	73674	97914	77989	47280	71804	74587	70563	77813	50242	60398
95662	83923	90790	49474	11901	30322	80254	99608	17019	17892	76813
97758	08206	54199	41327	01170	21745	71318	07978	35440	26128	10545
72154	86385	39490	57482	32921	33795	43155	30432	48384	85430	51828
25583	74101	87573	01556	89183	64830	16779	35724	82103	61658	20296

Table B.2 The z test: critical values for the standard normal distribution (abbreviated and adapted from *Geigy Scientific Tables*, 1982, with permission).

	Area in two tails (two-sided significance level)	0·10	0·05	0·02	0·01
	Area in one tail (one-sided significance level)	0·05	0·025	0·01	0·005
Critical value z_c		1·645	1·960	2·326	2·576

Significant result if $z \geqslant z_c$ or $z \leqslant -z_c$

Table B.3 The *t* test: critical values for the Student's *t* distribution (abbreviated and adapted from *Geigy Scientific Tables*, 1982, with permission).

	Area in two tails (two-sided significance level)	0·10	0·05	0·02	0·01
	Area in one tail (one-sided significance level)	0·05	0·025	0·01	0·005
d.f.	Critical value t_c				
1		6·314	12·706	31·821	63·657
2		2·920	4·303	6·965	9·925
3		2·353	3·182	4·541	5·841
4		2·132	2·776	3·747	4·604
5		2·015	2·571	3·365	4·032
6		1·943	2·447	3·143	3·707
7		1·895	2·365	2·998	3·499
8		1·860	2·306	2·896	3·355
9		1·833	2·262	2·821	3·250
10		1·812	2·228	2·764	3·169
11		1·796	2·201	2·718	3·106
12		1·782	2·179	2·681	3·055
13		1·771	2·160	2·650	3·012
14		1·761	2·145	2·624	2·977
15		1·753	2·131	2·602	2·947
16		1·746	2·120	2·583	2·921
17		1·740	2·110	2·567	2·898
18		1·734	2·101	2·552	2·878
19		1·729	2·093	2·539	2·861
20		1·725	2·086	2·528	2·845
21		1·721	2·080	2·518	2·831
22		1·717	2·074	2·508	2·819
23		1·714	2·069	2·500	2·807
24		1·711	2·064	2·492	2·797
25		1·708	2·060	2·485	2·787
30		1·697	2·042	2·457	2·750
40		1·684	2·021	2·423	2·704
60		1·671	2·000	2·390	2·660
80		1·664	1·990	2·374	2·639
100		1·660	1·984	2·364	2·626
∞		1·645	1·960	2·326	2·576

Significant result if $t \geqslant t_c$ or $t \leqslant -t_c$

Table B.4 The χ^2 test: critical values for the chi-square distribution (abbreviated and adapted from *Geigy Scientific Tables*, 1982, with permission).

Two-sided significance level	0·10	0·05	0·02	0·01
One-sided significance level	0·05	0·025	0·01	0·005
d.f.	Critical value χ^2_c			
1	2·706	3·841	5·412	6·635
2	4·605	5·991	7·824	9·210
3	6·251	7·815	9·837	11·345
4	7·779	9·488	11·668	13·277
5	9·236	11·070	13·388	15·086
6	10·645	12·592	15·033	16·812
7	12·017	14·067	16·622	18·475
8	13·362	15·507	18·168	20·090
9	14·684	16·919	19·679	21·666
10	15·987	18·307	21·161	23·209
11	17·275	19·675	22·618	24·725
12	18·549	21·026	24·054	26·217
13	19·812	22·362	25·472	27·688
14	21·064	23·685	26·873	29·141
15	22·307	24·996	28·259	30·578
16	23·542	26·296	29·633	32·000
17	24·769	27·587	30·995	33·409
18	25·989	28·869	32·346	34·805
19	27·204	30·144	33·687	36·191
20	28·412	31·410	35·020	37·566
21	29·615	32·671	36·343	38·932
22	30·813	33·924	37·659	40·289
23	32·007	35·172	38·968	41·638
24	33·196	36·415	40·270	42·980
25	34·382	37·652	41·566	44·314
26	35·563	38·885	42·856	45·642
27	36·741	40·113	44·140	46·963
28	37·916	41·337	45·419	48·278
29	39·087	42·557	46·693	49·588
30	40·256	43·773	47·962	50·892

Significant result if $\chi^2 \geqslant \chi^2_c$

Table B.5(a) The Wilcoxon two sample rank sum test for sample sizes $n_1 = 1$ to 9, $n_2 = 1$ to 35. Critical lower (T_l) and upper (T_u) values for the sum of ranks T_1 from sample sized n_1. (Abbreviated and adapted from *Geigy Scientific Tables*, 1982, with permission.)

Two-sided significance level: 0·10
One-sided significance level: 0·05

n_1	1	2	3	4	5	6	7	8	9
n_2	$T_l\ T_u$	$T_l\ T_u$	$T_l\ T_u$	$T_l\ T_u$	$T_l\ T_u$	$T_l\ T_u$	$T_l\ T_u$	$T_l\ T_u$	$T_l\ T_u$
1	–	–	–	–	–	–	–	–	–
2	–	–	–	–	15–25	21–33	28–42	37–51	46–62
3	–	–	6–15	10–22	16–29	23–37	30–47	39–57	49–68
4	–	–	6–18	11–25	17–33	24–42	32–52	41–63	51–75
5	–	3–13	7–20	12–28	19–36	26–46	34–57	44–68	54–81
6	–	3–15	8–22	13–31	20–40	28–50	36–62	46–74	57–87
7	–	3–17	8–25	14–34	21–44	29–55	39–66	49–79	60–93
8	–	4–18	9–27	15–37	23–47	31–59	41–71	51–85	63–99
9	–	4–20	10–29	16–40	24–51	33–63	43–76	54–90	66–105
10	–	4–22	10–32	17–43	26–54	35–67	45–81	56–96	69–111
11	–	4–24	11–34	18–46	27–58	37–71	47–86	59–101	72–117
12	–	5–25	11–37	19–49	28–62	38–76	49–91	62–106	75–123
13	–	5–27	12–39	20–52	30–65	40–80	52–95	64–112	78–129
14	–	6–28	13–41	21–55	31–69	42–84	54–100	67–117	81–135
15	–	6–30	13–44	22–58	33–72	44–88	56–105	69–123	84–141
16	–	6–32	14–46	24–60	34–76	46–92	58–110	72–128	87–147
17	–	6–34	15–48	25–63	35–80	47–97	61–114	75–133	90–153
18	–	7–35	15–51	26–66	37–83	49–101	63–119	77–139	93–159
19	1–20	7–37	16–53	27–69	38–87	51–105	65–124	80–144	96–165
20	1–21	7–39	17–55	28–72	40–90	53–109	67–129	83–149	99–171
21	1–22	8–40	17–58	29–75	41–94	55–113	69–134	85–155	102–177
22	1–23	8–42	18–60	30–78	43–97	57–117	72–138	88–160	105–183
23	1–24	8–44	19–62	31–81	44–101	58–122	74–143	90–166	108–189
24	1–25	9–45	19–62	32–84	45–105	60–126	76–148	93–171	111–195
25	1–26	9–47	20–67	33–87	47–108	62–130	78–153	96–176	114–201
26	1–27	9–49	21–69	34–90	48–112	64–134	81–157	98–182	117–207
27	1–28	10–50	21–72	35–93	50–115	66–138	83–162	101–187	120–213
28	1–29	10–52	22–74	36–96	51–119	67–143	85–167	104–192	123–219
29	1–30	10–54	23–76	37–99	53–122	69–147	87–172	106–198	127–224
30	1–31	10–56	23–79	38–102	54–126	71–151	89–177	109–203	130–230
31	1–32	11–57	24–81	39–105	55–130	73–155	92–181	112–208	133–236
32	1–33	11–59	25–83	40–108	57–133	75–159	94–186	114–214	136–242
33	1–34	11–61	25–86	41–111	58–137	77–163	96–191	117–219	139–248
34	1–35	12–62	26–88	42–114	60–140	78–168	98–196	120–224	142–254
35	1–36	12–64	27–90	43–117	61–144	80–172	101–200	122–230	145–260

Significant result if $T_1 \geqslant T_u$ or $T_1 \leqslant T_l$

Continued

Table B.5(a) The Wilcoxon two sample rank sum test for sample sizes $n_1 = 1$ to 9, $n_2 = 1$ to 35.
Critical lower (T_l) and upper (T_u) values for the sum of ranks T_1 from sample sized n_1.
(Abbreviated and adapted from *Geigy Scientific Tables*, 1982, with permission.)

Two-sided significance level: 0·05
One-sided significance level: 0·025

n_1	1	2	3	4	5	6	7	8	9
n_2	T_l T_u	T_l T_u	T_l T_u	T_l T_u	T_l T_u	T_l T_u	T_l T_u	T_l T_u	T_l T_u
1	–	–	–	–	–	–	–	–	–
2	–	–	–	–	–	–	–	36–52	45–63
3	–	–	–	–	15–30	22–38	29–48	38–58	47–70
4	–	–	–	10–26	16–34	23–43	31–53	40–64	49–77
5	–	–	6–21	11–29	17–38	24–48	33–58	42–70	52–83
6	–	–	7–23	12–32	18–42	26–52	34–64	44–76	55–89
7	–	–	7–26	13–35	20–45	27–57	36–69	46–82	57–96
8	–	3–19	8–28	14–38	21–49	29–61	38–74	49–87	60–102
9	–	3–21	8–31	14–42	22–53	31–65	40–79	51–93	62–109
10	–	3–23	9–33	15–45	23–57	32–70	42–84	53–99	65–115
11	–	3–25	9–36	16–48	24–61	34–74	44–89	55–105	68–121
12	–	4–26	10–38	17–51	26–64	35–79	46–94	58–110	71–127
13	–	4–28	10–41	18–54	27–68	37–83	48–99	60–116	73–134
14	–	4–30	11–43	19–57	28–72	38–88	50–104	62–122	76–140
15	–	4–32	11–46	20–60	29–76	40–92	52–109	65–127	79–146
16	–	4–34	12–48	21–63	30–80	42–96	54–114	67–133	82–152
17	–	5–35	12–51	21–67	32–83	43–101	56–119	70–138	84–159
18	–	5–37	13–53	22–70	33–87	45–105	58–124	72–144	87–165
19	–	5–39	13–56	23–73	34–91	46–110	60–129	74–150	90–171
20	–	5–41	14–58	24–76	35–95	48–114	62–134	77–155	93–177
21	–	6–42	14–61	25–79	37–98	50–118	64–139	79–161	95–184
22	–	6–44	15–63	26–82	38–102	51–123	66–144	81–167	98–190
23	–	6–46	15–66	27–85	39–106	53–127	68–149	84–172	101–196
24	–	6–48	16–68	27–89	40–110	54–132	70–154	86–178	104–202
25	–	6–50	16–71	28–92	42–113	56–136	72–159	89–183	107–208
26	–	7–51	17–73	29–95	43–117	58–140	74–164	91–189	109–215
27	–	7–53	17–76	30–98	44–121	59–145	76–169	93–195	112–221
28	–	7–55	18–78	31–101	45–125	61–149	78–174	96–200	115–227
29	–	7–57	19–80	32–104	47–128	63–153	80–179	98–206	118–233
30	–	8–58	19–83	33–107	48–132	64–158	82–184	101–211	121–239
31	–	8–60	20–85	34–110	49–136	66–162	84–189	103–217	123–246
32	–	8–62	20–88	34–114	50–140	67–167	86–194	105–223	126–252
33	–	8–64	21–90	35–117	52–143	69–171	88–199	108–228	129–258
34	–	8–66	21–93	36–120	53–147	71–175	90–204	110–234	132–264
35	–	9–67	22–95	37–123	54–151	72–180	92–209	113–239	134–271

Significant result if $T_1 \geqslant T_u$ or $T_1 \leqslant T_l$

Table B.5(a) (*Continued*)

Two-sided significance level: 0·02
One-sided significance level: 0·01

n_1	1	2	3	4	5	6	7	8	9
n_2	$T_l \ T_u$	$T_l \ T_u$	$T_l \ T_u$	$T_l \ T_u$	$T_l \ T_u$	$T_l \ T_u$	$T_l \ T_u$	$T_l \ T_u$	$T_l \ T_u$
1	–	–	–	–	–	–	–	–	–
2	–	–	–	–	–	–	–	–	–
3	–	–	–	–	–	–	28–49	36–60	46–71
4	–	–	–	–	15–35	22–44	29–55	38–66	48–78
5	–	–	–	10–30	16–39	23–49	31–60	40–72	50–85
6	–	–	–	11–33	17–43	24–54	32–66	42–78	52–92
7	–	–	6–27	11–37	18–47	25–59	34–71	43–85	54–99
8	–	–	6–30	12–40	19–51	27–63	35–77	45–91	56–106
9	–	–	7–32	13–43	20–55	28–68	37–82	47–97	59–112
10	–	–	7–35	13–47	21–59	29–73	39–87	49–103	61–119
11	–	–	7–38	14–50	22–63	30–78	40–93	51–109	63–126
12	–	–	8–40	15–53	23–67	32–82	42–98	53–115	66–132
13	–	3–29	8–43	15–57	24–71	33–87	44–103	56–120	68–139
14	–	3–31	8–46	16–60	25–75	34–92	45–109	58–126	71–145
15	–	3–33	9–48	17–63	26–79	36–96	47–114	60–132	73–152
16	–	3–35	9–51	17–67	27–83	37–101	49–119	62–138	76–158
17	–	3–37	10–53	18–70	28–87	39–105	51–124	64–144	78–165
18	–	3–39	10–56	19–73	29–91	40–110	52–130	66–150	81–171
19	–	4–40	10–59	19–77	30–95	41–115	54–135	68–156	83–178
20	–	4–42	11–61	20–80	31–99	43–119	56–140	70–162	85–185
21	–	4–44	11–64	21–83	32–103	44–124	58–145	72–168	88–191
22	–	4–46	12–66	21–87	33–107	45–129	59–151	74–174	90–198
23	–	4–48	12–69	22–90	34–111	47–133	61–156	76–180	93–204
24	–	4–50	12–72	23–93	35–115	48–138	63–161	78–186	95–211
25	–	4–52	13–74	23–97	36–119	50–142	64–167	81–191	98–217
26	–	4–54	13–77	24–100	37–123	51–147	66–172	83–197	100–224
27	–	5–55	13–80	25–103	38–127	52–152	68–177	85–203	103–230
28	–	5–57	14–82	26–106	39–131	54–156	70–182	87–209	105–237
29	–	5–59	14–85	26–110	40–135	55–161	71–188	89–215	108–243
30	–	5–61	15–87	27–113	41–139	56–166	73–193	91–221	110–250
31	–	5–63	15–90	28–116	42–143	58–170	75–198	93–227	113–256
32	–	5–65	15–93	28–120	43–147	59–175	77–203	95–233	115–263
33	–	5–67	16–95	29–123	44–151	61–179	78–209	97–239	118–269
34	–	6–68	16–98	30–126	45–155	62–184	80–214	100–244	120–276
35	–	6–70	17–100	30–130	46–159	63–189	82–219	102–250	123–282

Significant result if $T_1 \geqslant T_u$ or $T_1 \leqslant T_l$

Continued

Table B.5(a) The Wilcoxon two sample rank sum test for sample sizes $n_1 = 1$ to 9, $n_2 = 1$ to 35. Critical lower (T_l) and upper (T_u) values for the sum of ranks T_1 from sample sized n_1. (Abbreviated and adapted from *Geigy Scientific Tables*, 1982, with permission.)

Two-sided significance level: 0·01
One-sided significance level: 0·005

n_1	1	2	3	4	5	6	7	8	9
n_2	$T_l\ T_u$	$T_l\ T_u$	$T_l\ T_u$	$T_l\ T_u$	$T_l\ T_u$	$T_l\ T_u$	$T_l\ T_u$	$T_l\ T_u$	$T_l\ T_u$
1	–	–	–	–	–	–	–	–	–
2	–	–	–	–	–	–	–	–	–
3	–	–	–	–	–	–	–	–	45–72
4	–	–	–	–	–	21–45	28–56	37–67	46–80
5	–	–	–	–	15–40	22–50	29–62	38–74	48–87
6	–	–	–	10–34	16–44	23–55	31–67	40–80	50–94
7	–	–	–	10–38	16–49	24–60	32–73	42–86	52–101
8	–	–	–	11–41	17–53	25–65	34–78	43–93	54–108
9	–	–	6–33	11–45	18–57	26–70	35–84	45–99	56–115
10	–	–	6–36	12–48	19–61	27–75	37–89	47–105	58–122
11	–	–	6–39	12–52	20–65	28–80	38–95	49–111	61–128
12	–	–	7–41	13–55	21–69	30–84	40–100	51–117	63–135
13	–	–	7–44	13–59	22–73	31–89	41–106	53–123	65–142
14	–	–	7–47	14–62	22–78	32–94	43–111	54–130	67–149
15	–	–	8–49	15–65	23–82	33–99	44–117	56–136	69–156
16	–	–	8–52	15–69	24–86	34–104	46–122	58–142	72–162
17	–	–	8–55	16–72	25–90	36–108	47–128	60–148	74–169
18	–	–	8–58	16–76	26–94	37–113	49–133	62–154	76–176
19	–	3–41	9–60	17–79	27–98	38–118	50–139	64–160	78–183
20	–	3–43	9–63	18–82	28–102	39–123	52–144	66–166	81–189
21	–	3–45	9–66	18–86	29–106	40–128	53–150	68–172	83–196
22	–	3–47	10–68	19–89	29–111	42–132	55–155	70–178	85–203
23	–	3–49	10–71	19–93	30–115	43–137	57–160	71–185	88–209
24	–	3–51	10–74	20–96	31–119	44–142	58–166	73–191	90–216
25	–	3–53	11–76	20–100	32–123	45–147	60–171	75–197	92–223
26	–	3–55	11–79	21–103	33–127	46–152	61–177	77–203	94–230
27	–	4–56	11–82	22–106	34–131	48–156	63–182	79–209	97–236
28	–	4–58	11–85	22–110	35–135	49–161	64–188	81–215	99–243
29	–	4–60	12–87	23–113	36–139	50–166	66–193	83–221	101–250
30	–	4–62	12–90	23–117	37–143	51–171	68–198	85–227	103–257
31	–	4–64	12–93	24–120	37–148	53–175	69–204	87–233	106–263
32	–	4–66	13–95	24–124	38–152	54–180	71–209	89–239	108–270
33	–	4–68	13–98	25–127	39–156	55–185	72-215	91–245	110–277
34	–	4–70	13–101	26–130	40–160	56–190	74–220	93–251	113–283
35	–	4–72	14–103	26–134	41–164	58–194	75–226	95–257	115–290

Significant result if $T_1 \geq T_u$ or $T_1 \leq T_l$

Table B.5(b) The Wilcoxon two-sample rank sum test for sample sizes n_1 = 10 to 17, n_2 = 1 to 35. Critical lower (T_l) and upper (T_u) values for the sum of ranks T_1 from sample sized n_1. (Abbreviated and adapted from *Geigy Scientific Tables*, 1982, with permission.)

Two-sided significance level: 0·10
One-sided significance level: 0·05

n_1	10	11	12	13	14	15	16	17
n_2	$T_l\ T_u$	$T_l\ T_u$	$T_l\ T_u$	$T_l\ T_u$	$T_l\ T_u$	$T_l\ T_u$	$T_l\ T_u$	$T_l\ T_u$
1	–	–	–	–	–	–	–	–
2	56–74	67–87	80–100	93–115	108–130	123–147	139–165	156–184
3	59–81	71–94	83–109	97–124	112–140	127–158	144–176	162–195
4	62–88	74–102	87–117	101–133	116–150	132–168	150–186	168–206
5	66–94	78–109	91–125	106–141	121–159	138–177	155–197	173–218
6	69–101	82–116	95–133	110–150	126–168	143–187	161–207	179–229
7	72–108	85–124	99–141	115–158	131–177	148–197	166–218	186–239
8	75–115	89–131	104–148	119–167	136–186	153–207	172–228	192–250
9	79–121	93–138	108–156	124–175	141–195	159–216	178–238	198–261
10	82–128	97–145	112–164	128–184	146–204	164–226	184–248	204–272
11	86–134	100–153	116–172	133–192	151–213	170–235	190–258	210–283
12	89–141	104–160	120–180	138–200	156–222	175–245	196–268	217–293
13	92–148	108–167	125–187	142–209	161–231	181–254	201–279	223–304
14	96–154	112–174	129–195	147–217	166–240	186–264	207–289	230–314
15	99–161	116–181	133–203	152–225	171–249	192–273	213–299	236–325
16	103–167	120–188	138–210	156–234	176–258	197–283	219–309	242–336
17	106–174	123–196	142–218	161–242	182–266	203–292	225–319	249–346
18	110–180	127–203	146–266	166–250	187–275	208–302	231–329	255–357
19	113–187	131–210	150–234	171–258	192–284	214–311	237–339	262–367
20	117–193	135–217	155–241	175–267	197–293	220–320	243–349	268–378
21	120–200	135–224	159–249	180–275	202–302	225–330	249–359	274–389
22	123–207	143–231	163–257	185–283	207–311	231–339	255–369	281–399
23	127–213	147–238	168–264	189–292	212–320	236–349	261–379	287–410
24	130–220	151–245	172–272	194–300	218–328	242–358	267–389	294–420
25	134–226	155–252	176–280	199–308	223–337	248–367	273–399	300–431
26	137–233	158–260	181–287	204–316	228–346	253–377	279–409	307–441
27	141–239	162–267	185–295	208–325	233–355	259–386	285–419	313–452
28	144–246	166–274	189–303	213–333	238–364	264–396	292–428	320–462
29	148–252	170–281	194–310	218–341	243–373	270–405	298–438	326–473
30	151–259	174–288	198–318	223–349	249–381	276–414	304–448	333–483
31	155–265	178–295	202–326	227–358	254–390	281–424	310–458	339–494
32	158–272	182–302	206–334	232–366	259–399	287–433	316–468	346–504
33	162–278	186–309	211–341	237–374	264–408	292–443	322–478	352–515
34	165–285	190–316	215–349	242–382	269–417	298–452	328–488	359–525
35	169–291	194–323	219–357	247–390	275–425	304–461	334–498	365–536

Significant result if $T_1 \geqslant T_u$ or $T_1 \leqslant T_l$

Continued

Table B.5(b) The Wilcoxon two-sample rank sum test for sample sizes $n_1 = 10$ to 17, $n_2 = 1$ to 35. Critical lower (T_l) and upper (T_u) values for the sum of ranks T_1 from sample sized n_1. (Abbreviated and adapted from *Geigy Scientific Tables*, 1982, with permission.)

Two-sided significance level: 0·05
One-sided significance level: 0·025

n_1	10	11	12	13	14	15	16	17
n_2	T_l T_u	T_l T_u	T_l T_u	T_l T_u	T_l T_u	T_l T_u	T_l T_u	T_l T_u
1	–	–	–	–	–	–	–	–
2	55–75	66–88	79–101	92–116	106–132	121–149	137–167	155–185
3	58–82	69–96	82–110	95–126	110–142	125–160	142–178	159–198
4	60–90	72–104	85–119	99–135	114–152	130–170	147–189	164–210
5	63–97	75–112	89–127	103–144	118–162	134–181	151–201	170–221
6	66–104	79–119	92–136	107–153	122–172	139–191	157–211	175–233
7	69–111	82–127	96–144	111–162	127–181	144–201	162–222	181–244
8	72–118	85–135	100–152	115–171	131–191	149–211	167–233	187–255
9	75–125	89–142	104–160	119–180	136–200	154–221	173–243	192–267
10	78–132	92–150	107–169	124–188	141–209	159–231	178–254	198–278
11	81–139	96–157	111–177	128–197	145–219	164–241	183–265	204–289
12	84–146	99–165	115–185	132–206	150–228	169–251	189–275	210–300
13	88–152	103–172	119–193	136–215	155–237	174–261	195–285	216–311
14	91–159	106–180	123–201	141–223	160–246	179–271	200–296	222–322
15	94–166	110–187	127–209	145–232	164–256	184–281	206–306	228–333
16	97–173	113–195	131–217	150–240	169–265	190–290	211–317	234–344
17	100–180	117–202	135–225	154–249	174–274	195–300	217–327	240–355
18	103–187	121–209	139–233	158–258	179–283	200–310	222–338	246–366
19	107–193	124–217	143–241	163–266	183–293	205–320	228–348	252–377
20	110–200	128–224	147–249	167–275	188–302	210–330	234–358	258–388
21	113–207	131–232	151–257	171–284	193–311	216–339	239–369	264–399
22	116–214	135–239	155–265	176–292	198–320	221–349	245–379	270–410
23	119–221	139–246	159–273	180–301	203–329	226–359	251–389	276–421
24	122–228	142–254	163–281	185–309	207–339	231–369	256–400	282–432
25	126–234	146–261	167–289	189–318	212–348	237–378	262–410	288–443
26	129–241	149–269	171–297	193–327	217–357	242–388	268–420	294–454
27	132–248	153–276	175–305	198–335	222–366	247–398	273–431	300–465
28	135–255	156–284	179–313	202–344	227–375	252–408	279–441	307–475
29	138–262	160–291	183–321	207–352	232–384	258–417	285–451	313–486
30	142–268	164–298	187–329	211–361	236–394	263–427	290–462	319–497
31	145–275	167–306	191–337	216–369	241–403	268–437	296–472	325–508
32	148–282	171–313	195–345	220–378	246–412	273–447	302–482	331–519
33	151–289	174–321	199–353	224–387	251–421	279–456	307–493	337–530
34	154–296	178–328	203–361	229–395	256–430	284–466	313–503	343–541
35	158–302	182–335	207–369	233–404	261–439	289–476	319–513	349–552

Significant result if $T_1 \geqslant T_u$ or $T_1 \leqslant T_l$

Two-sided significance level: 0·02
One-sided significance level: 0·01

n_1	10	11	12	13	14	15	16	17
n_2	$T_l\ T_u$	$T_l\ T_u$	$T_l\ T_u$	$T_l\ T_u$	$T_l\ T_u$	$T_l\ T_u$	$T_l\ T_u$	$T_l\ T_u$
1	–	–	–	–	–	–	–	–
2	–	–	–	91–117	105–133	120–150	136–168	153–187
3	56–84	67–98	80–112	93–128	107–145	123–162	139–181	157–200
4	58–92	70–106	83–121	96–138	111–155	127–173	143–193	161–213
5	61–99	73–114	86–130	100–147	115–165	131–184	148–204	166–225
6	63–107	75–123	89–139	103–157	118–176	135–195	152–216	171–237
7	66–114	78–131	92–148	107–166	122–186	139–206	157–227	176–249
8	68–122	81–139	95–157	111–175	127–195	144–216	162–238	181–261
9	71–129	84–147	99–165	114–185	131–205	148–227	167–249	186–273
10	74–136	88–154	102–174	118–194	135–215	153–237	172–260	191–285
11	77–143	91–162	106–182	122–203	139–225	157–248	177–271	197–296
12	79–151	94–170	109–191	126–212	143–235	162–258	182–282	202–308
13	82–158	97–178	113–199	130–221	148–244	167–268	187–293	208–319
14	85–165	100–186	116–208	134–230	152–254	171–279	192–304	213–331
15	88–172	103–194	120–216	138–239	156–264	176–289	197–315	219–342
16	91–179	107–201	124–224	142–248	161–273	181–299	202–326	224–354
17	93–187	110–209	127–233	146–257	165–283	186–309	207–337	230–365
18	96–194	113–217	131–241	150–266	170–292	190–320	212–348	235–377
19	99–201	116–225	134–250	154–275	174–302	195–330	218–358	241–388
20	102–208	119–233	138–258	158–284	178–312	200–340	223–369	246–400
21	105–215	123–240	142–266	162–293	183–321	205–350	228–380	252–411
22	108–222	126–248	145–275	166–302	187–331	210–360	233–391	258–422
23	110–230	129–256	149–283	170–311	192–340	214–371	238–402	263–434
24	113–237	132–264	153–291	174–320	196–350	219–381	244–412	269–445
25	116–244	136–271	156–300	178–329	200–360	224–391	249–423	275–456
26	119–251	139–279	160–308	182–338	205–369	229–401	254–434	280–468
27	122–258	142–287	163–317	186–347	209–379	234–411	259–445	286–479
28	125–265	145–295	167–325	190–356	214–388	239–421	265–455	292–490
29	128–272	149–302	171–333	194–365	218–398	243–432	270–466	297–502
30	131–279	152–310	174–342	198–374	223–407	248–442	275–477	303–513
31	133–287	155–318	178–350	202–383	227–417	253–452	280–488	309–524
32	136–294	158–326	182–358	206–392	232–426	258–462	286–498	314–536
33	139–301	162–333	185–367	210–401	236–436	263–472	291–509	320–547
34	142–308	165–341	189–375	214–410	240–446	268–482	296–520	326–558
35	145–315	168–349	193–383	218–419	245–455	273–492	301–531	331–570

Significant result if $T_1 \geqslant T_u$ or $T_1 \leqslant T_l$

Continued

Table B.5(b) The Wilcoxon two-sample rank sum test for sample sizes $n_1 = 10$ to 17, $n_2 = 1$ to 35. Critical lower (T_l) and upper (T_u) values for the sum of ranks T_1 from sample sized n_1. (Abbreviated and adapted from *Geigy Scientific Tables*, 1982, with permission.)

Two-sided significance level: 0·01
One-sided significance level: 0·005

n_1	10	11	12	13	14	15	16	17
n_2	T_l T_u	T_l T_u	T_l T_u	T_l T_u	T_l T_u	T_l T_u	T_l T_u	T_l T_u
1	–	–	–	–	–	–	–	–
2	–	–	–	–	–	–	–	–
3	55–85	66–99	79–113	92–129	106–146	122–163	138–182	155–202
4	57–93	68–108	81–123	94–140	109–157	125–175	141–195	159–215
5	59–101	71–116	84–132	98–149	112–168	128–187	145–207	163–228
6	61–109	73–125	87–141	101–159	116–178	132–198	149–219	168–240
7	64–116	76–133	90–150	104–169	120–188	136–209	154–230	172–253
8	66–124	79–141	93–159	108–178	123–199	140–220	158–242	177–265
9	68–132	82–149	96–168	111–188	127–209	144–231	163–253	182–277
10	71–139	84–158	99–177	115–197	131–219	149–241	167–265	187–289
11	73–147	87–166	102–186	118–207	135–229	153–252	172–276	192–301
12	76–154	90–174	105–195	122–216	139–239	157–263	177–287	197–313
13	79–161	93–182	109–203	125–226	143–249	162–273	181–299	202–325
14	81–169	96–190	112–212	129–235	147–259	166–284	186–310	207–337
15	84–176	99–198	115–221	133–244	151–269	171–294	191–321	213–348
16	86–184	102–206	119–229	136–254	155–279	175–305	196–332	218–360
17	89–191	105–214	122–238	140–263	159–289	180–315	201–343	223–372
18	92–198	108–222	125–247	144–272	163–299	184–326	206–354	228–384
19	94–206	111–230	129–255	148–281	168–308	189–336	210–366	234–395
20	97–213	114–238	132–264	151–291	172–318	193–347	215–377	239–407
21	99–221	117–246	136–272	155–300	176–328	198–357	220–388	244–419
22	102–228	120–254	139–281	159–309	180–338	202–368	225–399	249–431
23	105–235	123–262	142–290	163–318	184–348	207–378	230–410	255–442
24	107–243	126–270	146–298	166–328	188–358	211–389	235–421	260–454
25	110–250	129–278	149–307	170–337	192–368	216–399	240–432	265–466
26	113–257	132–286	152–316	174–346	197–377	220–410	245–443	271–477
27	115–265	135–294	156–324	178–355	201–387	225–420	250–454	276–489
28	118–272	138–302	159–333	182–364	205–397	229–431	255–465	281–501
29	121–279	141–310	163–341	185–374	209–407	234–441	260–476	287–512
30	123–287	144–318	166–350	189–383	213–417	239–451	265–487	292–524
31	126–294	147–326	170–358	193–392	218–426	243–462	270–498	298–535
32	129–301	150–334	173–367	197–401	222–436	248–472	275–509	303–547
33	131–309	153–342	176–376	201–410	226–446	252–483	280–520	308–559
34	134–316	156–350	180–384	204–420	230–456	257–493	285–531	314–570
35	137–323	159–358	183–393	208–429	234–466	262–503	290–542	319–582

Significant result if $T_1 \geqslant T_u$ or $T_1 \leqslant T_l$

Table B.5(c) The Wilcoxon two-sample rank sum test for sample sizes $n_1 = 18$ to 25, $n_2 = 1$ to 35. Critical lower (T_l) and upper (T_u) values for the sum of ranks T_1 from sample sized n_1. (Abbreviated and adapted from *Geigy Scientific Tables*, 1982, with permission.)

Two-sided significance level: 0·10
One-sided significance level: 0·05

n_1	18	19	20	21	22	23	24	25
n_2	T_l T_u	T_l T_u	T_l T_u	T_l T_u	T_l T_u	T_l T_u	T_l T_u	T_l T_u
1	–	190–209	210–230	231–252	253–275	276–299	300–324	325–350
2	175–203	194–224	214–246	236–268	258–292	281–317	306–342	331–369
3	180–216	200–237	221–259	242–283	265–307	289–332	313–359	339–386
4	187–227	207–249	228–272	250–296	273–321	297–347	322–374	348–402
5	193–239	213–262	235–285	257–310	281–335	305–362	330–390	357–418
6	199–251	220–274	242–298	265–323	289–349	313–377	339–405	366–434
7	206–262	227–286	249–311	272–337	297–363	322–391	348–420	375–450
8	212–274	234–298	257–323	280–350	305–377	330–406	357–435	385–465
9	219–285	241–310	264–336	288–363	313–391	339–420	366–450	394–481
10	226–296	248–322	272–348	296–376	321–405	348–434	375–465	404–496
11	232–308	255–334	279–361	304–389	330–418	357–448	385–479	414–511
12	239–319	262–346	287–373	312–402	338–432	366–462	394–494	423–527
13	246–330	270–357	294–386	320–415	347–445	374–477	403–509	433–542
14	253–341	277–369	302–398	328–428	355–459	383–491	413–523	443–557
15	259–353	284–381	310–410	336–441	364–472	392–505	422–538	453–572
16	266–364	291–393	317–423	344–454	372–486	401–519	431–553	462–588
17	273–375	299–404	325–435	352–467	381–499	410–533	441–567	472–603
18	280–386	306–416	333–447	361–479	389–513	419–547	450–582	482–618
19	287–397	313–428	340–460	369–492	398–526	428–561	460–596	492–633
20	294–408	320–440	348–472	377–505	407–539	437–575	469–611	502–648
21	301–419	328–451	356–484	385–518	415–553	446–589	479–625	512–663
22	307–431	335–463	364–496	393–531	424–566	455–603	488–640	522–678
23	314–442	342–475	371–509	401–544	432–580	465–616	498–654	532–693
24	321–453	350–486	379–521	410–556	441–593	474–630	507–669	542–708
25	328–464	357–498	387–533	418–569	450–606	483–644	517–683	552–723
26	335–475	364–510	395–545	426–582	458–620	492–658	526–698	562–738
27	342–486	372–521	402–558	434–595	467–633	501–672	536–712	572–753
28	349–497	379–533	410–570	443–607	476–646	510–686	545–727	582–768
29	356–508	386–545	418–582	451–620	484–660	519–700	555–741	592–783
30	363–519	394–556	426–594	459–633	493–673	528–714	564–756	602–798
31	370–530	401–568	434–606	467–646	502–686	537–728	574–770	612–813
32	377–541	408–580	441–619	475–659	510–700	547–741	584–784	622–828
33	383–553	416–591	449–631	484–671	519–713	556–755	593–799	632–843
34	390–564	423–603	457–643	492–684	528–726	565–769	603–813	642–858
35	397–575	431–614	465–655	500–697	537–739	574–783	612–828	652–873

Significant result if $T_1 \geqslant T_u$ or $T_1 \leqslant T_l$

Continued

Table B.5(c) The Wilcoxon two-sample rank sum test for sample sizes $n_1 = 18$ to 25, $n_2 = 1$ to 35. Critical lower (T_l) and upper (T_u) values for the sum of ranks T_1 from sample sized n_1. (Abbreviated and adapted from *Geigy Scientific Tables*, 1982, with permission.)

Two-sided significance level: 0·05
One-sided significance level: 0·025

n_1	18	19	20	21	22	23	24	25
n_2	$T_l\ T_u$	$T_l\ T_u$	$T_l\ T_u$	$T_l\ T_u$	$T_l\ T_u$	$T_l\ T_u$	$T_l\ T_u$	$T_l\ T_u$
1	–	–	–	–	–	–	–	–
2	173–205	192–226	212–248	234–270	256–294	279–319	303–345	328–372
3	178–218	197–240	218–262	239–286	262–310	285–336	310–362	335–390
4	183–231	203–235	224–276	246–300	269–325	293–351	317–379	343–407
5	189–243	209–266	230–290	253–314	276–340	300–367	325–395	352–423
6	195–255	215–279	237–303	260–328	283–355	308–382	333–411	360–440
7	201–267	222–291	244–316	267–342	291–269	316–397	342–426	369–456
8	207–279	228–304	251–329	274–356	298–384	324–412	350–442	378–472
9	213–291	235–316	258–342	281–370	306–398	332–427	359–457	387–488
10	219–303	242–328	265–355	289–383	314–412	340–442	367–473	396–504
11	226–314	248–341	272–368	296–397	322–426	349–456	376–488	405–520
12	232–326	255–353	279–381	304–410	330–440	357–471	385–503	414–536
13	238–338	262–365	286–394	311–424	338–454	365–486	394–518	423–552
14	245–349	268–378	293–407	319–437	346–468	374–500	402–534	432–568
15	251–361	275–390	300–420	327–450	354–482	382–515	411–549	442–583
16	257–373	282–402	308–432	334–464	362–496	391–529	420–564	451–599
17	264–384	289–414	315–445	342–477	370–510	399–544	429–579	460–615
18	270–396	296–426	322–458	350–490	378–524	408–558	438–594	470–630
19	277–407	303–438	329–471	357–504	386–538	416–573	447–609	479–646
20	283–419	309–451	337–483	365–517	394–552	425–587	456–624	488–662
21	290–430	316–463	344–496	373–530	403–656	433–602	465–639	498–677
22	296–442	323–475	351–509	381–543	411–579	442–616	474–654	507–693
23	303–453	330–487	359–521	388–557	419–593	451–630	483–669	517–708
24	309–465	337–499	366–534	396–707	427–607	459–645	492–684	526–724
25	316–476	344–511	373–547	404–583	435–621	468–659	501–699	536–739
26	322–488	351–523	381–559	412–596	444–634	476–674	510–714	545–755
27	329–499	358–535	388–572	419–610	452–648	485–688	519–729	555–770
28	335–511	365–547	396–584	427–623	460–662	494–702	528–744	564–786
29	342–522	372–559	403–597	435–636	468–676	502–717	538–758	574–801
30	348–534	379–571	410–610	443–649	476–690	511–731	547–773	583–817
31	355–545	386–583	418–622	451–662	485–703	520–745	556–788	593–832
32	361–557	393–595	425–635	458–676	493–717	528–760	565–803	602–848
33	368–568	400–607	432–648	466–689	501–731	537–774	574–818	612–863
34	374–580	407–619	440–660	474–702	509–745	546–788	583–833	622–878
35	381–591	414–631	447–673	482–715	518–758	554–803	592–848	631–894

Significant result if $T_1 \geq T_u$ or $T_1 \leq T_l$

Two-sided significance level: 0·02
One-sided significance level: 0·01

n_1	18	19	20	21	22	23	24	25
n_2	$T_l\ T_u$	$T_l\ T_u$	$T_l\ T_u$	$T_l\ T_u$	$T_l\ T_u$	$T_l\ T_u$	$T_l\ T_u$	$T_l\ T_u$
1	–	–	–	–	–	–	–	–
2	171–207	191–227	211–249	232–272	254–296	277–321	301–347	326–374
3	175–221	194–243	215–265	236–289	259–313	282–339	306–366	332–393
4	180–234	199–257	220–280	242–304	264–330	288–356	313–383	338–412
5	185–247	205–270	226–294	248–319	271–345	295–372	320–400	346–429
6	190–260	210–284	232–308	254–334	277–361	302–388	327–417	354–446
7	195–273	216–297	238–322	261–348	284–376	309–404	335–433	361–464
8	201–285	222–310	244–336	267–363	291–391	316–420	342–450	370–480
9	207–297	228–323	250–350	274–377	298–406	324–435	350–466	378–497
10	212–310	234–336	257–363	281–391	306–420	331–451	358–482	386–514
11	218–322	240–349	263–377	288–405	313–435	339–466	366–498	395–530
12	224–334	246–362	270–390	295–419	320–450	347–481	375–513	403–547
13	230–346	253–374	277–403	302–433	328–464	355–496	383–529	412–563
14	236–358	259–387	283–417	309–447	335–479	363–511	391–545	420–580
15	241–371	265–400	290–430	316–461	343–493	370–527	399–561	429–596
16	247–383	272–412	297–443	323–475	350–508	378–542	408–576	438–612
17	253–395	278–425	303–457	330–489	358–522	386–557	416–592	447–628
18	259–407	284–438	310–470	337–503	365–537	394–572	424–608	455–645
19	265–419	291–450	317–483	344–517	373–551	402–587	433–623	464–661
20	271–431	297–463	324–496	352–530	380–566	410–602	441–639	473–677
21	277–443	303–476	331–509	359–544	388–580	418–617	450–654	482–693
22	283–455	310–488	337–523	366–558	396–594	426–632	458–670	491–709
23	289–467	316–501	344–536	373–572	403–609	434–647	467–685	500–725
24	295–479	323–513	351–549	381–585	411–623	443–661	475–701	509–741
25	301–491	329–526	358–562	388–599	419–637	451–676	484–716	517–758
26	307–503	336–538	365–575	395–613	426–652	459–691	492–732	526–774
27	313–515	342–551	372–588	402–627	434–666	467–706	501–747	535–790
28	320–526	349–563	379–601	410–640	442–680	475–721	509–763	544–806
29	326–538	355–576	386–614	417–654	450–694	483–736	518–778	553–822
30	332–550	362–588	392–628	424–668	457–709	491–751	526–794	562–838
31	338–562	368–601	399–641	432–681	465–723	499–766	535–809	571–854
32	344–574	375–613	406–654	439–695	473–737	508–780	543–825	580–870
33	350–586	381–626	413–667	446–709	481–751	516–795	552–840	589–886
34	356–598	388–638	420–680	454–722	488–766	524–810	561–855	598–902
35	362–610	394–651	427–693	461–736	496–780	532–825	569–871	607–918

Significant result if $T_1 \geqslant T_u$ or $T_1 \leqslant T_l$

Continued

Table B.5(c) The Wilcoxon two-sample rank sum test for sample sizes $n_1 = 18$ to 25, $n_2 = 1$ to 35. Critical lower (T_l) and upper (T_u) values for the sum of ranks T_1 from sample sized n_1. (Abbreviated and adapted from *Geigy Scientific Tables*, 1982, with permission.)

Two-sided significance level: 0·01
One-sided significance level: 0·005

n_1	18	19	20	21	22	23	24	25
n_2	T_l T_u	T_l T_u	T_l T_u	T_l T_u	T_l T_u	T_l T_u	T_l T_u	T_l T_u
1	–	–	–	–	–	–	–	–
2	–	190–228	210–250	231–273	253–297	276–322	300–348	325–375
3	173–223	193–244	213–267	234–291	257–315	280–341	304–368	330–395
4	177–237	197–259	218–282	239–307	262–332	285–359	310–386	335–415
5	182–250	202–273	223–297	245–322	267–349	291–376	316–404	342–433
6	187–263	207–287	228–312	250–338	274–364	298–392	323–421	349–451
7	192–276	212–301	234–326	256–353	280–380	305–408	330–438	357–468
8	197–289	218–314	240–340	263–367	287–395	311–425	337–455	364–486
9	202–302	223–328	246–354	269–382	293–411	319–440	345–471	372–503
10	208–314	229–341	252–368	275–397	300–426	326–456	352–488	380–520
11	213–327	235–354	258–382	282–411	307–441	333–472	360–504	388–537
12	218–340	241–367	264–396	289–425	314–456	340–488	368–520	396–554
13	224–352	247–380	270–410	295–440	321–471	348–503	375–537	404–571
14	229–365	253–393	277–423	302–454	328–486	355–519	383–553	412–588
15	235–377	259–406	283–437	309–468	335–501	363–534	391–569	421–604
16	241–389	264–420	289–451	315–483	342–516	370–550	399–585	429–621
17	246–402	271–432	296–464	322–497	349–531	378–565	407–601	437–638
18	252–414	277–445	302–478	329–511	357–545	385–581	415–617	446–654
19	258–426	283–458	309–491	336–525	364–560	393–596	423–633	454–671
20	263–439	289–471	315–505	343–539	371–575	401–611	431–649	463–687
21	269–451	295–484	322–518	349–554	378–590	408–627	439–665	471–704
22	275–463	301–497	328–532	356–568	386–604	416–642	447–681	480–720
23	280–476	307–510	335–545	363–582	393–619	424–657	455–697	488–737
24	286–488	313–523	341–559	370–596	400–634	431–673	464–712	497–753
25	292–500	319–536	348–572	377–610	408–648	439–688	472–728	505–770
26	298–512	325–549	354–586	384–624	415–663	447–703	480–744	514–786
27	303–525	332–561	361–599	391–638	422–678	455–718	488–760	522–803
28	309–537	338–574	367–613	398–652	430–692	462–734	496–776	531–819
29	315–549	344–587	374–626	405–666	437–707	470–749	504–792	540–835
30	321–561	350–600	380–640	412–680	444–722	478–764	513–807	548–852
31	326–574	356–613	387–653	419–694	452–736	486–779	521–823	557–868
32	332–586	362–626	394–666	426–708	459–751	494–794	529–839	565–885
33	338–598	369–638	400–680	433–722	467–765	501–810	537–855	574–901
34	344–610	375–651	407–693	440–736	474–780	509–825	545–871	583–917
35	350–622	381–664	413–707	447–750	482–794	517–840	554–886	591–934

Significant result if $T_1 \geqslant T_u$ or $T_1 \leqslant T_l$

Table B.6 (a) The sign test (paired data). Critical lower (S_l) and upper (S_u) values for the number of positive differences n_+ from a sample with n non-zero differences. (b) The exact test for correlated proportions. Critical values for the number of untied pairs 'c' in favour of one of the 'treatments' with n untied pairs altogether. (Abbreviated and adapted from *Geigy Scientific Tables*, 1982, with permission.)

Two-sided significance level	0·10	0·05	0·02	0·01
One-sided significance level	0·05	0·025	0·01	0·005
n	S_l S_u	S_l S_u	S_l S_u	S_l S_u
5	0–5	–	–	–
6	0–6	0–6	–	–
7	0–7	0–7	0–7	–
8	1–7	0–8	0–8	0–8
9	1–8	1–8	0–9	0–9
10	1–9	1–9	0–10	0–10
11	2–9	1–10	1–10	0–11
12	2–10	2–10	1–11	1–11
13	3–10	2–11	1–12	1–12
14	3–11	2–12	2–12	1–13
15	3–12	3–12	2–13	2–13
16	4–12	3–13	2–14	2–14
17	4–13	4–13	3–14	2–15
18	5–13	4–14	3–15	3–15
19	5–14	4–15	4–15	3–16
20	5–15	5–15	4–16	3–17
21	6–15	5–16	4–17	4–17
22	6–16	5–17	5–17	4–18
23	7–16	6–17	5–18	4–19
24	7–17	6–18	6–19	5–20
25	7–18	7–18	6–19	5–20
26	8–18	7–19	6–20	6–20
27	8–19	7–20	7–20	6–21
28	9–19	8–20	7–21	6–22
29	9–20	8–21	7–22	7–22
30	10–20	9–21	8–22	7–23
31	10–21	9–22	8–23	7–24
32	10–22	9–23	8–24	8–24
33	11–22	10–23	9–24	8–25
34	11–23	10–24	9–25	9–25
35	12–23	11–24	10–25	9–26
36	12–24	11–25	10–26	9–27
37	13–24	12–25	10–27	10–27
38	13–25	12–26	11–27	10–28
39	13–26	12–57	11–28	11–28
40	14–26	13–27	12–28	11–29
41	14–27	13–28	12–29	11–30
42	15–27	14–28	13–29	12–30
43	15–28	14–29	13–30	12–31
44	16–28	15–29	13–31	13–31
45	16–29	15–30	14–31	13–32
46	16–30	15–31	14–32	13–33
47	17–30	16–31	15–32	14–33

Significant result if (a) $n_+ \geqslant S_u$ or $n_+ \leqslant S_l$
(b) $c \geqslant S_u$ or $c \leqslant S_l$

Continued

Two-sided significance level	0·10	0·05	0·02	0·01
One-sided significance level	0·05	0·025	0·01	0·005
n	$S_l \ S_u$	$S_l \ S_u$	$S_l \ S_u$	$S_l \ S_u$
48	17–31	16–32	15–33	14–34
49	18–31	17–32	15–34	15–34
50	18–32	17–33	16–34	15–35
51	19–32	18–33	16–35	15–36
52	19–33	18–34	17–35	16–36
53	20–33	18–35	17–36	16–37
54	20–34	19–35	18–36	17–37
55	20–35	19–36	18–37	17–38
56	21–35	20–36	18–38	17–39
57	21–36	20–37	19–38	18–39
58	22–36	21–37	19–39	18–40
59	22–37	21–38	20–39	19–40
60	23–37	21–39	20–40	19–41
61	23–38	22–39	20–41	20–41
62	24–38	22–40	21–41	20–42
63	24–39	23–40	21–42	20–43
64	24–40	23–41	22–42	21–43
65	25–40	24–41	22–43	21–44
66	25–41	24–42	23–43	22–44
67	26–41	25–42	23–44	22–45
68	26–42	25–43	23–45	22–46
69	27–42	25–44	24–45	23–46
70	27–43	26–44	24–46	23–47
71	28–43	26–45	25–46	24–47
72	28–44	27–45	25–47	24–48
73	28–45	27–46	26–47	25–48
74	29–45	28–46	26–48	25–49
75	29–46	28–47	26–49	25–50
76	30–46	28–48	27–49	26–50
77	30–47	29–48	27–50	26–51
78	31–47	29–40	28–50	27–51
79	31–48	30–49	28–51	27–52
80	32–48	30–50	29–51	28–52
81	32–49	31–50	29–52	28–53
82	33–49	31–51	30–52	28–54
83	33–50	32–51	30–53	29–54
84	33–51	31–52	30–54	29–55
85	34–51	32–53	31–54	30–55
86	34–52	33–53	31–55	30–56
87	35–52	33–54	32–55	31–56
88	35–53	34–54	32–56	31–57
89	36–53	34–55	33–56	31–58
90	36–54	35–55	33–57	32–58

Significant result if (a) $n_+ \geqslant S_u$ or $n_+ \leqslant S_l$
(b) $c \geqslant S_u$ or $c \leqslant S_l$

Table B.6 (a) The sign test (paired data). Critical lower (S_l) and upper (S_u) values for the number of positive differences n_+ from a sample with n non-zero differences. (b) The exact test for correlated proportions. Critical values for the number of untied pairs 'c' in favour of one of the 'treatments' with n untied pairs altogether. (Abbreviated and adapted from *Geigy Scientific Tables*, 1982, with permission.)

Table B.6 (*Continued*)

Two-sided significance level	0·10	0·05	0·02	0·01
One-sided significance level	0·05	0·025	0·01	0·005
n	$S_l\ S_u$	$S_l\ S_u$	$S_l\ S_u$	$S_l\ S_u$
91	37–54	35–56	33–58	32–59
92	37–55	36–56	34–58	33–59
93	38–55	36–57	34–59	33–60
94	38–56	37–57	35–59	34–60
95	38–57	37–58	35–60	34–61
96	39–57	37–59	36–60	34–62
97	39–58	38–59	36–61	35–62
98	40–58	38–60	37–61	35–63
99	40–59	39–60	37–62	36–63
100	41–59	38–61	37–63	36–64

Significant result if (a) $n_+ \geqslant S_u$ or $n_+ \leqslant S_l$
(b) $c \geqslant S_u$ or $c \leqslant S_l$.

Table B.7 The Wilcoxon signed rank test (paired data). Critical lower (T_l) and upper (T_u) values for the sum of the positive ranks (T_+) from a study with n non-zero differences. (Abbreviated and adapted from *Geigy Scientific Tables*, 1982, with permission.)

Two-sided significance level	0·10	0·05	0·02	0·01
One-sided significance level	0·05	0·025	0·01	0·005
n	$T_l\ T_u$	$T_l\ T_u$	$T_l\ T_u$	$T_l\ T_u$
5	0–15	–	–	–
6	2–19	0–21	–	–
7	3–25	2–26	0–28	–
8	5–31	3–33	1–35	0–36
9	8–37	5–40	3–42	1–44
10	10–45	8–47	5–50	3–52
11	13–53	10–56	7–59	5–61
12	17–61	13–65	9–69	7–71
13	21–70	17–74	12–79	9–82
14	25–80	21–84	15–90	12–93
15	30–90	25–95	19–101	15–105
16	35–101	29–107	23–113	19–117
17	41–112	34–119	28–125	23–130
18	47–124	40–131	32–139	27–144
19	53–137	46–144	37–153	32–158
20	60–150	52–158	43–167	37–173
21	67–164	58–173	49–182	42–189
22	75–178	66–187	55–198	48–205
23	83–193	73–203	62–214	54–222
24	91–209	81–219	69–231	61–239
25	100–225	89–236	76–249	68–257

Significant result if $T_+ \geqslant T_u$ or $T_+ \leqslant T_l$

Table B.8 Logs of the factorials of $n = 0$ to 99 (abbreviated from *Geigy Scientific Tables*, 1982, with permission).

n	0	1	2	3	4	5	6	7	8	9
0	0·00000	0·00000	0·30103	0·77815	1·38021	2·07918	2·85733	3·70243	4·60552	5·55976
10	6·55976	7·60116	8·68034	9·79428	10·94041	12·11650	13·32062	14·55107	15·80634	17·08509
20	18·38612	19·70834	21·05077	22·41249	23·79271	25·19065	26·60562	28·03698	29·48414	30·94654
30	32·42366	33·91502	35·42017	36·93869	38·47016	40·01423	41·57054	43·13874	44·71852	46·30959
40	47·91165	49·52443	51·14768	52·78115	54·42460	56·07781	57·74057	59·41267	61·09391	62·78410
50	64·48307	66·19064	67·90665	69·63092	71·36332	73·10368	74·85187	76·60774	78·37117	80·14202
60	81·92017	83·70550	85·49790	87·29724	89·10342	90·91633	92·73587	94·56195	96·39446	98·23331
70	100·07841	101·92966	103·78700	105·65032	107·51955	109·39461	111·27543	113·16192	115·05401	116·95164
80	118·85473	120·76321	122·67703	124·59610	126·52038	128·44980	130·38430	132·32382	134·26830	136·21769
90	138·17194	140·13098	142·09476	144·06325	146·03638	148·01410	149·99637	151·98314	153·97437	155·97000

Table B.9 Antilogarithm table (reprinted from *Geigy Scientific Tables*, 1982, with permission).

	x										Proportional parts								
$\text{Log}_{10}x$	0	1	2	3	4	5	6	7	8	9	1	2	3	4	5	6	7	8	9
0·00	1000	1002	1005	1007	1009	1012	1014	1016	1019	1021	0	0	1	1	1	1	2	2	2
0·01	1023	1026	1028	1030	1033	1035	1038	1040	1042	1045	0	0	1	1	1	1	2	2	2
0·02	1047	1050	1052	1054	1057	1059	1062	1064	1067	1069	0	0	1	1	1	1	2	2	2
0·03	1072	1074	1076	1079	1081	1084	1086	1089	1091	1094	0	0	1	1	1	1	2	2	2
0·04	1096	1099	1102	1104	1107	1109	1112	1114	1117	1119	0	1	1	1	1	2	2	2	2
0·05	1122	1125	1127	1130	1132	1135	1138	1140	1143	1146	0	1	1	1	1	2	2	2	2
0·06	1148	1151	1153	1156	1159	1161	1164	1167	1169	1172	0	1	1	1	1	2	2	2	2
0·07	1175	1178	1180	1183	1186	1189	1191	1194	1197	1199	0	1	1	1	1	2	2	2	2
0·08	1202	1205	1208	1211	1213	1216	1219	1222	1225	1227	0	1	1	1	1	2	2	2	3
0·09	1230	1233	1236	1239	1242	1245	1247	1250	1253	1256	0	1	1	1	1	2	2	2	3
0·10	1259	1262	1265	1268	1271	1274	1276	1279	1282	1285	0	1	1	1	1	2	2	2	3
0·11	1288	1291	1294	1297	1300	1303	1306	1309	1312	1315	0	1	1	1	2	2	2	2	3
0·12	1318	1321	1324	1327	1330	1334	1337	1340	1343	1346	0	1	1	1	2	2	2	2	3
0·13	1349	1352	1355	1358	1361	1365	1368	1371	1374	1377	0	1	1	1	2	2	2	3	3
0·14	1380	1384	1387	1390	1393	1396	1400	1403	1406	1409	0	1	1	1	2	2	2	3	3
0·15	1413	1416	1419	1422	1426	1429	1432	1435	1439	1442	0	1	1	1	2	2	2	3	3
0·16	1445	1449	1452	1455	1459	1462	1466	1469	1472	1476	0	1	1	1	2	2	2	3	3
0·17	1479	1483	1486	1489	1493	1496	1500	1503	1507	1510	0	1	1	1	2	2	2	3	3
0·18	1514	1517	1521	1524	1528	1531	1535	1538	1542	1545	0	1	1	1	2	2	2	3	3
0·19	1549	1552	1556	1560	1563	1567	1570	1574	1578	1581	0	1	1	1	2	2	3	3	3
0·20	1585	1589	1592	1596	1600	1603	1607	1611	1614	1618	0	1	1	1	2	2	3	3	3
0·21	1622	1626	1629	1633	1637	1641	1644	1648	1652	1656	0	1	1	2	2	2	3	3	3
0·22	1660	1663	1667	1671	1675	1679	1683	1687	1690	1694	0	1	1	2	2	2	3	3	3
0·23	1698	1702	1706	1710	1714	1718	1722	1726	1730	1734	0	1	1	2	2	2	3	3	4
0·24	1738	1742	1746	1750	1754	1758	1762	1766	1770	1774	0	1	1	2	2	2	3	3	4
0·25	1778	1782	1786	1791	1795	1799	1803	1807	1811	1816	0	1	1	2	2	2	3	3	4
0·26	1820	1824	1828	1832	1837	1841	1845	1849	1854	1858	0	1	1	2	2	3	3	3	4
0·27	1862	1866	1871	1875	1879	1884	1888	1892	1897	1901	0	1	1	2	2	3	3	3	4
0·28	1905	1910	1914	1919	1923	1928	1932	1936	1941	1945	0	1	1	2	2	3	3	4	4
0·29	1950	1954	1959	1963	1968	1972	1977	1982	1986	1991	0	1	1	2	2	3	3	4	4
0·30	1995	2000	2004	2009	2014	2018	2023	2028	2032	2037	0	1	1	2	2	3	3	4	4
0·31	2042	2046	2051	2056	2061	2065	2070	2075	2080	2084	0	1	1	2	2	3	3	4	4
0·32	2089	2094	2099	2104	2109	2113	2118	2123	2128	2133	0	1	1	2	2	3	3	4	4

Table B.9 (*Continued*)

$\text{Log}_{10}x$	0	1	2	3	4	5	6	7	8	9		1	2	3	4	5	6	7	8	9
0·33	2138	2143	2148	2153	2158	2163	2168	2173	2178	2183	0	1	1	2	2	3	3	4	4
0·34	2188	2193	2198	2203	2208	2213	2218	2223	2228	2234	1	1	2	2	3	3	4	4	5
0·35	2239	2244	2249	2254	2259	2265	2270	2275	2280	2286	1	1	2	2	3	3	4	4	5
0·36	2291	2296	2301	2307	2312	2317	2323	2328	2333	2339	1	1	2	2	3	3	4	4	5
0·37	2344	2350	2355	2360	2366	2371	2377	2382	2388	2393	1	1	2	2	3	3	4	4	5
0·38	2399	2404	2410	2415	2421	2427	2432	2438	2443	2449	1	1	2	2	3	3	4	4	5
0·39	2455	2460	2466	2472	2477	2483	2489	2495	2500	2506	1	1	2	2	3	3	4	5	5
0·40	2512	2518	2523	2529	2535	2541	2547	2553	2559	2564	1	1	2	2	3	4	4	5	5
0·41	2570	2576	2582	2588	2594	2600	2606	2612	2618	2624	1	1	2	2	3	4	4	5	5
0·42	2630	2636	2642	2649	2655	2661	2667	2673	2679	2685	1	1	2	2	3	4	4	5	6
0·43	2692	2698	2704	2710	2716	2723	2729	2735	2742	2748	1	1	2	3	3	4	4	5	6
0·44	2754	2761	2767	2773	2780	2786	2793	2799	2805	2812	1	1	2	3	3	4	4	5	6
0·45	2818	2825	2831	2838	2844	2851	2858	2864	2871	2877	1	1	2	3	3	4	5	5	6
0·46	2884	2891	2897	2904	2911	2917	2924	2931	2938	2944	1	1	2	3	3	4	5	5	6
0·47	2951	2958	2965	2972	2979	2985	2992	2999	3006	3013	1	1	2	3	3	4	5	5	6
0·48	3020	3027	3034	3041	3048	3055	3062	3069	3076	3083	1	1	2	3	4	4	5	6	6
0·49	3090	3097	3105	3112	3119	3126	3133	3141	3148	3155	1	1	2	3	4	4	5	6	6
0·50	3162	3170	3177	3184	3192	3199	3206	3214	3221	3228	1	1	2	3	4	4	5	6	7
0·51	3236	3243	3251	3258	3266	3273	3281	3289	3296	3304	1	2	2	3	4	5	5	6	7
0·52	3311	3319	3327	3334	3342	3350	3357	3365	3373	3381	1	2	2	3	4	5	5	6	7
0·53	3388	3396	3404	3412	3420	3428	3436	3443	3451	3459	1	2	2	3	4	5	6	6	7
0·54	3467	3475	3483	3491	3499	3508	3516	3524	3532	3540	1	2	2	3	4	5	6	6	7
0·55	3548	3556	3565	3573	3581	3589	3597	3606	3614	3622	1	2	2	3	4	5	6	7	7
0·56	3631	3639	3648	3656	3664	3673	3681	3690	3698	3707	1	2	3	3	4	5	6	7	8
0·57	3715	3724	3733	3741	3750	3758	3767	3776	3784	3793	1	2	3	3	4	5	6	7	8
0·58	3802	3811	3819	3828	3837	3846	3855	3864	3873	3882	1	2	3	4	4	5	6	7	8
0·59	3890	3899	3908	3917	3926	3936	3945	3954	3963	3972	1	2	3	4	5	5	6	7	8
0·60	3981	3990	3999	4009	4018	4027	4036	4046	4055	4064	1	2	3	4	5	6	6	7	8
0·61	4074	4083	4093	4102	4111	4121	4130	4140	4150	4159	1	2	3	4	5	6	7	8	9
0·62	4169	4178	4188	4198	4207	4217	4227	4236	4246	4256	1	2	3	4	5	6	7	8	9
0·63	4266	4276	4285	4295	4305	4315	4325	4335	4345	4355	1	2	3	4	5	6	7	8	9
0·64	4365	4375	4385	4395	4406	4416	4426	4436	4446	4457	1	2	3	4	5	6	7	8	9
0·65	4467	4477	4487	4498	4508	4519	4529	4539	4550	4560	1	2	3	4	5	6	7	8	9
0·66	4571	4581	4592	4603	4613	4624	4634	4645	4656	4667	1	2	3	4	5	6	7	9	10
0·67	4677	4688	4699	4710	4721	4732	4742	4753	4764	4775	1	2	3	4	5	7	8	9	10
0·68	4786	4797	4808	4819	4831	4842	4853	4864	4875	4887	1	2	3	4	6	7	8	9	10
0·69	4898	4909	4920	4932	4943	4955	4966	4977	4989	5000	1	2	3	5	6	7	8	9	10
0·70	5012	5023	5035	5047	5058	5070	5082	5093	5105	5117	1	2	4	5	6	7	8	9	11
0·71	5129	5140	5152	5164	5176	5188	5200	5212	5224	5236	1	2	4	5	6	7	8	10	11
0·72	5248	5260	5272	5284	5297	5309	5321	5333	5346	5358	1	2	4	5	6	7	9	10	11
0·73	5370	5383	5395	5408	5420	5433	5445	5458	5470	5483	1	3	4	5	6	8	9	10	11
0·74	5495	5508	5521	5534	5546	5559	5572	5585	5598	5610	1	3	4	5	6	8	9	10	12
0·75	5623	5636	5649	5662	5675	5689	5702	5715	5728	5741	1	3	4	5	7	8	9	10	12
0·76	5754	5768	5781	5794	5808	5821	5834	5848	5861	5875	1	3	4	5	7	8	9	11	12
0·77	5888	5902	5916	5929	5943	5957	5970	5984	5998	6012	1	3	4	5	7	8	10	11	12
0·78	6026	6039	6053	6067	6081	6095	6109	6124	6138	6152	1	3	4	6	7	8	10	11	13
0·79	6166	6180	6194	6209	6223	6237	6252	6266	6281	6295	1	3	4	6	7	9	10	11	13

Continued

Table B.9 Antilogarithm table (reprinted from *Geigy Scientific Tables*, 1982, with permission).

$\log_{10}x$	0	1	2	3	4	5	6	7	8	9	1	2	3	4	5	6	7	8	9
0·80	6310	6324	6339	6353	6368	6383	6397	6412	6427	6442	1	3	4	6	7	9	10	12	13
0·81	6457	6471	6486	6501	6516	6531	6546	6561	6577	6592	2	3	5	6	8	9	11	12	14
0·82	6607	6622	6637	6653	6668	6683	6699	6714	6730	6745	2	3	5	6	8	9	11	12	14
0·83	6761	6776	6792	6808	6823	6839	6855	6871	6887	6902	2	3	5	6	8	9	11	13	14
0·84	6918	6934	6950	6966	6982	6998	7015	7031	7047	7063	2	3	5	6	8	10	11	13	15
0·85	7079	7096	7112	7129	7145	7161	7178	7194	7211	7228	2	3	5	7	8	10	12	13	15
0·86	7244	7261	7278	7295	7311	7328	7345	7362	7379	7396	2	3	5	7	8	10	12	13	15
0·87	7413	7430	7447	7464	7482	7499	7516	7534	7551	7568	2	3	5	7	9	10	12	14	16
0·88	7586	7603	7621	7638	7656	7674	7691	7709	7727	7745	2	4	5	7	9	11	12	14	16
0·89	7762	7780	7798	7816	7834	7852	7870	7889	7907	7925	2	4	5	7	9	11	13	14	16
0·90	7943	7962	7980	7998	8017	8035	8054	8072	8091	8110	2	4	6	7	9	11	13	15	17
0·91	8128	8147	8166	8185	8204	8222	8241	8260	8279	8299	2	4	6	8	9	11	13	15	17
0·92	8318	8337	8356	8375	8395	8414	8433	8453	8472	8492	2	4	6	8	10	12	14	15	17
0·93	8511	8531	8551	8570	8590	8610	8630	8650	8670	8690	2	4	6	8	10	12	14	16	18
0·94	8710	8730	8750	8770	8790	8810	8831	8851	8872	8892	2	4	6	8	10	12	14	16	18
0·95	8913	8933	8954	8974	8995	9016	9036	9057	9078	9099	2	4	6	8	10	12	15	17	19
0·96	9120	9141	9162	9183	9204	9226	9247	9268	9290	9311	2	4	6	8	11	13	15	17	19
0·97	9333	9354	9376	9397	9419	9441	9462	9484	9506	9528	2	4	7	9	11	13	15	17	20
0·98	9550	9572	9594	9616	9638	9661	9683	9705	9727	9750	2	4	7	9	11	13	16	18	20
0·99	9772	9795	9817	9840	9863	9886	9908	9931	9954	9977	2	5	7	9	11	14	16	18	20

The column group headed *x* spans columns 0–9; the column group headed *Proportional parts* spans columns 1–9.

Table B.10 Spearman's rank correlation coefficient: critical values for the correlation coefficient r_S calculated on n pairs of observations (abbreviated from *Geigy Scientific Tables*, 1982, with permission).

Two-sided significance level	0·10	0·05	0·02	0·01
One-sided significance level	0·05	0·025	0·01	0·005
n	Critical values r_c			
4	0·9999	–	–	–
5	0·9000	0·9999	0·9999	–
6	0·8286	0·8857	0·9429	0·9999
7	0·7143	0·7857	0·8929	0·9286
8	0·6429	0·7381	0·8333	0·8810
9	0·6000	0·6833	0·7833	0·8333
10	0·5636	0·6485	0·7333	0·7939
11	0·5364	0·6182	0·7000	0·7545
12	0·5035	0·5874	0·6783	0·7343
13	0·4835	0·5604	0·6484	0·7033
14	0·4637	0·5385	0·6264	0·6791
15	0·4464	0·5214	0·6036	0·6571
16	0·4294	0·5029	0·5853	0·6353
17	0·4142	0·4877	0·5662	0·6176
18	0·4014	0·4737	0·5501	0·5996
19	0·3912	0·4596	0·5351	0·5842
20	0·3805	0·4466	0·5218	0·5699
21	0·3701	0·4364	0·5091	0·5558
22	0·3608	0·4252	0·4975	0·5438
23	0·3528	0·4160	0·4862	0·5316
24	0·3443	0·4070	0·4757	0·5209
25	0·3369	0·3985	0·4662	0·5108
26	0·3306	0·3901	0·4571	0·5009
27	0·3242	0·3828	0·4487	0·4921
28	0·3180	0·3755	0·4406	0·4833
29	0·3118	0·3690	0·4325	0·4749
30	0·3063	0·3624	0·4256	0·4670

Significant result if $r_S \geqslant r_c$ or $r_S \leqslant -r_c$

Table B.11 Exact confidence limits for a binomial proportion: x events are observed in a sample sized n. $p = x/n$ is the observed proportion. p_l and p_u are the lower and upper confidence limits for the population proportion.

Confidence level			95%		99%	
n	x	p	p_l	p_u	p_l	p_u
2	0	0·0000	0·0000	0·8419	0·0000	0·9293
	1	0·5000	0·0126	0·9874	0·0025	0·9975
	2	1·0000	0·1581	1·0000	0·0707	1·0000
3	0	0·0000	0·0000	0·7076	0·0000	0·8290
	1	0·3333	0·0084	0·9057	0·0017	0·9586
	2	0·6667	0·0943	0·9916	0·0414	0·9983
	3	1·0000	0·2924	1·0000	0·1710	1·0000
4	0	0·0000	0·0000	0·6024	0·0000	0·7341
	1	0·2500	0·0063	0·8059	0·0013	0·8891
	2	0·5000	0·0676	0·9324	0·0294	0·9706
	3	0·7500	0·1941	0·9937	0·1109	0·9987
	4	1·0000	0·3976	1·0000	0·2659	1·0000
5	0	0·0000	0·0000	0·5218	0·0000	0·6534
	1	0·2000	0·0051	0·7164	0·0010	0·8149
	2	0·4000	0·0527	0·8534	0·0229	0·9172
	3	0·6000	0·1466	0·9473	0·0828	0·9771
	4	0·8000	0·2836	0·9949	0·1851	0·9990
	5	1·0000	0·4782	1·0000	0·3466	1·0000
6	0	0·0000	0·0000	0·4593	0·0000	0·5865
	1	0·1667	0·0042	0·6412	0·0008	0·7460
	2	0·3333	0·0433	0·7772	0·0187	0·8564
	3	0·5000	0·1181	0·8819	0·0663	0·9337
	4	0·6667	0·2228	0·9567	0·1436	0·9813
	5	0·8333	0·3588	0·9958	0·2540	0·9992
	6	1·0000	0·5407	1·0000	0·4135	1·0000
7	0	0·0000	0·0000	0·4096	0·0000	0·5309
	1	0·1429	0·0036	0·5787	0·0007	0·6849
	2	0·2857	0·0367	0·7096	0·0158	0·7970
	3	0·4286	0·0990	0·8159	0·0553	0·8823
	4	0·5714	0·1841	0·9010	0·1177	0·9447
	5	0·7143	0·2904	0·9633	0·2030	0·9842
	6	0·8571	0·4213	0·9964	0·3151	0·9993
	7	1·0000	0·5904	1·0000	0·4691	1·0000
8	0	0·0000	0·0000	0·3694	0·0000	0·4843
	1	0·1250	0·0032	0·5265	0·0006	0·6315
	2	0·2500	0·0319	0·6509	0·0137	0·7422
	3	0·3750	0·0852	0·7551	0·0475	0·8303
	4	0·5000	0·1570	0·8430	0·0999	0·9001
	5	0·6250	0·2449	0·9148	0·1697	0·9525
	6	0·7500	0·3491	0·9681	0·2578	0·9863
	7	0·8750	0·4735	0·9968	0·3685	0·9994
	8	1·0000	0·6306	1·0000	0·5157	1·0000
9	0	0·0000	0·0000	0·3363	0·0000	0·4450
	1	0·1111	0·0028	0·4825	0·0006	0·5850
	2	0·2222	0·0281	0·6001	0·0121	0·6926
	3	0·3333	0·0749	0·7007	0·0416	0·7809

Confidence level			95%		99%	
n	x	p	p_l	p_u	p_l	p_u
9	4	0·4444	0·1370	0·7880	0·0868	0·8539
	5	0·5556	0·2120	0·8630	0·1461	0·9132
	6	0·6667	0·2993	0·9251	0·2191	0·9584
	7	0·7778	0·3999	0·9719	0·3074	0·9879
	8	0·8889	0·5175	0·9972	0·4150	0·9994
	9	1·0000	0·6637	1·0000	0·5550	1·0000
10	0	0·0000	0·0000	0·3085	0·0000	0·4113
	1	0·1000	0·0025	0·4450	0·0005	0·5443
	2	0·2000	0·0252	0·5561	0·0109	0·6482
	3	0·3000	0·0667	0·6525	0·0370	0·7351
	4	0·4000	0·1216	0·7376	0·0768	0·8091
	5	0·5000	0·1871	0·8129	0·1283	0·8717
	6	0·6000	0·2624	0·8784	0·1909	0·9232
	7	0·7000	0·3475	0·9333	0·2649	0·9630
	8	0·8000	0·4439	0·9748	0·3518	0·9891
	9	0·9000	0·5550	0·9975	0·4557	0·9995
	10	1·0000	0·6915	1·0000	0·5887	1·0000
11	0	0·0000	0·0000	0·2849	0·0000	0·3822
	1	0·0909	0·0023	0·4128	0·0005	0·5086
	2	0·1818	0·0228	0·5178	0·0098	0·6085
	3	0·2727	0·0602	0·6097	0·0333	0·6933
	4	0·3636	0·1093	0·6921	0·0688	0·7668
	5	0·4545	0·1675	0·7662	0·1145	0·8307
	6	0·5455	0·2338	0·8325	0·1693	0·8855
	7	0·6364	0·3079	0·8907	0·2332	0·9312
	8	0·7273	0·3903	0·9398	0·3067	0·9667
	9	0·8182	0·4822	0·9772	0·3915	0·9902
	10	0·9091	0·5872	0·9977	0·4914	0·9995
	11	1·0000	0·7151	1·0000	0·6178	1·0000
12	0	0·0000	0·0000	0·2646	0·0000	0·3569
	1	0·0833	0·0021	0·3848	0·0004	0·4770
	2	0·1667	0·0209	0·4841	0·0090	0·5729
	3	0·2500	0·0549	0·5719	0·0303	0·6552
	4	0·3333	0·0992	0·6511	0·0624	0·7275
	5	0·4167	0·1517	0·7233	0·1034	0·7915
	6	0·5000	0·2109	0·7891	0·1522	0·8478
	7	0·5833	0·2767	0·8483	0·2085	0·8966
	8	0·6667	0·3489	0·9008	0·2725	0·9376
	9	0·7500	0·4281	0·9451	0·3448	0·9697
	10	0·8333	0·5159	0·9791	0·4271	0·9910
	11	0·9167	0·6152	0·9979	0·5230	0·9996
	12	1·0000	0·7354	1·0000	0·6431	1·0000
13	0	0·0000	0·0000	0·2471	0·0000	0·3347
	1	0·0769	0·0019	0·3603	0·0004	0·4490
	2	0·1538	0·0192	0·4545	0·0083	0·5410
	3	0·2308	0·0504	0·5381	0·0278	0·6206
	4	0·3077	0·0909	0·6143	0·0571	0·6913
	5	0·3846	0·1386	0·6842	0·0942	0·7546

Continued

Table B.11 Exact confidence limits for a binomial proportion: x events are observed in a sample sized n. $p = x/n$ is the observed proportion. p_l and p_u are the lower and upper confidence limits for the population proportion.

Confidence level			95%		99%	
n	x	p	p_l	p_u	p_l	p_u
13	6	0·4615	0·1922	0·7487	0·1383	0·8113
	7	0·5385	0·2513	0·8078	0·1887	0·8617
	8	0·6154	0·3158	0·8614	0·2454	0·9058
	9	0·6923	0·3857	0·9091	0·3087	0·9429
	10	0·7692	0·4619	0·9496	0·3794	0·9722
	11	0·8462	0·5455	0·9808	0·4590	0·9917
	12	0·9231	0·6397	0·9981	0·5510	0·9996
	13	1·0000	0·7529	1·0000	0·6653	1·0000
14	0	0·0000	0·0000	0·2316	0·0000	0·3151
	1	0·0714	0·0018	0·3387	0·0004	0·4240
	2	0·1429	0·0178	0·4281	0·0076	0·5123
	3	0·2143	0·0466	0·5080	0·0257	0·5892
	4	0·2857	0·0839	0·5810	0·0526	0·6579
	5	0·3571	0·1276	0·6486	0·0866	0·7201
	6	0·4286	0·1766	0·7114	0·1267	0·7766
	7	0·5000	0·2304	0·7696	0·1724	0·8276
	8	0·5714	0·2886	0·8234	0·2234	0·8733
	9	0·6429	0·3514	0·8724	0·2799	0·9134
	10	0·7143	0·4190	0·9161	0·3421	0·9474
	11	0·7857	0·4920	0·9534	0·4108	0·9743
	12	0·8571	0·5719	0·9822	0·4877	0·9924
	13	0·9286	0·6613	0·9982	0·5760	0·9996
	14	1·0000	0·7684	1·0000	0·6849	1·0000
15	0	0·0000	0·0000	0·2180	0·0000	0·2976
	1	0·0667	0·0017	0·3195	0·0003	0·4016
	2	0·1333	0·0166	0·4046	0·0071	0·4863
	3	0·2000	0·0433	0·4809	0·0239	0·5605
	4	0·2667	0·0779	0·5510	0·0488	0·6273
	5	0·3333	0·1182	0·6162	0·0801	0·6882
	6	0·4000	0·1634	0·6771	0·1170	0·7439
	7	0·4667	0·2127	0·7341	0·1587	0·7949
	8	0·5333	0·2659	0·7873	0·2051	0·8413
	9	0·6000	0·3229	0·8366	0·2561	0·8830
	10	0·6667	0·3838	0·8818	0·3118	0·9199
	11	0·7333	0·4490	0·9221	0·3727	0·9512
	12	0·8000	0·5191	0·9567	0·4395	0·9761
	13	0·8667	0·5954	0·9834	0·5137	0·9929
	14	0·9333	0·6805	0·9983	0·5984	0·9997
	15	1·0000	0·7820	1·0000	0·7024	1·0000
16	0	0·0000	0·0000	0·2059	0·0000	0·2819
	1	0·0625	0·0016	0·3023	0·0003	0·3814
	2	0·1250	0·0155	0·3835	0·0067	0·4628
	3	0·1875	0·0405	0·4565	0·0223	0·5344
	4	0·2500	0·0727	0·5238	0·0455	0·5991
	5	0·3125	0·1102	0·5866	0·0745	0·6585
	6	0·3750	0·1520	0·6457	0·1086	0·7132
	7	0·4375	0·1975	0·7012	0·1471	0·7638
	8	0·5000	0·2465	0·7535	0·1897	0·8103

Confidence level			95%		99%	
n	x	p	p_l	p_u	p_l	p_u
16	9	0·5625	0·2988	0·8025	0·2362	0·8529
	10	0·6250	0·3543	0·8480	0·2868	0·8914
	11	0·6875	0·4134	0·8898	0·3415	0·9255
	12	0·7500	0·4762	0·9273	0·4009	0·9545
	13	0·8125	0·5435	0·9595	0·4656	0·9777
	14	0·8750	0·6165	0·9845	0·5372	0·9933
	15	0·9375	0·6977	0·9984	0·6186	0·9997
	16	1·0000	0·7941	1·0000	0·7181	1·0000
17	0	0·0000	0·0000	0·1951	0·0000	0·2678
	1	0·0588	0·0015	0·2869	0·0003	0·3630
	2	0·1176	0·0146	0·3644	0·0063	0·4413
	3	0·1765	0·0380	0·4343	0·0209	0·5104
	4	0·2353	0·0681	0·4990	0·0426	0·5732
	5	0·2941	0·1031	0·5596	0·0697	0·6310
	6	0·3529	0·1421	0·6167	0·1014	0·6846
	7	0·4118	0·1844	0·6708	0·1371	0·7344
	8	0·4706	0·2298	0·7219	0·1764	0·7807
	9	0·5294	0·2781	0·7702	0·2193	0·8236
	10	0·5882	0·3292	0·8156	0·2656	0·8629
	11	0·6471	0·3833	0·8579	0·3154	0·8986
	12	0·7059	0·4404	0·8969	0·3690	0·9303
	13	0·7647	0·5010	0·9319	0·4268	0·9574
	14	0·8235	0·5657	0·9620	0·4896	0·9791
	15	0·8824	0·6356	0·9854	0·5587	0·9937
	16	0·9412	0·7131	0·9985	0·6370	0·9997
	17	1·0000	0·8049	1·0000	0·7322	1·0000
18	0	0·0000	0·0000	0·1853	0·0000	0·2550
	1	0·0556	0·0014	0·2729	0·0003	0·3463
	2	0·1111	0·0138	0·3471	0·0059	0·4217
	3	0·1667	0·0358	0·4142	0·0197	0·4884
	4	0·2222	0·0641	0·4764	0·0400	0·5492
	5	0·2778	0·0969	0·5348	0·0654	0·6055
	6	0·3333	0·1334	0·5901	0·0951	0·6579
	7	0·3889	0·1730	0·6425	0·1284	0·7068
	8	0·4444	0·2153	0·6924	0·1649	0·7526
	9	0·5000	0·2602	0·7398	0·2047	0·7953
	10	0·5556	0·3076	0·7847	0·2474	0·8351
	11	0·6111	0·3575	0·8270	0·2932	0·8716
	12	0·6667	0·4099	0·8666	0·3421	0·9049
	13	0·7222	0·4652	0·9031	0·3945	0·9346
	14	0·7778	0·5236	0·9359	0·4508	0·9600
	15	0·8333	0·5858	0·9642	0·5116	0·9803
	16	0·8889	0·6529	0·9862	0·5783	0·9941
	17	0·9444	0·7271	0·9986	0·6537	0·9997
	18	1·0000	0·8147	1·0000	0·7450	1·0000
19	0	0·0000	0·0000	0·1765	0·0000	0·2434
	1	0·0526	0·0013	0·2603	0·0003	0·3311
	2	0·1053	0·0130	0·3314	0·0056	0·4037
	3	0·1579	0·0338	0·3958	0·0186	0·4682

Continued

Table B.11 Exact confidence limits for a binomial proportion: x events are observed in a sample sized n. $p = x/n$ is the observed proportion. p_l and p_u are the lower and upper confidence limits for the population proportion.

Confidence level			95%		99%	
n	x	p	p_l	p_u	p_l	p_u
19	4	0·2105	0·0605	0·4557	0·0378	0·5271
	5	0·2632	0·0915	0·5120	0·0617	0·5818
	6	0·3158	0·1258	0·5655	0·0895	0·6329
	7	0·3684	0·1629	0·6164	0·1207	0·6809
	8	0·4211	0·2025	0·6650	0·1549	0·7260
	9	0·4737	0·2445	0·7114	0·1919	0·7684
	10	0·5263	0·2886	0·7555	0·2316	0·8081
	11	0·5789	0·3350	0·7975	0·2740	0·8451
	12	0·6316	0·3836	0·8371	0·3191	0·8793
	13	0·6842	0·4345	0·8742	0·3671	0·9105
	14	0·7368	0·4880	0·9085	0·4182	0·9383
	15	0·7895	0·5443	0·9395	0·4729	0·9622
	16	0·8421	0·6042	0·9662	0·5318	0·9814
	17	0·8974	0·6686	0·9870	0·5963	0·9944
	18	0·9474	0·7397	0·9987	0·6689	0·9997
	19	1·0000	0·8235	1·0000	0·7566	1·0000
20	0	0·0000	0·0000	0·1684	0·0000	0·2327
	1	0·0500	0·0013	0·2487	0·0003	0·3171
	2	0·1000	0·0123	0·3170	0·0053	0·3871
	3	0·1500	0·0321	0·3789	0·0176	0·4495
	4	0·2000	0·0573	0·4366	0·0358	0·5066
	5	0·2500	0·0866	0·4910	0·0583	0·5598
	6	0·3000	0·1189	0·5428	0·0846	0·6096
	7	0·3500	0·1539	0·5922	0·1139	0·6566
	8	0·4000	0·1912	0·6395	0·1460	0·7009
	9	0·4500	0·2306	0·6847	0·1806	0·7428
	10	0·5000	0·2720	0·7280	0·2177	0·7823
	11	0·5500	0·3153	0·7694	0·2572	0·8194
	12	0·6000	0·3605	0·8088	0·2991	0·8540
	13	0·6500	0·4078	0·8461	0·3434	0·8861
	14	0·7000	0·4572	0·8811	0·3904	0·9154
	15	0·7500	0·5090	0·9134	0·4402	0·9417
	16	0·8000	0·5634	0·9427	0·4934	0·9642
	17	0·8500	0·6211	0·9679	0·5505	0·9824
	18	0·9000	0·6830	0·9877	0·6129	0·9947
	19	0·9500	0·7513	0·9987	0·6829	0·9997
	20	1·0000	0·8316	1·0000	0·7673	1·0000
21	0	0·0000	0·0000	0·1611	0·0000	0·2230
	1	0·0476	0·0012	0·2382	0·0002	0·3043
	2	0·0952	0·0117	0·3038	0·0050	0·3718
	3	0·1429	0·0305	0·3634	0·0168	0·4322
	4	0·1905	0·0545	0·4191	0·0339	0·4876
	5	0·2381	0·0822	0·4717	0·0553	0·5392
	6	0·2857	0·1128	0·5218	0·0801	0·5878
	7	0·3333	0·1459	0·5697	0·1078	0·6337
	8	0·3810	0·1811	0·6156	0·1381	0·6772
	9	0·4286	0·2182	0·6598	0·1707	0·7185
	10	0·4762	0·2571	0·7022	0·2055	0·7576

Confidence level			95%		99%	
n	x	p	p_l	p_u	p_l	p_u
21	11	0·5238	0·2978	0·7429	0·2424	0·7945
	12	0·5714	0·3402	0·7818	0·2815	0·8293
	13	0·6190	0·3844	0·8189	0·3228	0·8619
	14	0·6667	0·4303	0·8541	0·3663	0·8922
	15	0·7143	0·4782	0·8872	0·4122	0·9199
	16	0·7619	0·5283	0·9178	0·4608	0·9447
	17	0·8095	0·5809	0·9455	0·5124	0·9661
	18	0·8571	0·6366	0·9695	0·5678	0·9832
	19	0·9048	0·6962	0·9883	0·6282	0·9950
	20	0·9524	0·7618	0·9988	0·6957	0·9998
	21	1·0000	0·8389	1·0000	0·7770	1·0000
22	0	0·0000	0·0000	0·1544	0·0000	0·2140
	1	0·0455	0·0012	0·2284	0·0002	0·2924
	2	0·0909	0·0112	0·2916	0·0048	0·3577
	3	0·1364	0·0291	0·3491	0·0160	0·4161
	4	0·1818	0·0519	0·4028	0·0323	0·4699
	5	0·2273	0·0782	0·4537	0·0526	0·5201
	6	0·2727	0·1073	0·5022	0·0761	0·5674
	7	0·3182	0·1386	0·5487	0·1024	0·6123
	8	0·3636	0·1720	0·5934	0·1310	0·6549
	9	0·4091	0·2071	0·6365	0·1618	0·6954
	10	0·4545	0·2439	0·6779	0·1946	0·7340
	11	0·5000	0·2822	0·7178	0·2293	0·7707
	12	0·5455	0·3221	0·7561	0·2660	0·8054
	13	0·5909	0·3635	0·7929	0·3046	0·8382
	14	0·6364	0·4066	0·8280	0·3451	0·8690
	15	0·6818	0·4513	0·8614	0·3877	0·8976
	16	0·7273	0·4978	0·8927	0·4326	0·9239
	17	0·7727	0·5463	0·9218	0·4799	0·9474
	18	0·8182	0·5972	0·9481	0·5301	0·9677
	19	0·8636	0·6509	0·9709	0·5839	0·9840
	20	0·9091	0·7084	0·9888	0·6423	0·9952
	21	0·9545	0·7716	0·9988	0·7076	0·9998
	22	1·0000	0·8456	0·0000	0·7860	1·0000
23	0	0·0000	0·0000	0·1482	0·0000	0·2058
	1	0·0435	0·0011	0·2195	0·0002	0·2814
	2	0·0870	0·0107	0·2804	0·0046	0·3446
	3	0·1304	0·0278	0·3359	0·0153	0·4012
	4	0·1739	0·0495	0·3878	0·0308	0·4534
	5	0·2174	0·0746	0·4370	0·0502	0·5022
	6	0·2609	0·1023	0·4841	0·0725	0·5483
	7	0·3043	0·1321	0·5292	0·0974	0·5921
	8	0·3478	0·1638	0·5727	0·1246	0·6338
	9	0·3913	0·1971	0·6146	0·1537	0·6736
	10	0·4348	0·2319	0·6551	0·1848	0·7116
	11	0·4783	0·2682	0·6941	0·2176	0·7479
	12	0·5217	0·3059	0·7318	0·2521	0·7824
	13	0·5652	0·3449	0·7681	0·2884	0·8152
	14	0·6087	0·3854	0·8029	0·3264	0·8463

Continued

Table B.11 Exact confidence limits for a binomial proportion: x events are observed in a sample sized n. $p = x/n$ is the observed proportion. p_l and p_u are the lower and upper confidence limits for the population proportion.

Confidence level			95%		99%	
n	x	p	p_l	p_u	p_l	p_u
23	15	0·6522	0·4273	0·8362	0·3662	0·8754
	16	0·6957	0·4708	0·8679	0·4079	0·9026
	17	0·7391	0·5159	0·8977	0·4517	0·9275
	18	0·7826	0·5630	0·9254	0·4978	0·9498
	19	0·8261	0·6122	0·9505	0·5466	0·9692
	20	0·8696	0·6641	0·9722	0·5988	0·9847
	21	0·9130	0·7196	0·9893	0·6554	0·9954
	22	0·9565	0·7805	0·9989	0·7186	0·9998
	23	1·0000	0·8518	1·0000	0·7942	1·0000
24	0	0·0000	0·0000	0·1425	0·0000	0·1981
	1	0·0417	0·0011	0·2112	0·0002	0·2713
	2	0·0833	0·0103	0·2700	0·0044	0·3324
	3	0·1250	0·0266	0·3236	0·0146	0·3873
	4	0·1667	0·0474	0·3738	0·0295	0·4379
	5	0·2083	0·0713	0·4215	0·0479	0·4855
	6	0·2500	0·0977	0·4671	0·0692	0·5304
	7	0·2917	0·1262	0·5109	0·0930	0·5732
	8	0·3333	0·1563	0·5532	0·1188	0·6140
	9	0·3750	0·1880	0·5941	0·1465	0·6530
	10	0·4167	0·2211	0·6336	0·1759	0·6904
	11	0·4583	0·2555	0·6718	0·2070	0·7262
	12	0·5000	0·2912	0·7088	0·2396	0·7604
	13	0·5417	0·3282	0·7445	0·2738	0·7930
	14	0·5833	0·3664	0·7789	0·3096	0·8241
	15	0·6250	0·4059	0·8120	0·3470	0·8535
	16	0·6667	0·4468	0·8437	0·3860	0·8812
	17	0·7083	0·4891	0·8738	0·4268	0·9070
	18	0·7500	0·5329	0·9023	0·4696	0·9308
	19	0·7917	0·5785	0·9287	0·5145	0·9521
	20	0·8333	0·6262	0·9526	0·5621	0·9705
	21	0·8750	0·6764	0·9734	0·6127	0·9854
	22	0·9167	0·7300	0·9897	0·6676	0·9956
	23	0·9583	0·7888	0·9989	0·7287	0·9998
	24	1·0000	0·8575	1·0000	0·8019	1·0000
25	0	0·0000	0·0000	0·1372	0·0000	0·1910
	1	0·0400	0·0010	0·2035	0·0002	0·2618
	2	0·0800	0·0098	0·2603	0·0042	0·3210
	3	0·1200	0·0255	0·3122	0·0140	0·3743
	4	0·1600	0·0454	0·3608	0·0282	0·4235
	5	0·2000	0·0683	0·4070	0·0459	0·4698
	6	0·2400	0·0936	0·4513	0·0663	0·5136
	7	0·2800	0·1207	0·4939	0·0889	0·5553
	8	0·3200	0·1495	0·5350	0·1135	0·5952
	9	0·3600	0·1797	0·5748	0·1399	0·6335
	10	0·4000	0·2113	0·6133	0·1679	0·6702
	11	0·4400	0·2440	0·6507	0·1974	0·7054
	12	0·4800	0·2780	0·6869	0·2283	0·7393
	13	0·5200	0·3131	0·7220	0·2607	0·7717

Confidence level			95%		99%	
n	x	p	p_l	p_u	p_l	p_u
25	14	0·5600	0·3493	0·7560	0·2946	0·8026
	15	0·6000	0·3867	0·7887	0·3298	0·8321
	16	0·6400	0·4252	0·8203	0·3665	0·8601
	17	0·6800	0·4650	0·8505	0·4048	0·8865
	18	0·7200	0·5061	0·8793	0·4447	0·9111
	19	0·7600	0·5487	0·9064	0·4864	0·9337
	20	0·8000	0·5930	0·9317	0·5302	0·9541
	21	0·8400	0·6392	0·9546	0·5765	0·9718
	22	0·8800	0·6878	0·9745	0·6257	0·9860
	23	0·9200	0·7397	0·9902	0·6790	0·9958
	24	0·9600	0·7965	0·9990	0·7382	0·9998
	25	1·0000	0·8628	1·0000	0·8090	1·0000
26	0	0·0000	0·0000	0·1323	0·0000	0·1844
	1	0·0385	0·0010	0·1964	0·0002	0·2529
	2	0·0769	0·0095	0·2513	0·0041	0·3104
	3	0·1154	0·0245	0·3015	0·0134	0·3621
	4	0·1538	0·0436	0·3487	0·0271	0·4100
	5	0·1923	0·0655	0·3935	0·0440	0·4550
	6	0·2308	0·0897	0·4365	0·0635	0·4977
	7	0·2692	0·1157	0·4779	0·0852	0·5385
	8	0·3077	0·1433	0·5179	0·1087	0·5775
	9	0·3462	0·1721	0·5567	0·1338	0·6150
	10	0·3846	0·2023	0·5943	0·1605	0·6510
	11	0·4231	0·2335	0·6308	0·1886	0·6857
	12	0·4615	0·2659	0·6663	0·2181	0·7191
	13	0·5000	0·2993	0·7007	0·2489	0·7511
	14	0·5385	0·3337	0·7341	0·2809	0·7819
	15	0·5769	0·3692	0·7665	0·3143	0·8114
	16	0·6154	0·4057	0·7977	0·3490	0·8395
	17	0·6538	0·4433	0·8279	0·3850	0·8662
	18	0·6923	0·4821	0·8567	0·4225	0·8913
	19	0·7308	0·5221	0·8843	0·4615	0·9148
	20	0·7692	0·5635	0·9103	0·5023	0·9365
	21	0·8077	0·6065	0·9345	0·5450	0·9560
	22	0·8462	0·6513	0·9564	0·5900	0·9729
	23	0·8846	0·6985	0·9775	0·6379	0·9866
	24	0·9231	0·7487	0·9905	0·6896	0·9959
	25	0·9615	0·8036	0·9990	0·7471	0·9998
	26	1·0000	0·8677	1·0000	0·8156	1·0000
27	0	0·0000	0·0000	0·1277	0·0000	0·1782
	1	0·0370	0·0009	0·1897	0·0002	0·2446
	2	0·0741	0·0091	0·2429	0·0039	0·3004
	3	0·1111	0·0235	0·2916	0·0129	0·3507
	4	0·1481	0·0419	0·3373	0·0260	0·3973
	5	0·1852	0·0630	0·3808	0·0423	0·4411
	6	0·2222	0·0862	0·4226	0·0610	0·4828
	7	0·2593	0·1111	0·4628	0·0817	0·5226
	8	0·2963	0·1375	0·5018	0·1042	0·5608
	9	0·3333	0·1652	0·5396	0·1283	0·5975

Continued

Table B.11 Exact confidence limits for a binomial proportion: x events are observed in a sample sized n. $p = x/n$ is the observed proportion. p_l and p_u are the lower and upper confidence limits for the population proportion.

Confidence level			95%		99%	
n	x	p	p_l	p_u	p_l	p_u
27	10	0·3704	0·1940	0·5763	0·1538	0·6328
	11	0·4074	0·2239	0·6120	0·1807	0·6669
	12	0·4444	0·2548	0·6467	0·2088	0·6998
	13	0·4815	0·2867	0·6805	0·2381	0·7314
	14	0·5185	0·3195	0·7133	0·2686	0·7619
	15	0·5556	0·3533	0·7452	0·3002	0·7912
	16	0·5926	0·3880	0·7761	0·3331	0·8193
	17	0·6296	0·4237	0·8060	0·3672	0·8462
	18	0·6667	0·4604	0·8348	0·4025	0·8717
	19	0·7037	0·4982	0·8625	0·4392	0·8958
	20	0·7407	0·5372	0·8889	0·4774	0·9183
	21	0·7778	0·5774	0·9138	0·5172	0·9390
	22	0·8148	0·6192	0·9370	0·5589	0·9577
	23	0·8519	0·6627	0·9581	0·6027	0·9740
	24	0·8889	0·7084	0·9765	0·6493	0·9871
	25	0·9259	0·7571	0·9909	0·6996	0·9961
	26	0·9630	0·8103	0·9991	0·7554	0·9998
	27	1·0000	0·8723	1·0000	0·8218	1·0000
28	0	0·0000	0·0000	0·1234	0·0000	0·1724
	1	0·0357	0·0009	0·1835	0·0002	0·2369
	2	0·0714	0·0088	0·2350	0·0038	0·2911
	3	0·1071	0·0227	0·2823	0·0124	0·3399
	4	0·1429	0·0403	0·3267	0·0251	0·3853
	5	0·1786	0·0606	0·3689	0·0407	0·4280
	6	0·2143	0·0830	0·4095	0·0586	0·4687
	7	0·2500	0·1069	0·4487	0·0786	0·5076
	8	0·2857	0·1322	0·4867	0·1002	0·5449
	9	0·3214	0·1588	0·5235	0·1232	0·5808
	10	0·3571	0·1864	0·5593	0·1477	0·6155
	11	0·3929	0·2150	0·5942	0·1733	0·6490
	12	0·4286	0·2446	0·6282	0·2002	0·6814
	13	0·4643	0·2751	0·6613	0·2282	0·7126
	14	0·5000	0·3065	0·6935	0·2572	0·7428
	15	0·5357	0·3387	0·7249	0·2874	0·7718
	16	0·5714	0·3718	0·7554	0·3186	0·7998
	17	0·6071	0·4058	0·7850	0·3510	0·8267
	18	0·6429	0·4407	0·8136	0·3845	0·8523
	19	0·6786	0·4765	0·8412	0·4192	0·8768
	20	0·7143	0·5133	0·8678	0·4551	0·8998
	21	0·7500	0·5513	0·8931	0·4924	0·9214
	22	0·7857	0·5905	0·9170	0·5313	0·9414
	23	0·8214	0·6311	0·9394	0·5720	0·9593
	24	0·8571	0·6733	0·9597	0·6147	0·9749
	25	0·8929	0·7177	0·9773	0·6601	0·9876
	26	0·9286	0·7650	0·9912	0·7089	0·9962
	27	0·9643	0·8165	0·9991	0·7631	0·9998
	28	1·0000	0·8766	1·0000	0·8276	1·0000
29	0	0·0000	0·0000	0·1194	0·0000	0·1670
	1	0·0345	0·0009	0·1776	0·0002	0·2296

n	x	p	95% p_l	p_u	99% p_l	p_u
29	2	0·0690	0·0085	0·2277	0·0036	0·2823
	3	0·1034	0·0219	0·2735	0·0120	0·3298
	4	0·1379	0·0389	0·3166	0·0242	0·3740
	5	0·1724	0·0585	0·3577	0·0392	0·4157
	6	0·2069	0·0799	0·3972	0·0565	0·4554
	7	0·2414	0·1030	0·4354	0·0756	0·4933
	8	0·2759	0·1273	0·4724	0·0964	0·5299
	9	0·3103	0·1528	0·5083	0·1185	0·5651
	10	0·3448	0·1794	0·5433	0·1420	0·5991
	11	0·3793	0·2069	0·5774	0·1666	0·6320
	12	0·4138	0·2352	0·6106	0·1923	0·6638
	13	0·4483	0·2645	0·6431	0·2191	0·6946
	14	0·4828	0·2945	0·6747	0·2469	0·7243
	15	0·5172	0·3253	0·7055	0·2757	0·7531
	16	0·5517	0·3569	0·7355	0·3054	0·7809
	17	0·5862	0·3894	0·7648	0·3362	0·8077
	18	0·6207	0·4226	0·7931	0·3680	0·8334
	19	0·6552	0·4567	0·8206	0·4009	0·8580
	20	0·6897	0·4917	0·8472	0·4349	0·8815
	21	0·7241	0·5276	0·8727	0·4701	0·9036
	22	0·7586	0·5646	0·8970	0·5067	0·9244
	23	0·7931	0·6028	0·9201	0·5446	0·9435
	24	0·8276	0·6423	0·9415	0·5843	0·9608
	25	0·8621	0·6834	0·9611	0·6260	0·9758
	26	0·8966	0·7265	0·9781	0·6702	0·9880
	27	0·9310	0·7723	0·9915	0·7177	0·9964
	28	0·9655	0·8224	0·9991	0·7704	0·9998
	29	1·0000	0·8806	1·0000	0·8330	1·0000
30	0	0·0000	0·0000	0·1157	0·0000	0·1619
	1	0·0333	0·0008	0·1722	0·0002	0·2228
	2	0·0667	0·0082	0·2207	0·0035	0·2740
	3	0·1000	0·0211	0·2653	0·0116	0·3203
	4	0·1333	0·0376	0·3072	0·0233	0·3634
	5	0·1667	0·0564	0·3472	0·0378	0·4040
	6	0·2000	0·0771	0·3857	0·0545	0·4428
	7	0·2333	0·0993	0·4228	0·0729	0·4799
	8	0·2667	0·1228	0·4589	0·0929	0·5156
	9	0·3000	0·1473	0·4940	0·1142	0·5501
	10	0·3333	0·1729	0·5281	0·1367	0·5834
	11	0·3667	0·1993	0·5614	0·1604	0·6157
	12	0·4000	0·2266	0·5940	0·1850	0·6470
	13	0·4333	0·2546	0·6257	0·2107	0·6773
	14	0·4667	0·2834	0·6567	0·2373	0·7067
	15	0·5000	0·3130	0·6870	0·2648	0·7352
	16	0·5333	0·3433	0·7166	0·2933	0·7627
	17	0·5667	0·3743	0·7454	0·3227	0·7893
	18	0·6000	0·4060	0·7734	0·3530	0·8150
	19	0·6333	0·4386	0·8007	0·3843	0·8396
	20	0·6667	0·4719	0·8271	0·4166	0·8633

Continued

Table B.11 Exact confidence limits for a binomial proportion: x events are observed in a sample sized n. $p = x/n$ is the observed proportion. p_l and p_u are the lower and upper confidence limits for the population proportion.

Confidence level			95%		99%	
n	x	p	p_l	p_u	p_l	p_u
30	21	0·7000	0·5060	0·8527	0·4499	0·8858
	22	0·7333	0·5411	0·8772	0·4844	0·9071
	23	0·7667	0·5772	0·9007	0·5201	0·9271
	24	0·8000	0·6143	0·9229	0·5572	0·9455
	25	0·8333	0·6528	0·9436	0·5960	0·9622
	26	0·8667	0·6928	0·9624	0·6366	0·9767
	27	0·9000	0·7347	0·9789	0·6797	0·9884
	28	0·9333	0·7793	0·9918	0·7260	0·9965
	29	0·9667	0·8278	0·9992	0·7772	0·9998
	30	1·0000	0·8843	1·0000	0·8381	1·0000
31	0	0·0000	0·0000	0·1122	0·0000	0·1571
	1	0·0323	0·0008	0·1670	0·0002	0·2163
	2	0·0645	0·0079	0·2142	0·0034	0·2662
	3	0·0968	0·0204	0·2575	0·0112	0·3113
	4	0·1290	0·0363	0·2983	0·0225	0·3533
	5	0·1613	0·0545	0·3373	0·0365	0·3930
	6	0·1935	0·0745	0·3747	0·0526	0·4308
	7	0·2258	0·0959	0·4110	0·0704	0·4671
	8	0·2581	0·1186	0·4461	0·0896	0·5021
	9	0·2903	0·1422	0·4804	0·1102	0·5358
	10	0·3226	0·1668	0·5137	0·1318	0·5685
	11	0·3548	0·1923	0·5463	0·1546	0·6002
	12	0·3871	0·2185	0·5781	0·1783	0·6309
	13	0·4194	0·2455	0·6092	0·2029	0·6608
	14	0·4516	0·2732	0·6397	0·2285	0·6898
	15	0·4839	0·3015	0·6694	0·2549	0·7179
	16	0·5161	0·3306	0·6985	0·2821	0·7451
	17	0·5484	0·3603	0·7268	0·3102	0·7715
	18	0·5806	0·3908	0·7545	0·3392	0·7971
	19	0·6129	0·4219	0·7815	0·3691	0·8217
	20	0·6452	0·4537	0·8077	0·3998	0·8454
	21	0·6774	0·4863	0·8332	0·4315	0·8682
	22	0·7097	0·5196	0·8578	0·4642	0·8898
	23	0·7419	0·5539	0·8814	0·4979	0·9104
	24	0·7742	0·5890	0·9041	0·5329	0·9296
	25	0·8065	0·6253	0·9255	0·5692	0·9474
	26	0·8387	0·6627	0·9455	0·6070	0·9635
	27	0·8710	0·7017	0·9637	0·6467	0·9775
	28	0·9032	0·7425	0·9796	0·6887	0·9888
	29	0·9355	0·7858	0·9921	0·7338	0·9966
	30	0·9677	0·8330	0·9992	0·7837	0·9998
	31	1·0000	0·8878	1·0000	0·8429	1·0000
32	0	0·0000	0·0000	0·1089	0·0000	0·1526
	1	0·0313	0·0008	0·1622	0·0002	0·2102
	2	0·0625	0·0077	0·2081	0·0033	0·2588
	3	0·0938	0·0198	0·2502	0·0108	0·3028
	4	0·1250	0·0351	0·2899	0·0218	0·3438
	5	0·1563	0·0528	0·3279	0·0353	0·3825

Table B.11 (*Continued*)

			95%		99%	
n	*x*	*p*	p_l	p_u	p_l	p_u
32	6	0·1875	0·0721	0·3644	0·0509	0·4195
	7	0·2188	0·0928	0·3997	0·0680	0·4550
	8	0·2500	0·1146	0·4340	0·0866	0·4892
	9	0·2813	0·1375	0·4675	0·1064	0·5223
	10	0·3125	0·1612	0·5001	0·1273	0·5543
	11	0·3438	0·1857	0·5319	0·1492	0·5854
	12	0·3750	0·2110	0·5631	0·1720	0·6156
	13	0·4063	0·2370	0·5936	0·1957	0·6450
	14	0·4375	0·2636	0·6234	0·2203	0·6735
	15	0·4688	0·2909	0·6526	0·2456	0·7013
	16	0·5000	0·3189	0·6811	0·2718	0·7282
	17	0·5313	0·3474	0·7091	0·2987	0·7544
	18	0·5625	0·3766	0·7364	0·3265	0·7797
	19	0·5938	0·4064	0·7630	0·3550	0·8043
	20	0·6250	0·4369	0·7890	0·3844	0·8280
	21	0·6563	0·4681	0·8143	0·4146	0·8508
	22	0·6875	0·4999	0·8388	0·4457	0·8727
	23	0·7188	0·5325	0·8625	0·4777	0·8936
	24	0·7500	0·5660	0·8854	0·5108	0·9134
	25	0·7813	0·6003	0·9072	0·5450	0·9320
	26	0·8125	0·6356	0·9279	0·5805	0·9491
	27	0·8438	0·6721	0·9472	0·6175	0·9647
	28	0·8750	0·7101	0·9649	0·6562	0·9782
	29	0·9063	0·7498	0·9802	0·6972	0·9892
	30	0·9375	0·7919	0·9923	0·7412	0·9967
	31	0·9688	0·8378	0·9992	0·7898	0·9998
	32	1·0000	0·8911	1·0000	0·8474	1·0000
33	0	0·0000	0·0000	0·1058	0·0000	0·1483
	1	0·0303	0·0008	0·1576	0·0002	0·2044
	2	0·0606	0·0074	0·2023	0·0032	0·2518
	3	0·0909	0·0192	0·2433	0·0105	0·2947
	4	0·1212	0·0340	0·2820	0·0211	0·3347
	5	0·1515	0·0511	0·3190	0·0342	0·3726
	6	0·1818	0·0698	0·3546	0·0492	0·4087
	7	0·2121	0·0898	0·3891	0·0658	0·4434
	8	0·2424	0·1109	0·4226	0·0838	0·4769
	9	0·2727	0·1330	0·4552	0·1029	0·5093
	10	0·3030	0·1559	0·4871	0·1231	0·5408
	11	0·3333	0·1796	0·5183	0·1442	0·5713
	12	0·3636	0·2040	0·5488	0·1662	0·6010
	13	0·3939	0·2291	0·5786	0·1890	0·6298
	14	0·4242	0·2548	0·6078	0·2127	0·6579
	15	0·4545	0·2811	0·6365	0·2371	0·6853
	16	0·4848	0·3080	0·6646	0·2622	0·7119
	17	0·5152	0·3354	0·6920	0·2881	0·7378
	18	0·5455	0·3635	0·7189	0·3147	0·7629
	19	0·5758	0·3922	0·7452	0·3421	0·7873
	20	0·6061	0·4214	0·7709	0·3702	0·8110
	21	0·6364	0·4512	0·7960	0·3990	0·8338
	22	0·6667	0·4817	0·8204	0·4287	0·8558

Continued

Table B.11 Exact confidence limits for a binomial proportion: x events are observed in a sample sized n. $p = x/n$ is the observed proportion. p_l and p_u are the lower and upper confidence limits for the population proportion.

Confidence level			95%		99%	
n	x	p	p_l	p_u	p_l	p_u
33	23	0·6970	0·5129	0·8441	0·4592	0·8769
	24	0·7273	0·5448	0·8670	0·4907	0·8971
	25	0·7576	0·5774	0·8891	0·5231	0·9162
	26	0·7879	0·6109	0·9102	0·5566	0·9342
	27	0·8182	0·6454	0·9302	0·5913	0·9508
	28	0·8485	0·6810	0·9489	0·6274	0·9658
	29	0·8788	0·7180	0·9660	0·6653	0·9789
	30	0·9091	0·7567	0·9808	0·7053	0·9895
	31	0·9394	0·7977	0·9926	0·7482	0·9968
	32	0·9697	0·8424	0·9992	0·7956	0·9998
	33	1·0000	0·8942	1·0000	0·8517	1·0000
34	0	0·0000	0·0000	0·1028	0·0000	0·1443
	1	0·0294	0·0007	0·1533	0·0001	0·1990
	2	0·0588	0·0072	0·1968	0·0031	0·2452
	3	0·0882	0·0186	0·2368	0·0102	0·2871
	4	0·1176	0·0330	0·2745	0·0205	0·3262
	5	0·1471	0·0495	0·3106	0·0332	0·3631
	6	0·1765	0·0676	0·3453	0·0477	0·3985
	7	0·2059	0·0870	0·3790	0·0638	0·4324
	8	0·2353	0·1075	0·4117	0·0811	0·4652
	9	0·2647	0·1288	0·4436	0·0996	0·4970
	10	0·2941	0·1510	0·4748	0·1191	0·5278
	11	0·3235	0·1739	0·5053	0·1395	0·5578
	12	0·3529	0·1975	0·5351	0·1607	0·5869
	13	0·3824	0·2217	0·5644	0·1828	0·6153
	14	0·4118	0·2465	0·5930	0·2056	0·6430
	15	0·4412	0·2719	0·6211	0·2291	0·6700
	16	0·4706	0·2978	0·6487	0·2533	0·6962
	17	0·5000	0·3243	0·6757	0·2782	0·7218
	18	0·5294	0·3513	0·7022	0·3038	0·7467
	19	0·5588	0·3789	0·7281	0·3300	0·7709
	20	0·5882	0·4070	0·7535	0·3570	0·7944
	21	0·6176	0·4356	0·7783	0·3847	0·8172
	22	0·6471	0·4649	0·8025	0·4131	0·8393
	23	0·6765	0·4947	0·8261	0·4422	0·8605
	24	0·7059	0·5252	0·8490	0·4722	0·8809
	25	0·7353	0·5564	0·8712	0·5030	0·9004
	26	0·7647	0·5883	0·8925	0·5348	0·9189
	27	0·7941	0·6210	0·9130	0·5676	0·9362
	28	0·8235	0·6547	0·9324	0·6015	0·9523
	29	0·8529	0·6894	0·9505	0·6369	0·9668
	30	0·8824	0·7255	0·9670	0·6738	0·9795
	31	0·9118	0·7632	0·9814	0·7129	0·9898
	32	0·9412	0·8032	0·9928	0·7548	0·9969
	33	0·9706	0·8467	0·9993	0·8010	0·9999
	34	1·0000	0·8972	1·0000	0·8557	1·0000
35	0	0·0000	0·0000	0·1000	0·0000	0·1405
	1	0·0286	0·0007	0·1492	0·0001	0·1938

Confidence level			95%		99%	
n	x	p	p_l	p_u	p_l	p_u
35	2	0·0571	0·0070	0·1916	0·0030	0·2389
	3	0·0857	0·0180	0·2306	0·0099	0·2798
	4	0·1143	0·0320	0·2674	0·0199	0·3180
	5	0·1429	0·0481	0·3026	0·0322	0·3542
	6	0·1714	0·0656	0·3365	0·0463	0·3887
	7	0·2000	0·0844	0·3694	0·0618	0·4220
	8	0·2286	0·1042	0·4014	0·0786	0·4541
	9	0·2571	0·1249	0·4326	0·0965	0·4852
	10	0·2857	0·1464	0·4630	0·1154	0·5155
	11	0·3143	0·1685	0·4929	0·1351	0·5449
	12	0·3429	0·1913	0·5221	0·1556	0·5735
	13	0·3714	0·2147	0·5508	0·1769	0·6014
	14	0·4000	0·2387	0·5789	0·1989	0·6287
	15	0·4286	0·2632	0·6065	0·2216	0·6552
	16	0·4571	0·2883	0·6335	0·2450	0·6811
	17	0·4857	0·3138	0·6601	0·2690	0·7064
	18	0·5143	0·3399	0·6862	0·2936	0·7310
	19	0·5429	0·3665	0·7117	0·3189	0·7550
	20	0·5714	0·3935	0·7368	0·3448	0·7784
	21	0·6000	0·4211	0·7613	0·3713	0·8011
	22	0·6286	0·4492	0·7853	0·3986	0·8231
	23	0·6571	0·4779	0·8087	0·4265	0·8444
	24	0·6857	0·5071	0·8315	0·4551	0·8649
	25	0·7143	0·5370	0·8536	0·4845	0·8846
	26	0·7429	0·5674	0·8751	0·5148	0·9035
	27	0·7714	0·5986	0·8958	0·5459	0·9214
	28	0·8000	0·6306	0·9156	0·5780	0·9382
	29	0·8286	0·6635	0·9344	0·6113	0·9537
	30	0·8571	0·6974	0·9519	0·6458	0·9678
	31	0·8857	0·7326	0·9680	0·6820	0·9801
	32	0·9143	0·7694	0·9820	0·7202	0·9901
	33	0·9429	0·8084	0·9930	0·7611	0·9970
	34	0·9714	0·8508	0·9993	0·8062	0·9999
	35	1·0000	0·9000	1·0000	0·8595	1·0000
36	0	0·0000	0·0000	0·0974	0·0000	0·1369
	1	0·0278	0·0007	0·1453	0·0001	0·1889
	2	0·0556	0·0068	0·1866	0·0029	0·2330
	3	0·0833	0·0175	0·2247	0·0096	0·2729
	4	0·1111	0·0311	0·2606	0·0193	0·3102
	5	0·1389	0·0467	0·2950	0·0312	0·3456
	6	0·1667	0·0637	0·3281	0·0449	0·3794
	7	0·1944	0·0819	0·3602	0·0600	0·4120
	8	0·2222	0·1012	0·3915	0·0763	0·4435
	9	0·2500	0·1212	0·4220	0·0936	0·4740
	10	0·2778	0·1420	0·4519	0·1119	0·5037
	11	0·3056	0·1635	0·4811	0·1310	0·5325
	12	0·3333	0·1856	0·5097	0·1509	0·5607
	13	0·3611	0·2082	0·5378	0·1714	0·5881
	14	0·3889	0·2314	0·5654	0·1927	0·6149
	15	0·4167	0·2551	0·5924	0·2146	0·6411

Continued

Table B.11 Exact confidence limits for a binomial proportion: x events are observed in a sample sized n. $p = x/n$ is the observed proportion. p_l and p_u are the lower and upper confidence limits for the population proportion.

Confidence level			95%		99%	
n	x	p	p_l	p_u	p_l	p_u
36	16	0·4444	0·2794	0·6190	0·2372	0·6666
	17	0·4722	0·3041	0·6451	0·2603	0·6916
	18	0·5000	0·3292	0·6708	0·2841	0·7159
	19	0·5278	0·3549	0·6959	0·3084	0·7397
	20	0·5556	0·3810	0·7206	0·3334	0·7628
	21	0·5833	0·4076	0·7449	0·3589	0·7854
	22	0·6111	0·4346	0·7686	0·3851	0·8073
	23	0·6389	0·4622	0·7918	0·4119	0·8286
	24	0·6667	0·4903	0·8144	0·4393	0·8491
	25	0·6944	0·5189	0·8365	0·4675	0·8690
	26	0·7222	0·5481	0·8580	0·4963	0·8881
	27	0·7500	0·5780	0·8788	0·5260	0·9064
	28	0·7778	0·6085	0·8988	0·5565	0·9237
	29	0·8056	0·6398	0·9181	0·5880	0·9400
	30	0·8333	0·6719	0·9363	0·6206	0·9551
	31	0·8611	0·7050	0·9533	0·6544	0·9688
	32	0·8889	0·7394	0·9689	0·6898	0·9807
	33	0·9167	0·7753	0·9825	0·7271	0·9904
	34	0·9444	0·8134	0·9932	0·7670	0·9971
	35	0·9722	0·8547	0·9993	0·8111	0·9999
	36	1·0000	0·9026	1·0000	0·8631	1·0000
37	0	0·0000	0·0000	0·0949	0·0000	0·1334
	1	0·0270	0·0007	0·1416	0·0001	0·1842
	2	0·0541	0·0066	0·1819	0·0028	0·2273
	3	0·0811	0·0170	0·2191	0·0093	0·2663
	4	0·1081	0·0303	0·2542	0·0188	0·3028
	5	0·1351	0·0454	0·2877	0·0304	0·3375
	6	0·1622	0·0619	0·3201	0·0436	0·3706
	7	0·1892	0·0796	0·3516	0·0583	0·4025
	8	0·2162	0·0983	0·3821	0·0741	0·4333
	9	0·2432	0·1177	0·4120	0·0909	0·4633
	10	0·2703	0·1379	0·4412	0·1086	0·4924
	11	0·2973	0·1587	0·4698	0·1271	0·5207
	12	0·3243	0·1801	0·4979	0·1464	0·5483
	13	0·3514	0·2021	0·5254	0·1663	0·5753
	14	0·3784	0·2246	0·5524	0·1869	0·6017
	15	0·4054	0·2475	0·5790	0·2081	0·6275
	16	0·4324	0·2710	0·6051	0·2299	0·6526
	17	0·4595	0·2949	0·6308	0·2522	0·6773
	18	0·4865	0·3192	0·6560	0·2752	0·7013
	19	0·5135	0·3440	0·6808	0·2987	0·7248
	20	0·5405	0·3692	0·7051	0·3227	0·7478
	21	0·5676	0·3949	0·7290	0·3474	0·7701
	22	0·5946	0·4210	0·7525	0·3725	0·7919
	23	0·6216	0·4476	0·7754	0·3983	0·8131
	24	0·6486	0·4746	0·7979	0·4247	0·8337
	25	0·6757	0·5021	0·8199	0·4517	0·8536
	26	0·7027	0·5302	0·8413	0·4793	0·8729
	27	0·7297	0·5588	0·8621	0·5076	0·8914

n	x	p	95% p_l	95% p_u	99% p_l	99% p_u
			Confidence level			
37	28	0·7568	0·5880	0·8823	0·5367	0·9091
	29	0·7838	0·6179	0·9017	0·5667	0·9259
	30	0·8108	0·6484	0·9204	0·5975	0·9417
	31	0·8378	0·6799	0·9381	0·6294	0·9564
	32	0·8649	0·7123	0·9546	0·6625	0·9696
	33	0·8919	0·7458	0·9697	0·6972	0·9812
	34	0·9189	0·7809	0·9830	0·7337	0·9907
	35	0·9459	0·8181	0·9934	0·7727	0·9972
	36	0·9730	0·8584	0·9993	0·8158	0·9999
	37	1·0000	0·9051	1·0000	0·8666	1·0000
38	0	0·0000	0·0000	0·0925	0·0000	0·1301
	1	0·0263	0·0007	0·1381	0·0001	0·1798
	2	0·0526	0·0064	0·1775	0·0028	0·2219
	3	0·0789	0·0166	0·2138	0·0091	0·2601
	4	0·1053	0·0294	0·2480	0·0183	0·2958
	5	0·1316	0·0441	0·2809	0·0295	0·3297
	6	0·1579	0·0602	0·3125	0·0424	0·3621
	7	0·1842	0·0774	0·3433	0·0567	0·3934
	8	0·2105	0·0955	0·3732	0·0720	0·4236
	9	0·2368	0·1144	0·4024	0·0883	0·4530
	10	0·2632	0·1340	0·4310	0·1055	0·4815
	11	0·2895	0·1542	0·4590	0·1235	0·5094
	12	0·3158	0·1750	0·4865	0·1421	0·5365
	13	0·3421	0·1963	0·5135	0·1614	0·5631
	14	0·3684	0·2181	0·5401	0·1814	0·5890
	15	0·3947	0·2404	0·5661	0·2019	0·6144
	16	0·4211	0·2631	0·5918	0·2230	0·6392
	17	0·4474	0·2862	0·6170	0·2447	0·6635
	18	0·4737	0·3098	0·6418	0·2668	0·6872
	19	0·5000	0·3338	0·6662	0·2895	0·7105
	20	0·5263	0·3582	0·6902	0·3128	0·7332
	21	0·5526	0·3830	0·7138	0·3365	0·7553
	22	0·5789	0·4082	0·7369	0·3608	0·7770
	23	0·6053	0·4339	0·7596	0·3856	0·7981
	24	0·6316	0·4599	0·7819	0·4110	0·8186
	25	0·6579	0·4865	0·8037	0·4369	0·8386
	26	0·6842	0·5135	0·8250	0·4635	0·8579
	27	0·7105	0·5410	0·8458	0·4906	0·8765
	28	0·7368	0·5690	0·8660	0·5185	0·8945
	29	0·7632	0·5976	0·8856	0·5470	0·9117
	30	0·7895	0·6268	0·9045	0·5764	0·9280
	31	0·8158	0·6567	0·9226	0·6066	0·9433
	32	0·8421	0·6875	0·9398	0·6379	0·9576
	33	0·8684	0·7191	0·9559	0·6703	0·9705
	34	0·8947	0·7520	0·9706	0·7042	0·9817
	35	0·9211	0·7862	0·9834	0·7399	0·9909
	36	0·9474	0·8225	0·9936	0·7781	0·9972
	37	0·9737	0·8619	0·9993	0·8202	0·9999
	38	1·0000	0·9075	1·0000	0·8699	1·0000
39	0	0·0000	0·0000	0·0903	0·0000	0·1270
	1	0·0256	0·0006	0·1348	0·0001	0·1756

Continued

Table B.11 Exact confidence limits for a binomial proportion: x events are observed in a sample sized n. $p = x/n$ is the observed proportion. p_l and p_u are the lower and upper confidence limits for the population proportion.

Confidence level			95%		99%	
n	x	p	p_l	p_u	p_l	p_u
39	2	0·0513	0·0063	0·1732	0·0027	0·2167
	3	0·0769	0·0162	0·2087	0·0089	0·2541
	4	0·1026	0·0287	0·2422	0·0178	0·2891
	5	0·1282	0·0430	0·2743	0·0287	0·3222
	6	0·1538	0·0586	0·3053	0·0413	0·3540
	7	0·1795	0·0754	0·3353	0·0551	0·3847
	8	0·2051	0·0930	0·3646	0·0700	0·4143
	9	0·2308	0·1113	0·3933	0·0859	0·4431
	10	0·2564	0·1304	0·4213	0·1026	0·4712
	11	0·2821	0·1500	0·4487	0·1200	0·4985
	12	0·3077	0·1702	0·4757	0·1381	0·5252
	13	0·3333	0·1909	0·5022	0·1569	0·5513
	14	0·3590	0·2120	0·5282	0·1762	0·5768
	15	0·3846	0·2336	0·5538	0·1961	0·6018
	16	0·4103	0·2557	0·5790	0·2166	0·6262
	17	0·4359	0·2781	0·6038	0·2375	0·6502
	18	0·4615	0·3009	0·6282	0·2590	0·6736
	19	0·4872	0·3242	0·6522	0·2810	0·6966
	20	0·5128	0·3478	0·6758	0·3034	0·7190
	21	0·5385	0·3718	0·6991	0·3264	0·7410
	22	0·5641	0·3962	0·7219	0·3498	0·7625
	23	0·5897	0·4210	0·7443	0·3738	0·7834
	24	0·6154	0·4462	0·7664	0·3982	0·8039
	25	0·6410	0·4718	0·7880	0·4232	0·8238
	26	0·6667	0·4978	0·8091	0·4487	0·8431
	27	0·6923	0·5243	0·8298	0·4748	0·8619
	28	0·7179	0·5513	0·8500	0·5015	0·8800
	29	0·7436	0·5787	0·8696	0·5288	0·8974
	30	0·7692	0·6067	0·8887	0·5569	0·9141
	31	0·7949	0·6354	0·9070	0·5857	0·9300
	32	0·8205	0·6647	0·9246	0·6153	0·9449
	33	0·8462	0·6947	0·9414	0·6460	0·9587
	34	0·8718	0·7257	0·9570	0·6778	0·9713
	35	0·8974	0·7578	0·9713	0·7109	0·9822
	36	0·9231	0·7913	0·9838	0·7459	0·9911
	37	0·9487	0·8268	0·9937	0·7833	0·9973
	38	0·9744	0·8652	0·9994	0·8244	0·9999
	39	1·0000	0·9097	1·0000	0·8730	1·0000
40	0	0·0000	0·0000	0·0881	0·0000	0·1241
	1	0·0250	0·0006	0·1316	0·0001	0·1715
	2	0·0500	0·0061	0·1692	0·0026	0·2118
	3	0·0750	0·0157	0·2039	0·0086	0·2484
	4	0·1000	0·0279	0·2366	0·0173	0·2826
	5	0·1250	0·0419	0·2680	0·0280	0·3151
	6	0·1500	0·0571	0·2984	0·0402	0·3463
	7	0·1750	0·0734	0·3278	0·0537	0·3763
	8	0·2000	0·0905	0·3565	0·0682	0·4054
	9	0·2250	0·1084	0·3845	0·0836	0·4337
	10	0·2500	0·1269	0·4120	0·0998	0·4612

Table B.11 (*Continued*)

Confidence level			95%		99%	
n	x	p	p_l	p_u	p_l	p_u
40	11	0·2750	0·1460	0·4389	0·1168	0·4881
	12	0·3000	0·1656	0·4653	0·1344	0·5143
	13	0·3250	0·1857	0·4913	0·1526	0·5400
	14	0·3500	0·2063	0·5168	0·1713	0·5651
	15	0·3750	0·2273	0·5420	0·1906	0·5897
	16	0·4000	0·2486	0·5667	0·2105	0·6138
	17	0·4250	0·2704	0·5911	0·2308	0·6374
	18	0·4500	0·2926	0·6151	0·2516	0·6605
	19	0·4750	0·3151	0·6387	0·2729	0·6832
	20	0·5000	0·3380	0·6620	0·2946	0·7054
	21	0·5250	0·3613	0·6849	0·3168	0·7271
	22	0·5500	0·3849	0·7074	0·3395	0·7484
	23	0·5750	0·4089	0·7296	0·3626	0·7692
	24	0·6000	0·4333	0·7514	0·3862	0·7895
	25	0·6250	0·4580	0·7727	0·4103	0·8094
	26	0·6500	0·4832	0·7937	0·4349	0·8287
	27	0·6750	0·5087	0·8143	0·4600	0·8474
	28	0·7000	0·5347	0·8344	0·4857	0·8656
	29	0·7250	0·5611	0·8540	0·5119	0·8832
	30	0·7500	0·5880	0·8731	0·5388	0·9002
	31	0·7750	0·6155	0·8916	0·5663	0·9164
	32	0·8000	0·6435	0·9095	0·5946	0·9318
	33	0·8250	0·6722	0·9266	0·6237	0·9463
	34	0·8500	0·7016	0·9429	0·6537	0·9598
	35	0·8750	0·7320	0·9581	0·6849	0·9720
	36	0·9000	0·7634	0·9721	0·7174	0·9827
	37	0·9250	0·7961	0·9843	0·7516	0·9914
	38	0·9500	0·8308	0·9939	0·7882	0·9974
	39	0·9750	0·8684	0·9994	0·8285	0·9999
	40	1·0000	0·9119	1·0000	0·8759	1·0000
41	0	0·0000	0·0000	0·0860	0·0000	0·1212
	1	0·0244	0·0006	0·1286	0·0001	0·1677
	2	0·0488	0·0060	0·1653	0·0026	0·2071
	3	0·0732	0·0154	0·1992	0·0084	0·2429
	4	0·0976	0·0272	0·2313	0·0169	0·2764
	5	0·1220	0·0408	0·2620	0·0273	0·3083
	6	0·1463	0·0557	0·2917	0·0392	0·3389
	7	0·1707	0·0715	0·3206	0·0523	0·3683
	8	0·1951	0·0882	0·3487	0·0664	0·3969
	9	0·2195	0·1056	0·3761	0·0814	0·4246
	10	0·2439	0·1236	0·4030	0·0972	0·4517
	11	0·2683	0·1422	0·4294	0·1137	0·4781
	12	0·2927	0·1613	0·4554	0·1308	0·5038
	13	0·3171	0·1808	0·4809	0·1485	0·5291
	14	0·3415	0·2008	0·5059	0·1667	0·5538
	15	0·3659	0·2212	0·5306	0·1855	0·5780
	16	0·3902	0·2420	0·5550	0·2047	0·6017
	17	0·4146	0·2632	0·5789	0·2244	0·6250
	18	0·4390	0·2847	0·6025	0·2446	0·6478
	19	0·4634	0·3066	0·6258	0·2652	0·6702

Continued

Table B.11 Exact confidence limits for a binomial proportion: x events are observed in a sample sized n. $p = x/n$ is the observed proportion. p_l and p_u are the lower and upper confidence limits for the population proportion.

Confidence level			95%		99%	
n	x	p	p_l	p_u	p_l	p_u
41	20	0·4878	0·3288	0·6487	0·2863	0·6922
	21	0·5122	0·3513	0·6712	0·3078	0·7137
	22	0·5366	0·3742	0·6934	0·3298	0·7348
	23	0·5610	0·3975	0·7153	0·3522	0·7554
	24	0·5854	0·4211	0·7368	0·3750	0·7756
	25	0·6098	0·4450	0·7580	0·3983	0·7953
	26	0·6341	0·4694	0·7788	0·4220	0·8145
	27	0·6585	0·4941	0·7992	0·4462	0·8333
	28	0·6829	0·5191	0·8192	0·4709	0·8515
	29	0·7073	0·5446	0·8387	0·4962	0·8692
	30	0·7317	0·5706	0·8578	0·5219	0·8863
	31	0·7561	0·5970	0·8764	0·5483	0·9028
	32	0·7805	0·6239	0·8944	0·5754	0·9186
	33	0·8049	0·6513	0·9118	0·6031	0·9336
	34	0·8293	0·6794	0·9285	0·6317	0·9477
	35	0·8537	0·7083	0·9443	0·6611	0·9608
	36	0·8780	0·7380	0·9592	0·6917	0·9727
	37	0·9024	0·7687	0·9728	0·7236	0·9831
	38	0·9268	0·8008	0·9846	0·7571	0·9916
	39	0·9512	0·8347	0·9940	0·7929	0·9974
	40	0·9756	0·8714	0·9994	0·8323	0·9999
	41	1·0000	0·9140	1·0000	0·8788	1·0000
42	0	0·0000	0·0000	0·0841	0·0000	0·1185
	1	0·0238	0·0006	0·1257	0·0001	0·1640
	2	0·0476	0·0058	0·1616	0·0025	0·2026
	3	0·0714	0·0150	0·1948	0·0082	0·2377
	4	0·0952	0·0266	0·2262	0·0165	0·2705
	5	0·1190	0·0398	0·2563	0·0266	0·3018
	6	0·1429	0·0543	0·2854	0·0382	0·3318
	7	0·1667	0·0697	0·3136	0·0510	0·3607
	8	0·1905	0·0860	0·3412	0·0647	0·3887
	9	0·2143	0·1030	0·3681	0·0794	0·4159
	10	0·2381	0·1205	0·3945	0·0947	0·4425
	11	0·2619	0·1386	0·4204	0·1108	0·4684
	12	0·2857	0·1572	0·4458	0·1274	0·4938
	13	0·3095	0·1762	0·4709	0·1446	0·5186
	14	0·3333	0·1957	0·4955	0·1623	0·5429
	15	0·3571	0·2155	0·5197	0·1806	0·5668
	16	0·3810	0·2357	0·5436	0·1993	0·5902
	17	0·4048	0·2563	0·5672	0·2184	0·6131
	18	0·4286	0·2772	0·5904	0·2380	0·6356
	19	0·4524	0·2985	0·6133	0·2580	0·6577
	20	0·4762	0·3200	0·6358	0·2785	0·6794
	21	0·5000	0·3419	0·6581	0·2993	0·7007
	22	0·5238	0·3642	0·6800	0·3206	0·7215
	23	0·5476	0·3867	0·7015	0·3423	0·7420
	24	0·5714	0·4096	0·7228	0·3644	0·7620
	25	0·5952	0·4328	0·7437	0·3869	0·7816
	26	0·6190	0·4564	0·7643	0·4098	0·8007

Confidence level			95%		99%	
n	x	p	p_l	p_u	p_l	p_u
42	27	0·6429	0·4803	0·7845	0·4332	0·8194
	28	0·6667	0·5045	0·8043	0·4571	0·8377
	29	0·6905	0·5291	0·8238	0·4814	0·8554
	30	0·7143	0·5542	0·8428	0·5062	0·8726
	31	0·7381	0·5796	0·8614	0·5316	0·8892
	32	0·7619	0·6055	0·8795	0·5575	0·9053
	33	0·7857	0·6319	0·8970	0·5841	0·9206
	34	0·8095	0·6588	0·9140	0·6113	0·9353
	35	0·8333	0·6864	0·9303	0·6393	0·9490
	36	0·8571	0·7146	0·9457	0·6682	0·9618
	37	0·8810	0·7437	0·9602	0·6982	0·9734
	38	0·9048	0·7738	0·9734	0·7295	0·9835
	39	0·9286	0·8052	0·9850	0·7623	0·9918
	40	0·9524	0·8384	0·9942	0·7974	0·9975
	41	0·9762	0·8743	0·9994	0·8360	0·9999
	42	1·0000	0·9159	1·0000	0·8815	1·0000
43	0	0·0000	0·0000	0·0822	0·0000	0·1159
	1	0·0233	0·0006	0·1229	0·0001	0·1604
	2	0·0465	0·0057	0·1581	0·0024	0·1982
	3	0·0698	0·0146	0·1906	0·0080	0·2327
	4	0·0930	0·0259	0·2214	0·0161	0·2649
	5	0·1163	0·0389	0·2508	0·0260	0·2955
	6	0·1395	0·0530	0·2793	0·0373	0·3249
	7	0·1628	0·0681	0·3070	0·0497	0·3533
	8	0·1860	0·0839	0·3340	0·0632	0·3808
	9	0·2093	0·1004	0·3604	0·0774	0·4076
	10	0·2326	0·1176	0·3863	0·0924	0·4337
	11	0·2558	0·1352	0·4117	0·1080	0·4592
	12	0·2791	0·1533	0·4367	0·1242	0·4841
	13	0·3023	0·1718	0·4613	0·1409	0·5085
	14	0·3256	0·1908	0·4854	0·1582	0·5325
	15	0·3488	0·2101	0·5093	0·1759	0·5559
	16	0·3721	0·2298	0·5327	0·1941	0·5790
	17	0·3953	0·2498	0·5559	0·2127	0·6016
	18	0·4186	0·2701	0·5787	0·2318	0·6238
	19	0·4419	0·2908	0·6012	0·2512	0·6456
	20	0·4651	0·3118	0·6235	0·2711	0·6670
	21	0·4884	0·3331	0·6454	0·2913	0·6880
	22	0·5116	0·3546	0·6669	0·3120	0·7087
	23	0·5349	0·3765	0·6882	0·3330	0·7289
	24	0·5581	0·3988	0·7092	0·3544	0·7488
	25	0·5814	0·4213	0·7299	0·3762	0·7682
	26	0·6047	0·4441	0·7502	0·3984	0·7873
	27	0·6279	0·4673	0·7702	0·4210	0·8059
	28	0·6512	0·4907	0·7899	0·4441	0·8241
	29	0·6744	0·5146	0·8092	0·4675	0·8418
	30	0·6977	0·5387	0·8282	0·4915	0·8591
	31	0·7209	0·5633	0·8467	0·5159	0·8758
	32	0·7442	0·5883	0·8648	0·5408	0·8920

Continued

Table B.11 Exact confidence limits for a binomial proportion: x events are observed in a sample sized n. $p = x/n$ is the observed proportion. p_l and p_u are the lower and upper confidence limits for the population proportion.

Confidence level			95%		99%	
n	x	p	p_l	p_u	p_l	p_u
43	33	0·7674	0·6137	0·8824	0·5663	0·9076
	34	0·7907	0·6396	0·8996	0·5924	0·9226
	35	0·8140	0·6660	0·9161	0·6192	0·9368
	36	0·8372	0·6930	0·9319	0·6467	0·9503
	37	0·8605	0·7207	0·9470	0·6751	0·9627
	38	0·8837	0·7492	0·9611	0·7045	0·9740
	39	0·9070	0·7786	0·9741	0·7351	0·9839
	40	0·9302	0·8094	0·9854	0·7673	0·9920
	41	0·9535	0·8419	0·9943	0·8018	0·9976
	42	0·9767	0·8771	0·9994	0·8396	0·9999
	43	1·0000	0·9178	1·0000	0·8841	1·0000
44	0	0·0000	0·0000	0·0804	0·0000	0·1134
	1	0·0227	0·0006	0·1202	0·0001	0·1570
	2	0·0455	0·0056	0·1547	0·0024	0·1941
	3	0·0682	0·0143	0·1866	0·0078	0·2279
	4	0·0909	0·0253	0·2167	0·0157	0·2595
	5	0·1136	0·0379	0·2456	0·0254	0·2895
	6	0·1364	0·0517	0·2735	0·0364	0·3184
	7	0·1591	0·0664	0·3007	0·0485	0·3463
	8	0·1818	0·0819	0·3271	0·0616	0·3733
	9	0·2045	0·0980	0·3530	0·0755	0·3996
	10	0·2273	0·1147	0·3784	0·0901	0·4252
	11	0·2500	0·1319	0·4034	0·1053	0·4503
	12	0·2727	0·1496	0·4279	0·1211	0·4748
	13	0·2955	0·1676	0·4520	0·1374	0·4988
	14	0·3182	0·1861	0·4758	0·1543	0·5224
	15	0·3409	0·2049	0·4992	0·1715	0·5455
	16	0·3636	0·2241	0·5223	0·1892	0·5682
	17	0·3864	0·2436	0·5450	0·2073	0·5905
	18	0·4091	0·2634	0·5675	0·2259	0·6124
	19	0·4318	0·2835	0·5897	0·2448	0·6339
	20	0·4545	0·3039	0·6115	0·2641	0·6551
	21	0·4773	0·3246	0·6331	0·2837	0·6758
	22	0·5000	0·3456	0·6544	0·3038	0·6962
	23	0·5227	0·3669	0·6754	0·3242	0·7163
	24	0·5455	0·3885	0·6961	0·3449	0·7359
	25	0·5682	0·4103	0·7165	0·3661	0·7552
	26	0·5909	0·4325	0·7366	0·3876	0·7741
	27	0·6136	0·4550	0·7564	0·4095	0·7927
	28	0·6364	0·4777	0·7759	0·4318	0·8108
	29	0·6591	0·5008	0·7951	0·4545	0·8285
	30	0·6818	0·5242	0·8139	0·4776	0·8457
	31	0·7045	0·5480	0·8324	0·5012	0·8626
	32	0·7273	0·5721	0·8504	0·5252	0·8789
	33	0·7500	0·5966	0·8681	0·5497	0·8947
	34	0·7727	0·6216	0·8853	0·5748	0·9099
	35	0·7955	0·6470	0·9020	0·6004	0·9245
	36	0·8182	0·6729	0·9181	0·6267	0·9384
	37	0·8409	0·6993	0·9336	0·6537	0·9515

Table B.11 (*Continued*)

Confidence level			95%		99%	
n	x	p	p_l	p_u	p_l	p_u
44	38	0·8636	0·7265	0·9483	0·6816	0·9636
	39	0·8864	0·7544	0·9621	0·7105	0·9746
	40	0·9091	0·7833	0·9747	0·7405	0·9843
	41	0·9318	0·8134	0·9857	0·7721	0·9922
	42	0·9545	0·8453	0·9944	0·8059	0·9976
	43	0·9773	0·8798	0·9994	0·8430	0·9999
	44	1·0000	0·9196	1·0000	0·8866	1·0000
45	0	0·0000	0·0000	0·0787	0·0000	0·1111
	1	0·0222	0·0006	0·1177	0·0001	0·1538
	2	0·0444	0·0054	0·1515	0·0023	0·1901
	3	0·0667	0·0140	0·1827	0·0077	0·2232
	4	0·0889	0·0248	0·2122	0·0153	0·2543
	5	0·1111	0·0371	0·2405	0·0248	0·2838
	6	0·1333	0·0505	0·2679	0·0356	0·3121
	7	0·1556	0·0649	0·2946	0·0474	0·3395
	8	0·1778	0·0800	0·3205	0·0602	0·3660
	9	0·2000	0·0958	0·3460	0·0737	0·3918
	10	0·2222	0·1120	0·3709	0·0880	0·4171
	11	0·2444	0·1288	0·3954	0·1028	0·4417
	12	0·2667	0·1460	0·4194	0·1182	0·4658
	13	0·2889	0·1637	0·4431	0·1341	0·4895
	14	0·3111	0·1817	0·4665	0·1505	0·5127
	15	0·3333	0·2000	0·4895	0·1673	0·5354
	16	0·3556	0·2187	0·5122	0·1846	0·5578
	17	0·3778	0·2377	0·5346	0·2022	0·5798
	18	0·4000	0·2570	0·5567	0·2202	0·6014
	19	0·4222	0·2766	0·5785	0·2386	0·6226
	20	0·4444	0·2964	0·6000	0·2574	0·6435
	21	0·4667	0·3166	0·6213	0·2765	0·6640
	22	0·4889	0·3370	0·6423	0·2960	0·6842
	23	0·5111	0·3577	0·6630	0·3158	0·7040
	24	0·5333	0·3787	0·6834	0·3360	0·7235
	25	0·5556	0·4000	0·7036	0·3565	0·7426
	26	0·5778	0·4215	0·7234	0·3774	0·7614
	27	0·6000	0·4433	0·7430	0·3986	0·7798
	28	0·6222	0·4654	0·7623	0·4202	0·7978
	29	0·6444	0·4878	0·7813	0·4422	0·8154
	30	0·6667	0·5105	0·8000	0·4646	0·8327
	31	0·6889	0·5335	0·8183	0·4873	0·8495
	32	0·7111	0·5569	0·8363	0·5105	0·8659
	33	0·7333	0·5806	0·8540	0·5342	0·8818
	34	0·7556	0·6046	0·8712	0·5583	0·8972
	35	0·7778	0·6291	0·8880	0·5829	0·9120
	36	0·8000	0·6540	0·9042	0·6082	0·9263
	37	0·8222	0·6795	0·9200	0·6340	0·9398
	38	0·8444	0·7054	0·9351	0·6605	0·9526
	39	0·8667	0·7321	0·9495	0·6879	0·9644
	40	0·8889	0·7595	0·9629	0·7162	0·9752
	41	0·9111	0·7878	0·9752	0·7457	0·9847
	42	0·9333	0·8173	0·9860	0·7768	0·9923

Continued

Table B.11 Exact confidence limits for a binomial proportion: x events are observed in a sample sized n. $p = x/n$ is the observed proportion. p_l and p_u are the lower and upper confidence limits for the population proportion.

Confidence level			95%		99%	
n	x	p	p_l	p_u	p_l	p_u
45	43	0·9556	0·8485	0·9946	0·8099	0·9977
	44	0·9778	0·8823	0·9994	0·8462	0·9999
	45	1·0000	0·9213	1·0000	0·8889	1·0000
46	0	0·0000	0·0000	0·0771	0·0000	0·1088
	1	0·0217	0·0006	0·1153	0·0001	0·1507
	2	0·0435	0·0053	0·1484	0·0023	0·1863
	3	0·0652	0·0137	0·1790	0·0075	0·2188
	4	0·0870	0·0242	0·2079	0·0150	0·2493
	5	0·1087	0·0362	0·2357	0·0242	0·2782
	6	0·1304	0·0494	0·2626	0·0347	0·3060
	7	0·1522	0·0634	0·2887	0·0463	0·3329
	8	0·1739	0·0782	0·3142	0·0588	0·3590
	9	0·1957	0·0936	0·3391	0·0720	0·3844
	10	0·2174	0·1095	0·3636	0·0859	0·4092
	11	0·2391	0·1259	0·3877	0·1004	0·4334
	12	0·2609	0·1427	0·4113	0·1154	0·4572
	13	0·2826	0·1599	0·4346	0·1310	0·4804
	14	0·3043	0·1774	0·4575	0·1469	0·5033
	15	0·3261	0·1953	0·4802	0·1633	0·5257
	16	0·3478	0·2135	0·5025	0·1801	0·5477
	17	0·3696	0·2321	0·5245	0·1973	0·5694
	18	0·3913	0·2509	0·5463	0·2149	0·5907
	19	0·4130	0·2700	0·5677	0·2328	0·6116
	20	0·4348	0·2893	0·5889	0·2511	0·6323
	21	0·4565	0·3090	0·6099	0·2697	0·6525
	22	0·4783	0·3289	0·6305	0·2886	0·6725
	23	0·5000	0·3490	0·6510	0·3079	0·6921
	24	0·5217	0·3695	0·6711	0·3275	0·7114
	25	0·5435	0·3901	0·6910	0·3475	0·7303
	26	0·5652	0·4111	0·7107	0·3677	0·7489
	27	0·5870	0·4323	0·7300	0·3884	0·7672
	28	0·6087	0·4537	0·7491	0·4093	0·7851
	29	0·6304	0·4755	0·7679	0·4306	0·8027
	30	0·6522	0·4975	0·7865	0·4523	0·8199
	31	0·6739	0·5198	0·8047	0·4743	0·8367
	32	0·6957	0·5425	0·8226	0·4967	0·8531
	33	0·7174	0·5654	0·8401	0·5196	0·8690
	34	0·7391	0·5887	0·8573	0·5428	0·8846
	35	0·7609	0·6123	0·8741	0·5666	0·8996
	36	0·7826	0·6364	0·8905	0·5908	0·9141
	37	0·8043	0·6609	0·9064	0·6156	0·9280
	38	0·8261	0·6858	0·9218	0·6410	0·9412
	39	0·8478	0·7113	0·9366	0·6671	0·9537
	40	0·8696	0·7374	0·9506	0·6940	0·9653
	41	0·8913	0·7643	0·9638	0·7218	0·9758
	42	0·9130	0·7921	0·9758	0·7507	0·9850
	43	0·9348	0·8210	0·9863	0·7812	0·9925
	44	0·9565	0·8516	0·9947	0·8137	0·9977

Confidence level			95%		99%	
n	*x*	*p*	p_l	p_u	p_l	p_u
46	45	0·9783	0·8847	0·9994	0·8493	0·9999
	46	1·0000	0·9229	1·0000	0·8912	1·0000
47	0	0·0000	0·0000	0·0755	0·0000	0·1066
	1	0·0213	0·0005	0·1129	0·0001	0·1477
	2	0·0426	0·0052	0·1454	0·0022	0·1827
	3	0·0638	0·0134	0·1754	0·0073	0·2145
	4	0·0851	0·0237	0·2038	0·0147	0·2444
	5	0·1064	0·0355	0·2310	0·0237	0·2729
	6	0·1277	0·0483	0·2574	0·0340	0·3002
	7	0·1489	0·0620	0·2831	0·0453	0·3266
	8	0·1702	0·0765	0·3081	0·0575	0·3523
	9	0·1915	0·0915	0·3326	0·0704	0·3773
	10	0·2128	0·1070	0·3566	0·0840	0·4016
	11	0·2340	0·1230	0·3803	0·0981	0·4255
	12	0·2553	0·1394	0·4035	0·1128	0·4488
	13	0·2766	0·1562	0·4264	0·1279	0·4717
	14	0·2979	0·1734	0·4489	0·1435	0·4942
	15	0·3191	0·1909	0·4712	0·1595	0·5163
	16	0·3404	0·2086	0·4931	0·1759	0·5380
	17	0·3617	0·2267	0·5148	0·1927	0·5594
	18	0·3830	0·2451	0·5362	0·2098	0·5804
	19	0·4043	0·2637	0·5573	0·2273	0·6011
	20	0·4255	0·2826	0·5782	0·2451	0·6214
	21	0·4468	0·3017	0·5988	0·2632	0·6414
	22	0·4681	0·3211	0·6192	0·2816	0·6611
	23	0·4894	0·3408	0·6394	0·3004	0·6805
	24	0·5106	0·3606	0·6592	0·3195	0·6996
	25	0·5319	0·3808	0·6789	0·3389	0·7184
	26	0·5532	0·4012	0·6983	0·3586	0·7368
	27	0·5745	0·4218	0·7174	0·3786	0·7549
	28	0·5957	0·4427	0·7363	0·3989	0·7727
	29	0·6170	0·4638	0·7549	0·4196	0·7902
	30	0·6383	0·4852	0·7733	0·4406	0·8073
	31	0·6596	0·5069	0·7914	0·4620	0·8241
	32	0·6809	0·5288	0·8091	0·4837	0·8405
	33	0·7021	0·5511	0·8266	0·5058	0·8565
	34	0·7234	0·5736	0·8438	0·5283	0·8721
	35	0·7447	0·5965	0·8606	0·5512	0·8872
	36	0·7660	0·6197	0·8770	0·5745	0·9019
	37	0·7872	0·6434	0·8930	0·5984	0·9160
	38	0·8085	0·6674	0·9085	0·6227	0·9296
	39	0·8298	0·6919	0·9235	0·6477	0·9425
	40	0·8511	0·7169	0·9380	0·6734	0·9547
	41	0·8723	0·7426	0·9517	0·6998	0·9660
	42	0·8936	0·7690	0·9645	0·7271	0·9763
	43	0·9149	0·7962	0·9763	0·7556	0·9853
	44	0·9362	0·8246	0·9866	0·7855	0·9927
	45	0·9574	0·8546	0·9948	0·8173	0·9978
	46	0·9787	0·8871	0·9995	0·8523	0·9999
	47	1·0000	0·9245	1·0000	0·8934	1·0000

Continued

Table B.11 Exact confidence limits for a binomial proportion: x events are observed in a sample sized n. $p = x/n$ is the observed proportion. p_l and p_u are the lower and upper confidence limits for the population proportion.

Confidence level			95%		99%	
n	x	p	p_l	p_u	p_l	p_u
48	0	0·0000	0·0000	0·0740	0·0000	0·1045
	1	0·0208	0·0005	0·1107	0·0001	0·1448
	2	0·0417	0·0051	0·1425	0·0022	0·1791
	3	0·0625	0·0131	0·1720	0·0072	0·2105
	4	0·0833	0·0232	0·1998	0·0144	0·2398
	5	0·1042	0·0347	0·2266	0·0232	0·2678
	6	0·1250	0·0473	0·2525	0·0332	0·2946
	7	0·1458	0·0607	0·2776	0·0443	0·3206
	8	0·1667	0·0748	0·3022	0·0562	0·3458
	9	0·1875	0·0895	0·3263	0·0689	0·3703
	10	0·2083	0·1047	0·3499	0·0821	0·3943
	11	0·2292	0·1203	0·3731	0·0959	0·4178
	12	0·2500	0·1364	0·3960	0·1103	0·4408
	13	0·2708	0·1528	0·4185	0·1251	0·4633
	14	0·2917	0·1695	0·4406	0·1403	0·4855
	15	0·3125	0·1866	0·4625	0·1559	0·5072
	16	0·3333	0·2040	0·4841	0·1719	0·5286
	17	0·3542	0·2216	0·5054	0·1883	0·5497
	18	0·3750	0·2395	0·5265	0·2050	0·5704
	19	0·3958	0·2577	0·5473	0·2220	0·5908
	20	0·4167	0·2761	0·5679	0·2393	0·6109
	21	0·4375	0·2948	0·5882	0·2570	0·6307
	22	0·4583	0·3137	0·6083	0·2750	0·6501
	23	0·4792	0·3329	0·6281	0·2933	0·6693
	24	0·5000	0·3523	0·6477	0·3118	0·6882
	25	0·5208	0·3719	0·6671	0·3307	0·7067
	26	0·5417	0·3917	0·6863	0·3499	0·7250
	27	0·5625	0·4118	0·7052	0·3693	0·7430
	28	0·5833	0·4321	0·7239	0·3891	0·7607
	29	0·6042	0·4527	0·7423	0·4092	0·7780
	30	0·6250	0·4735	0·7605	0·4296	0·7950
	31	0·6458	0·4946	0·7784	0·4503	0·8117
	32	0·6667	0·5159	0·7960	0·4714	0·8281
	33	0·6875	0·5375	0·8134	0·4928	0·8441
	34	0·7083	0·5594	0·8305	0·5145	0·8597
	35	0·7292	0·5815	0·8472	0·5367	0·8749
	36	0·7500	0·6040	0·8636	0·5592	0·8897
	37	0·7708	0·6269	0·8797	0·5822	0·9041
	38	0·7917	0·6501	0·8953	0·6057	0·9179
	39	0·8125	0·6737	0·9105	0·6297	0·9311
	40	0·8333	0·6978	0·9252	0·6542	0·9438
	41	0·8542	0·7224	0·9393	0·6794	0·9557
	42	0·8750	0·7475	0·9527	0·7054	0·9668
	43	0·8958	0·7734	0·9653	0·7322	0·9768
	44	0·9167	0·8002	0·9768	0·7602	0·9856
	45	0·9375	0·8280	0·9869	0·7895	0·9928
	46	0·9583	0·8575	0·9949	0·8209	0·9978
	47	0·9792	0·8893	0·9995	0·8552	0·9999
	48	1·0000	0·9260	1·0000	0·8955	1·0000

Table B.11 (*Continued*)

Confidence level			95%		99%	
n	x	p	p_l	p_u	p_l	p_u
49	0	0·0000	0·0000	0·0725	0·0000	0·1025
	1	0·0204	0·0005	0·1085	0·0001	0·1421
	2	0·0408	0·0050	0·1398	0·0021	0·1758
	3	0·0612	0·0128	0·1687	0·0070	0·2065
	4	0·0816	0·0227	0·1960	0·0141	0·2353
	5	0·1020	0·0340	0·2223	0·0227	0·2628
	6	0·1224	0·0463	0·2477	0·0325	0·2892
	7	0·1429	0·0594	0·2724	0·0434	0·3147
	8	0·1633	0·0732	0·2966	0·0550	0·3395
	9	0·1837	0·0876	0·3202	0·0674	0·3637
	10	0·2041	0·1024	0·3434	0·0803	0·3873
	11	0·2245	0·1177	0·3662	0·0939	0·4104
	12	0·2449	0·1334	0·3887	0·1079	0·4330
	13	0·2653	0·1495	0·4108	0·1223	0·4552
	14	0·2857	0·1658	0·4326	0·1372	0·4770
	15	0·3061	0·1825	0·4542	0·1524	0·4985
	16	0·3265	0·1995	0·4754	0·1681	0·5196
	17	0·3469	0·2167	0·4964	0·1840	0·5403
	18	0·3673	0·2342	0·5171	0·2003	0·5607
	19	0·3878	0·2520	0·5376	0·2169	0·5809
	20	0·4082	0·2700	0·5579	0·2339	0·6007
	21	0·4286	0·2882	0·5779	0·2511	0·6202
	22	0·4490	0·3067	0·5977	0·2686	0·6395
	23	0·4694	0·3253	0·6173	0·2864	0·6584
	24	0·4898	0·3442	0·6366	0·3045	0·6771
	25	0·5102	0·3634	0·6558	0·3229	0·6955
	26	0·5306	0·3827	0·6747	0·3416	0·7136
	27	0·5510	0·4023	0·6933	0·3605	0·7314
	28	0·5714	0·4221	0·7118	0·3798	0·7489
	29	0·5918	0·4421	0·7300	0·3993	0·7661
	30	0·6122	0·4624	0·7480	0·4191	0·7831
	31	0·6327	0·4829	0·7658	0·4393	0·7997
	32	0·6531	0·5036	0·7833	0·4597	0·8160
	33	0·6735	0·5246	0·8005	0·4804	0·8319
	34	0·6939	0·5458	0·8175	0·5015	0·8476
	35	0·7143	0·5674	0·8342	0·5230	0·8628
	36	0·7347	0·5892	0·8505	0·5448	0·8777
	37	0·7551	0·6113	0·8666	0·5670	0·8921
	38	0·7755	0·6338	0·8823	0·5896	0·9061
	39	0·7959	0·6566	0·8976	0·6127	0·9197
	40	0·8163	0·6798	0·9124	0·6363	0·9326
	41	0·8367	0·7034	0·9268	0·6605	0·9450
	42	0·8571	0·7276	0·9406	0·6853	0·9566
	43	0·8776	0·7523	0·9537	0·7108	0·9675
	44	0·8980	0·7777	0·9660	0·7372	0·9773
	45	0·9184	0·8040	0·9773	0·7647	0·9859
	46	0·9388	0·8313	0·9872	0·7935	0·9930
	47	0·9592	0·8602	0·9950	0·8242	0·9979
	48	0·9796	0·8915	0·9995	0·8579	0·9999
	49	1·0000	0·9275	1·0000	0·8975	1·0000

Continued

Table B.11 Exact confidence limits for a binomial proportion: x events are observed in a sample sized n. $p = x/n$ is the observed proportion. p_l and p_u are the lower and upper confidence limits for the population proportion.

Confidence level			95%		99%	
n	x	p	p_l	p_u	p_l	p_u
50	0	0·0000	0·0000	0·0711	0·0000	0·1005
	1	0·0200	0·0005	0·1065	0·0001	0·1394
	2	0·0400	0·0049	0·1371	0·0021	0·1725
	3	0·0600	0·0125	0·1655	0·0069	0·2027
	4	0·0800	0·0222	0·1923	0·0138	0·2311
	5	0·1000	0·0333	0·2181	0·0222	0·2580
	6	0·1200	0·0453	0·2431	0·0319	0·2840
	7	0·1400	0·0582	0·2674	0·0425	0·3091
	8	0·1600	0·0717	0·2911	0·0539	0·3335
	9	0·1800	0·0858	0·3144	0·0660	0·3573
	10	0·2000	0·1003	0·3372	0·0786	0·3805
	11	0·2200	0·1153	0·3596	0·0919	0·4032
	12	0·2400	0·1306	0·3817	0·1056	0·4255
	13	0·2600	0·1463	0·4034	0·1197	0·4474
	14	0·2800	0·1623	0·4249	0·1342	0·4689
	15	0·3000	0·1786	0·4461	0·1491	0·4900
	16	0·3200	0·1952	0·4670	0·1644	0·5108
	17	0·3400	0·2121	0·4877	0·1800	0·5312
	18	0·3600	0·2292	0·5081	0·1959	0·5514
	19	0·3800	0·2465	0·5283	0·2121	0·5713
	20	0·4000	0·2641	0·5482	0·2287	0·5908
	21	0·4200	0·2819	0·5679	0·2455	0·6101
	22	0·4400	0·2999	0·5875	0·2626	0·6291
	23	0·4600	0·3181	0·6068	0·2799	0·6478
	24	0·4800	0·3366	0·6258	0·2976	0·6663
	25	0·5000	0·3553	0·6447	0·3155	0·6845
	26	0·5200	0·3742	0·6634	0·3337	0·7024
	27	0·5400	0·3932	0·6819	0·3522	0·7201
	28	0·5600	0·4125	0·7001	0·3709	0·7374
	29	0·5800	0·4321	0·7181	0·3899	0·7545
	30	0·6000	0·4518	0·7359	0·4092	0·7713
	31	0·6200	0·4717	0·7535	0·4287	0·7879
	32	0·6400	0·4919	0·7708	0·4486	0·8041
	33	0·6600	0·5123	0·7879	0·4688	0·8200
	34	0·6800	0·5330	0·8048	0·4892	0·8356
	35	0·7000	0·5539	0·8214	0·5100	0·8509
	36	0·7200	0·5751	0·8377	0·5311	0·8658
	37	0·7400	0·5966	0·8537	0·5526	0·8803
	38	0·7600	0·6183	0·8694	0·5745	0·8944
	39	0·7800	0·6404	0·8847	0·5968	0·9081
	40	0·8000	0·6628	0·8997	0·6195	0·9214
	41	0·8200	0·6856	0·9142	0·6427	0·9340
	42	0·8400	0·7089	0·9283	0·6665	0·9461
	43	0·8600	0·7326	0·9418	0·6909	0·9575
	44	0·8800	0·7569	0·9547	0·7160	0·9681
	45	0·9000	0·7819	0·9667	0·7420	0·9778
	46	0·9200	0·8077	0·9778	0·7689	0·9862
	47	0·9400	0·8345	0·9875	0·7973	0·9931
	48	0·9600	0·8629	0·9951	0·8275	0·9979

n	x	p	95% p_l	p_u	99% p_l	p_u
50	49	0·9800	0·8935	0·9995	0·8606	0·9999
	50	1·0000	0·9289	1·0000	0·8995	1·0000
51	0	0·0000	0·0000	0·0698	0·0000	0·0987
	1	0·0196	0·0005	0·1045	0·0001	0·1368
	2	0·0392	0·0048	0·1346	0·0020	0·1694
	3	0·0588	0·0123	0·1624	0·0067	0·1990
	4	0·0784	0·0218	0·1888	0·0135	0·2269
	5	0·0980	0·0326	0·2141	0·0218	0·2535
	6	0·1176	0·0444	0·2387	0·0312	0·2790
	7	0·1373	0·0570	0·2626	0·0416	0·3037
	8	0·1569	0·0702	0·2859	0·0528	0·3277
	9	0·1765	0·0840	0·3087	0·0646	0·3511
	10	0·1961	0·0982	0·3312	0·0770	0·3739
	11	0·2157	0·1129	0·3532	0·0899	0·3963
	12	0·2353	0·1279	0·3749	0·1033	0·4182
	13	0·2549	0·1433	0·3963	0·1172	0·4398
	14	0·2745	0·1589	0·4174	0·1314	0·4610
	15	0·2941	0·1749	0·4383	0·1459	0·4818
	16	0·3137	0·1911	0·4589	0·1609	0·5023
	17	0·3333	0·2076	0·4792	0·1761	0·5225
	18	0·3529	0·2243	0·4993	0·1917	0·5423
	19	0·3725	0·2413	0·5192	0·2075	0·5619
	20	0·3922	0·2584	0·5389	0·2237	0·5813
	21	0·4118	0·2758	0·5583	0·2401	0·6003
	22	0·4314	0·2935	0·5775	0·2568	0·6191
	23	0·4510	0·3113	0·5966	0·2737	0·6376
	24	0·4706	0·3293	0·6154	0·2910	0·6558
	25	0·4902	0·3475	0·6340	0·3084	0·6738
	26	0·5098	0·3660	0·6525	0·3262	0·6916
	27	0·5294	0·3846	0·6707	0·3442	0·7090
	28	0·5490	0·4034	0·6887	0·3624	0·7263
	29	0·5686	0·4225	0·7065	0·3809	0·7432
	30	0·5882	0·4417	0·7242	0·3997	0·7599
	31	0·6078	0·4611	0·7416	0·4187	0·7763
	32	0·6275	0·4808	0·7587	0·4381	0·7925
	33	0·6471	0·5007	0·7757	0·4577	0·8083
	34	0·6667	0·5208	0·7924	0·4775	0·8239
	35	0·6863	0·5411	0·8089	0·4977	0·8391
	36	0·7059	0·5617	0·8251	0·5182	0·8541
	37	0·7255	0·5826	0·8411	0·5390	0·8686
	38	0·7451	0·6037	0·8567	0·5602	0·8828
	39	0·7647	0·6251	0·8721	0·5818	0·8967
	40	0·7843	0·6468	0·8871	0·6037	0·9101
	41	0·8039	0·6688	0·9018	0·6261	0·9230
	42	0·8235	0·6913	0·9160	0·6489	0·9354
	43	0·8431	0·7141	0·9298	0·6723	0·9472
	44	0·8627	0·7374	0·9430	0·6963	0·9584
	45	0·8824	0·7613	0·9556	0·7210	0·9688
	46	0·9020	0·7859	0·9674	0·7465	0·9782
	47	0·9216	0·8112	0·9782	0·7731	0·9865

Table B.11 Exact confidence limits for a binomial proportion: x events are observed in a sample sized n. $p = x/n$ is the observed proportion. p_l and p_u are the lower and upper confidence limits for the population proportion.

Confidence level			95%		99%	
n	x	p	p_l	p_u	p_l	p_u
51	48	0·9412	0·8376	0·9877	0·8010	0·9933
	49	0·9608	0·8654	0·9952	0·8306	0·9980
	50	0·9804	0·8955	0·9995	0·8632	0·9999
	51	1·0000	0·9302	1·0000	0·9013	1·0000
52	0	0·0000	0·0000	0·0685	0·0000	0·0969
	1	0·0192	0·0005	0·1026	0·0001	0·1344
	2	0·0385	0·0047	0·1321	0·0020	0·1663
	3	0·0577	0·0121	0·1595	0·0066	0·1955
	4	0·0769	0·0214	0·1854	0·0132	0·2229
	5	0·0962	0·0320	0·2103	0·0213	0·2490
	6	0·1154	0·0435	0·2344	0·0306	0·2741
	7	0·1346	0·0559	0·2579	0·0408	0·2984
	8	0·1538	0·0688	0·2808	0·0517	0·3220
	9	0·1731	0·0823	0·3033	0·0633	0·3451
	10	0·1923	0·0963	0·3253	0·0754	0·3676
	11	0·2115	0·1106	0·3470	0·0881	0·3896
	12	0·2308	0·1253	0·3684	0·1012	0·4112
	13	0·2500	0·1403	0·3895	0·1147	0·4324
	14	0·2692	0·1557	0·4102	0·1286	0·4533
	15	0·2885	0·1713	0·4308	0·1429	0·4738
	16	0·3077	0·1872	0·4510	0·1575	0·4940
	17	0·3269	0·2033	0·4711	0·1724	0·5139
	18	0·3462	0·2197	0·4909	0·1876	0·5336
	19	0·3654	0·2362	0·5104	0·2031	0·5529
	20	0·3846	0·2530	0·5298	0·2189	0·5720
	21	0·4038	0·2701	0·5490	0·2349	0·5908
	22	0·4231	0·2873	0·5680	0·2512	0·6093
	23	0·4423	0·3047	0·5867	0·2678	0·6276
	24	0·4615	0·3223	0·6053	0·2846	0·6457
	25	0·4808	0·3401	0·6237	0·3017	0·6635
	26	0·5000	0·3581	0·6419	0·3190	0·6810
	27	0·5192	0·3763	0·6599	0·3365	0·6983
	28	0·5385	0·3947	0·6777	0·3543	0·7154
	29	0·5577	0·4133	0·6953	0·3724	0·7322
	30	0·5769	0·4320	0·7127	0·3907	0·7488
	31	0·5962	0·4510	0·7299	0·4092	0·7651
	32	0·6154	0·4702	0·7470	0·4280	0·7811
	33	0·6346	0·4896	0·7638	0·4471	0·7969
	34	0·6538	0·5091	0·7803	0·4664	0·8124
	35	0·6731	0·5289	0·7967	0·4861	0·8276
	36	0·6923	0·5490	0·8128	0·5060	0·8425
	37	0·7115	0·5692	0·8287	0·5262	0·8571
	38	0·7308	0·5898	0·8443	0·5467	0·8714
	39	0·7500	0·6105	0·8597	0·5676	0·8853
	40	0·7692	0·6316	0·8747	0·5888	0·8988
	41	0·7885	0·6530	0·8894	0·6104	0·9119
	42	0·8077	0·6747	0·9037	0·6324	0·9246
	43	0·8269	0·6967	0·9177	0·6549	0·9367
	44	0·8462	0·7192	0·9312	0·6780	0·9483

Confidence level			95%		99%	
n	x	p	p_l	p_u	p_l	p_u
52	45	0·8654	0·7421	0·9441	0·7016	0·9592
	46	0·8846	0·7656	0·9565	0·7259	0·9694
	47	0·9038	0·7897	0·9680	0·7510	0·9787
	48	0·9231	0·8146	0·9786	0·7771	0·9868
	49	0·9423	0·8405	0·9879	0·8045	0·9934
	50	0·9615	0·8679	0·9953	0·8337	0·9980
	51	0·9808	0·8974	0·9995	0·8656	0·9999
	52	1·0000	0·9315	1·0000	0·9031	1·0000
53	0	0·0000	0·0000	0·0672	0·0000	0·0951
	1	0·0189	0·0005	0·1007	0·0001	0·1320
	2	0·0377	0·0046	0·1298	0·0020	0·1634
	3	0·0566	0·0118	0·1566	0·0065	0·1921
	4	0·0755	0·0209	0·1821	0·0130	0·2190
	5	0·0943	0·0313	0·2066	0·0209	0·2447
	6	0·1132	0·0427	0·2303	0·0300	0·2694
	7	0·1321	0·0548	0·2534	0·0400	0·2933
	8	0·1509	0·0675	0·2759	0·0507	0·3166
	9	0·1698	0·0807	0·2980	0·0620	0·3393
	10	0·1887	0·0944	0·3197	0·0739	0·3614
	11	0·2075	0·1084	0·3411	0·0863	0·3831
	12	0·2264	0·1228	0·3621	0·0992	0·4044
	13	0·2453	0·1376	0·3828	0·1124	0·4253
	14	0·2642	0·1526	0·4033	0·1260	0·4459
	15	0·2830	0·1679	0·4235	0·1400	0·4661
	16	0·3019	0·1834	0·4434	0·1543	0·4861
	17	0·3208	0·1992	0·4632	0·1689	0·5057
	18	0·3396	0·2152	0·4827	0·1837	0·5251
	19	0·3585	0·2314	0·5020	0·1989	0·5441
	20	0·3774	0·2479	0·5211	0·2143	0·5630
	21	0·3962	0·2645	0·5400	0·2300	0·5815
	22	0·4151	0·2814	0·5587	0·2459	0·5999
	23	0·4340	0·2984	0·5772	0·2621	0·6179
	24	0·4528	0·3156	0·5955	0·2786	0·6358
	25	0·4717	0·3330	0·6136	0·2952	0·6534
	26	0·4906	0·3506	0·6316	0·3121	0·6707
	27	0·5094	0·3684	0·6494	0·3293	0·6879
	28	0·5283	0·3864	0·6670	0·3466	0·7048
	29	0·5472	0·4045	0·6844	0·3642	0·7214
	30	0·5660	0·4228	0·7016	0·3812	0·7379
	31	0·5849	0·4413	0·7186	0·4001	0·7541
	32	0·6038	0·4600	0·7355	0·4185	0·7700
	33	0·6226	0·4789	0·7521	0·4370	0·7857
	34	0·6415	0·4980	0·7686	0·4559	0·8011
	35	0·6604	0·5173	0·7848	0·4749	0·8163
	36	0·6792	0·5368	0·8008	0·4943	0·8311
	37	0·6981	0·5566	0·8166	0·5139	0·8457
	38	0·7170	0·5765	0·8321	0·5339	0·8600
	39	0·7358	0·5967	0·8474	0·5541	0·8740
	40	0·7547	0·6172	0·8624	0·5747	0·8876

Continued

Table B.11 Exact confidence limits for a binomial proportion: x events are observed in a sample sized n. $p = x/n$ is the observed proportion. p_l and p_u are the lower and upper confidence limits for the population proportion.

Confidence level			95%		99%	
n	x	p	p_l	p_u	p_l	p_u
53	41	0·7736	0·6379	0·8772	0·5956	0·9008
	42	0·7925	0·6589	0·8916	0·6169	0·9137
	43	0·8113	0·6803	0·9056	0·6386	0·9261
	44	0·8302	0·7020	0·9193	0·6607	0·9380
	45	0·8491	0·7241	0·9325	0·6834	0·9493
	46	0·8679	0·7466	0·9452	0·7067	0·9600
	47	0·8868	0·7697	0·9573	0·7306	0·9700
	48	0·9057	0·7934	0·9687	0·7553	0·9791
	49	0·9245	0·8179	0·9791	0·7810	0·9870
	50	0·9434	0·8434	0·9882	0·8079	0·9935
	51	0·9623	0·8702	0·9954	0·8366	0·9980
	52	0·9811	0·8993	0·9995	0·8680	0·9999
	53	1·0000	0·9328	1·0000	0·9049	1·0000
54	0	0·0000	0·0000	0·0660	0·0000	0·0935
	1	0·0185	0·0005	0·0989	0·0001	0·1297
	2	0·0370	0·0045	0·1275	0·0019	0·1606
	3	0·0556	0·0116	0·1539	0·0064	0·1888
	4	0·0741	0·0206	0·1789	0·0127	0·2153
	5	0·0926	0·0308	0·2030	0·0205	0·2406
	6	0·1111	0·0419	0·2263	0·0294	0·2649
	7	0·1296	0·0537	0·2490	0·0392	0·2884
	8	0·1481	0·0662	0·2712	0·0497	0·3113
	9	0·1667	0·0792	0·2929	0·0608	0·3336
	10	0·1852	0·0925	0·3143	0·0725	0·3555
	11	0·2037	0·1063	0·3353	0·0846	0·3769
	12	0·2222	0·1204	0·3560	0·0972	0·3978
	13	0·2407	0·1349	0·3764	0·1102	0·4185
	14	0·2593	0·1496	0·3965	0·1235	0·4387
	15	0·2778	0·1646	0·4164	0·1372	0·4587
	16	0·2963	0·1798	0·4361	0·1512	0·4783
	17	0·3148	0·1952	0·4555	0·1655	0·4977
	18	0·3333	0·2109	0·4747	0·1800	0·5168
	19	0·3519	0·2268	0·4938	0·1948	0·5356
	20	0·3704	0·2429	0·5126	0·2099	0·5542
	21	0·3889	0·2592	0·5312	0·2253	0·5726
	22	0·4074	0·2757	0·5497	0·2409	0·5907
	23	0·4259	0·2923	0·5679	0·2567	0·6085
	24	0·4444	0·3092	0·5860	0·2727	0·6262
	25	0·4630	0·3262	0·6039	0·2890	0·6436
	26	0·4815	0·3434	0·6216	0·3055	0·6608
	27	0·5000	0·3608	0·6392	0·3223	0·6777
	28	0·5185	0·3784	0·6566	0·3392	0·6945
	29	0·5370	0·3961	0·6738	0·3564	0·7110
	30	0·5556	0·4140	0·6908	0·3738	0·7273
	31	0·5741	0·4321	0·7077	0·3915	0·7433
	32	0·5926	0·4503	0·7243	0·4093	0·7591
	33	0·6111	0·4688	0·7408	0·4274	0·7747
	34	0·6296	0·4874	0·7571	0·4458	0·7901
	35	0·6481	0·5062	0·7732	0·4644	0·8052

Confidence level			95%		99%	
n	x	p	p_l	p_u	p_l	p_u
54	36	0·6667	0·5253	0·7891	0·4832	0·8200
	37	0·6852	0·5445	0·8048	0·5023	0·8345
	38	0·7037	0·5639	0·8202	0·5217	0·8488
	39	0·7222	0·5836	0·8354	0·5413	0·8628
	40	0·7407	0·6035	0·8504	0·5613	0·8765
	41	0·7593	0·6236	0·8651	0·5815	0·8898
	42	0·7778	0·6440	0·8796	0·6022	0·9028
	43	0·7963	0·6647	0·8937	0·6231	0·9154
	44	0·8148	0·6857	0·9075	0·6445	0·9275
	45	0·8333	0·7071	0·9208	0·6664	0·9392
	46	0·8519	0·7288	0·9338	0·6887	0·9503
	47	0·8704	0·7510	0·9463	0·7116	0·9608
	48	0·8889	0·7737	0·9581	0·7351	0·9706
	49	0·9074	0·7970	0·9692	0·7594	0·9795
	50	0·9259	0·8211	0·9794	0·7847	0·9873
	51	0·9444	0·8461	0·9884	0·8112	0·9936
	52	0·9630	0·8725	0·9955	0·8394	0·9981
	53	0·9815	0·9011	0·9995	0·8703	0·9999
	54	1·0000	0·9340	1·0000	0·9065	1·0000
55	0	0·0000	0·0000	0·0649	0·0000	0·0918
	1	0·0182	0·0005	0·0972	0·0001	0·1275
	2	0·0364	0·0044	0·1253	0·0019	0·1579
	3	0·0545	0·0114	0·1512	0·0062	0·1856
	4	0·0727	0·0202	0·1759	0·0125	0·2117
	5	0·0909	0·0302	0·1995	0·0201	0·2366
	6	0·1091	0·0411	0·2225	0·0289	0·2605
	7	0·1273	0·0527	0·2448	0·0385	0·2837
	8	0·1455	0·0650	0·2666	0·0488	0·3062
	9	0·1636	0·0777	0·2880	0·0597	0·3282
	10	0·1818	0·0908	0·3090	0·0711	0·3497
	11	0·2000	0·1043	0·3297	0·0830	0·3708
	12	0·2182	0·1181	0·3501	0·0953	0·3915
	13	0·2364	0·1323	0·3702	0·1081	0·4118
	14	0·2545	0·1467	0·3900	0·1211	0·4318
	15	0·2727	0·1614	0·4096	0·1345	0·4515
	16	0·2909	0·1763	0·4290	0·1482	0·4708
	17	0·3091	0·1914	0·4481	0·1622	0·4900
	18	0·3273	0·2068	0·4671	0·1764	0·5088
	19	0·3455	0·2224	0·4858	0·1910	0·5274
	20	0·3636	0·2381	0·5044	0·2057	0·5457
	21	0·3818	0·2541	0·5227	0·2207	0·5639
	22	0·4000	0·2702	0·5409	0·2360	0·5817
	23	0·4182	0·2865	0·5589	0·2515	0·5994
	24	0·4364	0·3030	0·5768	0·2672	0·6168
	25	0·4545	0·3197	0·5945	0·2831	0·6340
	26	0·4727	0·3365	0·6120	0·2992	0·6510
	27	0·4909	0·3535	0·6293	0·3156	0·6678
	28	0·5091	0·3707	0·6465	0·3322	0·6844
	29	0·5273	0·3880	0·6635	0·3490	0·7008
	30	0·5455	0·4055	0·6803	0·3660	0·7169

Continued

Table B.11 Exact confidence limits for a binomial proportion: x events are observed in a sample sized n. $p = x/n$ is the observed proportion. p_l and p_u are the lower and upper confidence limits for the population proportion.

Confidence level			95%		99%	
n	x	p	p_l	p_u	p_l	p_u
55	31	0·5636	0·4232	0·6970	0·3832	0·7328
	32	0·5818	0·4411	0·7135	0·4006	0·7485
	33	0·6000	0·4591	0·7298	0·4183	0·7640
	34	0·6182	0·4773	0·7459	0·4361	0·7793
	35	0·6364	0·4956	0·7619	0·4543	0·7943
	36	0·6545	0·5142	0·7776	0·4726	0·8090
	37	0·6727	0·5329	0·7932	0·4912	0·8236
	38	0·6909	0·5519	0·8086	0·5100	0·8378
	39	0·7091	0·5710	0·8237	0·5292	0·8518
	40	0·7273	0·5904	0·8386	0·5485	0·8655
	41	0·7455	0·6100	0·8533	0·5682	0·8789
	42	0·7636	0·6298	0·8677	0·5882	0·8919
	43	0·7818	0·6499	0·8819	0·6085	0·9047
	44	0·8000	0·6703	0·8957	0·6292	0·9170
	45	0·8182	0·6910	0·9092	0·6503	0·9289
	46	0·8364	0·7120	0·9223	0·6718	0·9403
	47	0·8545	0·7334	0·9350	0·6938	0·9512
	48	0·8727	0·7552	0·9473	0·7163	0·9615
	49	0·8909	0·7775	0·9589	0·7395	0·9711
	50	0·9091	0·8005	0·9698	0·7634	0·9799
	51	0·9273	0·8241	0·9798	0·7883	0·9875
	52	0·9455	0·8488	0·9886	0·8144	0·9938
	53	0·9636	0·8747	0·9956	0·8421	0·9981
	54	0·9818	0·9028	0·9995	0·8725	0·9999
	55	1·0000	0·9351	1·0000	0·9082	1·0000
56	0	0·0000	0·0000	0·0638	0·0000	0·0903
	1	0·0179	0·0005	0·0955	0·0001	0·1253
	2	0·0357	0·0044	0·1231	0·0019	0·1552
	3	0·0536	0·0112	0·1487	0·0061	0·1825
	4	0·0714	0·0198	0·1729	0·0123	0·2082
	5	0·0893	0·0296	0·1962	0·0198	0·2327
	6	0·1071	0·0403	0·2188	0·0283	0·2563
	7	0·1250	0·0518	0·2407	0·0377	0·2791
	8	0·1429	0·0638	0·2622	0·0479	0·3013
	9	0·1607	0·0762	0·2833	0·0586	0·3230
	10	0·1786	0·0891	0·3040	0·0698	0·3442
	11	0·1964	0·1023	0·3243	0·0814	0·3649
	12	0·2143	0·1159	0·3444	0·0935	0·3853
	13	0·2321	0·1298	0·3642	0·1060	0·4053
	14	0·2500	0·1439	0·3837	0·1188	0·4250
	15	0·2679	0·1583	0·4030	0·1319	0·4445
	16	0·2857	0·1730	0·4221	0·1453	0·4636
	17	0·3036	0·1878	0·4410	0·1590	0·4824
	18	0·3214	0·2029	0·4596	0·1730	0·5010
	19	0·3393	0·2181	0·4781	0·1872	0·5194
	20	0·3571	0·2336	0·4964	0·2017	0·5375
	21	0·3750	0·2492	0·5145	0·2164	0·5554
	22	0·3929	0·2650	0·5325	0·2313	0·5731
	23	0·4107	0·2810	0·5502	0·2465	0·5905

Table B.11 (*Continued*)

Confidence level			95%		99%	
n	x	p	p_l	p_u	p_l	p_u
56	24	0·4286	0·2971	0·5678	0·2618	0·6077
	25	0·4464	0·3134	0·5853	0·2774	0·6248
	26	0·4643	0·3299	0·6026	0·2932	0·6416
	27	0·4821	0·3466	0·6197	0·3092	0·6582
	28	0·5000	0·3634	0·6366	0·3254	0·6746
	29	0·5179	0·3803	0·6534	0·3418	0·6908
	30	0·5357	0·3974	0·6701	0·3584	0·7068
	31	0·5536	0·4147	0·6866	0·3752	0·7226
	32	0·5714	0·4322	0·7029	0·3923	0·7382
	33	0·5893	0·4498	0·7190	0·4095	0·7535
	34	0·6071	0·4675	0·7350	0·4269	0·7687
	35	0·6250	0·4855	0·7508	0·4446	0·7836
	36	0·6429	0·5036	0·7664	0·4625	0·7983
	37	0·6607	0·5219	0·7819	0·4806	0·8128
	38	0·6786	0·5404	0·7971	0·4990	0·8270
	39	0·6964	0·5590	0·8122	0·5176	0·8410
	40	0·7143	0·5779	0·8270	0·5364	0·8547
	41	0·7321	0·5970	0·8417	0·5555	0·8681
	42	0·7500	0·6163	0·8561	0·5750	0·8812
	43	0·7679	0·6358	0·8702	0·5947	0·8940
	44	0·7857	0·6556	0·8841	0·6147	0·9065
	45	0·8036	0·6757	0·8977	0·6351	0·9186
	46	0·8214	0·6960	0·9109	0·6558	0·9302
	47	0·8393	0·7167	0·9238	0·6770	0·9414
	48	0·8571	0·7378	0·9362	0·6987	0·9521
	49	0·8750	0·7593	0·9482	0·7209	0·9623
	50	0·8929	0·7812	0·9597	0·7437	0·9717
	51	0·9107	0·8038	0·9704	0·7673	0·9802
	52	0·9286	0·8271	0·9802	0·7918	0·9877
	53	0·9464	0·8513	0·9888	0·8175	0·9939
	54	0·9643	0·8769	0·9956	0·8448	0·9981
	55	0·9821	0·9045	0·9995	0·8747	0·9999
	56	1·0000	0·9362	1·0000	0·9097	1·0000
57	0	0·0000	0·0000	0·0627	0·0000	0·0888
	1	0·0175	0·0004	0·0939	0·0001	0·1232
	2	0·0351	0·0043	0·1211	0·0018	0·1527
	3	0·0526	0·0110	0·1462	0·0060	0·1796
	4	0·0702	0·0195	0·1700	0·0120	0·2048
	5	0·0877	0·0291	0·1930	0·0194	0·2290
	6	0·1053	0·0396	0·2152	0·0278	0·2522
	7	0·1228	0·0508	0·2368	0·0371	0·2747
	8	0·1404	0·0626	0·2579	0·0470	0·2965
	9	0·1579	0·0748	0·2787	0·0575	0·3179
	10	0·1754	0·0875	0·2991	0·0685	0·3388
	11	0·1930	0·1005	0·3191	0·0799	0·3592
	12	0·2105	0·1138	0·3389	0·0918	0·3793
	13	0·2281	0·1274	0·3584	0·1040	0·3991
	14	0·2456	0·1413	0·3776	0·1166	0·4185
	15	0·2632	0·1554	0·3966	0·1294	0·4377
	16	0·2807	0·1697	0·4154	0·1426	0·4565

Continued

Table B.11 Exact confidence limits for a binomial proportion: x events are observed in a sample sized n. $p = x/n$ is the observed proportion. p_l and p_u are the lower and upper confidence limits for the population proportion.

Confidence level			95%		99%	
n	x	p	p_l	p_u	p_l	p_u
57	17	0·2982	0·1843	0·4340	0·1560	0·4751
	18	0·3158	0·1991	0·4524	0·1697	0·4935
	19	0·3333	0·2140	0·4706	0·1836	0·5116
	20	0·3509	0·2291	0·4887	0·1978	0·5295
	21	0·3684	0·2445	0·5066	0·2122	0·5472
	22	0·3860	0·2600	0·5243	0·2268	0·5646
	23	0·4035	0·2756	0·5418	0·2417	0·5819
	24	0·4211	0·2914	0·5592	0·2567	0·5989
	25	0·4386	0·3074	0·5764	0·2720	0·6157
	26	0·4561	0·3236	0·5934	0·2874	0·6324
	27	0·4737	0·3398	0·6103	0·3031	0·6488
	28	0·4912	0·3563	0·6271	0·3189	0·6651
	29	0·5088	0·3729	0·6437	0·3349	0·6811
	30	0·5263	0·3897	0·6602	0·3512	0·6969
	31	0·5439	0·4066	0·6764	0·3676	0·7126
	32	0·5614	0·4236	0·6926	0·3843	0·7280
	33	0·5789	0·4408	0·7086	0·4011	0·7433
	34	0·5965	0·4582	0·7244	0·4181	0·7583
	35	0·6140	0·4757	0·7400	0·4354	0·7732
	36	0·6316	0·4934	0·7555	0·4528	0·7878
	37	0·6491	0·5113	0·7709	0·4705	0·8022
	38	0·6667	0·5294	0·7860	0·4884	0·8164
	39	0·6842	0·5476	0·8009	0·5065	0·8303
	40	0·7018	0·5660	0·8157	0·5249	0·8440
	41	0·7193	0·5846	0·8303	0·5435	0·8574
	42	0·7368	0·6034	0·8446	0·5623	0·8706
	43	0·7544	0·6224	0·8587	0·5815	0·8834
	44	0·7719	0·6416	0·8726	0·6009	0·8960
	45	0·7895	0·6611	0·8862	0·6207	0·9082
	46	0·8070	0·6809	0·8995	0·6408	0·9201
	47	0·8246	0·7009	0·9125	0·6612	0·9315
	48	0·8421	0·7213	0·9252	0·6821	0·9425
	49	0·8596	0·7421	0·9374	0·7035	0·9530
	50	0·8772	0·7632	0·9492	0·7253	0·9629
	51	0·8947	0·7848	0·9604	0·7478	0·9722
	52	0·9123	0·8070	0·9709	0·7710	0·9806
	53	0·9298	0·8300	0·9805	0·7952	0·9880
	54	0·9474	0·8538	0·9890	0·8204	0·9940
	55	0·9649	0·8789	0·9957	0·8473	0·9982
	56	0·9825	0·9061	0·9996	0·8768	0·9999
	57	1·0000	0·9373	1·0000	0·9112	1·0000
58	0	0·0000	0·0000	0·0616	0·0000	0·0873
	1	0·0172	0·0004	0·0924	0·0001	0·1212
	2	0·0345	0·0042	0·1191	0·0018	0·1502
	3	0·0517	0·0108	0·1438	0·0059	0·1767
	4	0·0690	0·0191	0·1673	0·0118	0·2016
	5	0·0862	0·0286	0·1898	0·0191	0·2253
	6	0·1034	0·0389	0·2117	0·0273	0·2482
	7	0·1207	0·0499	0·2330	0·0364	0·2703

Table B.11 (*Continued*)

Confidence level			95%		99%	
n	x	p	p_l	p_u	p_l	p_u
58	8	0·1379	0·0615	0·2538	0·0461	0·2919
	9	0·1552	0·0735	0·2742	0·0564	0·3129
	10	0·1724	0·0859	0·2943	0·0672	0·3335
	11	0·1897	0·0987	0·3141	0·0785	0·3537
	12	0·2069	0·1117	0·3335	0·0901	0·3735
	13	0·2241	0·1251	0·3527	0·1021	0·3930
	14	0·2414	0·1387	0·3717	0·1144	0·4122
	15	0·2586	0·1526	0·3904	0·1270	0·4311
	16	0·2759	0·1666	0·4090	0·1399	0·4497
	17	0·2931	0·1809	0·4273	0·1531	0·4680
	18	0·3103	0·1954	0·4454	0·1665	0·4862
	19	0·3276	0·2101	0·4634	0·1802	0·5041
	20	0·3448	0·2249	0·4812	0·1941	0·5217
	21	0·3621	0·2399	0·4988	0·2082	0·5392
	22	0·3793	0·2551	0·5163	0·2225	0·5564
	23	0·3966	0·2705	0·5336	0·2370	0·5735
	24	0·4138	0·2860	0·5507	0·2518	0·5903
	25	0·4310	0·3016	0·5677	0·2667	0·6070
	26	0·4483	0·3174	0·5846	0·2818	0·6234
	27	0·4655	0·3334	0·6013	0·2972	0·6397
	28	0·4828	0·3495	0·6178	0·3127	0·6557
	29	0·5000	0·3658	0·6342	0·3284	0·6716
	30	0·5172	0·3822	0·6505	0·3443	0·6873
	31	0·5345	0·3987	0·6666	0·3603	0·7028
	32	0·5517	0·4145	0·6826	0·3766	0·7182
	33	0·5690	0·4323	0·6984	0·3930	0·7333
	34	0·5862	0·4493	0·7140	0·4097	0·7482
	35	0·6034	0·4664	0·7295	0·4265	0·7630
	36	0·6207	0·4837	0·7449	0·4436	0·7775
	37	0·6379	0·5012	0·7601	0·4608	0·7918
	38	0·6552	0·5188	0·7751	0·4783	0·8059
	39	0·6724	0·5366	0·7899	0·4959	0·8198
	40	0·6897	0·5546	0·8046	0·5138	0·8335
	41	0·7069	0·5727	0·8191	0·5320	0·8469
	42	0·7241	0·5910	0·8334	0·5503	0·8601
	43	0·7414	0·6096	0·8474	0·5689	0·8730
	44	0·7586	0·6283	0·8613	0·5878	0·8856
	45	0·7759	0·6473	0·8749	0·6070	0·8979
	46	0·7931	0·6665	0·8883	0·6265	0·9099
	47	0·8103	0·6859	0·9013	0·6463	0·9215
	48	0·8276	0·7057	0·9141	0·6665	0·9328
	49	0·8448	0·7258	0·9265	0·6871	0·9436
	50	0·8621	0·7462	0·9385	0·7081	0·9539
	51	0·8793	0·7670	0·9501	0·7297	0·9636
	52	0·8966	0·7883	0·9611	0·7518	0·9727
	53	0·9138	0·8102	0·9714	0·7747	0·9809
	54	0·9310	0·8327	0·9809	0·7984	0·9882
	55	0·9483	0·8562	0·9892	0·8233	0·9941
	56	0·9655	0·8809	0·9958	0·8498	0·9982
	57	0·9828	0·9076	0·9996	0·8788	0·9999
	58	1·0000	0·9384	1·0000	0·9127	1·0000

Continued

Table B.11 Exact confidence limits for a binomial proportion: x events are observed in a sample sized n. $p = x/n$ is the observed proportion. p_l and p_u are the lower and upper confidence limits for the population proportion.

Confidence level			95%		99%	
n	x	p	p_l	p_u	p_l	p_u
59	0	0·0000	0·0000	0·0606	0·0000	0·0859
	1	0·0169	0·0004	0·0909	0·0001	0·1193
	2	0·0339	0·0041	0·1171	0·0018	0·1478
	3	0·0508	0·0106	0·1415	0·0058	0·1739
	4	0·0678	0·0188	0·1646	0·0116	0·1984
	5	0·0847	0·0281	0·1868	0·0187	0·2218
	6	0·1017	0·0382	0·2083	0·0269	0·2443
	7	0·1186	0·0491	0·2293	0·0358	0·2662
	8	0·1356	0·0604	0·2498	0·0453	0·2874
	9	0·1525	0·0722	0·2699	0·0554	0·3082
	10	0·1695	0·0844	0·2897	0·0660	0·3284
	11	0·1864	0·0969	0·3091	0·0771	0·3483
	12	0·2034	0·1098	0·3283	0·0885	0·3679
	13	0·2203	0·1229	0·3473	0·1003	0·3871
	14	0·2373	0·1362	0·3659	0·1124	0·4060
	15	0·2542	0·1498	0·3844	0·1247	0·4247
	16	0·2712	0·1636	0·4027	0·1374	0·4430
	17	0·2881	0·1776	0·4208	0·1503	0·4612
	18	0·3051	0·1919	0·4387	0·1635	0·4791
	19	0·3220	0·2062	0·4564	0·1769	0·4967
	20	0·3390	0·2208	0·4739	0·1905	0·5142
	21	0·3559	0·2355	0·4913	0·2043	0·5314
	22	0·3729	0·2504	0·5085	0·2184	0·5484
	23	0·3898	0·2655	0·5256	0·2326	0·5653
	24	0·4068	0·2807	0·5425	0·2470	0·5819
	25	0·4237	0·2961	0·5593	0·2617	0·5984
	26	0·4407	0·3116	0·5760	0·2765	0·6147
	27	0·4576	0·3272	0·5925	0·2915	0·6308
	28	0·4746	0·3430	0·6088	0·3067	0·6467
	29	0·4915	0·3589	0·6250	0·3220	0·6624
	30	0·5085	0·3750	0·6411	0·3376	0·6780
	31	0·5254	0·3912	0·6570	0·3533	0·6933
	32	0·5424	0·4075	0·6728	0·3692	0·7085
	33	0·5593	0·4240	0·6884	0·3853	0·7235
	34	0·5763	0·4407	0·7039	0·4016	0·7383
	35	0·5932	0·4575	0·7193	0·4181	0·7530
	36	0·6102	0·4744	0·7345	0·4347	0·7674
	37	0·6271	0·4915	0·7496	0·4516	0·7816
	38	0·6441	0·5087	0·7645	0·4686	0·7957
	39	0·6610	0·5261	0·7792	0·4858	0·8095
	40	0·6780	0·5436	0·7938	0·5033	0·8231
	41	0·6949	0·5613	0·8081	0·5209	0·8365
	42	0·7119	0·5792	0·8224	0·5388	0·8497
	43	0·7288	0·5973	0·8364	0·5570	0·8626
	44	0·7458	0·6156	0·8502	0·5753	0·8753
	45	0·7627	0·6341	0·8638	0·5940	0·8876
	46	0·7797	0·6527	0·8771	0·6129	0·8997
	47	0·7966	0·6717	0·8902	0·6321	0·9115
	48	0·8136	0·6909	0·9031	0·6517	0·9229

Confidence level			95%		99%	
n	x	p	p_l	p_u	p_l	p_u
59	49	0·8305	0·7103	0·9156	0·6716	0·9340
	50	0·8475	0·7301	0·9278	0·6918	0·9446
	51	0·8644	0·7502	0·9396	0·7126	0·9547
	52	0·8814	0·7707	0·9509	0·7338	0·9642
	53	0·8983	0·7917	0·9618	0·7557	0·9731
	54	0·9153	0·8132	0·9719	0·7782	0·9813
	55	0·9322	0·8354	0·9812	0·8016	0·9884
	56	0·9492	0·8585	0·9894	0·8261	0·9942
	57	0·9661	0·8829	0·9959	0·8522	0·9982
	58	0·9831	0·9091	0·9996	0·8807	0·9999
	59	1·0000	0·9394	1·0000	0·9141	1·0000
60	0	0·0000	0·0000	0·0596	0·0000	0·0845
	1	0·0167	0·0004	0·0894	0·0001	0·1174
	2	0·0333	0·0041	0·1153	0·0017	0·1455
	3	0·0500	0·0104	0·1392	0·0057	0·1712
	4	0·0667	0·0185	0·1620	0·0114	0·1953
	5	0·0833	0·0276	0·1839	0·0184	0·2184
	6	0·1000	0·0376	0·2051	0·0264	0·2406
	7	0·1167	0·0482	0·2257	0·0351	0·2621
	8	0·1333	0·0594	0·2459	0·0445	0·2831
	9	0·1500	0·0710	0·2657	0·0545	0·3035
	10	0·1667	0·0829	0·2852	0·0649	0·3235
	11	0·1833	0·0952	0·3044	0·0757	0·3431
	12	0·2000	0·1078	0·3233	0·0869	0·3624
	13	0·2167	0·1207	0·3420	0·0985	0·3814
	14	0·2333	0·1338	0·3604	0·1104	0·4001
	15	0·2500	0·1472	0·3786	0·1225	0·4184
	16	0·2667	0·1607	0·3966	0·1349	0·4366
	17	0·2833	0·1745	0·4144	0·1476	0·4545
	18	0·3000	0·1885	0·4321	0·1605	0·4721
	19	0·3167	0·2026	0·4496	0·1737	0·4896
	20	0·3333	0·2169	0·4669	0·1870	0·5068
	21	0·3500	0·2313	0·4840	0·2006	0·5239
	22	0·3667	0·2459	0·5010	0·2144	0·5407
	23	0·3833	0·2607	0·5179	0·2283	0·5573
	24	0·4000	0·2756	0·5346	0·2425	0·5738
	25	0·4167	0·2907	0·5512	0·2568	0·5901
	26	0·4333	0·3059	0·5676	0·2713	0·6062
	27	0·4500	0·3212	0·5839	0·2860	0·6221
	28	0·4667	0·3367	0·6000	0·3009	0·6378
	29	0·4833	0·3523	0·6161	0·3160	0·6534
	30	0·5000	0·3681	0·6319	0·3312	0·6688
	31	0·5167	0·3839	0·6477	0·3466	0·6840
	32	0·5333	0·4000	0·6633	0·3622	0·6991
	33	0·5500	0·4161	0·6788	0·3779	0·7140
	34	0·5667	0·4324	0·6941	0·3938	0·7287
	35	0·5833	0·4488	0·7093	0·4099	0·7432
	36	0·6000	0·4654	0·7244	0·4262	0·7575
	37	0·6167	0·4821	0·7393	0·4427	0·7717
	38	0·6333	0·4990	0·7541	0·4593	0·7856

Continued

Table B.11 Exact confidence limits for a binomial proportion: x events are observed in a sample sized n. $p = x/n$ is the observed proportion. p_l and p_u are the lower and upper confidence limits for the population proportion.

Confidence level			95%		99%	
n	x	p	p_l	p_u	p_l	p_u
60	39	0·6500	0·5160	0·7687	0·4761	0·7994
	40	0·6667	0·5331	0·7831	0·4932	0·8130
	41	0·6833	0·5504	0·7974	0·5104	0·8263
	42	0·7000	0·5679	0·8115	0·5279	0·8395
	43	0·7167	0·5856	0·8255	0·5455	0·8524
	44	0·7333	0·6034	0·8393	0·5634	0·8651
	45	0·7500	0·6214	0·8528	0·5816	0·8775
	46	0·7667	0·6396	0·8662	0·5999	0·8896
	47	0·7833	0·6580	0·8793	0·6186	0·9015
	48	0·8000	0·6767	0·8922	0·6376	0·9131
	49	0·8167	0·6956	0·9048	0·6569	0·9243
	50	0·8333	0·7148	0·9171	0·6765	0·9351
	51	0·8500	0·7343	0·9290	0·6965	0·9455
	52	0·8667	0·7541	0·9406	0·7169	0·9555
	53	0·8833	0·7743	0·9518	0·7379	0·9649
	54	0·9000	0·7949	0·9624	0·7594	0·9736
	55	0·9167	0·8161	0·9724	0·7816	0·9816
	56	0·9333	0·8380	0·9815	0·8047	0·9886
	57	0·9500	0·8608	0·9896	0·8288	0·9943
	58	0·9667	0·8847	0·9959	0·8545	0·9983
	59	0·9833	0·9106	0·9996	0·8826	0·9999
	60	1·0000	0·9404	1·0000	0·9155	1·0000
61	0	0·0000	0·0000	0·0587	0·0000	0·0832
	1	0·0164	0·0004	0·0880	0·0001	0·1156
	2	0·0328	0·0040	0·1135	0·0017	0·1433
	3	0·0492	0·0103	0·1371	0·0056	0·1686
	4	0·0656	0·0182	0·1595	0·0112	0·1924
	5	0·0820	0·0272	0·1810	0·0181	0·2151
	6	0·0984	0·0370	0·2019	0·0259	0·2370
	7	0·1148	0·0474	0·2222	0·0345	0·2582
	8	0·1311	0·0584	0·2422	0·0438	0·2788
	9	0·1475	0·0698	0·2617	0·0535	0·2990
	10	0·1639	0·0815	0·2809	0·0638	0·3187
	11	0·1803	0·0936	0·2998	0·0744	0·3381
	12	0·1967	0·1060	0·3184	0·0854	0·3571
	13	0·2131	0·1186	0·3368	0·0968	0·3758
	14	0·2295	0·1315	0·3550	0·1084	0·3942
	15	0·2459	0·1446	0·3729	0·1204	0·4124
	16	0·2623	0·1580	0·3907	0·1326	0·4303
	17	0·2787	0·1715	0·4083	0·1450	0·4480
	18	0·2951	0·1852	0·4257	0·1577	0·4654
	19	0·3115	0·1990	0·4429	0·1706	0·4826
	20	0·3279	0·2131	0·4600	0·1837	0·4997
	21	0·3443	0·2273	0·4769	0·1970	0·5165
	22	0·3607	0·2416	0·4937	0·2105	0·5331
	23	0·3770	0·2561	0·5104	0·2242	0·5496
	24	0·3934	0·2707	0·5269	0·2381	0·5659
	25	0·4098	0·2855	0·5432	0·2521	0·5820
	26	0·4262	0·3004	0·5594	0·2664	0·5979

			95%		99%	
Confidence level						
n	x	p	p_l	p_u	p_l	p_u
61	27	0·4426	0·3155	0·5755	0·2808	0·6136
	28	0·4590	0·3306	0·5915	0·2954	0·6292
	29	0·4754	0·3460	0·6073	0·3101	0·6446
	30	0·4918	0·3614	0·6230	0·3250	0·6599
	31	0·5082	0·3770	0·6386	0·3401	0·6750
	32	0·5246	0·3927	0·6540	0·3554	0·6899
	33	0·5410	0·4085	0·6694	0·3708	0·7046
	34	0·5574	0·4245	0·6845	0·3864	0·7192
	35	0·5738	0·4406	0·6996	0·4021	0·7336
	36	0·5902	0·4568	0·7145	0·4180	0·7479
	37	0·6066	0·4731	0·7293	0·4341	0·7619
	38	0·6230	0·4896	0·7439	0·4504	0·7758
	39	0·6393	0·5063	0·7584	0·4669	0·7895
	40	0·6557	0·5231	0·7727	0·4835	0·8030
	41	0·6721	0·5400	0·7869	0·5003	0·8163
	42	0·6885	0·5571	0·8010	0·5174	0·8294
	43	0·7049	0·5743	0·8148	0·5346	0·8423
	44	0·7213	0·5917	0·8285	0·5520	0·8550
	45	0·7377	0·6093	0·8420	0·5697	0·8674
	46	0·7541	0·6271	0·8554	0·5876	0·8796
	47	0·7705	0·6450	0·8685	0·6058	0·8916
	48	0·7869	0·6632	0·8814	0·6242	0·9032
	49	0·8033	0·6816	0·8940	0·6429	0·9146
	50	0·8197	0·7002	0·9064	0·6619	0·9256
	51	0·8361	0·7191	0·9185	0·6813	0·9362
	52	0·8525	0·7383	0·9302	0·7010	0·9465
	53	0·8689	0·7578	0·9416	0·7212	0·9562
	54	0·8852	0·7778	0·9526	0·7418	0·9655
	55	0·9016	0·7981	0·9630	0·7630	0·9741
	56	0·9180	0·8190	0·9728	0·7849	0·9819
	57	0·9344	0·8405	0·9818	0·8076	0·9888
	58	0·9508	0·8629	0·9897	0·8314	0·9944
	59	0·9672	0·8865	0·9960	0·8567	0·9983
	60	0·9836	0·9120	0·9996	0·8844	0·9999
	61	1·0000	0·9413	1·0000	0·9168	1·0000
62	0	0·0000	0·0000	0·0578	0·0000	0·0819
	1	0·0161	0·0004	0·0866	0·0001	0·1138
	2	0·0323	0·0039	0·1117	0·0017	0·1411
	3	0·0484	0·0101	0·1350	0·0055	0·1660
	4	0·0645	0·0179	0·1570	0·0111	0·1895
	5	0·0806	0·0267	0·1783	0·0178	0·2119
	6	0·0968	0·0363	0·1988	0·0255	0·2335
	7	0·1129	0·0466	0·2189	0·0340	0·2544
	8	0·1290	0·0574	0·2385	0·0430	0·2747
	9	0·1452	0·0686	0·2578	0·0526	0·2946
	10	0·1613	0·0802	0·2767	0·0627	0·3141
	11	0·1774	0·0920	0·2953	0·0732	0·3332
	12	0·1935	0·1042	0·3137	0·0840	0·3520
	13	0·2097	0·1166	0·3318	0·0951	0·3704
	14	0·2258	0·1293	0·3497	0·1066	0·3886

Continued

Table B.11 Exact confidence limits for a binomial proportion: x events are observed in a sample sized n. $p = x/n$ is the observed proportion. p_l and p_u are the lower and upper confidence limits for the population proportion.

Confidence level			95%		99%	
n	x	p	p_l	p_u	p_l	p_u
62	15	0·2419	0·1422	0·3674	0·1183	0·4065
	16	0·2581	0·1553	0·3850	0·1303	0·4242
	17	0·2742	0·1685	0·4023	0·1425	0·4416
	18	0·2903	0·1820	0·4195	0·1549	0·4589
	19	0·3065	0·1956	0·4365	0·1676	0·4759
	20	0·3226	0·2094	0·4534	0·1805	0·4927
	21	0·3387	0·2233	0·4701	0·1935	0·5093
	22	0·3548	0·2374	0·4866	0·2068	0·5258
	23	0·3710	0·2516	0·5031	0·2202	0·5421
	24	0·3871	0·2660	0·5193	0·2338	0·5581
	25	0·4032	0·2805	0·5355	0·2476	0·5741
	26	0·4194	0·2951	0·5515	0·2616	0·5898
	27	0·4355	0·3099	0·5674	0·2757	0·6054
	28	0·4516	0·3248	0·5832	0·2900	0·6208
	29	0·4677	0·3398	0·5988	0·3045	0·6361
	30	0·4839	0·3550	0·6144	0·3191	0·6512
	31	0·5000	0·3702	0·6298	0·3339	0·6661
	32	0·5161	0·3856	0·6450	0·3488	0·6809
	33	0·5323	0·4012	0·6602	0·3639	0·6955
	34	0·5484	0·4168	0·6752	0·3792	0·7100
	35	0·5645	0·4326	0·6901	0·3946	0·7243
	36	0·5806	0·4485	0·7049	0·4102	0·7384
	37	0·5968	0·4645	0·7195	0·4259	0·7524
	38	0·6129	0·4807	0·7340	0·4419	0·7662
	39	0·6290	0·4969	0·7484	0·4579	0·7798
	40	0·6452	0·5134	0·7626	0·4742	0·7932
	41	0·6613	0·5299	0·7767	0·4907	0·8065
	42	0·6774	0·5466	0·7906	0·5073	0·8195
	43	0·6935	0·5635	0·8044	0·5241	0·8324
	44	0·7097	0·5805	0·8180	0·5411	0·8451
	45	0·7258	0·5977	0·8315	0·5584	0·8575
	46	0·7419	0·6150	0·8447	0·5758	0·8697
	47	0·7581	0·6326	0·8578	0·5935	0·8817
	48	0·7742	0·6503	0·8707	0·6114	0·8934
	49	0·7903	0·6682	0·8834	0·6296	0·9049
	50	0·8065	0·6863	0·8958	0·6480	0·9160
	51	0·8226	0·7047	0·9080	0·6668	0·9268
	52	0·8387	0·7233	0·9198	0·6859	0·9373
	53	0·8548	0·7422	0·9314	0·7054	0·9474
	54	0·8710	0·7615	0·9426	0·7253	0·9570
	55	0·8871	0·7811	0·9534	0·7456	0·9660
	56	0·9032	0·8012	0·9637	0·7665	0·9745
	57	0·9194	0·8217	0·9733	0·7881	0·9822
	58	0·9355	0·8430	0·9821	0·8105	0·9889
	59	0·9516	0·8650	0·9899	0·8340	0·9945
	60	0·9677	0·8883	0·9961	0·8589	0·9983
	61	0·9839	0·9134	0·9996	0·8862	0·9999
	62	1·0000	0·9422	1·0000	0·9181	1·0000

Confidence level			95%		99%	
n	x	p	p_l	p_u	p_l	p_u
63	0	0·0000	0·0000	0·0569	0·0000	0·0807
	1	0·0159	0·0004	0·0853	0·0001	0·1121
	2	0·0317	0·0039	0·1100	0·0017	0·1390
	3	0·0476	0·0099	0·1329	0·0054	0·1636
	4	0·0635	0·0176	0·1547	0·0109	0·1867
	5	0·0794	0·0263	0·1756	0·0175	0·2088
	6	0·0952	0·0358	0·1959	0·0251	0·2300
	7	0·1111	0·0459	0·2156	0·0334	0·2507
	8	0·1270	0·0565	0·2350	0·0423	0·2708
	9	0·1429	0·0675	0·2539	0·0518	0·2904
	10	0·1587	0·0788	0·2726	0·0617	0·3096
	11	0·1746	0·0905	0·2910	0·0719	0·3284
	12	0·1905	0·1025	0·3091	0·0826	0·3470
	13	0·2063	0·1147	0·3270	0·0935	0·3652
	14	0·2222	0·1272	0·3446	0·1048	0·3831
	15	0·2381	0·1398	0·3621	0·1163	0·4008
	16	0·2540	0·1527	0·3794	0·1281	0·4183
	17	0·2698	0·1657	0·3965	0·1401	0·4355
	18	0·2857	0·1789	0·4135	0·1523	0·4525
	19	0·3016	0·1923	0·4302	0·1647	0·4693
	20	0·3175	0·2058	0·4469	0·1774	0·4859
	21	0·3333	0·2195	0·4634	0·1902	0·5024
	22	0·3492	0·2334	0·4797	0·2032	0·5186
	23	0·3651	0·2473	0·4960	0·2164	0·5347
	24	0·3810	0·2615	0·5120	0·2297	0·5506
	25	0·3968	0·2757	0·5280	0·2433	0·5664
	26	0·4127	0·2901	0·5438	0·2570	0·5819
	27	0·4286	0·3046	0·5595	0·2708	0·5974
	28	0·4444	0·3192	0·5751	0·2849	0·6126
	29	0·4603	0·3339	0·5906	0·2990	0·6277
	30	0·4762	0·3488	0·6059	0·3134	0·6427
	31	0·4921	0·3638	0·6211	0·3279	0·6575
	32	0·5079	0·3789	0·6362	0·3425	0·6721
	33	0·5238	0·3941	0·6512	0·3573	0·6866
	34	0·5397	0·4094	0·6661	0·3723	0·7010
	35	0·5556	0·4249	0·6808	0·3874	0·7151
	36	0·5714	0·4405	0·6954	0·4026	0·7292
	37	0·5873	0·4562	0·7099	0·4181	0·7430
	38	0·6032	0·4720	0·7243	0·4336	0·7567
	39	0·6190	0·4880	0·7385	0·4494	0·7703
	40	0·6349	0·5040	0·7527	0·4653	0·7836
	41	0·6508	0·5203	0·7666	0·4814	0·7968
	42	0·6667	0·5366	0·7805	0·4976	0·8098
	43	0·6825	0·5531	0·7942	0·5141	0·8226
	44	0·6984	0·5698	0·8077	0·5307	0·8353
	45	0·7143	0·5865	0·8211	0·5475	0·8477
	46	0·7302	0·6035	0·8343	0·5645	0·8599
	47	0·7460	0·6206	0·8473	0·5817	0·8719
	48	0·7619	0·6379	0·8602	0·5992	0·8837
	49	0·7778	0·6554	0·8728	0·6169	0·8952
	50	0·7937	0·6730	0·8853	0·6348	0·9065

Continued

Table B.11 Exact confidence limits for a binomial proportion: x events are observed in a sample sized n. $p = x/n$ is the observed proportion. p_l and p_u are the lower and upper confidence limits for the population proportion.

Confidence level			95%		99%	
n	x	p	p_l	p_u	p_l	p_u
63	51	0·8095	0·6909	0·8975	0·6530	0·9174
	52	0·8254	0·7090	0·9095	0·6716	0·9281
	53	0·8413	0·7274	0·9212	0·6904	0·9383
	54	0·8571	0·7461	0·9325	0·7096	0·9482
	55	0·8730	0·7650	0·9435	0·7292	0·9577
	56	0·8889	0·7844	0·9541	0·7493	0·9666
	57	0·9048	0·8041	0·9642	0·7700	0·9749
	58	0·9206	0·8244	0·9737	0·7912	0·9825
	59	0·9365	0·8453	0·9824	0·8133	0·9891
	60	0·9524	0·8671	0·9901	0·8364	0·9946
	61	0·9683	0·8900	0·9961	0·8610	0·9983
	62	0·9841	0·9147	0·9996	0·8879	0·9999
	63	1·0000	0·9431	1·0000	0·9193	1·0000
64	0	0·0000	0·0000	0·0560	0·0000	0·0795
	1	0·0156	0·0004	0·0840	0·0001	0·1104
	2	0·0313	0·0038	0·1084	0·0016	0·1369
	3	0·0469	0·0098	0·1309	0·0053	0·1612
	4	0·0625	0·0173	0·1524	0·0107	0·1840
	5	0·0781	0·0259	0·1730	0·0172	0·2057
	6	0·0938	0·0352	0·1930	0·0247	0·2267
	7	0·1094	0·0451	0·2125	0·0329	0·2471
	8	0·1250	0·0555	0·2315	0·0416	0·2669
	9	0·1406	0·0664	0·2502	0·0509	0·2862
	10	0·1563	0·0776	0·2686	0·0606	0·3052
	11	0·1719	0·0890	0·2868	0·0708	0·3238
	12	0·1875	0·1008	0·3046	0·0812	0·3421
	13	0·2031	0·1128	0·3223	0·0920	0·3601
	14	0·2188	0·1251	0·3397	0·1030	0·3778
	15	0·2344	0·1375	0·3569	0·1144	0·3953
	16	0·2500	0·1502	0·3740	0·1259	0·4125
	17	0·2656	0·1630	0·3909	0·1377	0·4295
	18	0·2813	0·1760	0·4076	0·1497	0·4463
	19	0·2969	0·1891	0·4242	0·1619	0·4629
	20	0·3125	0·2024	0·4406	0·1743	0·4794
	21	0·3281	0·2159	0·4569	0·1869	0·4956
	22	0·3438	0·2295	0·4730	0·1997	0·5117
	23	0·3594	0·2432	0·4890	0·2127	0·5276
	24	0·3750	0·2570	0·5049	0·2258	0·5433
	25	0·3906	0·2710	0·5207	0·2391	0·5589
	26	0·4063	0·2851	0·5363	0·2525	0·5743
	27	0·4219	0·2994	0·5518	0·2661	0·5895
	28	0·4375	0·3137	0·5672	0·2799	0·6046
	29	0·4531	0·3282	0·5825	0·2938	0·6196
	30	0·4688	0·3428	0·5977	0·3079	0·6344
	31	0·4844	0·3575	0·6127	0·3221	0·6490
	32	0·5000	0·3723	0·6277	0·3364	0·6636
	33	0·5156	0·3873	0·6425	0·3510	0·6779
	34	0·5313	0·4023	0·6572	0·3656	0·6921
	35	0·5469	0·4175	0·6718	0·3804	0·7062

Table B.11 (*Continued*)

			95%		99%	
Confidence level						
n	x	p	p_l	p_u	p_l	p_u
64	36	0·5625	0·4328	0·6863	0·3954	0·7201
	37	0·5781	0·4482	0·7006	0·4105	0·7339
	38	0·5938	0·4637	0·7149	0·4257	0·7475
	39	0·6094	0·4793	0·7290	0·4411	0·7609
	40	0·6250	0·4951	0·7430	0·4567	0·7742
	41	0·6406	0·5110	0·7568	0·4724	0·7873
	42	0·6563	0·5270	0·7705	0·4883	0·8003
	43	0·6719	0·5431	0·7841	0·5044	0·8131
	44	0·6875	0·5594	0·7976	0·5206	0·8257
	45	0·7031	0·5758	0·8109	0·5371	0·8381
	46	0·7188	0·5924	0·8240	0·5537	0·8503
	47	0·7344	0·6091	0·8370	0·5705	0·8623
	48	0·7500	0·6260	0·8498	0·5875	0·8741
	49	0·7656	0·6431	0·8625	0·6047	0·8856
	50	0·7813	0·6603	0·8749	0·6222	0·8970
	51	0·7969	0·6777	0·8872	0·6399	0·9080
	52	0·8125	0·6954	0·8992	0·6579	0·9188
	53	0·8281	0·7132	0·9110	0·6762	0·9292
	54	0·8438	0·7314	0·9224	0·6948	0·9394
	55	0·8594	0·7498	0·9336	0·7138	0·9491
	56	0·8750	0·7685	0·9445	0·7331	0·9584
	57	0·8906	0·7875	0·9549	0·7529	0·9671
	58	0·9063	0·8070	0·9648	0·7733	0·9753
	59	0·9219	0·8270	9·9741	0·7943	0·9828
	60	0·9375	0·8476	0·9827	0·8160	0·9893
	61	0·9531	0·8691	0·9902	0·8388	0·9947
	62	0·9688	0·8916	0·9962	0·8631	0·9984
	63	0·9844	0·9160	0·9996	0·8896	0·9999
	64	1·0000	0·9440	1·0000	0·9205	1·0000
65	0	0·0000	0·0000	0·0552	0·0000	0·0783
	1	0·0154	0·0004	0·0828	0·0001	0·1088
	2	0·0308	0·0037	0·1068	0·0016	0·1349
	3	0·0462	0·0096	0·1290	0·0053	0·1588
	4	0·0615	0·0170	0·1501	0·0105	0·1813
	5	0·0769	0·0254	0·1705	0·0170	0·2028
	6	0·0923	0·0346	0·1902	0·0243	0·2235
	7	0·1077	0·0444	0·2094	0·0323	0·2436
	8	0·1231	0·0547	0·2282	0·0410	0·2631
	9	0·1385	0·0653	0·2466	0·0501	0·2822
	10	0·1538	0·0763	0·2648	0·0597	0·3009
	11	0·1692	0·0876	0·2827	0·0696	0·3193
	12	0·1846	0·0992	0·3003	0·0799	0·3373
	13	0·2000	0·1110	0·3177	0·0905	0·3551
	14	0·2154	0·1231	0·3349	0·1014	0·3726
	15	0·2308	0·1353	0·3519	0·1125	0·3899
	16	0·2462	0·1477	0·3687	0·1238	0·4069
	17	0·2615	0·1603	0·3854	0·1354	0·4237
	18	0·2769	0·1731	0·4019	0·1472	0·4403
	19	0·2923	0·1860	0·4183	0·1592	0·4567
	20	0·3077	0·1991	0·4345	0·1714	0·4729

Continued

Table B.11 Exact confidence limits for a binomial proportion: x events are observed in a sample sized n. $p = x/n$ is the observed proportion. p_l and p_u are the lower and upper confidence limits for the population proportion.

Confidence level			95%		99%	
n	x	p	p_l	p_u	p_l	p_u
65	21	0·3231	0·2123	0·4505	0·1838	0·4890
	22	0·3385	0·2257	0·4665	0·1964	0·5049
	23	0·3538	0·2392	0·4823	0·2091	0·5206
	24	0·3692	0·2528	0·4980	0·2220	0·5361
	25	0·3846	0·2665	0·5136	0·2350	0·5515
	26	0·4000	0·2804	0·5290	0·2482	0·5668
	27	0·4154	0·2944	0·5444	0·2616	0·5819
	28	0·4308	0·3085	0·5596	0·2751	0·5968
	29	0·4462	0·3227	0·5747	0·2888	0·6116
	30	0·4615	0·3370	0·5897	0·3026	0·6263
	31	0·4769	0·3515	0·6046	0·3165	0·6408
	32	0·4923	0·3660	0·6193	0·3306	0·6552
	33	0·5077	0·3807	0·6340	0·3448	0·6694
	34	0·5231	0·3954	0·6485	0·3592	0·6835
	35	0·5385	0·4103	0·6630	0·3737	0·6974
	36	0·5538	0·4253	0·6773	0·3884	0·7112
	37	0·5692	0·4404	0·6915	0·4032	0·7249
	38	0·5846	0·4556	0·7056	0·4181	0·7384
	39	0·6000	0·4710	0·7196	0·4332	0·7518
	40	0·6154	0·4864	0·7335	0·4485	0·7650
	41	0·6308	0·5020	0·7472	0·4639	0·7780
	42	0·6462	0·5177	0·7608	0·4794	0·7909
	43	0·6615	0·5335	0·7743	0·4951	0·8036
	44	0·6769	0·5495	0·7877	0·5110	0·8162
	45	0·6923	0·5655	0·8009	0·5271	0·8286
	46	0·7077	0·5817	0·8140	0·5433	0·8408
	47	0·7231	0·5981	0·8269	0·5597	0·8528
	48	0·7385	0·6146	0·8397	0·5763	0·8646
	49	0·7538	0·6313	0·8523	0·5931	0·8762
	50	0·7692	0·6481	0·8647	0·6101	0·8875
	51	0·7846	0·6651	0·8769	0·6274	0·8986
	52	0·8000	0·6823	0·8890	0·6449	0·9095
	53	0·8154	0·6997	0·9008	0·6627	0·9201
	54	0·8308	0·7173	0·9124	0·6807	0·9304
	55	0·8462	0·7352	0·9237	0·6991	0·9403
	56	0·8615	0·7534	0·9347	0·7178	0·9499
	57	0·8769	0·7718	0·9453	0·7369	0·9590
	58	0·8923	0·7906	0·9556	0·7564	0·9677
	59	0·9077	0·8098	0·9654	0·7765	0·9757
	60	0·9231	0·8295	0·9746	0·7972	0·9830
	61	0·9385	0·8499	0·9830	0·8187	0·9895
	62	0·9538	0·8710	0·9904	0·8412	0·9947
	63	0·9692	0·8932	0·9963	0·8651	0·9984
	64	0·9846	0·9172	0·9996	0·8912	0·9999
	65	1·0000	0·9448	1·0000	0·9217	1·0000
66	0	0·0000	0·0000	0·0544	0·0000	0·0771
	1	0·0152	0·0004	0·0816	0·0001	0·1072
	2	0·0303	0·0037	0·1052	0·0016	0·1330

Confidence level			95%		99%	
n	*x*	*p*	p_l	p_u	p_l	p_u
66	3	0·0455	0·0095	0·1271	0·0052	0·1566
	4	0·0606	0·0168	0·1480	0·0104	0·1788
	5	0·0758	0·0251	0·1680	0·0167	0·1999
	6	0·0909	0·0341	0·1874	0·0239	0·2204
	7	0·1061	0·0437	0·2064	0·0318	0·2402
	8	0·1212	0·0538	0·2249	0·0403	0·2595
	9	0·1364	0·0643	0·2431	0·0493	0·2783
	10	0·1515	0·0751	0·2610	0·0587	0·2968
	11	0·1667	0·0862	0·2787	0·0685	0·3149
	12	0·1818	0·0976	0·2961	0·0786	0·3327
	13	0·1970	0·1093	0·3132	0·0890	0·3503
	14	0·2121	0·1211	0·3302	0·0997	0·3675
	15	0·2273	0·1331	0·3470	0·1107	0·3846
	16	0·2424	0·1454	0·3636	0·1218	0·4014
	17	0·2576	0·1578	0·3801	0·1332	0·4180
	18	0·2727	0·1703	0·3964	0·1449	0·4344
	19	0·2879	0·1830	0·4125	0·1567	0·4506
	20	0·3030	0·1959	0·4285	0·1686	0·4667
	21	0·3182	0·2089	0·4444	0·1808	0·4825
	22	0·3333	0·2220	0·4601	0·1931	0·4982
	23	0·3485	0·2353	0·4758	0·2056	0·5138
	24	0·3636	0·2487	0·4913	0·2183	0·5292
	25	0·3788	0·2622	0·5066	0·2311	0·5444
	26	0·3939	0·2758	0·5219	0·2441	0·5595
	27	0·4091	0·2895	0·5371	0·2572	0·5744
	28	0·4242	0·3034	0·5521	0·2705	0·5892
	29	0·4394	0·3174	0·5670	0·2839	0·6039
	30	0·4545	0·3314	0·5819	0·2974	0·6184
	31	0·4697	0·3456	0·5966	0·3111	0·6328
	32	0·4848	0·3599	0·6112	0·3249	0·6470
	33	0·5000	0·3743	0·6257	0·3389	0·6611
	34	0·5152	0·3888	0·6401	0·3530	0·6751
	35	0·5303	0·4034	0·6544	0·3672	0·6889
	36	0·5455	0·4181	0·6686	0·3816	0·7026
	37	0·5606	0·4330	0·6826	0·3961	0·7161
	38	0·5758	0·4479	0·6966	0·4108	0·7295
	39	0·5909	0·4629	0·7105	0·4256	0·7428
	40	0·6061	0·4781	0·7242	0·4405	0·7559
	41	0·6212	0·4934	0·7378	0·4556	0·7689
	42	0·6364	0·5087	0·7513	0·4708	0·7817
	43	0·6515	0·5242	0·7647	0·4862	0·7944
	44	0·6667	0·5399	0·7780	0·5018	0·8069
	45	0·6818	0·5556	0·7911	0·5175	0·8192
	46	0·6970	0·5715	0·8041	0·5333	0·8314
	47	0·7121	0·5875	0·8170	0·5494	0·8433
	48	0·7273	0·6036	0·8297	0·5656	0·8551
	49	0·7424	0·6199	0·8422	0·5820	0·8668
	50	0·7576	0·6364	0·8546	0·5986	0·8782
	51	0·7727	0·6530	0·8669	0·6154	0·8893
	52	0·7879	0·6698	0·8789	0·6325	0·9003

Continued

Table B.11 Exact confidence limits for a binomial proportion: x events are observed in a sample sized n. $p = x/n$ is the observed proportion. p_l and p_u are the lower and upper confidence limits for the population proportion.

Confidence level			95%		99%	
n	x	p	p_l	p_u	p_l	p_u
66	53	0·8030	0·6868	0·8907	0·6497	0·9110
	54	0·8182	0·7039	0·9024	0·6673	0·9214
	55	0·8333	0·7213	0·9138	0·6851	0·9315
	56	0·8485	0·7390	0·9249	0·7032	0·9413
	57	0·8636	0·7569	0·9357	0·7217	0·9507
	58	0·8788	0·7751	0·9462	0·7405	0·9597
	59	0·8939	0·7936	0·9563	0·7598	0·9682
	60	0·9091	0·8126	0·9659	0·7796	0·9761
	61	0·9242	0·8320	0·9749	0·8001	0·9833
	62	0·9394	0·8520	0·9832	0·8212	0·9896
	63	0·9545	0·8729	0·9905	0·8434	0·9948
	64	0·9697	0·8948	0·9963	0·8670	0·9984
	65	0·9848	0·9184	0·9996	0·8928	0·9999
	66	1·0000	0·9456	1·0000	0·9229	1·0000
67	0	0·0000	0·0000	0·0536	0·0000	0·0760
	1	0·0149	0·0004	0·0804	0·0001	0·1057
	2	0·0299	0·0036	0·1037	0·0016	0·1311
	3	0·0448	0·0093	0·1253	0·0051	0·1544
	4	0·0597	0·0165	0·1459	0·0102	0·1763
	5	0·0746	0·0247	0·1656	0·0165	0·1972
	6	0·0896	0·0336	0·1848	0·0236	0·2173
	7	0·1045	0·0430	0·2035	0·0314	0·2369
	8	0·1194	0·0530	0·2218	0·0397	0·2559
	9	0·1343	0·0633	0·2397	0·0486	0·2745
	10	0·1493	0·0740	0·2574	0·0578	0·2928
	11	0·1642	0·0849	0·2748	0·0674	0·3107
	12	0·1791	0·0961	0·2920	0·0774	0·3282
	13	0·1940	0·1076	0·3089	0·0876	0·3456
	14	0·2090	0·1192	0·3257	0·0982	0·3626
	15	0·2239	0·1311	0·3422	0·1089	0·3795
	16	0·2388	0·1431	0·3586	0·1199	0·3961
	17	0·2537	0·1553	0·3749	0·1311	0·4125
	18	0·2687	0·1676	0·3910	0·1425	0·4287
	19	0·2836	0·1801	0·4069	0·1541	0·4447
	20	0·2985	0·1928	0·4227	0·1659	0·4606
	21	0·3134	0·2056	0·4384	0·1779	0·4763
	22	0·3284	0·2185	0·4540	0·1900	0·4918
	23	0·3433	0·2315	0·4694	0·2023	0·5072
	24	0·3582	0·2447	0·4847	0·2147	0·5224
	25	0·3731	0·2580	0·4999	0·2273	0·5374
	26	0·3881	0·2714	0·5150	0·2401	0·5524
	27	0·4030	0·2849	0·5300	0·2530	0·5672
	28	0·4179	0·2985	0·5448	0·2660	0·5818
	29	0·4328	0·3122	0·5596	0·2792	0·5963
	30	0·4478	0·3260	0·5742	0·2925	0·6107
	31	0·4627	0·3400	0·5888	0·3059	0·6249
	32	0·4776	0·3540	0·6033	0·3195	0·6390
	33	0·4925	0·3682	0·6176	0·3332	0·6530

Confidence level			95%		99%	
n	x	p	p_l	p_u	p_l	p_u
67	34	0·5075	0·3824	0·6318	0·3470	0·6668
	35	0·5224	0·3967	0·6460	0·3610	0·6805
	36	0·5373	0·4112	0·6600	0·3751	0·6941
	37	0·5522	0·4258	0·6740	0·3893	0·7075
	38	0·5672	0·4404	0·6878	0·4037	0·7208
	39	0·5821	0·4552	0·7015	0·4182	0·7340
	40	0·5970	0·4700	0·7151	0·4328	0·7470
	41	0·6119	0·4850	0·7286	0·4476	0·7599
	42	0·6269	0·5001	0·7420	0·4626	0·7727
	43	0·6418	0·5153	0·7553	0·4776	0·7853
	44	0·6567	0·5306	0·7685	0·4928	0·7977
	45	0·6716	0·5460	0·7815	0·5082	0·8100
	46	0·6866	0·5616	0·7944	0·5237	0·8221
	47	0·7015	0·5773	0·8072	0·5394	0·8341
	48	0·7164	0·5931	0·8199	0·5553	0·8459
	49	0·7313	0·6090	0·8324	0·5713	0·8575
	50	0·7463	0·6251	0·8447	0·5875	0·8689
	51	0·7612	0·6414	0·8569	0·6039	0·8801
	52	0·7761	0·6578	0·8689	0·6205	0·8911
	53	0·7910	0·6743	0·8808	0·6374	0·9018
	54	0·8060	0·6911	0·8924	0·6544	0·9124
	55	0·8209	0·7080	0·9039	0·6718	0·9226
	56	0·8358	0·7252	0·9151	0·6893	0·9326
	57	0·8507	0·7426	0·9260	0·7072	0·9422
	58	0·8657	0·7603	0·9367	0·7255	0·9514
	59	0·8806	0·7782	0·9470	0·7441	0·9603
	60	0·8955	0·7965	0·9570	0·7631	0·9686
	61	0·9104	0·8152	0·9664	0·7827	0·9764
	62	0·9254	0·8344	0·9753	0·8028	0·9835
	63	0·9403	0·8541	0·9835	0·8237	0·9898
	64	0·9552	0·8747	0·9907	0·8456	0·9949
	65	0·9701	0·8963	0·9964	0·8689	0·9984
	66	0·9851	0·9196	0·9996	0·8943	0·9999
	67	1·0000	0·9464	1·0000	0·9240	1·0000
68	0	0·0000	0·0000	0·0528	0·0000	0·0750
	1	0·0147	0·0004	0·0792	0·0001	0·1042
	2	0·0294	0·0036	0·1022	0·0015	0·1293
	3	0·0441	0·0092	0·1236	0·0050	0·1522
	4	0·0588	0·0163	0·1438	0·0101	0·1738
	5	0·0735	0·0243	0·1633	0·0162	0·1945
	6	0·0882	0·0331	0·1822	0·0232	0·2144
	7	0·1029	0·0424	0·2007	0·0309	0·2337
	8	0·1176	0·0522	0·2187	0·0391	0·2525
	9	0·1324	0·0623	0·2364	0·0478	0·2708
	10	0·1471	0·0728	0·2539	0·0569	0·2888
	11	0·1618	0·0836	0·2710	0·0664	0·3065
	12	0·1765	0·0947	0·2880	0·0762	0·3239
	13	0·1912	0·1059	0·3047	0·0863	0·3410
	14	0·2059	0·1174	0·3212	0·0966	0·3578
	15	0·2206	0·1290	0·3376	0·1072	0·3745

Table B.11 Exact confidence limits for a binomial proportion: x events are observed in a sample sized n. $p = x/n$ is the observed proportion. p_l and p_u are the lower and upper confidence limits for the population proportion.

Confidence level			95%		99%	
n	x	p	p_l	p_u	p_l	p_u
68	16	0·2353	0·1409	0·3538	0·1180	0·3909
	17	0·2500	0·1529	0·3698	0·1291	0·4071
	18	0·2647	0·1650	0·3857	0·1403	0·4231
	19	0·2794	0·1773	0·4015	0·1517	0·4390
	20	0·2941	0·1898	0·4171	0·1633	0·4546
	21	0·3088	0·2024	0·4326	0·1751	0·4702
	22	0·3235	0·2151	0·4479	0·1870	0·4855
	23	0·3382	0·2279	0·4632	0·1991	0·5007
	24	0·3529	0·2408	0·4783	0·2113	0·5158
	25	0·3676	0·2539	0·4933	0·2237	0·5307
	26	0·3824	0·2671	0·5082	0·2362	0·5454
	27	0·3971	0·2803	0·5230	0·2489	0·5600
	28	0·4118	0·2937	0·5377	0·2617	0·5745
	29	0·4265	0·3072	0·5523	0·2746	0·5889
	30	0·4412	0·3208	0·5668	0·2877	0·6031
	31	0·4559	0·3345	0·5812	0·3009	0·6172
	32	0·4706	0·3483	0·5955	0·3142	0·6312
	33	0·4853	0·3622	0·6097	0·3277	0·6450
	34	0·5000	0·3762	0·6238	0·3412	0·6588
	35	0·5147	0·3903	0·6378	0·3550	0·6723
	36	0·5294	0·4045	0·6517	0·3688	0·6858
	37	0·5441	0·4188	0·6655	0·3828	0·6991
	38	0·5588	0·4332	0·6792	0·3969	0·7123
	39	0·5735	0·4477	0·6928	0·4111	0·7254
	40	0·5882	0·4623	0·7063	0·4255	0·7383
	41	0·6029	0·4770	0·7197	0·4400	0·7511
	42	0·6176	0·4918	0·7329	0·4546	0·7638
	43	0·6324	0·5067	0·7461	0·4693	0·7763
	44	0·6471	0·5217	0·7592	0·4842	0·7887
	45	0·6618	0·5368	0·7721	0·4993	0·8009
	46	0·6765	0·5521	0·7849	0·5145	0·8130
	47	0·6912	0·5674	0·7976	0·5298	0·8249
	48	0·7059	0·5829	0·8102	0·5454	0·8367
	49	0·7206	0·5985	0·8227	0·5610	0·8483
	50	0·7353	0·6143	0·8350	0·5769	0·8597
	51	0·7500	0·6302	0·8471	0·5929	0·8709
	52	0·7647	0·6462	0·8591	0·6091	0·8820
	53	0·7794	0·6624	0·8710	0·6255	0·8928
	54	0·7941	0·6788	0·8826	0·6422	0·9034
	55	0·8088	0·6953	0·8941	0·6590	0·9137
	56	0·8235	0·7120	0·9053	0·6761	0·9238
	57	0·8382	0·7290	0·9164	0·6935	0·9336
	58	0·8529	0·7461	0·9272	0·7112	0·9431
	59	0·8676	0·7636	0·9377	0·7292	0·9522
	60	0·8824	0·7813	0·9478	0·7475	0·9609
	61	0·8971	0·7993	0·9576	0·7663	0·9691
	62	0·9118	0·8178	0·9669	0·7856	0·9768
	63	0·9265	0·8367	0·9757	0·8055	0·9838
	64	0·9412	0·8562	0·9837	0·8262	0·9899

Table B.11 (*Continued*)

Confidence level			95%		99%	
n	x	p	p_l	p_u	p_l	p_u
68	65	0·9559	0·8764	0·9908	0·8478	0·9950
	66	0·9706	0·8978	0·9964	0·8707	0·9985
	67	0·9853	0·9208	0·9996	0·8958	0·9999
	68	1·0000	0·9472	1·0000	0·9250	1·0000
69	0	0·0000	0·0000	0·0521	0·0000	0·0739
	1	0·0145	0·0004	0·0781	0·0001	0·1028
	2	0·0290	0·0035	0·1008	0·0015	0·1275
	3	0·0435	0·0091	0·1218	0·0050	0·1502
	4	0·0580	0·0160	0·1418	0·0099	0·1715
	5	0·0725	0·0239	0·1611	0·0160	0·1918
	6	0·0870	0·0326	0·1797	0·0229	0·2115
	7	0·1014	0·0418	0·1979	0·0304	0·2305
	8	0·1159	0·0514	0·2157	0·0385	0·2491
	9	0·1304	0·0614	0·2332	0·0471	0·2672
	10	0·1449	0·0717	0·2504	0·0561	0·2850
	11	0·1594	0·0824	0·2674	0·0654	0·3025
	12	0·1739	0·0932	0·2841	0·0750	0·3196
	13	0·1884	0·1043	0·3006	0·0850	0·3365
	14	0·2029	0·1156	0·3169	0·0951	0·3532
	15	0·2174	0·1271	0·3331	0·1056	0·3696
	16	0·2319	0·1387	0·3491	0·1162	0·3858
	17	0·2464	0·1505	0·3649	0·1271	0·4019
	18	0·2609	0·1625	0·3806	0·1381	0·4177
	19	0·2754	0·1746	0·3962	0·1493	0·4334
	20	0·2899	0·1869	0·4116	0·1607	0·4489
	21	0·3043	0·1992	0·4269	0·1723	0·4642
	22	0·3188	0·2117	0·4421	0·1840	0·4794
	23	0·3333	0·2244	0·4571	0·1959	0·4944
	24	0·3478	0·2371	0·4721	0·2080	0·5093
	25	0·3623	0·2499	0·4869	0·2201	0·5240
	26	0·3768	0·2629	0·5017	0·2324	0·5386
	27	0·3913	0·2760	0·5163	0·2449	0·5531
	28	0·4058	0·2891	0·5308	0·2575	0·5675
	29	0·4203	0·3024	0·5452	0·2702	0·5817
	30	0·4348	0·3158	0·5596	0·2830	0·5958
	31	0·4493	0·3292	0·5738	0·2960	0·6097
	32	0·4638	0·3428	0·5880	0·3091	0·6236
	33	0·4783	0·3565	0·6020	0·3223	0·6373
	34	0·4928	0·3702	0·6159	0·3357	0·6509
	35	0·5072	0·3841	0·6298	0·3491	0·6643
	36	0·5217	0·3980	0·6435	0·3627	0·6777
	37	0·5362	0·4120	0·6572	0·3764	0·6909
	38	0·5507	0·4262	0·6708	0·3903	0·7040
	39	0·5652	0·4404	0·6842	0·4042	0·7170
	40	0·5797	0·4548	0·6976	0·4183	0·7298
	41	0·5942	0·4692	0·7109	0·4325	0·7425
	42	0·6087	0·4837	0·7240	0·4469	0·7551
	43	0·6232	0·4983	0·7371	0·4614	0·7676
	44	0·6377	0·5131	0·7501	0·4760	0·7799
	45	0·6522	0·5279	0·7629	0·4907	0·7920

Continued

Table B.11 Exact confidence limits for a binomial proportion: x events are observed in a sample sized n. $p = x/n$ is the observed proportion. p_l and p_u are the lower and upper confidence limits for the population proportion.

Confidence level			95%		99%	
n	x	p	p_l	p_u	p_l	p_u
69	46	0·6667	0·5429	0·7756	0·5056	0·8041
	47	0·6812	0·5579	0·7883	0·5206	0·8160
	48	0·6957	0·5731	0·8008	0·5358	0·8277
	49	0·7101	0·5884	0·8131	0·5511	0·8393
	50	0·7246	0·6038	0·8254	0·5666	0·8507
	51	0·7391	0·6194	0·8375	0·5823	0·8619
	52	0·7536	0·6351	0·8495	0·5981	0·8729
	53	0·7681	0·6509	0·8613	0·6142	0·8838
	54	0·7826	0·6669	0·8729	0·6304	0·8944
	55	0·7971	0·6831	0·8844	0·6468	0·9049
	56	0·8116	0·6994	0·8957	0·6635	0·9150
	57	0·8261	0·7159	0·9068	0·6804	0·9250
	58	0·8406	0·7326	0·9176	0·6975	0·9346
	59	0·8551	0·7496	0·9283	0·7150	0·9439
	60	0·8696	0·7668	0·9386	0·7328	0·9529
	61	0·8841	0·7843	0·9486	0·7509	0·9615
	62	0·8986	0·8021	0·9582	0·7695	0·9696
	63	0·9130	0·8203	0·9674	0·7885	0·9771
	64	0·9275	0·8389	0·9761	0·8082	0·9840
	65	0·9420	0·8582	0·9840	0·8285	0·9901
	66	0·9565	0·8782	0·9909	0·8498	0·9950
	67	0·9710	0·8992	0·9965	0·8725	0·9985
	68	0·9855	0·9219	0·9996	0·8972	0·9999
	69	1·0000	0·9479	1·0000	0·9261	1·0000
70	0	0·0000	0·0000	0·0513	0·0000	0·0729
	1	0·0143	0·0004	0·0770	0·0001	0·1014
	2	0·0286	0·0035	0·0994	0·0015	0·1258
	3	0·0429	0·0089	0·1202	0·0049	0·1481
	4	0·0571	0·0158	0·1399	0·0098	0·1692
	5	0·0714	0·0236	0·1589	0·0157	0·1893
	6	0·0857	0·0321	0·1773	0·0225	0·2087
	7	0·1000	0·0412	0·1952	0·0300	0·2275
	8	0·1143	0·0507	0·2128	0·0380	0·2458
	9	0·1286	0·0605	0·2301	0·0464	0·2637
	10	0·1429	0·0707	0·2471	0·0552	0·2813
	11	0·1571	0·0811	0·2638	0·0644	0·2985
	12	0·1714	0·0918	0·2803	0·0739	0·3155
	13	0·1857	0·1028	0·2966	0·0837	0·3322
	14	0·2000	0·1139	0·3127	0·0937	0·3486
	15	0·2143	0·1252	0·3287	0·1040	0·3649
	16	0·2286	0·1367	0·3445	0·1145	0·3809
	17	0·2429	0·1483	0·3601	0·1251	0·3967
	18	0·2571	0·1601	0·3756	0·1360	0·4124
	19	0·2714	0·1720	0·3910	0·1471	0·4279
	20	0·2857	0·1840	0·4062	0·1583	0·4432
	21	0·3000	0·1962	0·4213	0·1697	0·4584
	22	0·3143	0·2085	0·4363	0·1812	0·4734
	23	0·3286	0·2209	0·4512	0·1929	0·4882
	24	0·3429	0·2335	0·4660	0·2047	0·5030

n	x	p	\(p_l\)	\(p_u\)	\(p_l\)	\(p_u\)
			95%		99%	
70	25	0·3571	0·2461	0·4807	0·2167	0·5176
	26	0·3714	0·2589	0·4952	0·2288	0·5320
	27	0·3857	0·2717	0·5097	0·2411	0·5463
	28	0·4000	0·2847	0·5241	0·2534	0·5605
	29	0·4143	0·2977	0·5383	0·2659	0·5746
	30	0·4286	0·3109	0·5525	0·2785	0·5886
	31	0·4429	0·3241	0·5666	0·2913	0·6024
	32	0·4571	0·3374	0·5806	0·3042	0·6161
	33	0·4714	0·3509	0·5945	0·3172	0·6297
	34	0·4857	0·3644	0·6083	0·3303	0·6432
	35	0·5000	0·3780	0·6220	0·3435	0·6565
	36	0·5143	0·3917	0·6356	0·3568	0·6697
	37	0·5286	0·4055	0·6491	0·3703	0·6828
	38	0·5429	0·4194	0·6626	0·3839	0·6958
	39	0·5571	0·4334	0·6759	0·3976	0·7087
	40	0·5714	0·4475	0·6891	0·4114	0·7215
	41	0·5857	0·4617	0·7023	0·4254	0·7341
	42	0·6000	0·4759	0·7153	0·4395	0·7466
	43	0·6143	0·4903	0·7283	0·4537	0·7589
	44	0·6286	0·5048	0·7411	0·4680	0·7712
	45	0·6429	0·5193	0·7539	0·4824	0·7833
	46	0·6571	0·5340	0·7665	0·4970	0·7953
	47	0·6714	0·5488	0·7791	0·5118	0·8071
	48	0·6857	0·5637	0·7915	0·5266	0·8188
	49	0·7000	0·5787	0·8038	0·5416	0·8303
	50	0·7143	0·5938	0·8160	0·5568	0·8417
	51	0·7286	0·6090	0·8280	0·5721	0·8529
	52	0·7429	0·6244	0·8399	0·5876	0·8640
	53	0·7571	0·6399	0·8517	0·6033	0·8749
	54	0·7714	0·6555	0·8633	0·6191	0·8855
	55	0·7857	0·6713	0·8748	0·6351	0·8960
	56	0·8000	0·6873	0·8861	0·6514	0·9063
	57	0·8143	0·7034	0·8972	0·6678	0·9163
	58	0·8286	0·7197	0·9082	0·6845	0·9261
	59	0·8429	0·7362	0·9189	0·7015	0·9356
	60	0·8571	0·7529	0·9293	0·7187	0·9448
	61	0·8714	0·7699	0·9395	0·7363	0·9536
	62	0·8857	0·7872	0·9493	0·7542	0·9620
	63	0·9000	0·8048	0·9588	0·7725	0·9700
	64	0·9143	0·8227	0·9679	0·7913	0·9775
	65	0·9286	0·8411	0·9764	0·8107	0·9843
	66	0·9429	0·8601	0·9842	0·8308	0·9902
	67	0·9571	0·8798	0·9911	0·8519	0·9951
	68	0·9714	0·9006	0·9965	0·8742	0·9985
	69	0·9857	0·9230	0·9996	0·8986	0·9999
	70	1·0000	0·9487	1·0000	0·9271	1·0000
71	0	0·0000	0·0000	0·0506	0·0000	0·0719
	1	0·0141	0·0004	0·0760	0·0001	0·1000
	2	0·0282	0·0034	0·0981	0·0015	0·1241
	3	0·0423	0·0088	0·1186	0·0048	0·1462

Continued

Table B.11 Exact confidence limits for a binomial proportion: x events are observed in a sample sized n. $p = x/n$ is the observed proportion. p_l and p_u are the lower and upper confidence limits for the population proportion.

Confidence level			95%		99%	
n	x	p	p_l	p_u	p_l	p_u
71	4	0·0563	0·0156	0·1380	0·0096	0·1669
	5	0·0704	0·0233	0·1567	0·0155	0·1868
	6	0·0845	0·0316	0·1749	0·0222	0·2059
	7	0·0986	0·0406	0·1926	0·0295	0·2245
	8	0·1127	0·0499	0·2100	0·0374	0·2426
	9	0·1268	0·0596	0·2270	0·0457	0·2603
	10	0·1408	0·0697	0·2438	0·0544	0·2777
	11	0·1549	0·0800	0·2603	0·0635	0·2947
	12	0·1690	0·0905	0·2766	0·0728	0·3114
	13	0·1831	0·1013	0·2927	0·0824	0·3279
	14	0·1972	0·1122	0·3086	0·0923	0·3442
	15	0·2113	0·1233	0·3244	0·1024	0·3602
	16	0·2254	0·1346	0·3400	0·1127	0·3761
	17	0·2394	0·1461	0·3554	0·1233	0·3917
	18	0·2535	0·1577	0·3708	0·1340	0·4072
	19	0·2676	0·1694	0·3859	0·1448	0·4225
	20	0·2817	0·1813	0·4010	0·1559	0·4377
	21	0·2958	0·1933	0·4159	0·1671	0·4527
	22	0·3099	0·2054	0·4308	0·1784	0·4675
	23	0·3239	0·2176	0·4455	0·1899	0·4822
	24	0·3380	0·2300	0·4601	0·2016	0·4968
	25	0·3521	0·2424	0·4746	0·2134	0·5112
	26	0·3662	0·2550	0·4890	0·2253	0·5256
	27	0·3803	0·2676	0·5033	0·2373	0·5397
	28	0·3944	0·2803	0·5175	0·2495	0·5538
	29	0·4085	0·2932	0·5316	0·2618	0·5677
	30	0·4225	0·3061	0·5456	0·2742	0·5815
	31	0·4366	0·3191	0·5595	0·2867	0·5952
	32	0·4507	0·3323	0·5734	0·2994	0·6088
	33	0·4648	0·3455	0·5871	0·3122	0·6223
	34	0·4789	0·3588	0·6008	0·3250	0·6356
	35	0·4930	0·3722	0·6144	0·3380	0·6488
	36	0·5070	0·3856	0·6278	0·3512	0·6620
	37	0·5211	0·3992	0·6412	0·3644	0·6750
	38	0·5352	0·4129	0·6545	0·3777	0·6878
	39	0·5493	0·4266	0·6677	0·3912	0·7006
	40	0·5634	0·4405	0·6809	0·4048	0·7133
	41	0·5775	0·4544	0·6939	0·4185	0·7258
	42	0·5915	0·4684	0·7068	0·4323	0·7382
	43	0·6056	0·4825	0·7197	0·4462	0·7505
	44	0·6197	0·4967	0·7324	0·4603	0·7627
	45	0·6338	0·5110	0·7450	0·4744	0·7747
	46	0·6479	0·5254	0·7576	0·4888	0·7866
	47	0·6620	0·5399	0·7700	0·5032	0·7984
	48	0·6761	0·5545	0·7824	0·5178	0·8101
	49	0·6901	0·5692	0·7946	0·5325	0·8216
	50	0·7042	0·5841	0·8067	0·5473	0·8329
	51	0·7183	0·5990	0·8187	0·5623	0·8441
	52	0·7324	0·6141	0·8306	0·5775	0·8552

Table B.11 (*Continued*)

n	x	p	95% p_l	p_u	99% p_l	p_u
71	53	0·7465	0·6292	0·8423	0·5928	0·8660
	54	0·7606	0·6446	0·8539	0·6083	0·8767
	55	0·7746	0·6600	0·8654	0·6239	0·8873
	56	0·7887	0·6756	0·8767	0·6398	0·8976
	57	0·8028	0·6914	0·8878	0·6558	0·9077
	58	0·8169	0·7073	0·8987	0·6721	0·9176
	59	0·8310	0·7234	0·9095	0·6886	0·9272
	60	0·8451	0·7397	0·9200	0·7053	0·9365
	61	0·8592	0·7562	0·9303	0·7223	0·9456
	62	0·8732	0·7730	0·9404	0·7397	0·9543
	63	0·8873	0·7900	0·9501	0·7574	0·9626
	64	0·9014	0·8074	0·9594	0·7755	0·9705
	65	0·9155	0·8251	0·9684	0·7941	0·9778
	66	0·9296	0·8433	0·9767	0·8132	0·9845
	67	0·9437	0·8620	0·9844	0·8331	0·9904
	68	0·9577	0·8814	0·9912	0·8538	0·9952
	69	0·9718	0·9019	0·9966	0·8759	0·9985
	70	0·9859	0·9240	0·9996	0·9000	0·9999
	71	1·0000	0·9494	1·0000	0·9281	1·0000
72	0	0·0000	0·0000	0·0499	0·0000	0·0709
	1	0·0139	0·0004	0·0750	0·0001	0·0987
	2	0·0278	0·0034	0·0968	0·0014	0·1225
	3	0·0417	0·0087	0·1170	0·0047	0·1442
	4	0·0556	0·0153	0·1362	0·0095	0·1648
	5	0·0694	0·0229	0·1547	0·0153	0·1844
	6	0·0833	0·0312	0·1726	0·0219	0·2033
	7	0·0972	0·0400	0·1901	0·0291	0·2216
	8	0·1111	0·0492	0·2072	0·0369	0·2395
	9	0·1250	0·0588	0·2241	0·0451	0·2570
	10	0·1389	0·0687	0·2406	0·0536	0·2741
	11	0·1528	0·0788	0·2569	0·0626	0·2909
	12	0·1667	0·0892	0·2730	0·0718	0·3075
	13	0·1806	0·0998	0·2889	0·0812	0·3238
	14	0·1944	0·1106	0·3047	0·0910	0·3399
	15	0·2083	0·1216	0·3202	0·1009	0·3557
	16	0·2222	0·1327	0·3356	0·1111	0·3714
	17	0·2361	0·1440	0·3509	0·1214	0·3869
	18	0·2500	0·1554	0·3660	0·1320	0·4022
	19	0·2639	0·1670	0·3810	0·1427	0·4173
	20	0·2778	0·1786	0·3959	0·1536	0·4323
	21	0·2917	0·1905	0·4107	0·1646	0·4471
	22	0·3056	0·2024	0·4253	0·1758	0·4618
	23	0·3194	0·2144	0·4399	0·1871	0·4764
	24	0·3333	0·2266	0·4543	0·1986	0·4908
	25	0·3472	0·2388	0·4686	0·2101	0·5051
	26	0·3611	0·2512	0·4829	0·2219	0·5192
	27	0·3750	0·2636	0·4970	0·2337	0·5333
	28	0·3889	0·2762	0·5111	0·2457	0·5472
	29	0·4028	0·2888	0·5250	0·2578	0·5610

Continued

Table B.11 Exact confidence limits for a binomial proportion: x events are observed in a sample sized n. $p = x/n$ is the observed proportion. p_l and p_u are the lower and upper confidence limits for the population proportion.

Confidence level			95%		99%	
n	x	p	p_l	p_u	p_l	p_u
72	30	0·4167	0·3015	0·5389	0·2700	0·5747
	31	0·4306	0·3143	0·5527	0·2823	0·5882
	32	0·4444	0·3272	0·5664	0·2948	0·6017
	33	0·4583	0·3402	0·5800	0·3073	0·6150
	34	0·4722	0·3533	0·5935	0·3200	0·6282
	35	0·4861	0·3665	0·6069	0·3328	0·6413
	36	0·5000	0·3798	0·6202	0·3457	0·6543
	37	0·5139	0·3931	0·6335	0·3587	0·6672
	38	0·5278	0·4065	0·6467	0·3718	0·6800
	39	0·5417	0·4200	0·6598	0·3850	0·6927
	40	0·5556	0·4336	0·6728	0·3983	0·7052
	41	0·5694	0·4473	0·6857	0·4118	0·7177
	42	0·5833	0·4611	0·6985	0·4253	0·7300
	43	0·5972	0·4750	0·7112	0·4390	0·7422
	44	0·6111	0·4889	0·7238	0·4528	0·7543
	45	0·6250	0·5030	0·7364	0·4667	0·7663
	46	0·6389	0·5171	0·7488	0·4808	0·7781
	47	0·6528	0·5314	0·7612	0·4949	0·7899
	48	0·6667	0·5457	0·7734	0·5092	0·8014
	49	0·6806	0·5601	0·7856	0·5236	0·8129
	50	0·6944	0·5747	0·7976	0·5382	0·8242
	51	0·7083	0·5893	0·8095	0·5529	0·8354
	52	0·7222	0·6041	0·8214	0·5677	0·8464
	53	0·7361	0·6190	0·8330	0·5827	0·8573
	54	0·7500	0·6340	0·8446	0·5978	0·8680
	55	0·7639	0·6491	0·8560	0·6131	0·8786
	56	0·7778	0·6644	0·8673	0·6286	0·8889
	57	0·7917	0·6798	0·8784	0·6443	0·8991
	58	0·8056	0·6953	0·8894	0·6601	0·9090
	59	0·8194	0·7111	0·9002	0·6762	0·9188
	60	0·8333	0·7270	0·9108	0·6925	0·9282
	61	0·8472	0·7431	0·9212	0·7091	0·9374
	62	0·8611	0·7594	0·9313	0·7259	0·9464
	63	0·8750	0·7759	0·9412	0·7430	0·9549
	64	0·8889	0·7928	0·9508	0·7605	0·9631
	65	0·9028	0·8099	0·9600	0·7784	0·9709
	66	0·9167	0·8274	0·9688	0·7967	0·9781
	67	0·9306	0·8453	0·9771	0·8156	0·9847
	68	0·9444	0·8638	0·9847	0·8352	0·9905
	69	0·9583	0·8830	0·9913	0·8558	0·9953
	70	0·9722	0·9032	0·9966	0·8775	0·9986
	71	0·9861	0·9250	0·9996	0·9013	0·9999
	72	1·0000	0·9501	1·0000	0·9291	1·0000
73	0	0·0000	0·0000	0·0493	0·0000	0·0700
	1	0·0137	0·0003	0·0740	0·0001	0·0974
	2	0·0274	0·0033	0·0955	0·0014	0·1209
	3	0·0411	0·0086	0·1154	0·0047	0·1424
	4	0·0548	0·0151	0·1344	0·0094	0·1626

Confidence level			95%		99%	
n	x	p	p_l	p_u	p_l	p_u
73	5	0·0685	0·0226	0·1526	0·0151	0·1820
	6	0·0822	0·0308	0·1704	0·0216	0·2007
	7	0·0959	0·0394	0·1876	0·0287	0·2188
	8	0·1096	0·0485	0·2046	0·0363	0·2365
	9	0·1233	0·0580	0·2212	0·0444	0·2537
	10	0·1370	0·0677	0·2375	0·0529	0·2707
	11	0·1507	0·0777	0·2536	0·0617	0·2873
	12	0·1644	0·0879	0·2695	0·0707	0·3037
	13	0·1781	0·0984	0·2853	0·0801	0·3198
	14	0·1918	0·1090	0·3008	0·0897	0·3357
	15	0·2055	0·1198	0·3162	0·0995	0·3513
	16	0·2192	0·1308	0·3314	0·1095	0·3668
	17	0·2329	0·1419	0·3465	0·1197	0·3821
	18	0·2466	0·1532	0·3614	0·1301	0·3973
	19	0·2603	0·1645	0·3762	0·1406	0·4122
	20	0·2740	0·1761	0·3909	0·1513	0·4271
	21	0·2877	0·1877	0·4055	0·1622	0·4417
	22	0·3014	0·1994	0·4200	0·1732	0·4563
	23	0·3151	0·2113	0·4344	0·1843	0·4707
	24	0·3288	0·2233	0·4487	0·1956	0·4849
	25	0·3425	0·2353	0·4628	0·2070	0·4991
	26	0·3562	0·2475	0·4769	0·2186	0·5131
	27	0·3699	0·2597	0·4909	0·2302	0·5270
	28	0·3836	0·2721	0·5048	0·2420	0·5407
	29	0·3973	0·2845	0·5186	0·2539	0·5544
	30	0·4110	0·2971	0·5323	0·2659	0·5679
	31	0·4247	0·3097	0·5459	0·2780	0·5814
	32	0·4384	0·3224	0·5595	0·2903	0·5947
	33	0·4521	0·3352	0·5730	0·3026	0·6079
	34	0·4658	0·3480	0·5863	0·3151	0·6210
	35	0·4795	0·3610	0·5996	0·3277	0·6340
	36	0·4932	0·3740	0·6128	0·3403	0·6469
	37	0·5068	0·3872	0·6260	0·3531	0·6597
	38	0·5205	0·4004	0·6390	0·3660	0·6723
	39	0·5342	0·4137	0·6520	0·3790	0·6849
	40	0·5479	0·4270	0·6648	0·3921	0·6974
	41	0·5616	0·4405	0·6776	0·4053	0·7097
	42	0·5753	0·4541	0·6903	0·4186	0·7220
	43	0·5890	0·4677	0·7029	0·4321	0·7341
	44	0·6027	0·4814	0·7155	0·4456	0·7461
	45	0·6164	0·4952	0·7279	0·4593	0·7580
	46	0·6301	0·5091	0·7403	0·4730	0·7698
	47	0·6438	0·5231	0·7525	0·4869	0·7814
	48	0·6575	0·5372	0·7647	0·5009	0·7930
	49	0·6712	0·5513	0·7767	0·5151	0·8044
	50	0·6849	0·5656	0·7887	0·5293	0·8157
	51	0·6986	0·5800	0·8006	0·5437	0·8268
	52	0·7123	0·5945	0·8123	0·5583	0·8378
	53	0·7260	0·6091	0·8239	0·5729	0·8487
	54	0·7397	0·6238	0·8355	0·5878	0·8594

Continued

Table B.11 Exact confidence limits for a binomial proportion: x events are observed in a sample sized n. $p = x/n$ is the observed proportion. p_l and p_u are the lower and upper confidence limits for the population proportion.

Confidence level			95%		99%	
n	x	p	p_l	p_u	p_l	p_u
73	55	0·7534	0·6386	0·8468	0·6027	0·8699
	56	0·7671	0·6535	0·8581	0·6179	0·8803
	57	0·7808	0·6686	0·8692	0·6332	0·8905
	58	0·7945	0·6838	0·8802	0·6487	0·9005
	59	0·8082	0·6992	0·8910	0·6643	0·9103
	60	0·8219	0·7147	0·9016	0·6802	0·9199
	61	0·8356	0·7305	0·9121	0·6963	0·9293
	62	0·8493	0·7464	0·9223	0·7127	0·9383
	63	0·8630	0·7625	0·9323	0·7293	0·9471
	64	0·8767	0·7788	0·9420	0·7463	0·9556
	65	0·8904	0·7954	0·9515	0·7635	0·9637
	66	0·9041	0·8124	0·9606	0·7812	0·9713
	67	0·9178	0·8296	0·9692	0·7993	0·9784
	68	0·9315	0·8474	0·9774	0·8180	0·9849
	69	0·9452	0·8656	0·9849	0·8374	0·9906
	70	0·9589	0·8846	0·9914	0·8576	0·9953
	71	0·9726	0·9045	0·9967	0·8791	0·9986
	72	0·9863	0·9260	0·9997	0·9026	0·9999
	73	1·0000	0·9507	1·0000	0·9300	1·0000
74	0	0·0000	0·0000	0·0486	0·0000	0·0691
	1	0·0135	0·0003	0·0730	0·0001	0·0962
	2	0·0270	0·0033	0·0942	0·0014	0·1193
	3	0·0405	0·0084	0·1139	0·0046	0·1406
	4	0·0541	0·0149	0·1327	0·0092	0·1606
	5	0·0676	0·0223	0·1507	0·0149	0·1797
	6	0·0811	0·0303	0·1682	0·0213	0·1981
	7	0·0946	0·0389	0·1852	0·0283	0·2160
	8	0·1081	0·0478	0·2020	0·0358	0·2335
	9	0·1216	0·0571	0·2184	0·0438	0·2506
	10	0·1351	0·0668	0·2345	0·0521	0·2673
	11	0·1486	0·0766	0·2504	0·0608	0·2837
	12	0·1622	0·0867	0·2661	0·0697	0·2999
	13	0·1757	0·0970	0·2817	0·0789	0·3158
	14	0·1892	0·1075	0·2970	0·0884	0·3315
	15	0·2027	0·1181	0·3122	0·0980	0·3470
	16	0·2162	0·1289	0·3272	0·1079	0·3624
	17	0·2297	0·1399	0·3421	0·1180	0·3775
	18	0·2432	0·1510	0·3569	0·1282	0·3925
	19	0·2568	0·1622	0·3716	0·1386	0·4073
	20	0·2703	0·1735	0·3861	0·1491	0·4219
	21	0·2838	0·1850	0·4005	0·1598	0·4364
	22	0·2973	0·1966	0·4148	0·1707	0·4508
	23	0·3108	0·2083	0·4290	0·1816	0·4651
	24	0·3243	0·2200	0·4432	0·1927	0·4792
	25	0·3378	0·2319	0·4572	0·2040	0·4932
	26	0·3514	0·2439	0·4711	0·2153	0·5070
	27	0·3649	0·2560	0·4849	0·2268	0·5208
	28	0·3784	0·2681	0·4987	0·2384	0·5344
	29	0·3919	0·2804	0·5123	0·2501	0·5479

Table B.11 (*Continued*)

n	x	p	95%		99%	
			p_l	p_u	p_l	p_u
74	30	0·4054	0·2927	0·5259	0·2620	0·5614
	31	0·4189	0·3051	0·5394	0·2739	0·5747
	32	0·4324	0·3177	0·5528	0·2859	0·5879
	33	0·4459	0·3302	0·5661	0·2981	0·6010
	34	0·4595	0·3429	0·5793	0·3103	0·6139
	35	0·4730	0·3557	0·5925	0·3227	0·6268
	36	0·4865	0·3685	0·6056	0·3352	0·6396
	37	0·5000	0·3814	0·6186	0·3477	0·6523
	38	0·5135	0·3944	0·6315	0·3604	0·6648
	39	0·5270	0·4075	0·6443	0·3732	0·6773
	40	0·5405	0·4207	0·6571	0·3861	0·6897
	41	0·5541	0·4339	0·6698	0·3990	0·7019
	42	0·5676	0·4472	0·6823	0·4121	0·7141
	43	0·5811	0·4606	0·6949	0·4253	0·7261
	44	0·5946	0·4741	0·7073	0·4386	0·7380
	45	0·6081	0·4877	0·7196	0·4521	0·7499
	46	0·6216	0·5013	0·7319	0·4656	0·7616
	47	0·6351	0·5151	0·7440	0·4792	0·7732
	48	0·6486	0·5289	0·7561	0·4930	0·7847
	49	0·6622	0·5428	0·7681	0·5068	0·7960
	50	0·6757	0·5568	0·7800	0·5208	0·8073
	51	0·6892	0·5710	0·7917	0·5349	0·8184
	52	0·7027	0·5852	0·8034	0·5492	0·8293
	53	0·7162	0·5995	0·8150	0·5636	0·8402
	54	0·7297	0·6139	0·8265	0·5781	0·8509
	55	0·7432	0·6284	0·8378	0·5927	0·8614
	56	0·7568	0·6431	0·8490	0·6075	0·8718
	57	0·7703	0·6579	0·8601	0·6225	0·8820
	58	0·7838	0·6728	0·8711	0·6376	0·8921
	59	0·7973	0·6878	0·8819	0·6530	0·9020
	60	0·8108	0·7030	0·8925	0·6685	0·9116
	61	0·8243	0·7183	0·9030	0·6842	0·9211
	62	0·8378	0·7339	0·9133	0·7001	0·9303
	63	0·8514	0·7496	0·9234	0·7163	0·9392
	64	0·8649	0·7655	0·9332	0·7327	0·9479
	65	0·8784	0·7816	0·9429	0·7494	0·9562
	66	0·8919	0·7980	0·9522	0·7665	0·9642
	67	0·9054	0·8148	0·9611	0·7840	0·9717
	68	0·9189	0·8318	0·9697	0·8019	0·9787
	69	0·9324	0·8493	0·9777	0·8203	0·9851
	70	0·9459	0·8673	0·9851	0·8394	0·9908
	71	0·9595	0·8861	0·9916	0·8594	0·9954
	72	0·9730	0·9058	0·9967	0·8807	0·9986
	73	0·9865	0·9270	0·9997	0·9038	0·9999
	74	1·0000	0·9514	1·0000	0·9309	1·0000
75	0	0·0000	0·0000	0·0480	0·0000	0·0682
	1	0·0133	0·0003	0·0721	0·0001	0·0949
	2	0·0267	0·0032	0·0930	0·0014	0·1178
	3	0·0400	0·0083	0·1125	0·0046	0·1388
	4	0·0533	0·0147	0·1310	0·0091	0·1585

Continued

Table B.11 Exact confidence limits for a binomial proportion: x events are observed in a sample sized n. $p = x/n$ is the observed proportion. p_l and p_u are the lower and upper confidence limits for the population proportion.

Confidence level			95%		99%	
n	x	p	p_l	p_u	p_l	p_u
75	5	0·0667	0·0220	0·1488	0·0147	0·1774
	6	0·0800	0·0299	0·1660	0·0210	0·1957
	7	0·0933	0·0384	0·1829	0·0279	0·2134
	8	0·1067	0·0472	0·1994	0·0353	0·2306
	9	0·1200	0·0564	0·2156	0·0432	0·2475
	10	0·1333	0·0658	0·2316	0·0514	0·2640
	11	0·1467	0·0756	0·2473	0·0599	0·2803
	12	0·1600	0·0855	0·2628	0·0688	0·2963
	13	0·1733	0·0957	0·2781	0·0778	0·3120
	14	0·1867	0·1060	0·2933	0·0871	0·3275
	15	0·2000	0·1165	0·3083	0·0967	0·3429
	16	0·2133	0·1271	0·3232	0·1064	0·3580
	17	0·2267	0·1379	0·3379	0·1163	0·3730
	18	0·2400	0·1489	0·3525	0·1264	0·3878
	19	0·2533	0·1599	0·3670	0·1366	0·4024
	20	0·2667	0·1711	0·3814	0·1470	0·4169
	21	0·2800	0·1824	0·3956	0·1575	0·4313
	22	0·2933	0·1938	0·4098	0·1682	0·4455
	23	0·3067	0·2053	0·4238	0·1790	0·4596
	24	0·3200	0·2169	0·4378	0·1900	0·4736
	25	0·3333	0·2286	0·4517	0·2010	0·4874
	26	0·3467	0·2404	0·4654	0·2122	0·5011
	27	0·3600	0·2523	0·4791	0·2235	0·5148
	28	0·3733	0·2643	0·4927	0·2349	0·5283
	29	0·3867	0·2764	0·5062	0·2465	0·5416
	30	0·4000	0·2885	0·5196	0·2581	0·5549
	31	0·4133	0·3008	0·5330	0·2699	0·5681
	32	0·4267	0·3131	0·5462	0·2817	0·5812
	33	0·4400	0·3255	0·5594	0·2937	0·5942
	34	0·4533	0·3379	0·5725	0·3057	0·6070
	35	0·4667	0·3505	0·5855	0·3179	0·6198
	36	0·4800	0·3631	0·5985	0·3302	0·6325
	37	0·4933	0·3758	0·6114	0·3425	0·6450
	38	0·5067	0·3886	0·6242	0·3550	0·6575
	39	0·5200	0·4015	0·6369	0·3675	0·6698
	40	0·5333	0·4145	0·6495	0·3802	0·6821
	41	0·5467	0·4275	0·6621	0·3930	0·6943
	42	0·5600	0·4406	0·6745	0·4058	0·7063
	43	0·5733	0·4538	0·6869	0·4188	0·7183
	44	0·5867	0·4670	0·6992	0·4319	0·7301
	45	0·6000	0·4804	0·7115	0·4451	0·7419
	46	0·6133	0·4938	0·7236	0·4584	0·7535
	47	0·6267	0·5073	0·7357	0·4717	0·7651
	48	0·6400	0·5209	0·7477	0·4852	0·7765
	49	0·6533	0·5346	0·7596	0·4989	0·7878
	50	0·6667	0·5483	0·7714	0·5126	0·7990
	51	0·6800	0·5622	0·7831	0·5264	0·8100
	52	0·6933	0·5762	0·7947	0·5404	0·8210
	53	0·7067	0·5902	0·8062	0·5545	0·8318

Table B.11 (*Continued*)

			95%		99%	
n	x	p	p_l	p_u	p_l	p_u
75	54	0·7200	0·6044	0·8176	0·5687	0·8425
	55	0·7333	0·6186	0·8289	0·5831	0·8530
	56	0·7467	0·6330	0·8401	0·5976	0·8634
	57	0·7600	0·6475	0·8511	0·6122	0·8736
	58	0·7733	0·6621	0·8621	0·6270	0·8837
	59	0·7867	0·6768	0·8729	0·6420	0·8936
	60	0·8000	0·6917	0·8835	0·6571	0·9033
	61	0·8133	0·7067	0·8940	0·6725	0·9129
	62	0·8267	0·7219	0·9043	0·6880	0·9222
	63	0·8400	0·7372	0·9145	0·7037	0·9312
	64	0·8533	0·7527	0·9244	0·7197	0·9401
	65	0·8667	0·7684	0·9342	0·7360	0·9486
	66	0·8800	0·7844	0·9436	0·7525	0·9568
	67	0·8933	0·8006	0·9528	0·7694	0·9647
	68	0·9067	0·8171	0·9616	0·7866	0·9721
	69	0·9200	0·8340	0·9701	0·8043	0·9790
	70	0·9333	0·8512	0·9780	0·8226	0·9853
	71	0·9467	0·8690	0·9853	0·8415	0·9909
	72	0·9600	0·8875	0·9917	0·8612	0·9954
	73	0·9733	0·9070	0·9968	0·8822	0·9986
	74	0·9867	0·9279	0·9997	0·9051	0·9999
	75	1·0000	0·9520	1·0000	0·9318	1·0000

Table B.12 Confidence limits for a median in a sample sized n. The lower confidence limit is the R_lth observation counting from low to high; the upper confidence limit is the R_uth observation where $R_u = n + 1 - R_l$. The upper confidence limit is also the R_lth observation counting from high to low. The nominal confidence level is approximate and the actual (nearest attainable) level of confidence is also tabulated.

Nominal confidence level	95%		99%	
n	R_l	Exact level	R_l	Exact level
5	1	93·8	1	93·8
6	1	96·9	1	96·9
7	1	98·4	1	98·4
8	2	93·0	1	99·2
9	2	96·1	1	99·6
10	2	97·9	1	99·8
11	3	93·5	2	98·8
12	3	96·1	2	99·4
13	3	97·8	2	99·7
14	4	94·3	3	98·7
15	4	96·5	3	99·3
16	5	92·3	3	99·6
17	5	95·1	4	98·7
18	5	96·9	4	99·2
19	6	93·6	4	99·6
20	6	95·9	5	98·8
21	6	97·3	5	99·3
22	7	94·8	5	99·6

Continued

Nominal confidence level	95%		99%	
n	R_l	Exact level	R_l	Exact level
23	7	96·5	6	98·9
24	8	93·6	6	99·3
25	8	95·7	7	98·5
26	8	97·1	7	99·1
27	9	94·8	7	99·4
28	9	96·4	8	98·7
29	10	93·9	8	99·2
30	10	95·7	8	99·5
31	10	97·1	9	98·9
32	11	95·0	9	99·3
33	11	96·5	10	98·6
34	12	94·2	10	99·1
35	12	95·9	10	99·4
36	13	93·5	11	98·9
37	13	95·3	11	99·2
38	13	96·6	12	98·6
39	14	94·7	12	99·1
40	14	96·2	12	99·4
41	15	94·0	13	98·8
42	15	95·6	13	99·2
43	16	93·4	14	98·6
44	16	95·1	14	99·0
45	16	96·4	14	99·3
46	17	94·6	15	98·9
47	17	96·0	15	99·2
48	18	94·1	16	98·7
49	18	95·6	16	99·1
50	19	93·5	16	99·3
51	19	95·1	17	98·9
52	19	96·4	17	99·2
53	20	94·7	18	98·7
54	20	96·0	18	99·1
55	21	94·2	18	99·4
56	21	95·6	19	99·0
57	22	93·7	19	99·2
58	22	95·2	20	98·8
59	22	96·4	20	99·1
60	23	94·8	21	98·7
61	23	96·0	2i	99·0
62	24	94·4	21	99·3
63	24	95·7	22	98·9
64	25	94·0	22	99·2
65	25	95·4	23	98·7
66	26	93·6	23	99·1
67	26	95·0	23	99·3
68	26	96·2	24	99·0
69	27	94·7	24	99·2
70	27	95·9	25	98·8
71	28	94·3	25	99·1
72	28	95·6	26	98·7

Table B.12 Confidence limits for a median in a sample sized n. The lower confidence limit is the R_lth observation counting from low to high; the upper confidence limit is the R_uth observation where $R_u = n + 1 - R_l$. The upper confidence limit is also the R_lth observation counting from high to low. The nominal confidence level is approximate and the actual (nearest attainable) level of confidence is also tabulated.

Table B.12 (*Continued*)

Nominal confidence level	95%		99%	
n	R_l	Exact level	R_l	Exact level
73	29	94·0	26	99·0
74	29	95·3	26	99·3
75	29	96·3	27	98·9
76	30	95·0	27	99·2
77	30	96·0	28	98·8
78	31	94·6	28	99·1
79	31	95·8	29	98·7
80	32	94·3	29	99·0
81	32	95·5	29	99·3
82	33	94·0	30	98·9
83	33	95·2	30	99·2
84	33	96·2	31	98·8
85	34	95·0	31	99·1
86	34	96·0	32	98·7
87	35	94·7	32	99·0
88	35	95·8	32	99·3
89	36	94·4	33	98·9
90	36	95·5	33	99·2
91	37	94·1	34	98·9
92	37	95·3	34	99·1
93	38	93·9	35	98·8
94	38	95·1	35	99·0
95	38	96·0	35	99·3
96	39	94·8	36	99·0
97	39	95·8	36	99·2
98	40	94·6	37	98·9
99	40	95·6	37	99·1
100	41	94·3	38	98·8

Table B.13 Exact confidence limits for a Poisson count: x is an observed Poisson count, x_l and x_u are the lower and upper limits for the population count.

Confidence level	95%		99%	
x	x_l	x_u	x_l	x_u
0	0·000	3·689	0·000	5·298
1	0·025	5·572	0·005	7·430
2	0·242	7·225	0·103	9·274
3	0·619	8·767	0·338	10·977
4	1·090	10·242	0·672	12·594
5	1·623	11·668	1·078	14·150
6	2·202	13·059	1·537	15·660
7	2·814	14·423	2·037	17·134
8	3·454	15·763	2·571	18·578
9	4·115	17·085	3·132	19·998
10	4·795	18·390	3·717	21·398

Continued

Table B.13 Exact confidence limits for a Poisson count: x is an observed Poisson count, x_l and x_u are the lower and upper limits for the population count.

Confidence level	95%		99%	
x	x_l	x_u	x_l	x_u
11	5·491	19·682	4·321	22·779
12	6·201	20·962	4·943	24·145
13	6·922	22·230	5·580	25·497
14	7·654	23·490	6·231	26·836
15	8·395	24·740	6·893	28·164
16	9·145	25·983	7·567	29·482
17	9·903	27·219	8·251	30·791
18	10·668	28·448	8·943	32·091
19	11·439	29·671	9·644	33·383
20	12·217	30·888	10·353	34·668
21	12·999	32·101	11·069	35·946
22	13·787	33·308	11·792	37·218
23	14·580	34·511	12·521	38·484
24	15·377	35·710	13·255	39·745
25	16·179	36·905	13·995	41·000
26	16·984	38·096	14·741	42·251
27	17·793	39·284	15·491	43·497
28	18·606	40·468	16·245	44·738
29	19·422	41·649	17·004	45·976
30	20·241	42·827	17·767	47·209
31	21·063	44·002	18·534	48·439
32	21·888	45·174	19·305	49·665
33	22·716	46·344	20·079	50·888
34	23·546	47·512	20·857	52·107
35	24·379	48·677	21·638	53·324
36	25·214	49·839	22·422	54·537
37	26·051	51·000	23·208	55·748
38	26·891	52·158	23·998	56·955
39	27·733	53·314	24·791	58·161
40	28·577	54·469	25·586	59·363
41	29·422	55·621	26·384	60·563
42	30·270	56·772	27·184	61·761
43	31·119	57·921	27·986	62·956
44	31·970	59·068	28·791	64·149
45	32·823	60·214	29·598	65·341
46	33·678	61·358	30·407	66·530
47	34·534	62·500	31·218	67·717
48	35·391	63·641	32·032	68·902
49	36·250	64·781	32·847	70·085
50	37·111	65·919	33·664	71·266
51	37·973	67·056	34·483	72·446
52	38·836	68·191	35·303	73·624
53	39·701	69·325	36·125	74·800
54	40·566	70·458	36·949	75·974
55	41·434	71·590	37·775	77·147

Confidence level	95%		99%	
x	x_l	x_u	x_l	x_u
56	42·302	72·721	38·602	78·319
57	43·171	73·850	39·431	79·489
58	44·042	74·978	40·261	80·657
59	44·914	76·106	41·093	81·824
60	45·786	77·232	41·926	82·990
61	46·660	78·357	42·760	84·154
62	47·535	79·481	43·596	85·317
63	48·411	80·604	44·433	86·479
64	49·288	81·727	45·272	87·639
65	50·166	82·848	46·111	88·798
66	51·044	83·968	46·952	89·956
67	51·924	85·088	47·794	91·113
68	52·805	86·206	48·637	92·269
69	53·686	87·324	49·482	93·423
70	54·568	88·441	50·327	94·577
71	55·452	89·557	51·174	95·729
72	56·336	90·672	52·022	96·881
73	57·220	91·787	52·871	98·031
74	58·106	92·900	53·720	99·180
75	58·992	94·013	54·571	100·328
76	59·879	95·125	55·423	101·476
77	60·767	96·237	56·276	102·622
78	61·656	97·348	57·129	103·767
79	62·545	98·458	57·984	104·912
80	63·435	99·567	58·840	106·056
81	64·326	100·676	59·696	107·198
82	65·217	101·784	60·553	108·340
83	66·109	102·891	61·412	109·481
84	67·002	103·998	62·271	110·621
85	67·895	105·104	63·131	111·761
86	68·789	106·209	63·991	112·899
87	69·683	107·314	64·853	114·037
88	70·579	108·418	65·715	115·174
89	71·474	109·522	66·578	116·310
90	72·371	110·625	67·442	117·445
91	73·268	111·728	68·307	118·580
92	74·165	112·830	69·172	119·714
93	75·063	113·931	70·038	120·847
94	75·962	115·032	70·905	121·980
95	76·861	116·133	71·773	123·112
96	77·760	117·232	72·641	124·243
97	78·660	118·332	73·510	125·373
98	79·561	119·431	74·379	126·503
99	80·462	120·529	75·250	127·632
100	81·364	121·627	76·120	128·761

Table B.14(a) The F test: critical values for F distribution. For ANOVA $F = S_1^2/S_2^2$. d.f.$_1$ = degrees of freedom for S_1^2. d.f.$_2$ = degrees of freedom for S_2^2 ($S_1^2 > S_2^2$).

One-sided significance level: 0·05

d.f.$_1$	1	2	3	4	5	6	7	8	9	10
d.f.$_2$	Critical value F_c									
1	161	200	216	225	230	234	237	239	241	242
2	18·51	19·00	19·16	19·25	19·30	19·33	19·35	19·37	19·38	19·40
3	10·13	9·55	9·28	9·12	9·01	8·94	8·89	8·85	8·81	8·79
4	7·71	6·94	6·59	6·39	6·26	6·16	6·09	6·04	6·00	5·96
5	6·61	5·79	5·41	5·19	5·05	4·95	4·88	4·82	4·77	4·74
6	5·99	5·14	4·76	4·53	4·39	4·28	4·21	4·15	4·10	4·06
7	5·59	4·74	4·35	4·12	3·97	3·87	3·79	3·73	3·68	3·64
8	5·32	4·46	4·07	3·84	3·69	3·58	3·50	3·44	3·39	3·35
9	5·12	4·26	3·86	3·63	3·48	3·37	3·29	3·23	3·18	3·14
10	4·96	4·10	3·71	3·48	3·33	3·22	3·14	3·07	3·02	2·98
11	4·84	3·98	3·59	3·36	3·20	3·09	3·01	2·95	2·90	2·85
12	4·75	3·89	3·49	3·26	3·11	3·00	2·91	2·85	2·80	2·75
13	4·67	3·81	3·41	3·18	3·03	2·92	2·83	2·77	2·71	2·67
14	4·60	3·74	3·34	3·11	2·96	2·85	2·76	2·70	2·65	2·60
15	4·54	3·68	3·29	3·06	2·90	2·79	2·71	2·64	2·59	2·54
16	4·49	3·63	3·24	3·01	2·85	2·74	2·66	2·59	2·54	2·49
17	4·45	3·59	3·20	2·96	2·81	2·70	2·61	2·55	2·49	2·45
18	4·41	3·55	3·16	2·93	2·77	2·66	2·58	2·51	2·46	2·41
19	4·38	3·52	3·13	2·90	2·74	2·63	2·54	2·48	2·42	2·38
20	4·35	3·49	3·10	2·87	2·71	2·60	2·51	2·45	2·39	2·35
30	4·17	3·32	2·92	2·69	2·53	2·42	2·33	2·27	2·21	2·16
40	4·08	3·23	2·84	2·61	2·45	2·34	2·25	2·18	2·12	2·08
50	4·03	3·18	2·79	2·56	2·40	2·29	2·20	2·13	2·07	2·03
60	4·00	3·15	2·76	2·53	2·37	2·25	2·17	2·10	2·04	1·99
70	3·98	3·13	2·74	2·50	2·35	2·23	2·14	2·07	2·02	1·97
80	3·96	3·11	2·72	2·49	2·33	2·21	2·13	2·06	2·00	1·95
90	3·95	3·10	2·71	2·47	2·32	2·20	2·11	2·04	1·99	1·94
100	3·94	3·09	2·70	2·46	2·31	2·19	2·10	2·03	1·97	1·93
200	3·89	3·04	2·65	2·42	2·26	2·14	2·06	1·98	1·93	1·88
300	3·87	3·03	2·63	2·40	2·24	2·13	2·04	1·97	1·91	1·86
400	3·86	3·02	2·63	2·39	2·24	2·12	2·03	1·96	1·90	1·85
500	3·86	3·01	2·62	2·39	2·23	2·12	2·03	1·96	1·90	1·85

Significant result if $F \geqslant F_c$

Table B.14(b) The F test: critical values for F distribution. For ANOVA $F = S_1^2/S_2^2$. d.f.$_1$ = degrees of freedom for S_1^2. d.f.$_2$ = degrees of freedom for S_2^2 ($S_1^2 > S_2^2$).

One-sided significance level: 0·01

d.f.$_1$	1	2	3	4	5	6	7	8	9	10
d.f.$_2$	Critical value F_c									
1	4052	5000	5403	5625	5764	5859	5928	5981	6023	6056
2	98·50	99·00	99·17	99·25	99·30	99·33	99·36	99·37	99·39	99·40
3	34·12	30·82	29·46	28·71	28·24	27·91	27·67	27·49	27·35	27·23
4	21·20	18·00	16·69	15·98	15·52	15·21	14·98	14·80	14·66	14·55
5	16·26	13·27	12·06	11·39	10·97	10·67	10·46	10·29	10·16	10·05
6	13·75	10·92	9·78	9·15	8·75	8·47	8·26	8·10	7·98	7·87
7	12·25	9·55	8·45	7·85	7·46	7·19	6·99	6·84	6·72	6·62
8	11·26	8·65	7·59	7·01	6·63	6·37	6·18	6·03	5·91	5·81
9	10·56	8·02	6·99	6·42	6·06	5·80	5·61	5·47	5·35	5·26
10	10·04	7·56	6·55	5·99	5·64	5·39	5·20	5·06	4·94	4·85
11	9·65	7·21	6·22	5·67	5·32	5·07	4·89	4·74	4·63	4·54
12	9·33	6·93	5·95	5·41	5·06	4·82	4·64	4·50	4·39	4·30
13	9·07	6·70	5·74	5·21	4·86	4·62	4·44	4·30	4·19	4·10
14	8·86	6·51	5·56	5·04	4·69	4·46	4·28	4·14	4·03	3·94
15	8·68	6·36	5·42	4·89	4·56	4·32	4·14	4·00	3·89	3·80
16	8·53	6·23	5·29	4·77	4·44	4·20	4·03	3·89	3·78	3·69
17	8·40	6·11	5·18	4·67	4·34	4·10	3·93	3·79	3·68	3·59
18	8·29	6·01	5·09	4·58	4·25	4·01	3·84	3·71	3·60	3·51
19	8·18	5·93	5·01	4·50	4·17	3·94	3·77	3·63	3·52	3·43
20	8·10	5·85	4·94	4·43	4·10	3·87	3·70	3·56	3·46	3·37
30	7·56	5·39	4·51	4·02	3·70	3·47	3·30	3·17	3·07	2·98
40	7·31	5·18	4·31	3·83	3·51	3·29	3·12	2·99	2·89	2·80
50	7·17	5·06	4·20	3·72	3·41	3·19	3·02	2·89	2·78	2·70
60	7·08	4·98	4·13	3·65	3·34	3·12	2·95	2·82	2·72	2·63
70	7·01	4·92	4·07	3·60	3·29	3·07	2·91	2·78	2·67	2·59
80	6·96	4·88	4·04	3·56	3·26	3·04	2·87	2·74	2·64	2·55
90	6·93	4·85	4·01	3·53	3·23	3·01	2·84	2·72	2·61	2·52
100	6·90	4·82	3·98	3·51	3·21	2·99	2·82	2·69	2·59	2·50
200	6·76	4·71	3·88	3·41	3·11	2·89	2·73	2·60	2·50	2·41
300	6·72	4·68	3·85	3·38	3·08	2·86	2·70	2·57	2·47	2·38
400	6·70	4·66	3·83	3·37	3·06	2·85	2·68	2·56	2·45	2·37
500	6·69	4·65	3·82	3·36	3·05	2·84	2·68	2·55	2·44	2·36

Significant result if $F \geqslant F_c$

Appendix C A 'Cookbook' for Hypothesis Tests and Confidence Intervals

C.1 Introduction

The purpose of this appendix is to summarize the statistical techniques discussed in the book by outlining their area of applicability and by providing step-by-step guides to their calculation.

Statistical analysis can be approached either by using confidence intervals to estimate relevant parameters or by hypothesis tests. A confidence interval gives, at a particular confidence level (usually 95% or 99%), a range of values within which the parameter being estimated is likely to lie.

Nearly all hypothesis tests follow the same general structure. A null hypothesis is postulated specifying a particular value for a relevant parameter. This null value is usually related to a lack of association between the variables being studied. A test statistic (e.g. t or χ^2), which is known to have a particular theoretical distribution if the null hypothesis is true, is calculated from the observed results. If, on the assumption of the null hypothesis, the probability of obtaining the value of this statistic, or one even more extreme, is less than a specified level—the significance level of the test—this is considered as evidence to reject the null hypothesis.

This probability is determined by referring the test statistic to a table that gives the critical values appropriate to the test and to the chosen one- or two-sided significance level (usually 5% or 1%). These critical values determine the acceptance and rejection regions for the test. If the test statistic lies in the acceptance region, the null hypothesis is not rejected and a non-significant result obtains. If, on the other hand, the test statistic lies in the rejection region—in the tail(s) of the particular distribution—the null hypothesis can be rejected and a significant result declared.

The simplest situation encountered is that of a single variable in one group or sample. In this case, simple population parameters can be estimated using confidence intervals, or one-sample hypothesis tests can be performed. Table C.1 lists the different techniques in this area and indicates where they are discussed in the body of the book and where they are to be found in this appendix.

Usually, however, analysis relates to a more complex situation than the one-group/one-variable case. Medical research, in essence, is concerned with examining associations between variables and, as has been emphasized before, group membership can be considered a variable. Thus, one could examine the association or relationship of treatment to survival by comparing a treatment and control group. Such two-group comparisons are particularly common in medical research and much emphasis in this book has been on this situation. Table C.2 outlines the different techniques discussed. The significance tests for a null hypothesis of no group difference are given, together with various comparative measures that can summarize that difference. These are either *difference* measures (such as the mean in one group minus the mean in the other group) or *ratio* measures (such as the relative risk).

When more than two groups are being compared, somewhat different

Table C.1 Statistical analysis in the one-group/one-variable situation (section and appendix numbers where the procedures are discussed are given in parentheses).

	Single-group analysis	
	Confidence intervals	Hypothesis tests
Proportions	(4.4; C.2)	z test (5.9; C.2) χ^2 test (5.10; C.6)
Means	(4.6; C.3)	z test (5.6; C.3) t test (5.8; C.3)
Geometric means	(4.7; C.3)	Use t test on transformed data (5.8; C.3)
Medians	(4.8; C.4)	–
Counts or rates	(4.9; C.5)	z test (5.11; C.5)

techniques are employed, and Table C.3 indicates the methods discussed. Gaps in the coverage are apparent but such situations do not arise that commonly in medical comparisons.

If an association between two quantitative variables is being analysed, then regression or correlation is the appropriate technique and these are considered in Chapter 10 and Sections C.20 and C.21 below. When more than two variables are involved in an analysis the statistical techniques become much more complex. Usually, there is a single dependent variable, and there are two possible motives for the investigation. Interest may centre on the association between the dependent variable and a single explanatory variable, with the other variables being potential confounders of the association whose influence is to be adjusted for. Alternatively, the joint effects of the explanatory variables on the dependent variable may be of concern. These methods are all considered in Chapter 11 and Table C.4 (a repeat of the summary box at the end of

Table C.2 Hypothesis tests and summary measures of association (in italics) in the comparison of two groups (section and appendix numbers where the tests or relevant confidence intervals are discussed are given in parentheses).

	Two-group comparisons		
	Independent	Frequency matched	Paired
Means	t test (7.4.1; C.7) *Difference* (7.4.2; C.7)	Two-way ANOVA (11.2.2)* *Difference* (11.2.2)*	Paired t test (7.8.1; C.9) *Difference* (7.8.2; C.9)
Geometric means	t test (7.6.1; C.7) *Ratio* (7.6.2; C.7)	Use two-way ANOVA on transformed data (11.2.2)* *Ratio* (7.6.2)*	–
Medians	Wilcoxon rank sum test - (7.7.1; C.8)	–	Sign test (7.9.1; C.10) Wilcoxon signed rank test (7.9.2; C.11)
Proportions	z test (7.10.1; C.12) χ^2 test (7.10.3; C.13) Fisher's test (7.10.4; C.14) *Difference* (7.10.2; C.12) *Relative risk* (7.10.5; C.13) *Odds ratio* (7.10.5; C.13)	Mantel–Haenzel χ^2 (11.3.1) *Relative risk* (11.3.1) *Odds ratio* (11.3.1)	McNemar's χ^2 (7.12.1; C.16) Exact test (7.12.2; C.16) *Difference* (7.12.3; C.16) *Odds ratio* (7.12.4; C.16)
Counts	z test (7.13.1; C.17) *Difference* (7.13.2; C.17)		–
Rates	z test (7.14.1; C.17) *Difference* (7.14.2; C.17) *Ratio* (7.14.3; C.17)	*Direct standardization* (11.5.2) *Indirect standardization* (11.5.3) *Population life tables* (11.5.5) *CMF* (11.5.2) *SMR* (11.5.3; 11.5.4)	
Life table survival (mortality)	Logrank test (7.15.6) *Difference* (7.15.5) *Ratio* (7.15.7)	Logrank test (11.3.3)* *Ratio* (11.3.3)*	–

* Computational details not given in this text.
CMF, comparative mortality figure; SMR, standardized mortality ratio.

Table C.3 Summary of techniques for multigroup comparisons (section and appendix numbers where the procedures are discussed are given in parentheses).

	Multigroup comparisons	
	Independent	Frequency matched
Means	One-way ANOVA (9.2; C.18)	Two-way ANOVA (11.2.2)*
Proportions	χ^2 test (9.3.1; C.15)	
	χ^2 test for trend (9.3.2; C.19)	

* Computational details not given in this text.

Table C.4 Summary of multivariate techniques for the control of confounding and examination of the effects of explanatory variables (section numbers where the procedures are discussed are given in parentheses).

	Dependent variable			
Explanatory or confounding variable(s)	Mean	Binary proportion (risk)	Rate	Life table survival (mortality)
Qualitative only	ANOVA (9.2; 11.2.2)	Mantel–Haenzel techniques (11.3.1)	Direct and indirect standardization (11.5) Current life tables (11.5.5)	Logrank methods (7.15; 11.3.3)
Quantitative and/or qualitative	Multiple regression (11.2.1) Analysis of covariance (11.2.3)	Logistic regression (11.3.2)	–	Cox regression (11.3.3)

Chapter 11) outlines the material covered. In this text, the computations necessary to control confounding in 2×2 tables, using the Mantel–Haenzel methods, were described fully, while the other approaches, which really require computerized analysis, were discussed from the point of view of interpretation without computational detail.

The remaining sections of this appendix detail, in step-by-step form, the computations for the majority of the analytic techniques considered in this book. Life tables (Section 7.15) and the methods of Chapter 11 are not included, however, since these are best understood by following the text itself. It is hoped that this entire appendix will prove useful as a quick reference to the common techniques likely to be encountered by the medical researcher in analysing his or her own data.

C.2 The z test for a single proportion. Confidence intervals for a proportion

These procedures are discussed in Sections 4.3, 4.4 and 5.9.

Situation

Random sample size n from a population; qualitative binary variable with unknown proportion π in one category.

Assumptions/requirements

That $n\pi$ and $n(1 - \pi)$ are both greater than 5.

Null hypothesis

That the proportion π in the population is equal to π_0 (a numerical value).

Method

1 Calculate the proportion p observed in the sample ($p = x/n$).
2 Calculate the z statistic:

$$z = \frac{p - \pi_0}{\sqrt{\dfrac{\pi_0(1 - \pi_0)}{n}}}$$

3 Look up the critical value z_c of the normal distribution at the required one- or two-sided significance level (Table B.2).

One-sided test
If $z \geqslant z_c$ conclude $\pi > \pi_0$
If $z \leqslant -z_c$ conclude $\pi < \pi_0$
If $-z_c < z < z_c$ conclude $\pi = \pi_0$

Two-sided test
If $z \geqslant z_c$ or $z \leqslant -z_c$ conclude $\pi \neq \pi_0$
If $-z_c < z < z_c$ conclude $\pi = \pi_0$

Confidence intervals

Exact 95% and 99% confidence limits for a proportion are given in Table B.11 for sample sizes up to $n = 75$.

Look up n in the column on the left and find x, the number of events in the next column. Succeeding columns give p and the lower (p_l) and upper (p_u) 95% and 99% limits for π.

Approximate 95% and 99% confidence intervals for π are calculated as:

$$p \pm z_c \sqrt{p(1 - p)/n}$$

where z_c is the two-sided 5% or 1% critical value for the normal distribution. (See Section 4.4.3 on the accuracy of this approximation.)

C.3 The z and t tests for a single mean. Confidence intervals for a mean or geometric mean

These procedures are discussed in Sections 4.6.1, 4.6.4, 5.6 and 5.8.

Situation

Random sample size n from a population; quantitative variable of unknown mean μ. To satisfy the assumptions, the variable may be based on a transformation of the original data.

Assumptions/requirements

That the distribution of the variable in the population is not markedly skewed.

Null hypothesis

That the mean μ of the population is equal to μ_0 (a numerical value).

Method

1 Calculate the mean, $\bar{x}$, and the standard deviation, S, in the sample.
2 If the standard deviation σ in the population is known, calculate the z statistic (equivalent to the t statistic on infinite degrees of freedom):

$$z = \frac{\bar{x} - \mu_0}{\sigma/\sqrt{n}}$$

If the standard deviation in the population is not known, calculate the t statistic on $n - 1$ degrees of freedom:

$$t = \frac{\bar{x} - \mu_0}{S/\sqrt{n}}.$$

3 Look up the critical value t_c of the t distribution for degrees of freedom $n - 1$ or infinity at the required one- or two-sided significance level (Table B.3).

One-sided test
If $t \geqslant t_c$	conclude $\mu > \mu_0$
If $t \leqslant -t_c$	conclude $\mu < \mu_0$
If $-t_c < t < t_c$	conclude $\mu = \mu_0$

Two-sided test
If $t \geqslant t_c$ or $t \leqslant -t_c$	conclude $\mu \neq \mu_0$
If $-t_c < t < t_c$	conclude $\mu = \mu_0$

Confidence intervals for a mean

95% and 99% confidence intervals for μ are calculated as:

$$\bar{x} \pm t_c\, \sigma/\sqrt{n} \quad (\sigma \text{ known})$$

or:

$$\bar{x} \pm t_c\, S/\sqrt{n} \quad (\sigma \text{ unknown})$$

where t_c on $n-1$ (σ unknown) or infinite (σ known) degrees of freedom is the two-sided 5% or 1% critical value for the t distribution.

Confidence intervals for a geometric mean

95% and 99% confidence intervals for the geometric mean are calculated from:

$$10^{\bar{x}' \pm t_c (S'/\sqrt{n})}$$

where $\bar{x}'$ and S' are the mean and standard deviation of the log-transformed data, and:

$$GM(x) = 10^{\bar{x}'}$$

C.4 Confidence intervals for a single median

This procedure is discussed in Section 4.8.

Situation

A single sample size n from a population; quantitative variable of unknown median.

Assumptions/requirements

None.

Confidence intervals for a median

95% and 99% confidence limits for a median are based on Table B.12 for sample sizes up to 100. Order the data from lowest to highest, and assign a rank to each observation from 1 to n. Table B.12 gives the rank of the observation corresponding to the lower confidence limit R_l. The lower limit is the R_lth observation counting from low to high. The upper limit is the $R_u = n+1-R_l$th observation. This is the same as the R_lth observation counting from high to low.

If $n > 100$, then:

$$R_l = \text{smallest integer} \geq \left(\frac{n}{2} - z_\text{c} \frac{\sqrt{n}}{2} \right)$$

where z_c is the two-sided 5% or 1% critical value for the normal distribution. The upper confidence limit is the observation with rank of $n + 1 - R_l$ counting from low to high, or is the R_lth observation counting backwards from the highest value.

C.5 The z test for a single count or rate. Confidence intervals for a count or rate

These procedures are discussed in Sections 4.9 and 5.11.

Situation

A single sample on which a count x has been determined; a rate r calculated as a count divided by person-years at risk or person-years of follow-up ($r = x/PYRS$).

Assumptions/requirements

That the count is based on independent events, and that, for the z test, the count is above 10.

Null hypotheses

1 That the underlying population count μ is μ_0 (a numerical value).
2 That the population rate θ is θ_0.

Method—null hypothesis (1)

1 Calculate the z statistic:

$$z = \frac{x - \mu_0}{\sqrt{\mu_0}}$$

2 Look up the critical value z_c of the normal distribution at the required one- or two-sided significance level (Table B.2).

One-sided test
If $z \geq z_\text{c}$ conclude $\mu > \mu_0$
If $z \leq -z_\text{c}$ conclude $\mu < \mu_0$
If $-z_\text{c} < z < z_\text{c}$ conclude $\mu = \mu_0$

Two-sided test
If $z \geq z_\text{c}$ or $z \leq -z_\text{c}$ conclude $\mu \neq \mu_0$
If $-z_\text{c} < z < z_\text{c}$ conclude $\mu = \mu_0$

Method—null hypothesis (2)

1 Calculate the z statistic

$$z = \frac{r - \theta_0}{\sqrt{\theta_0/PYRS}}$$

2 Look up the critical value z_c of the normal distribution at the required one- or two-sided significance level (Table B.2).

One-sided test

If $z \geq z_c$	conclude $\theta > \theta_0$
If $z \leq -z_c$	conclude $\theta < \theta_0$
If $-z_c < z < z_c$	conclude $\theta = \theta_0$

Two-sided test

If $z \geq z_c$ or $z \leq -z_c$	conclude $\theta \neq \theta_0$
If $-z_c < z < z_c$	conclude $\theta = \theta_0$

Confidence intervals for a count

Exact 95% and 99% confidence limits for a count are given in Table B.13 for counts up to 100. Look up the observed count x in the left-hand column. Succeeding columns give the lower (x_l) and upper (x_u) 95% and 99% limits for μ.

Approximate 95% and 99% confidence intervals are calculated as:

$$x \pm z_c \sqrt{x}$$

where z_c is the two-sided 5% or 1% critical value for the normal distribution. (This approximation should only be used for observed counts above 100.)

Confidence intervals for a rate

Confidence intervals for a rate ($r = x/PYRS$) can be obtained by calculating the limits for x as described above and dividing by $PYRS$. An alternative approximate formula for the 95% and 99% limits directly is:

$$r \pm z_c \sqrt{\frac{r}{PYRS}}$$

where z_c is the two-sided 5% or 1% critical value for the normal distribution. Note that $PYRS$ should be in the same units as the rate. (This approximation should only be used for observed counts above 100.)

C.6 The χ^2 test for many proportions (in one group)

This procedure is discussed in Section 5.10.

Situation

Random sample size n from a population; qualitative variable with two or more categories.

Assumptions/requirements

That not more than 20% of the expected numbers (see below) in the categories are less than 5, and that no expected number is less than 1.

Null hypothesis

That the proportions in each category of the variable in the population have certain values defined independently of the data.

Method

1 Calculate the expected numbers (E) in each category of the variable by multiplying the sample size n by each of the hypothesized proportions.
2 Calculate the χ^2 statistic on degrees of freedom one less than the number of categories:

$$\chi^2 = \sum \frac{(O - E)^2}{E}$$

where O is the observed numbers in each category of the variable, and the summation is over all the categories.
3 Look up the critical value χ_c^2 of the chi-square distribution for the appropriate degrees of freedom at the required two-sided significance level (Table B.4):

If $\chi^2 \geqslant \chi_c^2$ reject the null hypothesis
If $\chi^2 < \chi_c^2$ do not reject the null hypothesis

C.7 The *t* test for two independent means. Confidence intervals for the difference between two means and for a ratio of geometric means

These procedures are discussed in Sections 7.4.1, 7.4.2, 7.6.1 and 7.6.2.

Situation

Two independent random samples size n_1 and n_2 from two populations; quantitative variable with means μ_1 and μ_2 in the two populations. To satisfy the assumptions, the variable can be based on a transformation of the original data.

Assumptions/requirements

That the distribution of the variable is not markedly skewed in either of the populations and either (a) that the population variances σ_1^2 and σ_2^2 are equal, or (b) that these variances are unequal and the sample size in both groups combined is greater than 60, with numbers in each group roughly the same.

Null hypothesis

That the means μ_1 and μ_2 of the two populations are equal or, equivalently, that the mean difference is zero.

Method

1 Calculate the means $\bar{x}_1$ and $\bar{x}_2$ and the standard deviations S_1 and S_2 in the two samples.

2 Assumption a: calculate the pooled variance

$$S_P^2 = \frac{(n_1 - 1)S_1^2 + (n_2 - 1)S_2^2}{n_1 + n_2 - 2}$$

and the t statistic on $n_1 + n_2 - 2$ degrees of freedom:

$$t = \frac{\bar{x}_1 - \bar{x}_2}{\sqrt{\dfrac{S_P^2}{n_1} + \dfrac{S_P^2}{n_2}}}$$

3 Assumption b: calculate the z statistic (equivalent to the t statistic on infinite degrees of freedom):

$$z = \frac{\bar{x}_1 - \bar{x}_2}{\sqrt{\dfrac{S_1^2}{n_1} + \dfrac{S_2^2}{n_2}}}$$

4 Look up the critical value t_c of the t distribution for degrees of freedom $n_1 + n_2 - 2$ (assumption a) or infinity (assumption b) at the required one- or two-sided significance level (Table B.3):

One-sided test
If $t \geqslant t_c$ conclude $\mu_1 > \mu_2$
If $t \leqslant -t_c$ conclude $\mu_1 < \mu_2$
If $-t_c < t < t_c$ conclude $\mu_1 = \mu_2$

Two-sided test
If $t \geqslant t_c$ or $t \leqslant -t_c$ conclude $\mu_1 \neq \mu_2$
If $-t_c < t < t_c$ conclude $\mu_1 = \mu_2$

Confidence intervals for a difference between means (independent data)

95% and 99% confidence intervals for the difference $\mu_1 - \mu_2$ between the population means are calculated from:

$$(\bar{x}_1 - \bar{x}_2) \pm t_c \, SE(\bar{x}_1 - \bar{x}_2)$$

where SE $(\bar{x}_1 - \bar{x}_2)$ is the denominator of the t test statistic above, and t_c on $n_1 + n_2 - 2$ (assumption a) or infinity (assumption b) degrees of freedom is the two-sided 5% or 1% critical value for the t distribution.

Confidence intervals for a ratio of geometric means (independent data)

95% and 99% confidence intervals for the ratio of two geometric means are based on the confidence interval for the difference between means of log-transformed data. Assuming all estimates are of the transformed data, the ratio of the geometric means is:

$$10^{\bar{x}'_1 - \bar{x}'_2}$$

with lower and upper confidence limits of:

$$10^{(\bar{x}'_1 - \bar{x}'_2) \pm t_c \, SE(\bar{x}'_1 - \bar{x}'_2)}$$

with SE $(\bar{x}'_1 - \bar{x}'_2)$ defined as above on the log-transformed data.

C.8 The Wilcoxon rank sum test for two independent medians

This procedure is discussed in Section 7.7.1.

Situation

Two independent random samples size n_1 and n_2 from two populations; quantitative or ordinal variable with medians m_1 and m_2 in the two populations.

Assumptions/requirements

That there is an underlying continuous distribution of the variable, even if it is only measured on an ordinal scale; that there are not too many tied observations.

Null hypothesis

That the medians m_1 and m_2 in the two populations are equal.

Method

1 Combine the observations from the two groups and order them from lowest to highest, while still noting which observation came from which group. Assign a rank to each observation, giving the smallest observation rank 1. If there are tied observations, assign the mean of the ranks in the positions concerned.

2 Calculate the sum of the ranks assigned to the observations in the group with sample size n_1. Call this T_1.

3 Locate the pages of the rank sum test table (Table B.5) corresponding to the sample size in group 1 (n_1). Choose the page that corresponds to the required one- or two-sided significance level, and look in the table for the entries corresponding to the sample sizes n_1 (in the row) and n_2 (in the column). These give the lower (T_l) and upper (T_u) critical values for the sum of ranks in group 1 (T_1). Relabel the groups, if necessary, to use the table:

One-sided test
If $T_1 \geqslant T_u$	conclude $m_1 > m_2$
If $T_1 \leqslant T_l$	conclude $m_1 < m_2$
If $T_l < T_1 < T_u$	conclude $m_1 = m_2$

Two-sided test
If $T_1 \geqslant T_u$ or $T_1 \leqslant T_l$	conclude $m_1 \neq m_2$
If $T_l < T_1 < T_u$	conclude $m_1 = m_2$

C.9 The *t* test for paired means. Confidence intervals for a mean difference

These procedures are discussed in Sections 7.8.1 and 7.8.2.

Situation

Two individually matched samples each of sample size n (n pairs of observations); quantitative variable with population means μ_1 and μ_2.

Assumptions/requirements

That the distribution of the differences between pairs in the population is not too skewed.

Null hypothesis

That the population means μ_1 and μ_2 are equal or, equivqlently, that the mean difference is zero.

Method

1 Calculate the difference between each pair of values, $d = x_1 - x_2$, and compute the mean, $\bar{d}$, and standard deviation, S_d, of these n differences (include zero values of d).

2 Compute the t statistic on $n - 1$ degrees of freedom:

$$t = \frac{\bar{d}}{S_d/\sqrt{n}}$$

3 Look up the critical value t_c of the t distribution for degrees of freedom $n - 1$ at the required one- or two-sided significance level (Table B.3):

One-sided test
If $t \geqslant t_c$	conclude $\mu_1 > \mu_2$
If $t \leqslant -t_c$	conclude $\mu_1 < \mu_2$
If $-t_c < t < t_c$	conclude $\mu_1 = \mu_2$

Two-sided test
If $t \geqslant t_c$ or $t \leqslant -t_c$	conclude $\mu_1 \neq \mu_2$
If $-t_c < t < t_c$	conclude $\mu_1 = \mu_2$

Confidence intervals for a mean difference (paired data)

95% and 99% confidence intervals for the mean difference between the two populations are calculated from:

$$\bar{d} \pm t_c S_d/\sqrt{n}$$

where t_c on $n - 1$ degrees of freedom is the two-sided 5% or 1% critical value for the t distribution.

C.10 The sign test for paired medians

This procedure is discussed in Section 7.9.1.

Situation

Two individually matched samples each of sample size N (N pairs of observations); quantitative or ordinal variable (in that one can determine which individual in each pair has a higher value than the other).

Assumptions/requirements

That there is an underlying continuous distribution of the variable, even if it is only measured on an ordinal scale.

Null hypothesis

That the medians m_1 and m_2 in the two populations are equal.

Method

1 Calculate the sign (+ or −) of the differences $x_1 - x_2$ between each pair of values. If some pairs have the same value, the difference is zero. Count the number of non-zero differences and call it n. If there are no ties, $N = n$.

2 Count the number of positive (+) differences and call it n_+.

3 Look up the table for the sign test (Table B.6) corresponding to the chosen one- or two-sided significance level and the number of non-zero differences n. The entry gives the lower (S_l) and upper (S_u) critical values for the number of positive differences n_+:

One-sided test

If $n_+ \geqslant S_u$	conclude $m_1 > m_2$
If $n_+ \leqslant S_l$	conclude $m_1 < m_2$
If $S_l < n_+ < S_u$	conclude $m_1 = m_2$

Two-sided test

If $n_+ \geqslant S_u$ or $n_+ \leqslant S_l$	conclude $m_1 \neq m_2$
If $S_l < n_+ < S_u$	conclude $m_1 = m_2$

C.11 The Wilcoxon signed rank test for paired medians

This procedure is discussed in Section 7.9.2.

Situation

Two individually matched samples each of sample size N (N pairs of observations); quantitative or ordinal variable, in that the differences between each pair can be ordered.

Assumptions/requirements

That there is an underlying continuous distribution of the variable, even if it is only measured on an ordinal scale; that there are not too many ties among the differences.

Null hypothesis

That the medians m_1 and m_2 in the two populations are equal.

Method

1 Calculate the differences between each pair of values, $d = x_1 - x_2$. Let n equal the number of non-zero differences.

2 Rank these non-zero differences from smallest to highest, ignoring the sign of the difference. Assign a rank to each of these differences, giving the smallest a rank of 1. If two differences have the same magnitude, assign the mean of the ranks in the positions concerned. Now affix to each rank the sign (+ or −) of the difference it represents.

3 Add up the positive (+) ranks and call the sum T_+.

4 Look up the table for this test (Table B.7), and find the lower (T_l) and upper (T_u) critical values for T_+ corresponding to the number of non-zero differences n and the chosen one- or two-sided significance level:

One-sided test

If $T_+ \geqslant T_u$	conclude $m_1 > m_2$
If $T_+ \leqslant T_l$	conclude $m_1 < m_2$
If $T_l < T_+ < T_u$	conclude $m_1 = m_2$

Two-sided test

If $T_+ \geqslant T_u$ or $T_+ \leqslant T_l$	conclude $m_1 \neq m_2$
If $T_l < T_+ < T_u$	conclude $m_1 = m_2$

C.12 The z test for two independent proportions. Confidence intervals for a difference between proportions

These procedures are discussed in Sections 7.10.1 and 7.10.2.

Situation

Two independent random samples size n_1 and n_2 from two populations; qualitative binary variable with unknown population proportions, π_1 and π_2, in one category of the variable.

Assumptions/requirements

That for total sample size, $n_1 + n_2$, less than 40, the four quantities obtained by multiplying n_1 and n_2 by p and $1 - p$ are all greater than 5, where p is the pooled proportion in the two samples combined (see below). Thus, this test should not be used for total sample sizes less than 20.

Null hypothesis

That the proportions π_1 and π_2 in the populations are equal.

Method

1 Calculate the proportions p_1 and p_2 in each of the samples. Also calculate the overall sample proportion p in the two groups combined (the pooled value).

2 Calculate the z statistic:

$$z = \frac{p_1 - p_2}{\sqrt{pq\left(\dfrac{1}{n_1} + \dfrac{1}{n_2}\right)}}$$

where $q = 1 - p$.

3 Look up the critical value z_c of the normal distribution at the required one- or two-sided significance level (Table B.2).

One-sided test

If $z \geqslant z_c$ conclude $\pi_1 > \pi_2$

If $z \leqslant -z_c$ conclude $\pi_1 < \pi_2$

If $-z_c < z < z_c$ conclude $\pi_1 = \pi_2$

Two-sided test

If $z \geqslant z_c$ or $z \leqslant -z_c$ conclude $\pi_1 \neq \pi_2$

If $-z_c < z < z_c$ conclude $\pi_1 = \pi_2$

Confidence intervals for a difference between proportions

95% and 99% confidence intervals for the difference between the population proportions $\pi_1 - \pi_2$ are calculated from:

$$(p_1 - p_2) \pm z_c \sqrt{\frac{p_1 q_1}{n_1} + \frac{p_2 q_2}{n_2}}$$

where $q_1 = 1 - p_1$, $q_2 = 1 - p_2$ and z_c is the two-sided 5% or 1% critical value for the normal distribution.

C.13 The χ^2 test for a 2 × 2 table. Confidence intervals for a relative risk (ratio of proportions) and for an odds ratio

These procedures are discussed in Sections 7.10.3, 7.10.5 and A.3.

Situation

A 2 × 2 table with independent data laid out as below:

a	b	r_1
c	d	r_2
c_1	c_2	n

where r_1, r_2, c_1 and c_2 are the row and column totals and n is the total sample size. Often the columns represent disease/non-disease and the rows represent exposed/non-exposed.

Assumptions

That none of the expected numbers (see below) be less than 5. (However, this may be too stringent a requirement.)

Null hypothesis

That the population proportions in the two groups are the same or, equivalently, that the two variables defining group membership are independent or not associated.

Method

1 Calculate the expected numbers in each cell (E). These are obtained by multiplying the corresponding row and column totals and dividing by n.
2 Calculate the χ^2 statistic on 1 degree of freedom:

$$\chi^2 = \sum \frac{(O - E)^2}{E}$$

where O are the observed numbers in the table and summation is over the four table cells. An equivalent formula is:

$$\chi^2 = \frac{(ad - bc)^2 n}{r_1 r_2 c_1 c_2}$$

3 Look up the critical value χ_c^2 of the chi-square distribution on 1 degree of freedom at the required two-sided significance level (one-sided tests are difficult to interpret):

$$\text{If } \chi^2 \geq \chi_c^2 \quad \text{reject the null hypothesis}$$
$$\text{If } \chi^2 < \chi_c^2 \quad \text{do not reject the null hypothesis}$$

Confidence intervals for a relative risk (ratio of independent proportions)

95% and 99% confidence intervals for the relative risk:

$$\text{RR} = \frac{a/r_1}{c/r_2}$$

are calculated as:

$$\text{RR}^{(1 \pm z_c/\chi)}$$

where χ is the square root of χ^2 and z_c is the critical two-sided 5% or 1% value of the normal distribution.

Confidence intervals for an odds ratio (independent data)

95% and 99% confidence intervals for the odds ratio:

$$OR = \frac{a/b}{c/d}$$

are calculated as:

$$OR^{(1\pm z_c/\chi)}$$

where χ is the square root of χ^2 and z_c is the critical two-sided 5% or 1% value of the normal distribution.

C.14 Fisher's test for a 2 × 2 table

This procedure is discussed in Section 7.10.4.

Situation

Independent data laid out in a 2×2 table.

Assumptions/requirements

That the row and column totals are fixed.

Null hypothesis

That the row and column variables are not associated or, equivalently, that a binary variable is not associated with group membership in a two-sample situation.

Method

1 Rearrange the table so that the smallest cell frequency is in the top left-hand corner.

2 Create a new table by reducing the number in the top left cell by 1 (unless it is zero to start with) and fill in the rest of the table so that it has the same row and column totals as the original.

3 Repeat step 2 until a table with a zero in the top left cell is obtained. There should now be a total of $V + 1$ tables, including the original, where V is the smallest cell frequency in the original. Label these tables from set 0 to set V according to the number in the top left cell. The table in set i has the form:

a_i	b_i	r_1
c_i	d_i	r_2
s_1	s_2	n

where, of course, r_1, r_2, s_1 and s_2 are the row and column totals, which are the same for each table. $a_0 = 0$ and $a_i = i$.

4 Calculate the probability of the table in set 0, directly or using logs (Tables B.8 and B.9):

$$P_0 = \frac{r_2! s_2!}{d_0! n!}$$

5 Calculate the probability of the table in the next set (if there is one), using:

$$P_{i+1} = P_i \times \frac{b_i \times c_i}{a_{i+1} \times d_{i+1}}$$

6 Repeat the last step until all the probabilities from P_0 to P_V have been calculated.

7 Sum these $V + 1$ probabilities. This is the one-sided p value for the test. Multiply this by 2 to obtain the two-sided value. If the (one- or two-sided) p value is less than 5%, the null hypothesis can be rejected.

8 For a mid-p value, sum the V probabilities for tables other than the original one and add half the probability for set V. Multiply by two to obtain the two-sided value.

C.15 The χ^2 test for a general $I \times J$ table

This procedure is discussed in Sections 7.10.3, 7.11.1 and 9.3.1.

Situation

Independent random samples from two or more populations; qualitative variable with two or more categories. The data are usually laid out in an $I \times J$ table, where I is the number of rows and J is the number of columns. The number of observations in each cell of the table must be known. The situation also arises when two qualitative variables are being examined in a single sample.

Assumptions

That not more than 20% of the expected values in the cells (see below) should be less than 5 and no cell should have an expected value of less than 1.

Null hypothesis

That the distributions of the qualitative variable in the different populations are the same or, equivalently, that two qualitative variables in a single sample are not associated.

Method

1 Calculate the expected values (E) in each cell in the table. The expected value for the cell in the ith row and jth column is obtained by multiplying the totals of the corresponding row, r_i, and column, s_j, and dividing by the total sample size in all groups combined (n).

2 Calculate the χ^2 statistic on $(I - 1)(J - 1)$ degrees of freedom:

$$\chi^2 = \sum \frac{(O - E)^2}{E}$$

where the O is the observed numbers in each cell and summation is over all cells in the table. (Equation 9.18 may be computationally simpler for a $2 \times k$ table.)

3 Look up the critical value χ_c^2 of the chi-square distribution for degrees of freedom $(I - 1)(J - 1)$ at the required two-sided significance level (Table B.4):

If $\chi^2 \geqslant \chi_c^2$ reject the null hypothesis
If $\chi^2 < \chi_c^2$ do not reject the null hypothesis

C.16 The McNemar and exact tests for paired proportions. Confidence intervals for a difference between proportions and for an odds ratio

These procedures are discussed in Sections 7.12.1, 7.12.2, 7.12.3 and 7.12.4.

Situation

Two individually matched groups, each of size N (N pairs of observations); qualitative binary variable with unknown population proportions π_1 and π_2 in one category of the variable. This category is denoted by a plus sign below. Often the groups are cases and controls in a pair-matched case–control study, and the binary variable is exposure/non-exposure to a risk factor.

Assumptions/requirements

None.

Null hypothesis

That the proportions π_1 and π_2 in the two paired populations are equal.

1 Lay out the data in a 2×2 table as:

	Group 2	Group 1	
		+	−
+		*a*	*b*
−		*c*	*d*

where the classification is based on the N pairs of observations, and the plus and minus refer to the categories of the binary variable.

2 For small sample sizes, refer c (number of untied pairs in favour of group 1) to Table B.6, which gives the lower (S_l) and upper (S_u) critical values for the test, entered at $n = b + c$, which is the total number of untied pairs:

One-sided test

If $c \geqslant S_u$	conclude $\pi_1 > \pi_2$
If $c \leqslant S_l$	conclude $\pi_1 < \pi_2$
If $S_l < c < S_u$	conclude $\pi_1 = \pi_2$

Two-sided test

If $c \geqslant S_u$ or $c \leqslant S_l$	conclude $\pi_1 \neq \pi_2$
If $S_l < c < S_u$	conclude $\pi_1 = \pi_2$

3 For large sample sizes, calculate:

$$\chi^2 = \frac{(c-b)^2}{b+c}$$

on 1 degree of freedom.

4 Look up the critical value χ_c^2 of the chi-square distribution on 1 degree of freedom at the required two-sided significance level (Table B.4):

If $\chi^2 \geqslant \chi_c^2$	conclude $\pi_1 \neq \pi_2$
If $\chi^2 < \chi_c^2$	conclude $\pi_1 = \pi_2$

Confidence intervals for a difference between paired proportions

95% and 99% confidence intervals for the difference between the population proportions $\pi_1 - \pi_2$ are calculated from:

$$(p_1 - p_2) \pm z_c \frac{1}{N} \sqrt{c + b - \frac{(c-b)^2}{N}}$$

where $p_1 = (a + c)/N$ and $p_2 = (a + b)/N$ are the observed proportions and z_c is the two-sided 5% or 1% critical value for the normal distribution.

Confidence interval for an odds ratio (paired data)

95% and 99% confidence intervals for the odds ratio from a pair-matched study:

$$OR = c/b$$

are given by:

$$OR^{(1 \pm z_c/\chi)}$$

where χ is the square root of χ^2, and z_c is the critical two-sided 5% or 1% value of the normal distribution.

C.17 The *z* test for two independent counts or rates. Confidence intervals for a difference between counts or rates, and for a ratio of counts or rates

These procedures are discussed in Sections 7.13 and 7.14.

Situation

Two independent samples, over the same time period or spatial area, on which two counts x_1 and x_2 are observed; rates r_1 and r_2 based on counts per person-years at risk or person-years of follow-up in two groups ($r_1 = x_1/PYRS_1$, $r_2 = x_2/PYRS_2$).

Assumptions/requirements

That the counts are independent and greater than about 10 in each group.

Null hypotheses

1 That the underlying population counts μ_1 and μ_2 are equal.
2 That the underlying population rates θ_1 and θ_2 are equal.

Method—null hypothesis (1)

1 Calculate the *z* statistic

$$z = \frac{x_1 - x_1}{\sqrt{(x_1 + x_2)}}$$

where x_1 and x_2 are the two counts.
2 Look up the critical value z_c of the normal distribution at the required one- or two-sided significance level (Table B.2):

One-sided test

If $z \geqslant z_c$	conclude $\mu_1 > \mu_2$
If $z \leqslant -z_c$	conclude $\mu_1 < \mu_2$
If $-z_c < z < z_c$	conclude $\mu_1 = \mu_2$

Two-sided test

If $z \geqslant z_c$ or $z \leqslant -z_c$	conclude $\mu_1 \neq \mu_2$
If $-z_c < z < z_c$	conclude $\mu_1 = \mu_2$

Method — null hypothesis (2)

1 Calculate the rates in the two populations $r_1 = x_1/\text{PYRS}_1$, $r_2 = x_2/\text{PYRS}_2$.
2 Calculate the overall (pooled) rate in the two populations combined:

$$r = \frac{\text{PYRS}_1(r_1) + \text{PYRS}_2(r_2)}{\text{PYRS}_1 + \text{PYRS}_2}$$

3 Calculate the z statistic

$$z = \frac{r_1 - r_2}{\sqrt{\dfrac{r}{\text{PYRS}_1} + \dfrac{r}{\text{PYRS}_2}}}$$

4 Look up the critical value z_c of the normal distribution at the required one-
or two-sided significance level (Table B.2):

One-sided test

If $z \geqslant z_c$	conclude $\theta_1 > \theta_2$
If $z \leqslant -z_c$	conclude $\theta_1 < \theta_2$
If $-z_c < z < z_c$	conclude $\theta_1 = \theta_2$

Two-sided test

If $z \geqslant z_c$ or $z \leqslant -z_c$	conclude $\theta_1 \neq \theta_2$
If $-z_c < z < z_c$	conclude $\theta_1 = \theta_2$

Confidence interval for a difference in counts

95% and 99% confidence intervals for the difference between two population
counts μ_1 and μ_2 (if based on the same time period or spatial area) are calculated from:

$$(x_1 - x_2) \pm z_c \sqrt{(x_1 + x_2)}$$

where z_c is the two-sided 5% or 1% critical value of the normal distribution.

Confidence interval for a difference between rates

95% and 99% confidence intervals for the difference between the population
rates θ_1 and θ_2 are calculated from:

$$(r_1 - r_2) \pm z_c \sqrt{\frac{r_1}{PYRS_1} + \frac{r_2}{PYRS_2}}$$

where z_c is the two-sided 5% or 1% critical value of the normal distribution.

Confidence intervals for a ratio of counts

Exact 95% and 99% confidence intervals for the ratio of two population counts μ_1/μ_2 (not necessarily from the same time periods or spatial areas) can be obtained by considering $p = x_1/(x_1 + x_2)$ as a binomial proportion. The lower (p_l) and upper (p_u) limits for this proportion can be obtained using the method described in Section C.2. The lower and upper limits for the population ratio of the counts are then:

$$\frac{p_l}{1 - p_l} \quad \text{and} \quad \frac{p_u}{1 - p_u}$$

Confidence intervals for ratio of rates

The ratio of rates is $RR = (x_1/x_2)(PYRS_2/PYRS_1)$ and lower (RR_l) and upper (RR_u) confidence limits are obtained by multiplying the confidence limits for the ratio of the counts x_1/x_2 by $PYRS_2/PYRS_1$ (see above):

$$RR_l = \frac{p_l}{1 - p_l} \frac{PYRS_2}{PYRS_1}$$

$$RR_u = \frac{p_u}{1 - p_u} \frac{PYRS_2}{PYRS_1}$$

C.18 One-way analysis of variance for means in more than two groups. Confidence intervals for means and mean differences

These procedures are discussed in Sections 9.2 and A.5.

Situation

Independent random samples from k groups. Sample size in group i is n_i and total sample size is N. Quantitative variable with population mean in group i of μ_i.

Assumptions/requirements

That the population variances in the k groups are equal and that the distribution of the variable is approximately normal in each group.

Null hypotheses

1 That the k population means μ_i are all equal.
2 That two particular population means μ_1 and μ_2 are equal (if a significant F value was obtained and the comparison was pre-specified).

Method — null hypothesis (1)

1 Calculate the within- and between-groups SSq using the methods of Section A.4. Also calculate the sample means $\bar{x}_i$ in each group.
2 Calculate:

$$S_W^2 = \text{Within-groups SSq}/N - k$$
$$S_B^2 = \text{Between-groups SSq}/k - 1$$

3 Calculate the F statistic on $k - 1$ and $N - k$ degrees of freedom:

$$F = S_B^2/S_W^2$$

4 Look up the critical value F_c of the F distribution on $k - 1$ and $N - k$ degrees of freedom at the required (one-sided) significance level (Table B.14):

If $F \geqslant F_c$ conclude that the μ_i are not all equal
If $F < F_c$ conclude that the μ_i are all equal

Method — null hypothesis (2)

1 Calculate the t statistic on $N - k$ degrees of freedom:

$$t = \frac{\bar{x}_1 - \bar{x}_2}{\sqrt{\dfrac{S_W^2}{n_1} + \dfrac{S_W^2}{n_2}}}$$

2 Look up the critical value t_c of the t distribution for degrees of freedom $N - k$:

One-sided test
If $t \geqslant t_c$ conclude $\mu_1 > \mu_2$
If $t \leqslant -t_c$ conclude $\mu_1 < \mu_2$
If $-t_c < t < t_c$ conclude $\mu_1 = \mu_2$

Two-sided test
If $t \geqslant t_c$ or $t \leqslant -t_c$ conclude $\mu_1 \neq \mu_2$
If $-t_c < t < t_c$ conclude $\mu_1 = \mu_2$

Confidence interval for a single mean

95% and 99% confidence for a particular population mean μ_i are calculated from:

$$\bar{x}_i \pm t_c \frac{S_W}{\sqrt{n_i}}$$

where t_c on $N - k$ degrees of freedom is the two-sided 5% or 1% critical value for the t distribution.

Confidence intervals for a mean difference

95% and 99% confidence intervals for the mean difference $\mu_1 - \mu_2$ between the two corresponding populations are calculated from:

$$(\bar{x}_1 - \bar{x}_2) \pm t_c \sqrt{\frac{S_W^2}{n_1} + \frac{S_W^2}{n_2}}$$

where t_c on $N - k$ degrees of freedom is the two-sided 5% or 1% critical value for the t distribution.

C.19 The χ^2 test for a trend in proportions in a $2 \times k$ table

This procedure is discussed in Section 9.3.2.

Situation

Independent random samples from k groups that have some intrinsic order. Sample size in group i is n_i and total sample size is N. Binary variable with a proportion d_i/n_i in each group and a total number of 'events' $D = \Sigma d_i$.

Assumptions/requirements

That not more than 20% of the expected numbers in the cells should fall below 5 or any fall below 1.

Null hypothesis

That there is no linear trend in the population proportions with group membership.

Method

1 Assign a score x_i to each group that reflects the relative ordering of the groups.

2 Calculate the following quantities from the data:

$$\mathcal{B} = \Sigma n_i x_i$$
$$\mathcal{C} = \Sigma d_i x_i$$
$$\mathcal{D} = \Sigma n_i x_i^2$$

3 Calculate the χ^2_{TR} statistic for trend on 1 degree of freedom:

$$\chi^2_{TR} = \frac{N(N\mathscr{C} - D\mathscr{B})^2}{D(N-D)(N\mathscr{D} - \mathscr{B}^2)}$$

4 Calculate the usual χ^2 statistic for the $2 \times k$ table (see Section C.15), and obtain the χ^2_{DEP} for a departure from a linear trend on $k-2$ degrees of freedom using:

$$\chi^2_{DEP} = \chi^2 - \chi^2_{TR}$$

5 Look up the critical value χ^2_c of the χ^2 distribution for 1 degree of freedom at the required two-sided significance level:

If $\chi^2_{TR} \geq \chi^2_c$ conclude there is a linear trend
If $\chi^2_{TR} < \chi^2_c$ conclude there is no linear trend

6 Look up the critical value χ^2_c of the χ^2 distribution for $k-2$ degrees of freedom at the required two-sided significance level:

If $\chi^2_{DEP} \geq \chi^2_c$ conclude there is a departure from a linear trend
If $\chi^2_{DEP} < \chi^2_c$ conclude there is no departure from a linear trend

C.20 Tests for regression and correlation

These procedures are discussed in Sections 10.5.4 and A.4.

Situation

Random samples of a y variable at different values of an x variable; both variables quantitative; often assumed in random sampling from a single group; n pairs of values in all.

Assumptions/requirements

That the population distribution of y at each fixed x is normal and that the variances of these y distributions are all equal; that the means of the y distributions are linearly related to x.

Null hypotheses

1 That the population regression coefficient β is equal to a fixed value β_0 (usually zero).
2 That the population correlation coefficient ρ is equal to zero.

Method—null hypothesis (1)

1 Calculate the regression coefficient b, the sum of squares $\Sigma(x - \bar{x})^2$ and the standard error of the estimate, $S_{y.x}$, using the methods outlined in Section A.4.

2 Calculate the t statistic on $n-2$ degrees of freedom:

$$t = \frac{b - \beta_0}{SE(b)}$$

where:

$$SE(b) = \frac{S_{y.x}}{\sqrt{\sum (x - \bar{x})^2}}$$

3 Look up the critical value t_c of the t distribution on $n-2$ degrees of freedom at the required two-sided (usually) significance level (Table B.3):

$$
\begin{aligned}
&\text{If } t \geqslant t_c \text{ or } t \leqslant -t_c && \text{conclude } \beta \neq \beta_0 \\
&\text{If } -t_c < t < t_c && \text{conclude } \beta = \beta_0
\end{aligned}
$$

Confidence intervals

95% and 99% confidence intervals for β are calculated from:

$$b \pm t_c SE(b)$$

where t_c is the appropriate critical value of the t distribution on $n-1$ degrees of freedom.

Method—null hypothesis (2)

1 Calculate the correlation coefficient r (see Section A.4).
2 Calculate the t statistic on $n-2$ degrees of freedom:

$$t = r\sqrt{\frac{n-2}{1-r^2}}$$

3 Look up the critical value t_c of the t distribution on $n-2$ degrees of freedom at the required two-sided (usually) significance level (Table B.3):

$$
\begin{aligned}
&\text{If } t \geqslant t_c \text{ or } t \leqslant -t_c && \text{conclude } \rho \neq 0 \\
&\text{If } -t_c < t < t_c && \text{conclude } \rho = 0
\end{aligned}
$$

C.21 Spearman's rank order correlation coefficient

This procedure is discussed in Section 10.6.4.

Situation

n pairs of observations on an x and y variable. Both variables quantitative or ordered.

Assumptions/requirements

That there are not too many ties in the ranks of the variables.

Null hypothesis

That the population correlation ρ_S between the two variables is zero.

Method

1 Assign ranks to the x and y variables separately, from lowest to highest, giving the average rank to tied observations.
2 For each pair, subtract the rank of variable y from the rank of variable x and call the result d.
3 Square each d and add to obtain Σd^2.
4 Spearman's rank correlation coefficient is calculated as:

$$r_S = 1 - \frac{6\sum d^2}{n(n^2 - 1)}.$$

5 Look up the critical value r_c for Spearman's rank correlation coefficient in Table B.10 for n equal to the number of pairs at the appropriate (usually) two-sided significance level:

$$\begin{array}{ll} \text{If } r_S \geqslant r_c \text{ or } r_S \leqslant -r_c & \text{conclude } \rho_S \neq 0 \\ \text{If } -r_c < r_S < r_c & \text{conclude } \rho_S = 0 \end{array}$$

Appendix D   World Medical Association Declaration of Helsinki

Recommendations guiding physicians in biomedical research involving human subjects

Adopted by the 18th World Medical Assembly, Helsinki, Finland, June 1964, and amended by the 29th World Medical Assembly, Tokyo, Japan, October 1975, the 35th World Medical Assembly, Venice, Italy, October 1983, the 41st World Medical Assembly, Hong Kong, September 1989, and the 48th General Assembly, Somerset West, Republic of South Africa, October 1996.

(Reprinted with the permission of the World Medical Association.)

Introduction

It is the mission of the physician to safeguard the health of the people. His or her knowledge and conscience are dedicated to the fulfilment of this mission.

The Declaration of Geneva of the World Medical Association binds the physician with the words, 'The health of my patient will be my first consideration,' and the International Code of Medical Ethics declares that, 'A physician shall act only in the patient's interest when providing medical care which might have the effect of weakening the physical and mental condition of the patient.'

The purpose of biomedical research involving human subjects must be to improve diagnostic, therapeutic and prophylactic procedures and the understanding of the aetiology and pathogenesis of disease.

In current medical practice most diagnostic, therapeutic or prophylactic procedures involve hazards. This applies especially to biomedical research.

Medical progress is based on research, which ultimately must rest in part on experimentation involving human subjects.

In the field of biomedical research, a fundamental distinction must be recognized between medical research in which the aim is essentially diagnostic or therapeutic for a patient, and medical research the essential object of which is purely scientific and without implying direct diagnostic or therapeutic value to the person subjected to the research.

Special caution must be exercised in the conduct of research that may affect the environment, and the welfare of animals used for research must be respected.

Because it is essential that the results of laboratory experiments be applied to human beings to further scientific knowledge and to help suffering humanity, the World Medical Association has prepared the following recommendations as a guide to every physician in biomedical research involving human subjects. They should be kept under review in the future. It must be stressed that the standards as drafted are only a guide to physicians all over the world. Physicians are not relieved from criminal, civil and ethical responsibilities under the laws of their own countries.

I. Basic principles

1 Biomedical research involving human subjects must conform to generally accepted scientific principles and should be based on adequately performed laboratory and animal experimentation and on a thorough knowledge of the scientific literature.

2 The design and performance of each experimental procedure involving human subjects should be clearly formulated in an experimental protocol, which should be transmitted for consideration, comment and guidance to a specially appointed committee independent of the investigator and the sponsor, provided that this independent committee is in conformity with the laws and regulations of the country in which the research experiment is performed.

3 Biomedical research involving human subjects should be conducted only by scientifically qualified persons and under the supervision of a clinically competent medical person. The responsibility for the human subject must always rest with a medically qualified person and never rest on the subject of the research, even though the subject has given his or her consent.

4 Biomedical research involving human subjects cannot legitimately be carried out unless the importance of the objective is in proportion to the inherent risk to the subject.

5 Every biomedical research project involving human subjects should be preceded by careful assessment of predictable risks in comparison with foreseeable benefits to the subject or to others. Concern for the interests of the subject must always prevail over the interests of science and society.

6 The right of the research subject to safeguard his or her integrity must always be respected. Every precaution should be taken to respect the privacy of the subject and to minimize the impact of the study on the subject's physical and mental integrity and on the personality of the subject.

7 Physicians should abstain from engaging in research projects involving human subjects unless they are satisfied that the hazards involved are believed to be predictable. Physicians should cease any investigation if the hazards are found to outweigh the potential benefits.

8 In publication of the results of his or her research, the physician is obliged to preserve the accuracy of the results. Reports of experimentation not in accordance with the principles laid down in this Declaration should not be accepted for publication.

9 In any research on human beings, each potential subject must be ade-

quately informed of the aims, methods, anticipated benefits and potential hazards of the study and the discomfort it may entail. He or she should be informed that he or she is at liberty to abstain from participation in the study and that he or she is free to withdraw his or her consent to participation at any time. The physician should then obtain the subject's freely given informed consent, preferably in writing.

10 When obtaining informed consent for the research project, the physician should be particularly cautious if the subject is in a dependent relationship to him or her or may consent under duress. In that case, the informed consent should be obtained by a physician who is not engaged in the investigation and who is completely independent of this official relationship.

11 In case of legal incompetence, informed consent should be obtained from the legal guardian in accordance with national legislation. Where physical or mental incapacity makes it impossible to obtain informed consent, or when the subject is a minor, permission from the responsible relative replaces that of the subject in accordance with national legislation.

Whenever the minor child is in fact able to give a consent, the minor's consent must be obtained in addition to the consent of the minor's legal guardian.

12 The research protocol should always contain a statement of the ethical considerations involved and should indicate that the principles enunciated in the present Declaration are complied with.

II. Medical research combined with professional care (clinical research)

1 In the treatment of the sick person, the physician must be free to use a new diagnostic and therapeutic measure, if in his or her judgement it offers hope of saving life, re-establishing health or alleviating suffering.

2 The potential benefits, hazards and discomfort of a new method should be weighed against the advantages of the best current diagnostic and therapeutic methods.

3 In any medical study, every patient—including those of a control group, if any—should be assured of the best proved diagnostic and therapeutic method. This does not exclude the use of inert placebo in studies where no proved diagnostic or therapeutic method exists.

4 The refusal of the patient to participate in a study must never interfere with the physician–patient relationship.

5 If the physician considers it essential not to obtain informed consent, the specific reasons for this proposal should be stated in the experimental protocol for transmission to the independent committee (I, 2).

6 The physician can combine medical research with professional care, the objective being the acquisition of new medical knowledge, only to the extent that medical research is justified by its potential diagnostic or therapeutic value for the patient.

III. Non-therapeutic biomedical research involving human subjects (non-clinical biomedical research)

1 In the purely scientific application of medical research carried out on a human being, it is the duty of the physician to remain the protector of the life and health of that person on whom biomedical research is being carried out.

2 The subjects should be volunteers—either healthy persons or patients for whom the experimental design is not related to the patient's illness.

3 The investigator or the investigating team should discontinue the research if in his/her or their judgement it may, if continued, be harmful to the individual.

4 In research on humans, the interest of science and society should never take precedence over considerations related to the well-being of the subject.

Bibliography and References

The bibliography lists a number of books or articles for further reading. Some, but not all, have already been referred to. They are works that extend the coverage of the present text to a more advanced level. Of course, the choice is not comprehensive and is quite subjective. However, none of the books or articles listed would be out of place on the bookshelves of any investigator involved in the design or analysis of epidemiological or clinical research projects.

The reference list includes all other publications cited in the main text. Included are the original descriptions of some of the statistical procedures discussed and the source of the illustrative examples. Reproduction of tables or figures from any of these works was by kind permission of the authors, editors and publishers concerned.

Bibliography

Abramson, J.H. & Abramson, Z.H. (1999) *Survey Methods in Community Medicine* 5th edn. Churchill Livingstone, Edinburgh. A comprehensive textbook on the planning and performance of medical surveys and clinical trials.

Altman, D.G. (1991) *Practical Statistics for Medical Research*, 1st edn. Chapman & Hall, Altman *et al.* from p 549 London. A textbook at a slightly more advanced level than this book.

Altman, D.G., Machin, D., Bryant, T.N. & Gardner, M.J. (ed.) (2000) *Statistics with Confidence*, 2nd edn. BMJ Books, London. Reprints and expansions of articles from the *British Medical Journal* on the use of confidence intervals in the analysis of data. A truly excellent book which details the calculations required in most situations. Much of the material in this textbook is covered, but confidence interval calculations are described for many of the non-parametric tests also. A computer program implementing the techniques is available.

Armitage, P. & Berry, G. (1994) *Statistical Methods in Medical Research*, 3rd edn. Blackwell Science, Oxford. A standard reference work in medical statistics which includes details of many of the more complex techniques used in medical research. A good deal more advanced than this book.

Begg, C., Cho, M. *et al.* (1996) Improving the quality of reporting of randomized controlled trials: the CONSORT statement. *Journal of the American Medical Association* **276**, 637–639. A widely accepted proposal on what should be included in the published description of a randomized trial.

Breslow, N.E. & Day, N.E. (1980, 1987) *Statistical Methods in Cancer Research*, Vols I and II. International Agency for Research on Cancer, Lyons. An excellent exposition of case–control and cohort studies, including a detailed discussion of design and implementation. Heavy emphasis is placed on the analytic techniques for the control of confounders. Appropriate multiple regression techniques are described in detail.

Cancer Research Campaign Working Party in Breast Conservation (1983) Informed consent: ethical, legal, and medical implications for doctors and patients who participate in randomised clinical trials. *British Medical Journal* **286**, 1117–21. An excellent exposition of some of the ethical problems that arise in the context of the randomized controlled trial.

Chalmers, I. & Altman, D.G. (eds) (1995) *Systematic Reviews*. British Medical Journal, London. A good exposition of the strengths and weaknesses of meta analysis.

Clayton, D. & Hills, M. (1993) *Statistical Methods in Epidemiology*. Oxford University Press, Oxford. This book approaches statistical analysis in epidemiology through the ideas of statistical modelling. A good bit more advanced than the present text.

Cohen, J. (1988) *Statistical Power Analysis for the Behavioral Sciences*, 2nd edn. Lawrence Erlbaum, Mahwah, New Jersey. A classic text for the calculation of sample sizes for many types of investigations. Extensive tables are given.

Conover, W.J. (1998) *Practical Nonparametric Statistics*, 3rd edn. John Wiley & Sons, New York.

A classic textbook detailing the non-parametric approach to statistical analysis. Most non-parametric significance tests in common use are discussed.

Dunn, G. (1989) *Design and Analysis of Reliability Studies*. Oxford University Press, New York. A clear but somewhat mathematical text on the techniques to quantify measurement error.

Esteve, J., Benhamou, E. & Raymond, L. (1994) *Statistical Methods in Cancer Research*, Vol. IV. *Descriptive Epidemiology*. International Agency for Research on Cancer, Lyons. An excellent and comprehensive introduction to descriptive epidemiology and the underlying statistics. It should be of use to anyone involved in the analysis of routine data or disease rates in general.

Feinstein, A.R. (1977) *Clinical Biostatistics*. C.V. Mosby, St Louis. A collection of articles on various topics in biostatistics, which originally appeared as essays in the *Journal of Clinical Pharmacology and Therapeutics*. This is a very readable book which discusses many of the problems and pitfalls to be encountered in epidemiological research.

Fleiss, J.L. (1981) *Statistical Methods for Rates and Proportions*, 2nd edn. John Wiley & Sons, New York. A standard reference work on the analysis of categorical or qualitative data.

Geigy Scientific Tables (1982) Vol. 2, *Introduction to Statistics, Statistical Tables, Mathematical Formulae*, 8th edn. Ciba-Geigy, Basle. A useful and comprehensive handbook of statistical tables with a summary section outlining a large body of statistical theory and significance tests.

Giesecke, J. (1996) *Modern Infectious Disease Epidemiology*. Oxford University Press, Oxford. An excellent introduction to this important topic, which is not covered in the present book.

Kalbfleisch, J.D. & Prentice, R.L. (1980) *The Statistical Analysis of Failure Time Data*. John Wiley & Sons, New York. A standard reference on the techniques for the analysis of censored data. A difficult and theoretical book.

Kleinbaum, D.G. (1994) *Logistic Regression: A Self-Learning Text*. Springer-Verlag, New York. If you want to really learn how to use logistic regression, this text has to be one of the best.

Last, J.M. (1995) *A Dictionary of Epidemiology*, 3rd edn. Oxford University Press, Oxford. A dictionary of the terms used in epidemiology. Includes many statistical terms also. An essential reference work.

McDowell, I. & Newell, C. (1996) *Measuring Health: A Guide to Rating Scales and Question-naires*, 2nd edn. Oxford University Press, New York. An indispensable book for anyone involved in health or illness surveys. It is the most comprehensive source of available health-related questionnaires and nearly all the instruments are given in full in the text.

Machin, D., Campbell, M.J., Fayers, P.M. & Pinol. A.P.Y. (1997) *Sample Size Tables for Clinical Studies*, 2nd edn. Blackwell Science, Oxford. A comprehensive set of sample size tables. More medically orientated than the book by Cohen (1988). Includes discussion, theoretical back-ground and formulae.

Peto, R., Pike, M.C., Armitage, P. *et al.* (1976) Design and analysis of randomized clinical trials requiring prolonged observation of each patient. I. Introduction and design. *British Journal of Cancer* 34, 585–612.

Peto, R., Pike, M.C., Armitage, P. *et al.* (1977) Design and analysis of randomized clinical trials requiring prolonged observation of each patient. II. Analysis and examples. *British Journal of Cancer* 35, 1–39. Two articles on the design and analysis of clinical trials with particular emphasis on survival as an end-point. This article describes life tables and the logrank test in a readily understandable manner and is required reading for those interested in this area.

Rothman, K.J. & Greenland, S. (1998) *Modern Epidemiology*, 2nd edn. Lippincott-Raven, Philadelphia, Pennsylvania. A text that no one involved in epidemiology should be without. A superb exposition of the field that is quite thought-provoking.

Sackett, D.L. (1979) Bias in analytic research. *Journal of Chronic Disease* 32, 51–63. A catalogue of biases in medical research with references to their occurrence in the literature.

Sackett, D.L., Haynes, R.B., Guyatt, G.H. & Tugwell, P. (1991) *Clinical Epidemiology: A Basic Science for Clinical Medicine*, 2nd edn. Little, Brown & Co. Boston, Massachusetts. This is a practical book that avoids overuse of mathematics and puts epidemiological principles and practice into a bedside context. An essential book for every clinician.

Streiner, D.L. & Norman, G.R. (1995) *Health Measurement Scales: A Practical Guide to their Development and Use*. Oxford University Press, Oxford. A good introduction to the problems that arise in trying to measure aspects of health and illness. An essential read for someone involved in designing questionnaires in medical research.

Tufte, E.R. (1983) *The Visual Display of Quantitative Information*. Graphics Press, Cheshire, Connecticut.

Tufte, E.R. (1990) *Envisioning Information*. Graphics Press, Cheshire, Connecticut. These two beautifully produced books show how to use graphics to explain, rather than to confuse. They are the definitive works on communicating with graphs and diagrams.

Tukey, J.W. (1977) *Exploratory Data Analysis*. Addison-Wesley, Reading, Massachusetts. This classic text shows how to discover what a wealth of information may be in a set of data.

References

Altman, D.G. (1994) The scandal of poor medical research [editorial]. *British Medical Journal* 308, 283–4.

Apgar, V. (1953) Proposal for new method of evaluation of newborn infants. *Anesthesia and Analgesia* 32, 260–7.

Barry, J. & Daly, L. (1988) *The Travellers' Health Status Study: Census of Travelling People, November 1986*. Health Research Board, Dublin.

Barry, J., Herity, B. & Solan, J. (1989) *The Travellers' Health Status Study: Vital Statistics of Travelling People, 1987*. Health Research Board, Dublin.

Bland, J.M. & Altman, D.G. (1986) Statistical methods for assessing agreement between two methods of clinical measurement. *Lancet* i, 307–10.

Bland, J.M. & Altman, D.G. (1996) Measurement error proportional to the mean. *British Medical Journal* 313, 106.

Cox, D.R. (1972) Regression models and life tables (with discussion). *Journal of the Royal Statistical Association* B34, 187–220.

D'Agostino, R.B., Chase, W. & Belanger, A. (1988) The appropriateness of some common procedures for testing the equality of two independent binomial populations. *American Statistician* 42, 198–201.

Daly, L.E. (1991a) The first international urokinase/warfarin trial in colo-rectal carcinoma. *Clinical and Experimental Metastases* 9, 3–12.

Daly, L. (1991b) Confidence intervals and sample sizes: don't throw out all your old sample size tables. *British Medical Journal* 302, 333–6.

Daly, L.E., Mulcahy, R., Graham, I. & Hickey, N. (1983) Long term effect on mortality of stopping smoking after unstable angina and myocardial infarction. *British Medical Journal* 287, 324–6.

Dawber, T.R. (1980) *The Framingham Study: The Epidemiology of Atherosclerotic Disease*. Harvard University Press, Cambridge, Massachusetts.

Department of Health (1987) *Report on Vital Statistics*. Stationery Office, Dublin.

Department of Health (1997) *Report on Vital Statistics*. Stationery Office, Dublin.

Doll, R., Peto R., Wheatley, K., Gray, R. & Sutherland, I. (1994) Mortality in relation to smoking: 40 years' observations on male British doctors. *British Medical Journal* 309, 901–11.

Ederer, F. & Mantel, N. (1974) Confidence limits on the ratio of two Poisson variables. *American Journal of Epidemiology* 100, 165–7.

Frigge, M., Hoaglin, D.C. & Iglewicz, B. (1989) Some implementations of the boxplot. *American Statistician* 43, 50–4.

Geigy Scientific Tables (1984) Vol. 3, *Physical Chemistry, Composition of Blood, Hematology, Somatometric Data*, 8th edn. Ciba-Geigy, Basle.

Gormally, S.M., Kierce, B.M., Daly, L.E. *et al.* (1996) Gastric metaplasia and duodenal ulcer disease in children infected by *Helicobacter pylori*. *Gut* 38, 513–17.

Gottlieb, M.S., Schroff, R., Schanker, H.M. *et al.* (1981) *Pneumocystis carinii* pneumonia and mucosal candidiasis in previously healthy homosexual men. *New England Journal of Medicine* 305, 1425–31.

Graham, I.M., Daly, L., Refsum, H.M. *et al.* (1997) Plasma homocysteine as a risk factor for vascular disease. *Journal of the American Medical Association* 277, 1775–81.

Green, T.P., Thompson, T.R., Johnson, D.E. & Lock, J.E. (1983) Furosemide promotes patent ductus arteriosus in premature infants with the respiratory-distress syndrome. *New England Journal of Medicine* 308, 743–8.

Gregg, N.M. (1941) Congenital cataract following German measles in the mother. *Transactions of the Ophthalmological Society of Australia* 3, 35–46.

Hayes, A., Daly, L., O'Brien, N.G. & MacDonald, D. (1983) Anthropometric standards for Irish newborn. *Irish Medical Journal* 76, 60–70.

Herity, B., Moriarty, M., Bourke, G.J. & Daly, L. (1981) A case–control study of head and neck cancer in the Republic of Ireland. *British Journal of Cancer* 43, 177–82.

Hickey, N., Mulchay, R., Daly, L., Bourke, G. & Moriarty, J. (1979) The relationship between blood glucose and prevalence of coronary heart disease: a study in the Republic of Ireland. *Journal of Chronic Diseases* 32, 767–72.

Hill, A.B. (1965) The environment and disease: association or causation? *Proceedings of the Royal Society of Medicine* 58, 295–300.

Kaplan, E.L. & Meier, P. (1958) Nonparametric estimation from incomplete observations. *Journal of the American Statistical Association* 53, 457–81.

Mantel, N. & Haenzel, W. (1959) Statistical aspects of the analysis of data from retrospective studies of disease. *Journal of the National Cancer Institute* 22, 719–48.

Miettinen, O.S. (1976) Estimability and estimation in case-referent studies. *American Journal of Epidemiology* 103, 226–35.

Mitchell, J.R.A. (1981) Timolol after myocardial infarction: an answer or a new set of questions? *British Medical Journal* 282, 1565–70.

Newcombe, R.G. (1998a) Two-sided confidence intervals for the single proportion: comparison of seven methods. *Statistics in Medicine* 17, 857–72.

Newcombe, R.G. (1998b) Interval estimation for the difference between independent proportions: comparison of eleven methods. *Statistics in Medicine* 17, 873–90.

Newcombe, R.G. (1998c) Improved confidence intervals for the difference between binomial proportions based on paired data. *Statistics in Medicine* 17, 2635–50.

Norwegian Multicentre Study Group (1981) Timolol-induced reduction in mortality and reinfarction in patients surviving acute myocardial infarction. *New England Journal of Medicine* 304, 801–7.

O'Connor, J. & Daly, M. (1983) *Smoking and Drinking Behaviour*, Vol. 1. Health Education Bureau, Dublin.

Palmeri, S.T., Harrison, D.G., Cobb, F.R. *et al.* (1982) A QRS scoring system for assessing left ventricular function after myocardial infarction. *New England Journal of Medicine* 306, 4–9.

Parks, J.H., Coe, F.L. & Strauss, A.L. (1982) Calcium nephrolithiasis and medullary sponge kidney in women. *New England Journal of Medicine* 306, 1088–91.

Peto, R. & Peto, J. (1972) Asymptotically efficient rank invariant test procedures. *Journal of the Royal Statistical Society (Series A)* 135, 185–207.

Pollock, E., Wines, W. & Hall, D. (1981) A survey of blood pressure in 10-year-old children of a health district together with a consideration of screening policy for hypertension. *Community Medicine* 3, 199–204.

Puska, P., Tuomilehto, J., Salonen, J. *et al.* (1981) *Community Control of Cardiovascular Diseases: The North Karelia Project*. World Health Organization, Copenhagen.

Salonen, J.T. & Vohlonen, I. (1982) Longitudinal cross-national analysis of coronary mortality. *International Journal of Epidemiology* 11, 229–38.

Smoking and Health (1964) *A Report of the Advisory Committee to the Surgeon General of the Public Health Service*. US Department of Health, Education and Welfare, Washington, DC.

Wald, N.J. & Watt, H.C. (1997) Prospective study of effect of switching from cigarettes to pipes or cigars on mortality from three smoking related diseases *British Medical Journal* 314, 1860–1863.

Zelen, M. (1979) A new design for randomized clinical trials. *New England Journal of Medicine* 300, 1242–6.

Index

Please note: page references in *italics* indicate figures; those in **bold** indicate tables. The index entries are arranged in word-by-word alphabetical order.